Enteric Infection 2

Enteric Infection 2

INTESTINAL HELMINTHS

Edited by

M. J. G. Farthing MD, FRCP

Department of Gastroenterology,
St Bartholomew's Hospital,
London, UK

G. T. Keusch

Division of Geographic Medicine and Infectious Diseases,
New England Medical Center and
Tufts University School of Medicine,
Boston, USA

and

D. Wakelin

Department of Life Science,
University Park,
Nottingham, UK

CHAPMAN & HALL MEDICAL

London · Glasgow · Weinheim · New York · Tokyo · Melbourne · Madras

Published by Chapman & Hall, 2–6 Boundary Row, London SE1 8HN, UK

Chapman & Hall, 2–6 Boundary Row, London SE1 8HN, UK

Blackie Academic & Professional, Wester Cleddens Road, Bishopbriggs, Glasgow G64 2NZ, UK

Chapman & Hall GmbH, Pappelallee 3, 69469 Weinheim, Germany

Chapman & Hall, USA, One Penn Plaza, 41st Floor, New York NY 10119, USA

Chapman & Hall Japan, ITP-Japan, Kyowa Building, 3F, 2–2–1, Hirakawacho, Chiyoda-ku, Tokyo 102, Japan

Chapman & Hall Australia, Thomas Nelson Australia, 102 Dodds Street, South Melbourne, Victoria 3205, Australia

Chapman & Hall India, R. Seshadri, 32 Second Main Road, CIT East, Madras 600 035, India

First edition 1995

Typeset in 10/12pt Palatino by Photoprint, Torquay, Devon
Printed in England by Alden Press, Oxford

ISBN 0 412 39140 6

A catalogue record for this book is available from the British Library

∞ Printed on acid-free text paper, manufactured in accordance with ANSI/NISO Z39.48–1922 (Permanence of Paper).

Contents

Contributors

E. E. Billett
Department of Life Science, Trent University, Clifton Lane, Nottingham NG11 8NS, UK

D. A. P. Bundy
Centre for the Epidemiology of Infectious Diseases, University of Oxford, South Parks Road, Oxford OX1 3PS, UK

A. Dean Befus, PhD
Astra Chair in Asthma Research, Research Director, Alberta Asthma Center, University of Alberta, Heritage Medical Research Center, Suite 559, Edmonton, AB T6G252, Canada

Gilbert A. Castro, PhD
Department of Physiology and Cell Biology, University of Texas, Medical School at Houston, PO Box 20708, Houston, TX, 77225, USA

G. C. Cook, MD, DSc, FRCP, FRACP, FLS
Department of Clinical Sciences, Hospital for Tropical Diseases, St Pancras Way, London NW1 0PE, UK

Edward S. Cooper, MBBS, FRCP
Tropical Metabolism Research Unit, University of the West Indies, Mona, Kingston 7, Jamaica, West Indies

John H. Cross, PhD
Department of Preventive Medicine and Biometrics, Uniformed Services University of the Health Sciences, 4301 Jones Bridge Road, Bethesda, Maryland 20814, USA

Dickson Despommier, PhD
School of Public Health, Divisions of Tropical Medicine and Environmental Sciences, and the Department of Microbiology, Columbia University, 630 W 168th Street, New York, NY 10032, USA

J. S. Edirisinghe, MB BS, MSc, PhD, MD
Centre for International Child Health, Institute of Child Health, 30 Guildford Street, London WC1N 1EH, UK and Department of Medical Parasitology, Faculty of Medicine, University of Peradiniya, Sri Lanka

Michael, J. G. Farthing, MD, FRCP
Department of Gastroenterology, St Bartholomew's Hospital, West Smithfield, London EC1A 7BE, UK

Anna Flisser, Biol., DS
Facultad de Medicina, UNAM, Depto. de Microbiología y Parasitología, Edificio A, 2° piso, Cd. Universitaria 04510 Mexico DF

Peter Hotez, MD, PhD
Departments of Pediatrics (Infectious Diseases) and Epidemiology and Public Health, Yale University School of Medicine, Cedar Street, PO Box 3333, New Haven, CT 06510, USA

Peter Katelaris, MD, FRACP
Department of Gastroenterology, St Bartholomew's Hospital, West Smithfield, London EC1A 7BE, UK

James W. Kazura, MD
Division of Geographic Medicine, School of Medicine, Case Western Reserve University, 10900 Euclid Avenue, Cleveland, Ohio 44106–4983, USA

G. T. Keusch, MD
Division of Geographic Medicine and Infectious Diseases, Tufts University School of Medicine, Boston, USA

Pedro Morera
Institute of Health Research and School of Medicine, University of Costa Rica, PO Box 2117, San José-1000, Costa Rica

Franklin Neva, MD
Laboratory of Parasitic Diseases, National Institute of Allergy and Infectious Diseases, National Institutes of Health, Bethesda, MD 20892, USA

Peter O'Hanley, MD, PhD
Veterans Administration Hospital, Palo Albo, California USA

G. Richard Olds, MD
Department of Medicine, MetroHealth Medical Center Campus, Case Western Reserve University, 2500 MetroHealth Drive, Cleveland, Ohio 44109, USA

Thomas Pool, DVM, MPH
Tropical Medicine Navy Medical Research Unit-2, Jakarta, Indonesia

D. I. Pritchard, PLD
Department of Life Science, University of Nottingham NG7 2RD

P. I. Tighe, PLD
Department of Immunology, University of Nottingham, Queen's Medical Centre

Sui Zhang
Department of Pediatrics, University of Texas Medical Branch, Galveston, TX 77555–0352, USA

A. M. Tomkins, MB BS, FRCP
Centre for International Child Health, Institute of Child Health, 30 Guildford Street, London WC1N 1EH, UK

Hugo Vanden Bossche
Department of Comparative Biochemistry, Janssen Research Foundation, Turnhoutseweg 30, B 2340 Beerse, Belgium

D. Wakelin, PhD, DSc, FRCPath
Department of Life Science, University Park, Nottingham NG7 2RD, UK

Kenneth S. Warren, MD, DTM&H
Picower Institute for Medical Research, 350 Community Drive, Manhasset, New York, NY 11030, USA

Peter M. Wiest, MD
Program in International Health, MetroHealth Medical Center Campus, Case Western Reserve University, 2500 MetroHealth Drive, Cleveland, Ohio 44109, USA

Preface

Intestinal infection continues to be a major problem worldwide to which helminths make an enormous contribution with billions of individuals currently infected. The major burden of disease falls on those living in the developing world although the increase in foreign travel during the last 3–4 decades has brought a number of helminth infections closer to home for those living in industrialized societies. Similar to *Enteric Infection* Part 1 which covered bacterial, viral and protozoan infections of the gut, this book aims to bring together important basic science developments in the pathogenesis of intestinal helminth infection with clinical descriptions of disease and up-to-date guidance on management. The contributors are a truly international panel of experts all of whom have a first class reputation as laboratory and clinical investigators and many of whom have a continuing active research interest in those parts of the world where these infections are most common.

We hope that this mix of basic science and clinical medicine will make the volume useful to clinicians, particularly those working in the fields of infectious diseases and gastroenterology who may want to update their knowledge about the scientific underpinning of their specialty, to laboratory scientists who wish to broaden their perspective on the clinical aspects of intestinal infection and to students of biology, medicine and microbiology.

M. J. G. Farthing
G. T. Keusch
D. Wakelin

December 1994

ONE

Global impact of intestinal helminth infection

G. T. Keusch
and
M. J. G. Farthing

Nobody likes worms except other worms, fishermen, and parasitologists.

Anonymous

Intestinal helminths undoubtedly were the first enteric pathogens to be seen by the human eye and to be associated with intestinal disease many thousands of years ago. Indeed, there is a close relationship between the size of an enteropathogen and the point in history when it was first discovered by humans (Figure 1.1). None the less, an inverse relationship prevails between the first sighting of these worms and the depth of our current knowledge of the mechanisms by which they cause disease, in particular molecular pathogenesis and host immune responses.

It is impossible to estimate accurately the global prevalence of intestinal helminthic infections, because surveillance data are incomplete, being available from some but not all countries, from some communities or populations but not others, and at different times in each (Walsh, 1989). The presence of certain helminth infections can be documented by microscopical examination of stools (Goka *et al.*, 1990), but even for these agents there has never been (and probably never will be) a global survey conducted at the same time in ecologically representative groups of large enough sample size to enable extrapolation to the entire human population. However, whether the real proportion of humans harbouring an intestinal worm is one-third or two-thirds (or more) of the population is irrelevant, because the lowest estimate is staggering enough to gain attention (Pawlowski, 1983).

The epidemiology and transmission of intestinal helminths is intrinsically linked to the behaviour of humans and the application of technology to the protection of water supplies, the sanitary disposal of faeces, and personal hygiene (Udonsi and Ogan, 1993) (Chapter 2). Behavioural modification alone could dramatically reduce the prevalence of these infections, but not necessarily eradicate them (Feachem *et al.*, 1983). While such changes, coupled with improved environmental sanitation, provision of clean water, and protected food supplies have eradicated some helminths in some places, their continued presence in the poorest groups of the developing world in whom population growth proceeds unchecked, means that the

Enteric Infection 2. Intestinal helminths. Edited by M.J.G. Farthing, G.T. Keusch and D. Wakelin. Published in 1995 by Chapman and Hall, London. ISBN 0 412 39140 6

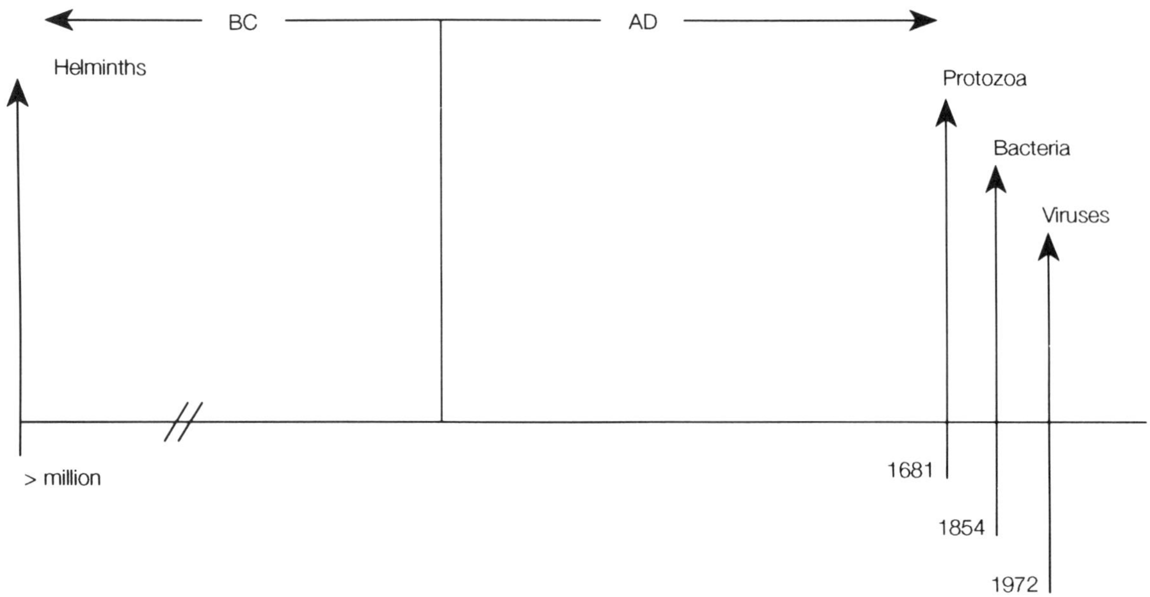

Figure 1.1 Discovery of enteropathogens.

global prevalence of helminthic infection will more likely increase than decrease, let alone remain level, albeit perhaps somewhat more geographically restricted.

In the chapters to follow, the brilliant biological strategies for survival of helminths will be carefully detailed (Chapter 3), pathogenesis will be described (Chapters 4–6), their capacity for causing clinically recognizable disease symptoms will be elaborated (Chapters 7–19), and diagnostic, treatment and control measures reviewed (Chapters 20–23). In the course of the discussions, a great many of the episodes of infection will be said to be clinically inapparent, but it is probably more correct to say that these infections are clinically unrecognized because their impact may be subtle or manifested entirely outside the gastrointestinal tract (Nokes *et al.*, 1992).

It is well known that the likelihood of symptoms due to intestinal helminths is directly related to the burden of infection, and that this accumulates over time as exposure continues and behaviour facilitates transmission (Guyatt and Bundy, 1991). Children are, in general, the most heavily infected and bear the greatest clinical burden (Anderson and May, 1982). However, major clinical manifestations associated with some of these organisms may be long delayed (e.g. in schistosomiasis), becoming recognized only in adulthood. Some of the more important biological impacts of helminthic infections can be mediated indirectly through the nutritional consequences of infection (Chapter 6). Thus, blood loss due to hookworms leads to iron deficiency anaemia and results in a significant reduction in work productivity in adults, a unique and reliable measure of the functional impact of the infection (Prasad and Prasad, 1991; Dallman, 1989). Iron deficiency is also associated with impaired host defence mechanisms for other infections (Sherman and Kelyar, 1988), and thus contributes to the cycle of infection and malnutrition (Farthing and Keusch, 1986). More subtle still are the effects of nutritional deficiencies on learning and neuropsychological development (Lozoff, 1988; Kvalsvig, Cooppan and Connolly, 1991). While early childhood delays in cognitive development may be overcome in later childhood (Grantham-McGregor, Schofield and Powell, 1987), wherever educational opportunities are limited and the social environment is not supportive, as is often the case in economically disadvantaged developing country populations, the likelihood of permanent effects increases. Lost intellectual growth is neither easily measurable nor translatable into lost economic growth of a nation, but is surely an issue of significance that must be included in any assessment of a global impact of intestinal helminths. These latter issues are the hidden agenda of this volume, a more subdued counterpart to the acute and, more commonly, chronic morbidity and the generally low mortality attributed to intestinal helminths. Yet because of the extremely high prevalence of helminths, their associated morbidity and the direct cost to the health care system or to individuals is also high (Pawlowski, 1984).

Of late, however, considerable progress has been made in understanding the aetiology and specific manifestations of these infections, and new therapeutic approaches have revolutionized their management. The purpose of this book is to provide this information in a comprehensive and readily accessible manner. We give our thanks to the many contributors to this volume, and we proudly present to you, the reader, *Enteric Infections. Volume 2: Intestinal Helminths.*

REFERENCES

Anderson, R. M. and May, R. M. (1982) Population dynamics of human helminth infections: control by chemotherapy. *Nature*, **297**, 557–63.

Dallman, P. R. (1989) Iron deficiency: does it matter? *J. Int. Med.*, **226**, 367–72.

Farthing, M. J. G. and Keusch, G. T. (1986) Nutrition and infection. *Ann. Rev. Nutr.*, **6**, 131–54.

Feachem, R. G., Guy, M. W., Harrison, S. *et al.* (1983) Excreta disposal facilities and intestinal parasitism in urban Africa: preliminary studies in Botswana, Ghana and Zambia. *Trans. Roy. Soc. Trop. Med. Hyg.*, **77**, 4515–21.

Goka, A. K., Rolston, D. D., Mathan, V. I. and Farthing, M. J. (1990) Diagnosis of strongyloides and hookworm infections: comparison of faecal and duodenal fluid microscopy. *Trans. Roy. Soc. Trop. Med. Hyg.,*, **84**, 829–31.

Grantham-McGregor, S. M., Schofield, W. and Powell, C. (1987) Development of severely malnourished children who received psychosocial stimulation: six year follow-up. *Pediatrics*, **79**, 247–54.

Guyatt, H. L. and Bundy, D. A. (1991) Estimating prevalence of community morbidity due to intestinal helminths: prevalence of infection as an indicator of the prevalence of disease. *Trans. Roy. Soc. Trop. Med. Hyg.*, **85**, 778–82.

Kvalsvig, J. D., Cooppan, R. M. and Connolly, K. J. (1991) The effects of parasite infections on cognitive processes in children. *Ann. Trop. Med. Parasit.*, **85**, 551–68.

Lozoff, B. (1988) Behavioral alterations in iron deficiency. *Adv. Pediatr.*, **35**, 331–59.

Nokes, C., Grantham-McGregor, S. M., Sawyer, A. W. *et al.* (1992) Parasitic helminth infection and cognitive function in school children. *Proc. Roy. Soc. (London) Series B*, **247**, 77–81.

Pawlowski, Z. S. (1983) Intestinal parasitic infections as a public health problem. *Parasitologia*, **25**, 141–50.

Pawlowski, Z. S. (1984) Implications of parasite–nutrition interactions from a world perspective. *Fed. Proc.*, **43**, 2565–609.

Prasad, A. N. and Prasad, C. (1991) Iron deficiency; non-hematological manifestations. *Prog. Food Nutr. Sci.*, **145**, 255–83.

Sherman, A. R. and Kelyar, L. (1988) Iron deficiency, immunity, and disease resistance in early life, in *Nutrition and Immunology* (ed. R. K. Chandra), Alan R. Liss, N. Y., pp. 169–95.

Udonsi, J. K. and Ogan, V. N. (1993) Assessment of the effectiveness of primary health care interventions in the control of three intestinal nematode infections in rural communities. *Public Health*, **107**, 53–60.

Walsh, J. A. (1989) Disease problems in the Third World. *Ann. N. Y. Acad. Sci.*, **569**, 1–16.

TWO

Epidemiology and transmission of intestinal helminths

D. A. P. Bundy

Understanding the epidemiology of helminth infections requires a fundamentally different approach from that required for all other infectious agents. Indeed, Anderson and May (1979) have suggested that, for epidemiological purposes, infectious agents can be usefully divided into macroparasites (the helminths) and microparasites (a taxonomically highly diverse group including viruses, bacteria and protozoa). The characteristic which requires this separation is helminth reproductive behaviour: while most helminth species reproduce within the definitive host, in the sense of producing stages which are infective to other hosts, only a very small minority of helminth species (e.g. *Strongyloides* and *Capillaria*, see Chapters 8 and 12) multiply within the same host individual. Thus each worm establishing in a host is the result of a separate infection event, and the number of infective stages shed (the infectiousness of the host) is a function of the number of worms present. This contrasts with the situation in microparasites, where infection is typically an all-or-nothing event that leads to colonization of the host individual, and where the subsequent infectiousness of the host is largely unrelated to the degree of prior exposure. In population dynamic terms this implies that the individual worm is the unit of transmission for helminths, while the individual host is the unit for microparasites (Anderson and May, 1982).

The size of the worm burden (the intensity of infection) is therefore a central determinant of helminth transmission dynamics. This variable is of further significance to helminth epidemiology since it is also the major determinant of morbidity. The relationship between infection and disease is another area in which helminthiases differ significantly from microparasitic infections. With the latter there is usually close correspondence between infection and disease, whereas with helminths the pathology is related to the size of the worm burden, usually in a non-linear fashion (Stephenson, 1987; Cooper and Bundy, 1989). Since the size of the worm burden varies considerably between individuals, and infection implies only that worms are present, a population of 'infected' people will exhibit considerable variation in the severity of disease manifestations. The intuitive assumption that all infections are equal may help to explain the historical confusion over the pathogenicity

Enteric Infection 2. Intestinal helminths. Edited by M.J.G. Farthing, G.T. Keusch and D. Wakelin. Published in 1995 by Chapman and Hall, London. ISBN 0 412 39140 6

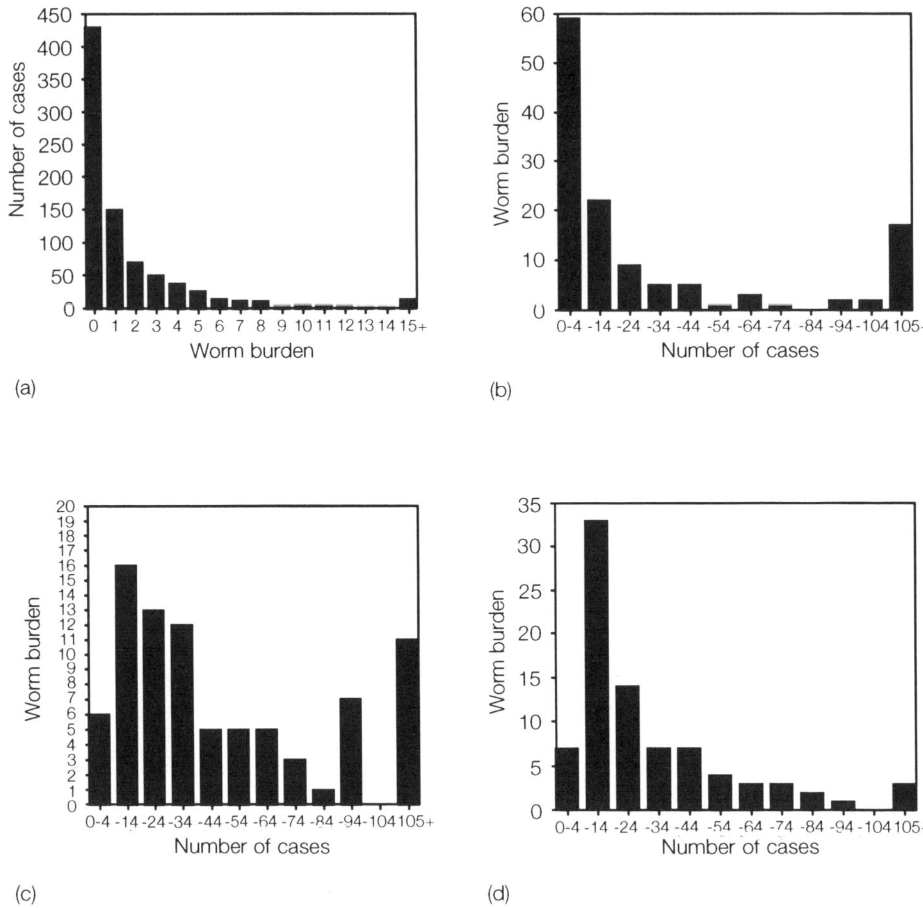

Figure 2.1 Frequency distributions of (a) *Ascaris* (Korea); (b) *Trichuris* (St Lucia); (c) *Necator* (India) and (d) *Ancylostoma* (India) in humans. All the distributions are markedly overdispersed. (Source: Seo, Cho and Chai, 1979; Bundy, 1986; Schad and Anderson, 1985).

and public health significance of helminth infection (Bundy, 1988; Cooper and Bundy, 1990).

From these considerations it is apparent that an understanding of helminth epidemiology centres around an understanding of the patterns and determinants of infection intensity (Bundy and Cooper, 1988a). This chapter examines how worm burdens differ between individuals and how these patterns change with time and hence age, before considering the relationship between worm burden and both morbidity and transmission.

2.1 WORM BURDEN DISTRIBUTIONS

Worm burdens are neither uniformly nor randomly distributed amongst individuals, but are highly overdispersed distributions such that most individuals have few worms while a few hosts harbour disproportionately large worm burdens (Figure 2.1). This pattern has been described for *Ascaris lumbricoides* (Croll *et al.*, 1982, Holland *et al.*, 1989), both species of hookworm (Schad and Anderson, 1985), *Trichuris trichiura* (Bundy *et al.*, 1985), *Schistosoma mansoni* (Cheever, 1968), *Enterobius vermicularis* (Haswell-Elkins *et al.*, 1987) and the false hookworm *Ternidens diminutus* (Bradley, 1990). Most studies suggest that approximately 70% of the worm population is harboured by 15% of the host population. These few heavily infected individuals – the 'wormy people' described by Croll and Ghadirian (1981) – are simultaneously at highest risk of disease and the major source of environmental contamination.

Studies of reinfection suggest that individuals are predisposed to a high or low intensity of infection; the size of the worm burden reacquired after successful treatment is positively associated with the intensity of infection before treatment (Figure 2.2). This association has been shown for all the major geohelminths (Anderson, 1986; Elkins, Haswell-Elkins and Anderson, 1986; Bundy and Cooper, 1988b; Holland *et al.*, 1990), *S. mansoni* (Bensted-Smith *et al.*, 1987) and *E. vermicularis* (Haswell-Elkins *et al.*, 1987). With geohelminths this trend persists over at least two reinfection periods (Chan, Kan and Bundy, 1991). Longitudinal studies of *T. trichiura* (Bundy *et al.*, 1988) and *A. lumbricoides* (Forrester *et al.*, 1990) confirm that this positive association reflects a direct relation between the rate of reinfection and initial infection status (Figure 2.3). Thus in an endemic community it appears that there is a consistent trend for an individual to have an above (or below) average intensity of infection. This trend is more apparent in children with *A. lumbricoides* (Haswell-Elkins, Elkins and Anderson 1987), *T. trichiura* (Bundy and Cooper, 1988b) and *S. mansoni* (Bensted-Smith *et al.*, 1987) infection, and more apparent in adults with *Necator americanus* (Bradley and Chandiwana, 1990) and *E. vermicularis* (Haswell-Elkins *et al.*, 1987) infection, perhaps reflecting the different age-intensity patterns of these species (see section 2.3).

This pattern is also apparent at the family level. In endemic areas more families tend to have a majority of family members with heavy (or light) infections of *T. trichiura* and

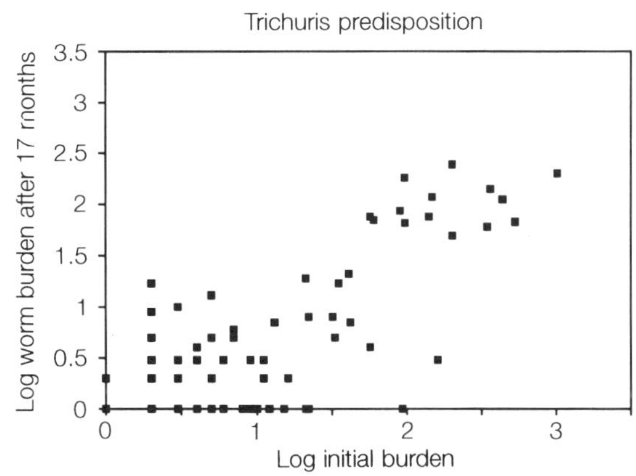

(a)

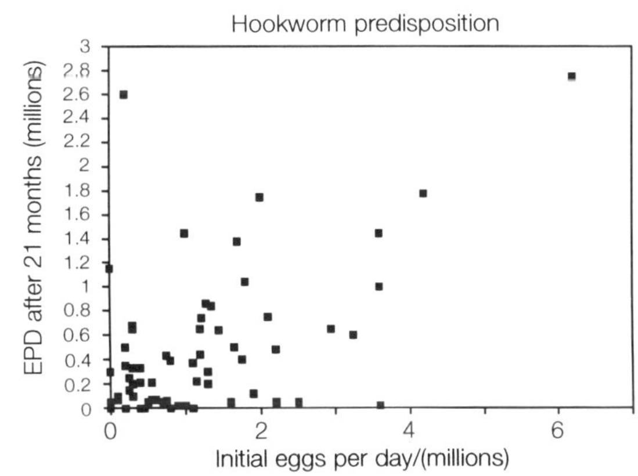

(b)

Figure 2.2 Evidence for predisposition to (a) *Trichuris trichiura* and (b) mixed hookworm infection. The data indicate, for each individual, the initial intensity of infection, and that acquired after successful treatment and a period of reinfection. There is a significant rank correlation between initial and reinfection worm burdens in individuals. (Source: Bundy, Cooper and Thompson, 1987b; Schad and Anderson, 1985.)

A. lumbricoides than would be expected by chance, whereas families with a mixture of both heavy and lightly infected individuals are less common than would be predicted; heavily infected individuals tend to be aggregated in families (Chai *et al.*, 1985; Forrester *et al.*, 1988). Studies of these parasites in Mexico and Malaysia indicate that families also exhibit predisposition to infection (For-

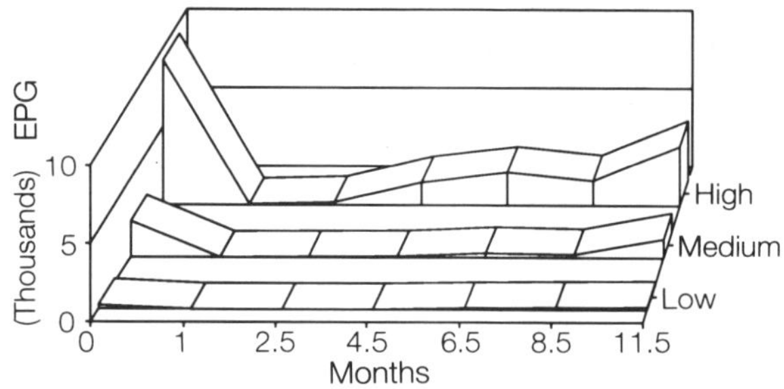

Figure 2.3 Relationship between initial infection intensity and rate of reacquisition of *T. trichiura* infection. The mean worm burdens of the children (mean age 4.5 years) in each intensity class (n=10) at the start of the study were: high, 295.5 worms; medium, 36.9; low, 5.3. Initial worm burdens were determined by anthelmintic expulsion. The same cohort of children was examined at each time point, and infection intensity expressed as eggs per g. stool (epg). (Source: Bundy *et al.*, 1988.)

rester *et al.*, 1990; Chan, Kan and Bundy, 1991)

A critical review of the data on predisposition (Keymer and Pagel, 1989) indicated that the rank status between initial and reinfection worm burden was retained by only 30 to 60% of individuals. This theme has also been examined using probability theory (McCallum, 1990) which indicated that the observed covariance was less than that predicted if predisposition was considered to be a fixed characteristic of the individual. These analyses suggest that the mechanisms of predisposition involve both underlying long-term factors and factors which vary on a sufficiently short time scale to affect the outcome of a reinfection study (Guyatt and Bundy, 1991).

Heterogeneity in exposure to infection may have both long- and short-term effects (Anderson and Gordon, 1982). Human exposure to parasitic infection is notoriously difficult to quantify since it usually depends on detailed behavioural study (Bundy and Blumenthal, 1990). Measurement of the rate of soil ingestion has been proposed as a proxy measure of exposure to soil-borne geohelminths (Wong, Bundy and Golden,

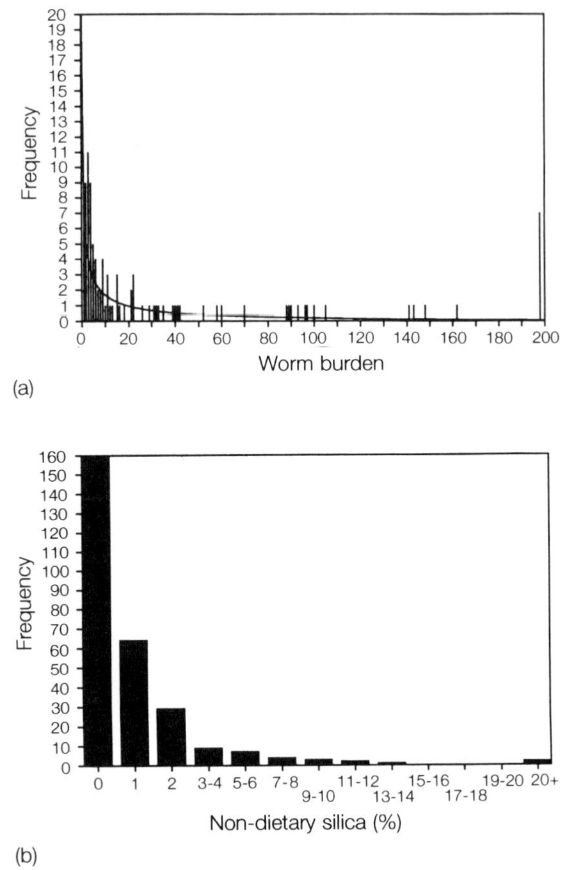

Figure 2.4 Comparison between the frequency distributions of (a) *T. trichiura* infection intensity and (b) the practice of geophagia in children, as assessed by levels of soil-derived silica in stool. The distribution of the infection and exposure parameters are similarly overdispersed. (Source: Cooper and Bundy, 1988; Bundy, 1988.)

1988), and it has been shown that the overdispersed distribution of geophagia within a community closely mirrors observed distributions of geohelminth infection intensity (Figure 2.4). Since pica is in part dependent on social circumstances (Singhi, Singhi and Adwani, 1981) the practice could operate as a long-term determinant of predisposition. In contrast, the patchy distribution of geohelminth eggs in the environment (Beaver, 1975; Wong and Bundy, 1990) could generate short-term heterogeneity. Such an interaction between long- and short-term factors is suggested by the observation that geophagia and geohelminth infection intensity in children are covariants in an environment where the parasite eggs are uniformly distributed, but not where the infective stages have an overdispersed distribution (Wong, Bundy and Golden, 1991).

Individual behaviours appear also to influence exposure to hookworm infection. In some endemic areas, communal defaecation grounds appear to act as foci for transmission (Schad, Nawalinski and Kochar, 1983). Individual children and young adults, particularly males who disregard behavioural norms and defaecate in previously contaminated areas, tend to have significantly higher intensities of infection (Hominick, Dean and Schad, 1987).

Exposure to schistosome infection results from contact with water containing infective intermediate host snails. The interpretation of water-contact studies has proved controversial (Barbour, 1985), but studies using indices of exposure indicate that intensity of infection with *S. haematobium* is related to exposure in children (Wilkins *et al.*, 1987; Bundy and Blumenthal, 1990), although not in adults (see section 2.3).

Heterogeneity in individual susceptibility is an alternative, or counterpart, to variability in exposure as a determinant of predisposition. Susceptibility might be modified by nutritional status; malnutrition, whether gross or involving single nutrients, has been shown to have a major impact on the human immune and inflammatory responses (Suskind, 1980). Individuals with low levels of plasma zinc, a trace element that is essential to thymus-mediated immune responses (Beisel, 1982) tend to have above-average *T. trichiura* worm burdens (Bundy and Golden, 1987), although diet and infection may merely be covariates of poverty. Susceptibility to helminths may also be modified by concurrent infection, as is seen in animal models (Behnke, Ali and Jenkins, 1983; Hannah and Pritchard, 1984). There is evidence that HTLV-I infection (Nakada *et al.*, 1984), and less convincingly HIV infection (Gompels *et al.*, 1991), predispose to disseminated strongyloidiasis.

Another potential candidate for generating long-term heterogeneity in susceptibility to helminths is genetic restriction (see Wakelin and Blackwell (1988) for discussion of this issue). Studies of laboratory mice have demonstrated MHC-H2 restriction of susceptibility to helminths (Wassom, Krco and David, 1987). Studies of a West Indian population exposed to *A. lumbricoides* and *T. trichiura* infection have shown that the MHC-HLA A20-C7-DR18 haplotype is significantly more frequent in individuals with intense infection with either parasite (Bundy and Medley, 1992). The implications of this correlation are, however, far from clear. The haplotype is not known to be associated with any specific immunological defect and occurred in less than 50% of heavily infected individuals. Furthermore, animal studies suggest that the response to helminths is unlikely to depend only on the MHC; while immunorecognition, as assessed by immunoblots, is highly correlated with MHC(H-2) haplotype (Wassom *et al.*, 1984), the expression of an effector response is heavily modified by the background genome (Else and Wakelin, 1988). Interpretation of the human response is likely to be similarly confounded by polygenic responses, as well as by Type II statistical errors.

Studies of the human MHC in schistosomiasis have focused on the relationship with disease. It has been shown that HLA-DQ is epistatic to DR in mediating the immuno-pathological response to *Schistosoma japonicum* antigen (Hirayama *et al.*, 1987; Sasazuki *et al.*, 1980), but correlates with resistance or susceptibility to infection have not been sought.

A family-based study of predisposition to *T. trichiura* and *A. lumbricoides* in Malaysia has used a novel approach to dissect out the potential role of genetics (Chan, Kan and

Bundy, 1992). The study showed that covariance between initial and reinfection worm burdens was significantly stronger if the data were analysed using family units rather than randomly assigned groups of individuals, thus confirming the existence of a familial affect. However, further analysis showed that there was equally strong evidence for a correlation between the worm burdens of parents as for a correlation between the worm burdens of parents and those of their children. Since parents are unrelated genetically, but related to their children, this is evidence against rather than for a genetic basis for predisposition. It does indicate strongly, however, the importance of the household unit and thus the potential role of the local environment and family-specific practices and behaviours.

2.2 WORM BURDEN AND HOST AGE

Overdispersed distributions of infection intensity are observed in the community as a whole and also in individual age classes. The degree of overdispersion, however, shows some age dependency. In hookworm infection the distribution becomes more overdispersed in adults (Bradley and Chandiwana, 1990), while in *A. lumbricoides* and *T. trichiura* there is evidence that dispersion increases to a peak in the child age classes (Bundy *et al.*, 1988) and then declines in adults (Chan, Kan and Bundy, 1991; Bundy, Kan and Rose, 1988). These changes reflect age-specific trends in the proportion infected (the size of the zero class in the frequency distribution) and in the mean intensity of infection (the mean of the distribution).

The age-dependent pattern of infection prevalence is generally rather similar amongst the major helminth species, exhibiting a rise in childhood to a relatively stable asymptote in adulthood (Figure 2.5). Maximum prevalence is usually attained before 5 years of age for *A. lumbricoides*, *T. trichiura* and *E. vermicularis*, between 5 and 10 years for the schistosomes, and in young adults with hookworm infection. In *A. lumbricoides* and schistosome infection, there is often a slight decline in prevalence during adulthood, but this is less common with the other major nematode species.

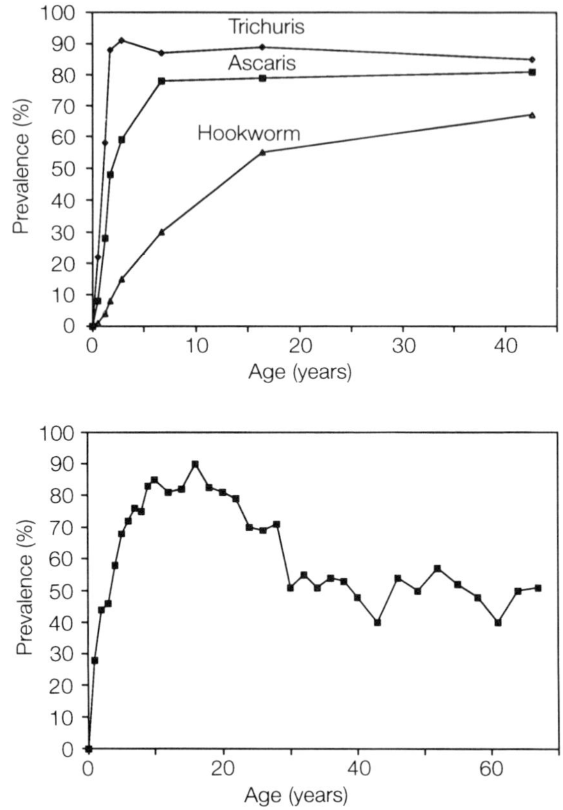

Figure 2.5 Age-prevalence profiles for (a) geohelminths and (b) *Schistosoma haematobium*. (Source: Hsieh, 1970; Bradley and McCullough, 1974; Bundy *et al.*, 1987a.)

The two species of *Strongyloides* infecting humans exhibit age-prevalence patterns which are quite different from each other and unique amongst nematodes infecting humans. *S. stercoralis* is typically rare in children, and studies from endemic foci in Japan and Poland indicate that the majority of infections occur in people over 40 years of age (Soroczan, 1976; Sato, 1986). In contrast, the *S. fulleborni*-like parasite in Papua New Guinea is most prevalent in children under 5 years of age, and in one study 65% of children had patent infections by 3 months of age (Ashford and Barnish, 1989).

Helminths transmitted by ingestion of an intermediate host, or of an intermediate stage attached to food, tend to have age-prevalence patterns which reflect anthropological factors. *Fasciolopsis buski* infection is said to be more prevalent in the child age classes because children are more likely to eat raw the water caltrop (*Trapa* spp.) to which the metacercariae attach (Sadun and Maiphoon, 1953). *Angiostrongylus* infection is also more prevalent in children, in this case because children are more likely to ingest the molluscan intermediate host (Morera, 1987). *Capillaria philippinensis*, in contrast, is most prevalent in adult males who eat the fish intermediate host (Cross and Basaca-Sevilla, 1987).

Data on the age-specific prevalence patterns of cestodes are rare. Infection with adult *Taenia saginata* or *T. solium* appears to occur in all age groups that eat infected meat (Cruz *et al.*, 1989); *Hymenolepis nana* is most prevalent in young children (Sahba, Arfaa and Bijan, 1967).

Prevalence data indicate the proportion of individuals infected, and do not provide a simple indication of the number of worms harboured. Figure 2.6a shows the relationship between prevalence and worm burden for *A. lumbricoides*. The marked non-linearity of this relationship is a direct statistical consequence of the overdispersed pattern of intensity. If worm burdens were uniformly (normally) distributed there would be a linear relationship between prevalence and intensity (see Anderson and May, 1985a for further discussion of this issue).

The intensity data for Figure 2.6a are derived by anthelmintic expulsion and enumeration of adult worms, a procedure which can provide a 90% accurate estimate of actual worm burden (Bundy *et al.*, 1985). Similarly detailed data are unavailable for other species and it is therefore necessary to use the density of parasite eggs in stool as a proxy measure of intensity. This measure, usually expressed as eggs per g stool (epg), provides a practically useful, but only approximate estimate of intensity because the *per capita* fecundity of female worms is itself density dependent (see Anderson, 1986 and Keymer and Slater, 1987 for contrasting views on this issue). Despite these limitations on the interpretation of egg count data, it is apparent from Figure 2.6b–e that the non-linear relationship between prevalence and intensity is characteristic of schistosomes and all the major nematode species.

It is apparent from Figure 2.6 that prevalence provides a reasonable estimate of mean intensity at low average worm burdens (e.g. < 5 *A. lumbricoides* worms), but not at higher values. This has the important practical consequence that very large changes in mean worm burden (e.g. from 30 to 5 *A. lumbricoides* worms) are hardly reflected in changing prevalence, and thus that even successful control measures in hyperendemic areas are unlikely to be detected by prevalence measures (Guyatt *et al.*, 1990).

The lack of simple correspondence between prevalence and intensity has the additional consequence that the observed age-prevalence profiles provide little indication of the underlying profiles of age-intensity. For most helminth species the initial rise in intensity with age closely mirrors that of prevalence but occurs at a slightly slower rate (Figure 2.7). Maximum intensity occurs at a host age which is parasite species-specific and dependent on parasite longevity, but independent of local transmission rates (Anderson, 1986). For *A. lumbricoides* and *T. trichiura* maximum worm burdens occur in human populations at 5–10 years of age, for schistosomes at 10–15 years, and for hookworms 20–25 years.

The most important differences in the age-intensity profiles of these species become

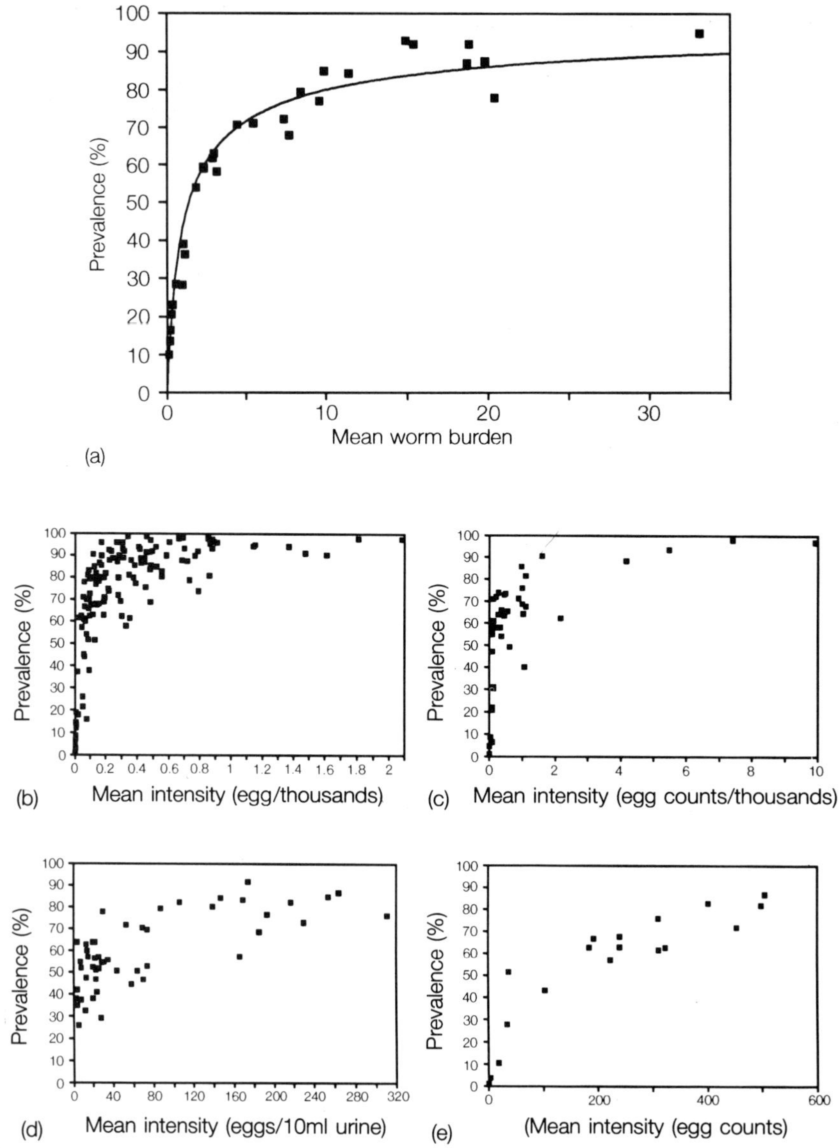

Figure 2.6 Non-linear relationship between infection prevalence and intensity for (a) *Ascaris lumbricoides*, (b) mixed hookworm infection, (c) *Trichuris trichiura*, (d) *Schistosoma haematobium* and (e) *S. mansoni*. Data for (a) based on anthelmintic expulsion as a measure of intensity, and epg for all others. (Redrawn from Guyatt *et al.*, 1990.)

apparent after peak intensity has been attained. The schistosomes, *A. lumbricoides* and *T. trichiura* all exhibit a marked decline in intensity to a low level which then persists throughout adulthood (Figure 2.7). Age-profiles based on egg density in stool had suggested that there was considerable variation in the patterns seen in hookworm infec-

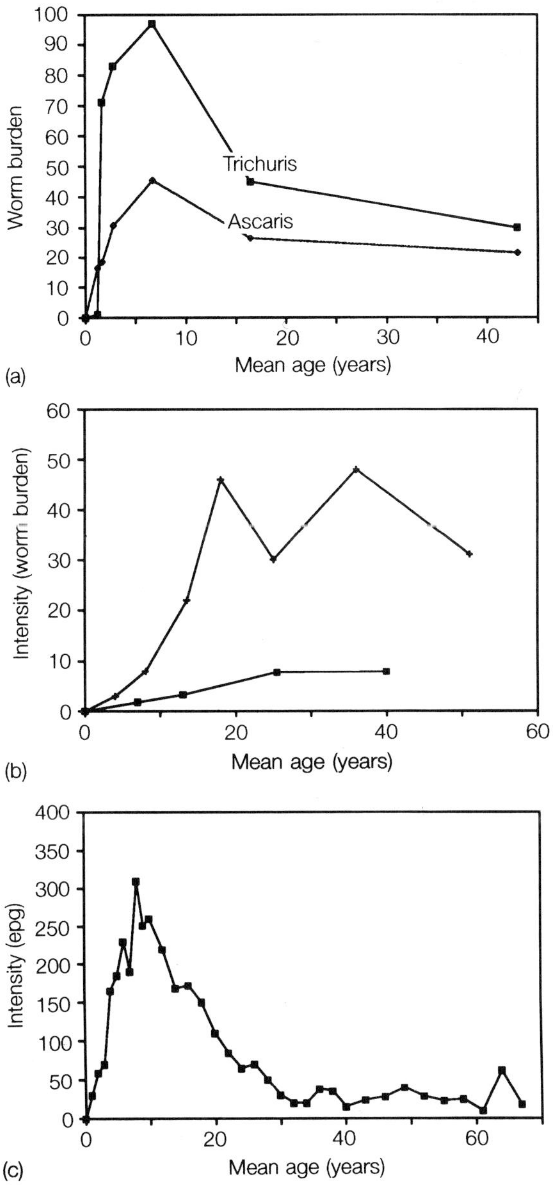

Figure 2.7 Age-intensity profiles for (a) *A. lumbricoides* (× 7) and *T. trichiura*, (b) *Necator americanus* and (c) *Schistosoma haematobium*. (Source for (a) Bundy, 1988, (b) Bradley *et al.*, 1991; Pritchard *et al.*, 1990; (c) Bradley and McCullough, 1974.)

tions (Behnke, 1987; Bundy, 1990a), but it now appears, from studies where burdens have been enumerated by anthelmintic expulsion, that the intensity attains a stable asymptote, or rises marginally, in adulthood (Pritchard *et al.*, 1990; Bradley *et al.*, 1992) (Figure 2.7b).

Thus, for those species with convex age-intensity profiles, but asymptotic age-prevalence profiles, a similar proportion of children and adults are infected but the adults have substantially smaller worm burdens. With hookworm infection, where both prevalence and intensity are asymptotic, more adults are infected and they have larger worm burdens.

With *Enterobius vermicularis* a biphasic age-intensity pattern is typically observed (Haswell-Elkins *et al.*, 1987a). The pattern initially resembles that of *A. lumbricoides* and *T. trichiura* with a peak in the child age classes, but a secondary peak occurs in adults. This has been attributed to familial transmission with intense infection occurring simultaneously in children and their parents (Pawlowski, 1989).

In order to explain these patterns it is necessary to examine again the relationship between prevalence and intensity (Figure 2.6). For those species which exhibit a convex age-intensity pattern the form of the prevalence profile is dependent on the absolute magnitude of the change in worm burden. From Figure 2.6a it can be seen that a decline in mean burden from 30 to 25 worms has a negligible effect on prevalence, whereas a decline from 10 to 5 reduces the prevalence dramatically. Thus there can be a major reduction in intensity in those species of parasite which typically have large worm burdens (such as *T. trichiura*, where mean burdens are often in the range of 50–100 worms) without this being reflected in a detectable reduction in prevalence. This explains why age-prevalence profiles of schistosomes and *A. lumbricoides* often decline in adulthood, but those of *T. trichiura* and other worms in very large worm burdens do so only rarely (Bundy, 1986). It also indicates why prevalence is an inadequate measure of macroparasite infection status.

It does not, however, explain why the profiles are convex in some species, or why they are not in others. Studies of reinfection with schistosomes (Wilkins *et al.*, 1987; Bensted–Smith *et al.*, 1987), *A. lumbricoides* (Cabrera, 1981) and *T. trichiura* (Bundy *et al.*, 1988) demonstrate that the rate of reacquisition of infection after treatment is markedly age-dependent, with children reacquiring worm burdens at a substantially higher rate than adults. Since the rate of acquisition of infection reflects a balance between exposure and resistance to infection, these results imply, for the species other than hookworm, that either children are more exposed to infection or adults are less susceptible, or some combination of both processes.

Soil ingestion, which enhances exposure to the soil-borne nematodes *A. lumbricoides* and *T. trichiura*, is a significantly more common practice in children than adults (Wong, Bundy and Golden, 1988) (Figure 2.8a). This suggests that the childhood peak in intensity of infection with these nematodes may be related to age-dependent changes in behaviour. No analogous studies of exposure to hookworm have been undertaken and claims that exposure is occupationally related, and thus higher in adults, appear to be anecdotal. It is perhaps worth mentioning in this context that the wearing of shoes, a widely promoted control measure against hookworm infection, would appear to be most prevalent in the adult age group that harbours the most intense infections. Quantitative studies of exposure to hookworm infection are clearly necessary.

The relation between exposure, host age and schistosome infection has been extensively examined (see Bundy and Blumenthal, 1990, for a recent review of this literature). Individuals within an endemic population who have similar indices of exposure do not all acquire the same intensity of infection after treatment, but instead exhibit a trend for the reinfection rate to decrease with increasing age (Wilkins *et al.*, 1987; Butterworth

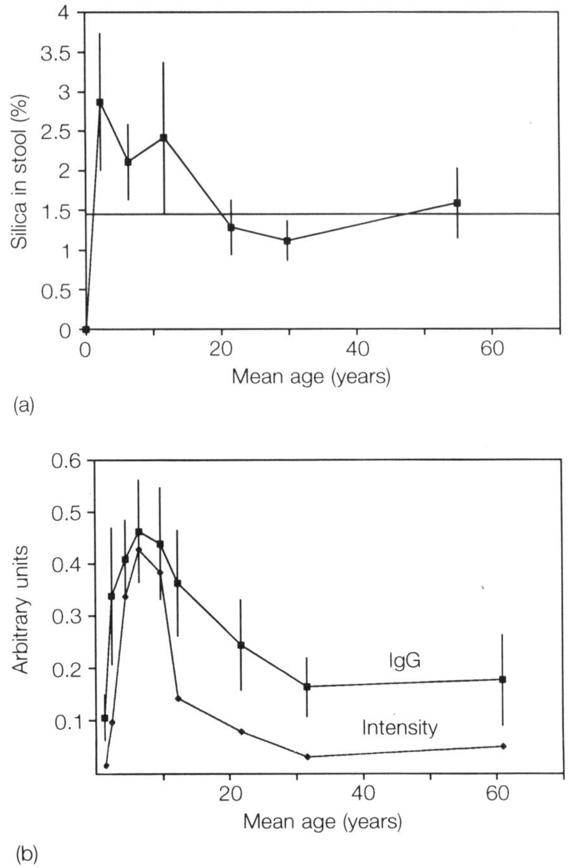

Figure 2.8 Age dependency of exposure, immune response and *T. trichiura* infection intensity. (a) Age-pattern of the practice of geophagia, as assessed by the proportion of soil-derived silica in stool. Children have higher levels of stool silica than adults, whose silica levels are largely attributable to dietary sources (horizontal line represents a normative silica level owing to the diet); (b) *T. trichiura*-specific IgG antibody levels rise and fall in concert with the intensity of *T. trichiura* infection. (Redrawn from Bundy, 1988.)

et al., 1985). This may suggest that host resistance to infection increases with past exposure to infection and hence age.

Convex age-intensity profiles are likely to arise if rates of parasite establishment and survival decrease in a manner related to the host's accumulated past experience of infection (Anderson and May, 1985a,b). An effect-

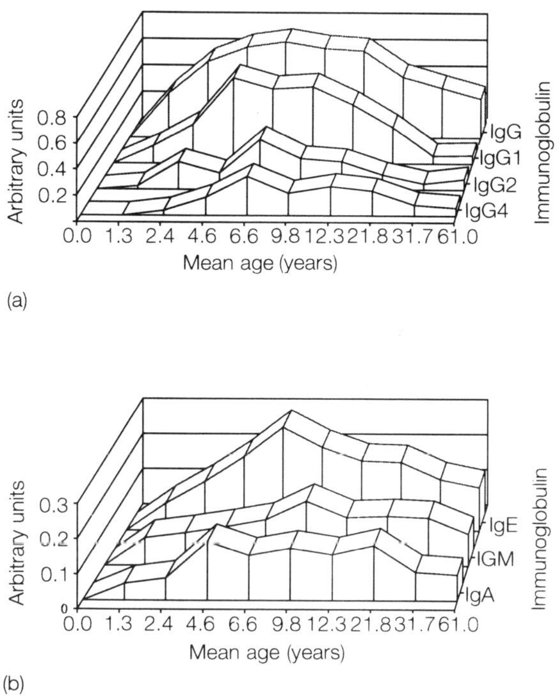

Figure 2.9 Age profiles of *T. trichiura*-specific antibody levels (E492nm) measured by ELISA against an extract of adult worm. (a) IgG subclass, (b) IgE, IgM and IgA. All isotypes exhibit age convexity. There was a negligible IgG_3 response (data not plotted). (Redrawn from Bundy *et al.*, 1991a.)

ive acquired immune response would therefore provide an appropriate mechanism for the development of age-dependent resistance.

Immuno-epidemiological studies of geohelminths have only recently been attempted, and data on *A. lumbricoides* remain inadequate (discussed by Kennedy *et al.*, 1987). The human humoral response to *T. trichiura* ES and whole worm antigen involves IgG (all subgroups except IgG_3), IgA, IgM and IgE (Lillywhite *et al.*, 1991). Examination by ELISA of sera from an endemic community indicates that the mean level of all these isotypes rises with age in childhood and then declines in adulthood (Bundy *et al.*, 1991b) (Figure 2.9). The peak parasite-specific antibody level coincides with the peak of infection intensity (Figure 2.8b), and sera from this age class recognize the widest spectrum of antigens in immunoblots, as is also the case for *A. lumbricoides* infection (Haswell–Elkins *et al.*, 1989). In children, all the isotypes exhibit a significant correlation with infection intensity. These results suggest that antibody level reflects current infection status. However, in hosts above 30 years of age, after the worm burdens have already declined to a low level, evidence suggestive of an effector response emerges. In this age class, parasite-specific IgG_4 correlates positively with intensity, perhaps indicating competitive immune blockade as has been suggested for other chronic nematode infections of humans (Hussein and Ottesen, 1986), although this result would also be compatible with a simple intensity-related response. Levels of IgA, in contrast, exhibit a negative correlation with intensity in adults, as might be expected if secretory antibody were involved in a protective response. The relevance of this observation awaits clarification of the relative roles of dimeric and monomeric IgA in this response. It is also difficult to envisage how these responses, which are only detectable in adulthood, might contribute to the observed age convexity of *T. trichiura* intensity.

It has been recognized for some time that humans mount an antibody response to hookworm infection (Ogilvie *et al.*, 1978). A recent series of studies has examined the age dependency of this response in *Necator americanus* infection (Pritchard *et al.*, 1990). Antibody responses to surface antigen increase steadily with age, while the response to ES antigen correlates with both age and infection intensity, mirroring the response of *T. trichiura*. Thus, in *N. americanus* infection, where intensity increases monotonically with age, and in *T. trichiura* and *A. lumbricoides* infection, where intensity exhibits particularly marked age convexity, the human humoral response is most prominent in the hosts harbouring the most intense infection.

On the basis of the available data, therefore, there is no clear evidence that the human antibody response plays a major role in modifying susceptibility to infection with age. Given the demonstrated importance of the immune response to helminthic infection in animal models (see, for example, Else and Grencis, 1991; Wakelin and Lee, 1987), and the apparent importance of cell-mediated immunity in these hosts, the apparent absence of a response in humans may simply indicate that the studies to date have examined the inappropriate component of the immune response. On the other hand, the phenomenon of predisposition, which indicates that those with most prior experience of infection are the most susceptible to reinfection, may suggest that the existing studies of mean antibody level and mean worm burden fail to take appropriate account of underlying heterogeneity in susceptibility to infection.

The role of acquired immunity as a determinant of the convex age-intensity profiles of schistosome infection has been the subject of extensive investigation (Wilkins *et al.*, 1987; Butterworth *et al.*, 1987). Epidemiological evidence has now been provided for a mechanism in human *S. haematobium* infection (Hagan *et al.*, 1991), and supportive evidence for a similar mechanism in *S. mansoni* (Butterworth *et al.*, 1992). It is suggested that susceptibility is determined by the balance between a protective IgE response and the blocking activity of specific IgG_4. IgE levels increase with age, while IgG_4 is maximal in the susceptible child age classes and declines thereafter. Studies *in vitro* indicate that the interaction of IgE through specific receptors with inflammatory cells can result in parasite killing, with amplification by chemotactic agents released by IgE binding to mast cells (Capron *et al.*, 1989). In susceptible humans IgG_4 may block mast-cell degranulation by competing with specific antiparasite IgE for allergenic worm antigens (Iskander, Das and Aalberse, 1981). The early production of specific IgG_4 and later production of specific IgE could be indicative of immunoglobulin class switching caused by the sequential involvement of different lymphokines.

2.3 WORM BURDEN AND MORBIDITY

For most infectious diseases, as the name would suggest, there is a close and simple correspondence between infection and disease. In contrast, for most helminthiases the relationship between infection and disease is non-linear and complex. If we accept, for the moment, the simple premise that only heavy worm burdens cause illness, then it is apparent that disease will be age-dependent, since intensity is age-dependent, and also that disease will have an overdispersed pattern even within the susceptible age classes. The relationship is further complicated by the non-linear relationship between the severity of disease and the intensity of infection, and by the interaction between symptomatology and the chronicity of infection. Helminthic infection does not inevitably lead to disease: a failure to appreciate this has led to apparently contradictory results from morbidity studies and may be the major contributor to the under-recognition of the public health significance of helminthiasis (Cooper and Bundy, 1989).

There is a general acceptance of the simple view that very intense infection results in illness, a view that reflects both clinical experience of overwhelming infection and, perhaps equally importantly, an atavistic repugnance at the insidious invasion of the body by large numbers of worms. Such extremes of infection result in the severe anaemia of necatoriasis (Stephenson, 1987), the hepatomegaly and oesophageal varices of schistosomiasis (Jordan and Webbe, 1982), and the chronic colitis of classical trichuris dysentery syndrome (Cooper and Bundy, 1988). That helminth morbidity is dependent on infection intensity is, from this perspective, uncontroversial. An understanding of the pattern of relationship between infection intensity and clinical signs has proven more elusive. This appears to be due to two main factors.

Firstly, intensity and pathogenesis are non-linearly related. Studies of the anaemia associated with hookworm infection indicate that there is a disproportionate reduction in plasma haemoglobin concentration after some threshold worm burden is exceeded (Figure 2.10a). Although profound anaemia is associated with thousands of worms, a clinically important anaemia can be induced by a few hundred worms, the precise threshold depending on host iron status (Lwambo, Bundy and Medley, 1991). Note that this occurs despite the constant *per capita* blood loss due to hookworm feeding (Martinez-Torres *et al.*, 1967) which might intuitively be expected to give a linear relationship between burden and anaemia. Studies of protein-losing enteropathy in trichuriasis also indicate a non-linear relationship with worm burden (Cooper *et al.*, 1992). The rate of gut clearance of α-1-antitrypsin at first rises rapidly with increasing worm burden to a threshold and rises more slowly thereafter (Figure 2.10b). This implies that significant intralumenal leakage of protein can occur with *T. trichiura* burdens of a few hundred worms. The clinical consequences of this loss will be determined by the nutritional and dietary status of the host and by the chronicity of infection (Cooper, Bundy and Henry, 1986). In one study, children with the classical trichuriasis dysentery syndrome had all experienced mucoid dysentery and rectal prolapse for more than three years (Cooper and Bundy, 1989).

The second reason for the lack of understanding of the relationship between intensity and disease is the difficulty of measuring and attributing morbidity. This is in part the classical epidemiological problem of identifying specific morbidity in an endemic popula-

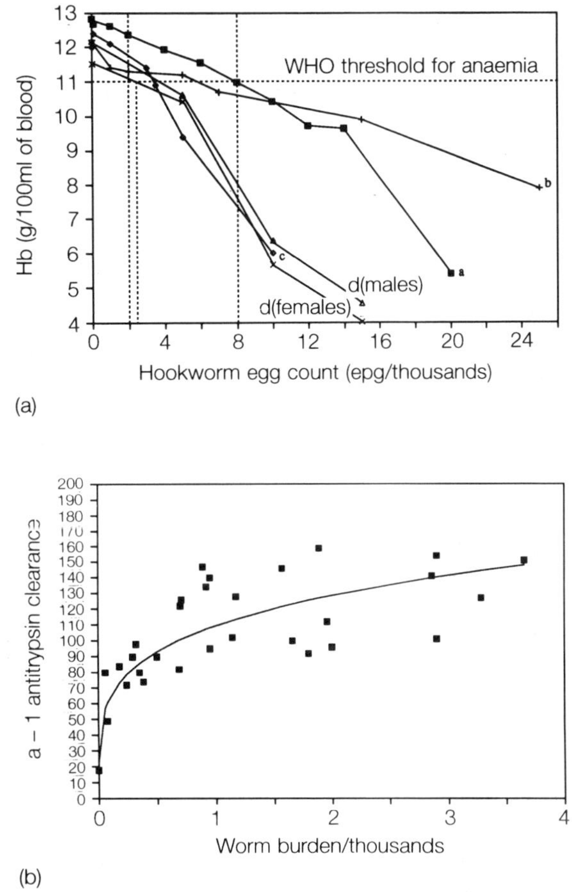

Figure 2.10 Non-linearity in the relationship between worm burden and morbidity. (a) Anaemia and hookworm infection. (Redrawn from Lwambo, Bundy and Medley, 1991); (b) α-1 antitrypsin clearance as a measure of intestinal permeability in trichuriasis dysentery syndrome. (Redrawn from Cooper *et al.*, 1992).

tion subjected to multiple insults (Walsh, 1984). It is exacerbated for helminth infection, however, by the absence of pathognomonic signs in moderate, but clinically significant, infection. This problem has been addressed by intervention trials using specific anthelmintic therapy. Such studies have shown, for example, significant improvements in linear growth after treatment of moderately infected and stunted children with hookworm, schistosome and, most spectacularly, *T. trichiura* infection (Stephenson, 1987; Stephenson *et al.*, 1989; Cooper *et al.*, 1990). Even more subtle consequences of infection are suggested by recent double-blind placebo trials which show significant improvement in the cognitive ability of schoolchildren moderately infected with *T. trichiura* (Nokes *et al.*, 1991a,b). These results suggest that even moderate helminthic infection may have insidious consequences that are unlikely to be attributed to helminthiasis in public health statistics. In one study of a village population with hyperendemic geohelminthiasis (Cooper, Bundy and Henry, 1986), only 2% of actual morbidity had been reported to the health authorities.

Some insights into the relationship between infection and disease can be provided by data analytical procedures (Guyatt *et al.*, 1990). If it is assumed that a threshold number of worms is associated with disease (see above), then based on the relationship between infection intensity and prevalence shown in Figure 2.6 it is possible to estimate the proportion of individuals which exceed the threshold worm burden (i.e. are likely to suffer morbidity) at a given prevalence of infection. This relationship between the prevalence of infection and the estimated prevalence of disease is shown for a range of thresholds of *A. lumbricoides* in Figure 2.11. Since the morbidity threshold for ascariasis is unknown, one of the fortunate conclusions of this analysis is that the threshold need not be precisely defined since the form of the relationship between infection and disease is relatively insensitive to the threshold value, provided the value is relatively large (> 20 worms in the present case). These analyses indicate that disease prevalence increases dramatically as infection prevalence rises. For example, if 25 *A. lumbricoides* worms are assumed to be associated with disease, then almost half the population will suffer morbidity at an infection prevalence of 90%, and less than 2% at an infection prevalence of 70%.

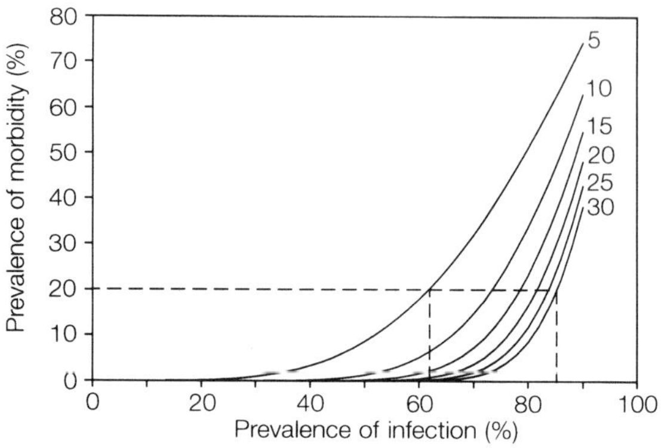

Figure 2.11 Non-linear relationship between predicted prevalence of morbidity and prevalence of *Ascaris lumbricoides* infection. Each line represents the theoretical form of the relationship (for k=0.54), assuming different threshold worm burdens (from 5 to 30 worms) at which infection is assumed to be associated with disease. (Redrawn from Guyatt and Bundy, 1991.)

Since both these infection prevalences could reasonably be considered to be high, it is not surprising that studies of morbidity in 'high' prevalence areas often reach very different conclusions about the public health significance of helminthiasis (see, for example, Keusch, 1982). There is obviously a need for quantitative rigour in defining the prevalence of disease, particularly where this is used to develop policy for disease control (Guyatt and Bundy, 1991).

2.4 WORM BURDEN AND TRANSMISSION

There is a positive, although again non-linear, relationship between worm burden and production of infective stages (Figure 2.12). The non-linearity arises because the *per capita* fecundity of female worms is density dependent, and thus the total egg output of a large worm burden is less than would be intuitively expected. Nevertheless, the larger the worm burden the greater the potential contribution to transmission.

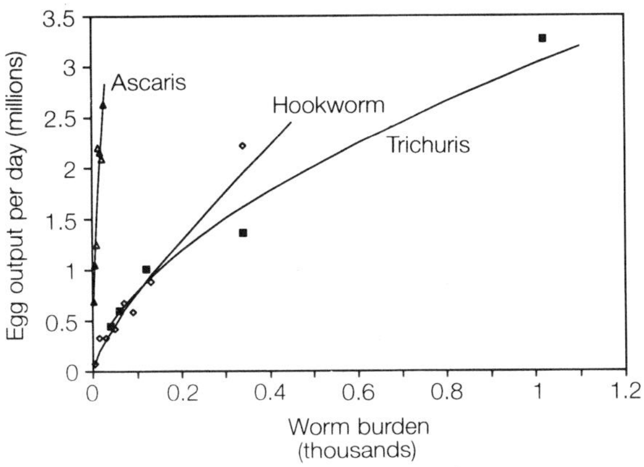

Figure 2.12 The relationship between worm burden and total daily egg output per infected host, for *A. lumbricoides*, *T. trichiura* and mixed hookworm infection. (Source: Anderson and Schad, 1985; Bundy *et al.*, 1985; Elkins, Haswell-Elkins and Anderson, 1986.)

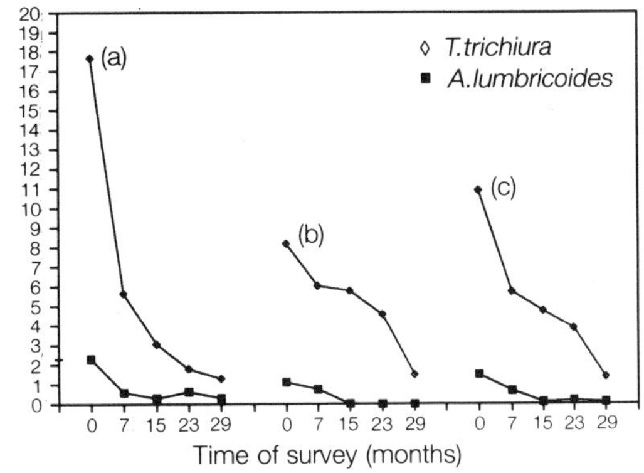

Figure 2.13 The effect of school-based chemotherapy (3× per annum) targeted at children (2–12 years) on the prevalence of *T. trichiura* and *A. lumbricoides* infection in the population of the island of Montserrat. (a) Target age classes; (b) adult age classes; (c) overall. Infection prevalence fell, as expected, in the treated age class, but also in the adult age class which did not receive treatment. The programme resulted in a significant decline in the (age-standardized) prevalence of infection in the population overall. (Source: Bundy *et al.*, 1990.)

This relationship has led to the suggestion that heavily infected individuals and intensely infected age groups contribute disproportionately to transmission (Anderson and May, 1982). This conclusion has recently been subjected to experimental proof by studies in which anthelmintic treatment is targeted at the most intensely infected age class of an environmentally isolated population and the effects on transmission to other age classes monitored. A study of the population (n=12 000) of the island of Monserrat in the Caribbean (Bundy *et al.*, 1990) showed that age-targeting treatment of more than 90% of schoolchildren resulted in a significant decline in *A. lumbricoides* and *T. trichiura* infection in the untreated adult population (Figure 2.13). Treatment of children in villages in Burma also resulted in a significant decline in *A. lumbricoides* worm burden in adults (Thien-Hlaing *et al.*, 1991) while age targeting of children infected with *S. mansoni* in a Kenyan village produced a decline in schistosomiasis in adults (Butterworth, 1991). These large-scale longitudinal studies provide clear evidence of the role of worm burden as a determinant of transmission.

2.5 CONCLUSIONS

This review of the epidemiology of intestinal helminths suggests important, but quite different, conclusions to the health planner and the physician.

From the perspective of the health policy maker, it is now recognized that community-wide programmes are required if reduction in transmission is to be achieved, that community chemotherapy can have a long-term impact on transmission, and that a significant reduction in morbidity can be achieved by a reduction in intensity that falls short of eradication. Although there remains some debate about the logistics of implementation (Anderson and Medley, 1985; Mott, 1989; Bundy, 1990c) it is clear that age-targeted programmes, which deliver chemotherapy through schools, rank amongst the most cost-effective of public health interventions

(Warren *et al.*, 1993). This has led to a range of new control initiatives (Bundy, 1990b) and has stimulated research into strategies which are targeted at multiple species infections (Bundy *et al.*, 1991a).

From the perspective of the clinician, the recognition of the importance of infection intensity and predisposition is of considerable practical relevance. All patients are not equal; the mere presence of infection has little prognostic value and diagnosis should include some measure of the intensity of infection. The lightly infected patient is unlikely to suffer clinical consequences and has a low probability of acquiring more intense infection. Whether this justifies withholding the relatively benign treatment now available is a matter of debate (Cooper and Bundy, 1989; Pawlowski and Davis, 1989), but will presumably depend on competing demands for limited health resources. The heavily infected patient is both more likely to suffer morbidity and to re-present, not because of relapse but because of reinfection. Such patients require long-term monitoring and, since intense infection is a familial phenomenon, the monitoring should involve all members of the patient's household.

In reviewing the epidemiology of intestinal helminthiasis it is apparent there is greater understanding of schistosomiasis and geohelminthiasis than of other helminthiases. This is, perhaps, appropriate since these are also the most globally prevalent infections. There are, however, some clinically important infections of primarily local importance, such as cysticercosis, or of general but low prevalence, such as strongyloidiasis, which clearly deserve greater attention from the research community. Indeed, creating a greater breadth of understanding may be essential to the future development of control approaches. With the advent of benign and broad-spectrum anthelmintics, and the move away from vertical, single-species control strategies, the current challenge to the parasite epidemiologist is to develop novel strategies for the control of multiple-species infection in the community.

REFERENCES

Anderson, R. M. (1986) The population dynamics and epidemiology of intestinal nematode infections. *Trans. Roy. Soc. Trop. Med. Hyg.*, **80**, 686–96.

Anderson, R. M. and Gordon, D. M. (1982) Processes influencing the distribution of parasite numbers within host population with special emphasis on parasite-induced host mortalities. *Parasitology*, **85**, 373–98.

Anderson, R. M. and May, R. M. (1979) Population biology of infectious diseases. Part I. *Nature, Lond.*, **280**, 361–7.

Anderson, R. M. and May, R. M. (1982) Population dynamics of human helminth infections: control by chemotherapy. *Nature*, **297**, 557–63.

Anderson, R. M. and May, R. M. (1985a) Helminth infections of humans: mathematical models, population dynamics and control. *Adv. Parasit.*, **24**, 1–101.

Anderson, R. M. and May, R. M. (1985b) Herd immunity to helminth infections: implications for parasite control. *Nature*, **315**, 493–6.

Anderson, R. M. and Medley, G. F. (1985) Community control of helminth infections of man by mass and selective chemotherapy. *Parasitology*, **90**, 629–60.

Anderson, R. M. and Schad, G. A. (1986) Hookworm burdens and faecal egg counts: an analysis of the biological basis of variation. *Trans. Roy. Soc. Trop. Med. Hyg.*, **79**, 812–25.

Ashford, R. W. and Barnish, G. (1989). *Strongyloides fulleborni* and similar parasites in animals and man, in *Strongyloidiasis, a Major Roundworm Infection of Man* (ed. D. I. Grove), Taylor & Francis: London, pp. 271–86.

Barbour, A. D. (1985) The importance of age and water contact patterns in relation to *Schistosoma haematobium* infection. *Trans. Roy. Soc. Trop. Med. Hyg.*, **79**, 151–3.

Beaver, P. C. (1975) Biology of soil-transmitted helminths: the massive infection. *Health Lab. Sci.*, **12** (2), 116–25.

Behnke, J. M. (1987) Do hookworms elicit protective immunity in man? *Parasit. Today*, **3**, 200–6.

Behnke, J. M., Ali, N. M. H. and Jenkins, S. N. (1984) Survival to patency of low-level infections with *Trichuris muris* in mice concurrently infected with *Nematospiroides dubius*. *Ann. Trop. Med. Parasit.*, **78**, 509–17.

Behnke, J. M., Hannah, J. and Pritchard, D. I. (1983) *Nematospiroides dubius* in the mouse:

evidence that adult worms depress the expression of homologous immunity. *Parasite Immunol.*, **5**, 397–408.

Beisel, W. R. (1982) Single nutrients and immunity. *Am. J. Clin. Nutr.*, **35**, 417–68.

Bensted-Smith, R., Anderson, R. M., Butterworth, A. E. *et al.* (1987) Evidence for predisposition of individual patients to reinfection with *Schistosoma mansoni*: after treatment. *Trans. Roy. Soc. Trop. Med. Hyg.*, **81**, 651–4.

Bradley, D. J. and McCullough, F. S. (1974) Egg output stability and the epidemiology of *Schistosoma haematobium*. II. An analysis of the epidemiology of endemic *S. haematobium*. *Trans. Roy. Soc. Trop. Med. Hyg.*, **80**, 706–18.

Bradley, M. (1990) Rate of expulsion of *Necator americanus* and the false hookworm *Ternidens deminutus* Railliet and Henry 1909 (Nematoda) from humans following albendazole treatment (Short Report). *Trans. Roy. Soc. Trop. Med. Hyg.*, **84**, 611–754.

Bradley, M. and Chandiwana, S. K. (1990) Age-dependency in predisposition to hookworm infection in the Burma valley area of Zimbabwe. *Trans. Roy. Soc. Trop. Med. Hyg.*, **84**, 826–8.

Bradley, M., Chandiwana, S. K., Medley, G. F. and Bundy, D. A. P. (1992) The epidemiology and population biology of *Necator americanus* in a rural community in Zimbabwe. *Trans. Roy. Soc. Trop. Med. Hyg.*, **86**, 73–6.

Bundy, D. A. P. (1986) Epidemiological aspects of *Trichuris* and trichuriasis in Caribbean communities. *Trans. Roy. Soc. Trop. Med. Hyg.*, **80**, 706–18.

Bundy, D. A. P. (1988) Population ecology of intestinal helminth infections in human communities. *Phil. Trans. Roy. Soc. London, Series B*, **321**, 405–20.

Bundy, D. A. P. (1990a) Is the hookworm just another geohelminth?, in *Hookworm Disease: Current Status and New Directions* (eds G. A. Schad and K. S. Warren), Taylor and Francis, London pp. 147–64.

Bundy, D. A. P. (1990b) New initiatives in the control of helminths. *Trans. Roy. Soc. Trop. Med. Hyg.*, **84**, 467–8.

Bundy, D. A. P. (1990c) Control of intestinal nematode infections by chemotherapy: mass treatment versus diagnostic screening. *Trans. Roy. Soc. Trop. Med. Hyg.*, **84**, 622–5.

Bundy, D. A. P. and Blumenthal, U. (1990) Human behaviour and epidemiology of helminth infection, in: *Parasitism and Host Behaviour* (eds C. Barnard and J. M. Behnke), Taylor and Francis, London; pp. 264–89.

Bundy, D. A. P. and Cooper, E. S. (1988a) Human *Trichuris* and trichuriasis. *Adv. Parasit.*, **28**, 107–73.

Bundy, D. A. P. and Cooper, E. S. (1988b) The evidence for predisposition to trichuriasis in humans: comparison of institutional and community studies. *Ann. Trop. Med. Parasit.*, **82**, 251–6.

Bundy, D. A. P. and Golden, M. H. N. (1987) The impact of host nutrition on gastro-intestinal helminth populations. *Parasitology*, **95**, 623–35.

Bundy, D. A. P., Kan, S. P. and Rose, R. (1988) age-related prevalence, intensity and frequency distribution of gastrointestinal helminth infection in urban slum children from Kuala Lumpur, Malaysia. *Trans. Roy. Soc. Trop. Med. Hyg.*, **82**, 298–4.

Bundy, D. A. P., Thompson, D. E., Golden, M. H. N. *et al.* (1985) Population distribution of *Trichuris trichiura* in a community of Jamaican children. *Trans. Roy. Soc. Trop. Med. Hyg.*, **79**, 232–7.

Bundy, D. A. P., Cooper, E. S., Thompson, D. E. *et al.* (1988) Effect of age and initial infection status on the rate of reinfection with *Trichuris trichiura* after treatment. *Parasitology*, **97**, 469–76.

Bundy, D. A. P., Cooper, E. S., Thompson, D. E. *et al.* (1987a) Age-related prevalence and intensity of *Trichuris trichiura* infection in a St Lucian community. *Trans. Roy. Soc. Trop. Med. Hyg.*, **88**, 85–94.

Bundy, D. A. P., Cooper, E. S., Thompson, D. E. *et al.* (1987b) Predisposition to *Trichuris trichiura* infections in humans. *Epidem. Infec.*, **98**, 65–71.

Bundy, D. A. P., Wong, M. S., Lewis, L. and Horton, J. (1990) Control of gastrointestinal helminths by age-targeted chemotherapy delivered through schools. *Trans. Roy. Soc. Trop. Med. Hyg.*, **84**, 115–20.

Bundy, D. A. P., Chandiwana, S. K., Homeida, M. M. A. *et al.* (1991a) The epidemiological implications of a multiple-infection approach to the control of human helminth infections. *Trans. Roy. Soc. Trop. Med. Hyg.*, **85**, 274–6.

Bundy, D. A. P., Lillywhite, J. E., Didier, J. M. *et al.* (1991b) Age-dependency of infection status and serum antibody levels in human whipworm (*Trichuris trichiura*) infection. *Clin. Exp. Immunol.* (in press).

Butterworth, A. E. (1991) The immunology and epidemiology of *Schistosoma mansoni* in Kenya. *Trans. Roy. Soc. Trop. Med. Hyg.* (in press).

Butterworth, A. E., Capron, M., Cordingley, J. S. *et al.* (1985) Immunity after treatment of human schistosomiasis mansoni. II. Identification of resistant individuals, and analysis of their immune responses. *Trans. Roy. Soc. Trop. Med. Hyg.*, **79**, 393–408.

Butterworth, A. E., Bensted-Smith, R., Capron, A. *et al.* (1987) Immunity in human schistosomiasis mansoni. Prevention by blocking antibodies of the expression of immunity in young children. *Parasitology*, **94**, 281–300.

Cabrera, B. D. (1981) Reinfection and infection rate studies of soil-transmitted helminthiasis in Juban, Sorsogon, in *Collected Papers on the Control of Soil-Transmitted Helminthiases*, Vol. 1, Asian Parasitic Control Organisation, Tokyo, Japan, pp. 181–91.

Capron, A., Capron, M., Grangette, C. and Dessaint, J.-P. (1989) *CIBA Fdn Symp.*, **147**, 153–60.

Chai, J. Y., Kim, K. S., Hong, S. T. *et al.* (1985) Prevalence, worm burden and other epidemiological parameters of *Ascaris lumbricoides* infection in rural communities in Korea. *Korean J. Parasit.*, **23**, 241–6.

Chan, L. L., Kan, S. P. and Bundy, D. A. P. (1992) Predisposition to *Ascaris lumbricoides* and *Trichuris trichiura* in an urban slum area of Kuala Lumpur, Malaysia. *Parasitology*, **104**, 371–7.

Cheever, A. W. (1968) A quantitative post mortem study of schistosomiasis mansoni in man. *Am. J. Trop. Med. Hyg.*, **17**, 38–64.

Cooper, E. S. and Bundy, D. A. P. (1988) Trichuriasis, in *Intestinal Helminthic Infections* (ed. Z. S. Pawlowski), Baillière's Clinical Tropical Medicine and Communicable Disease, **2** (3), 629–43.

Cooper, E. S. and Bundy, D. A. P. (1989) *Trichuris* is not trivial. *Parasit. Today*, **4**, 301–6.

Cooper, E. S., Bundy, D. A. P. and Henry, F. J. (1986) Chronic dysentery, stunting and whipworm infestation. *Lancet* **ii**, 280–1.

Cooper, E. S., Bundy, D. A. P., MacDonald, T. T. and Golden, M. H. N. (1990) Growth suppression in the trichuris dysentery syndrome. *Europ. J. Clin. Nutr.*, **44**, 285–91.

Cooper, E. S., Whyte-Alleng, C. A. M., Finzi-Smith, J. S. and MacDonald, T. T. (1992) Intestinal nematode infection in children: the pathophysiological price paid. *Parasitology*, **104**, S91–S103.

Croll, N. A. and Ghandirian, E. (1981) Wormy persons: contributions to the nature and patterns of overdispersion with *Ascaris lumbricoides, Ancylostoma duodenale, Necator americanus* and *Trichuris trichiura*. *Trop. Geog. Med.*, **33**, 241–8.

Croll, N. A., Anderson, R. M., Gyorkos, T. W. and Ghadirian, E. (1982) The population biology and control of *Ascaris lumbricoides* in a rural community in Iran. *Trans. Roy. Soc. Trop. Med. Hyg.*, **76**, 187–97.

Cross, J. H. and Basaca–Sevilla, V. (1987) Intestinal capillariasis, in *Intestinal Helminthic Infections* (ed. Z. S. Pawlowski), *Baillière's Clinical Tropical Medicine and Communicable Diseases*, **2**, 735–46.

Cruz, M., Davis, A., Dixon, H. *et al.* (1989) Operational studies on the control of *Taenia solium* taeniasis/cysticercosis in Ecuador. *Bull. Wld. Hlth. Org.*, **67**, 401–7.

Elkins, D. B., Haswell–Elkins, M. and Anderson, R. M. (1986) The epidemiology and control of intestinal helminths in the Pulicat Lake region of Southern India. I. Study design and pre- and post-treatment observations on *Ascaris lumbricoides* infection. *Trans. Roy. Soc. Trop. Med. Hyg.*, **80**, 774–92.

Else, K. J. and Grencis, R. K. (1991) Cellular immune responses to the murine nematode parasite *Trichuris muris*. I. Differential cytokine production during acute or chronic infection. *Immunology*, **72**, 508–13.

Else, K. and Wakelin, D. (1988) The effects of H-2 and non-H-2 genes on the expulsion of the nematode *Trichuris muris* from inbred and congenic mice. *Parasitology*, **96**, 543–50.

Forrester, J. E., Scott, M. E., Bundy, D. A. P. and Golden, M. H. N. (1988) Clustering of *Ascaris lumbricoides* and *Trichuris trichiura* infections within households. *Trans. Roy. Soc. Trop. Med. Hyg.*, **82**, 282–289.

Forrester, J. E., Scott, M. E., Bundy, D. A. P. and Golden, M. H. N. (1990) Predisposition of individuals and families in Mexico to heavy infection with *Ascaris lumbricoides* and *Trichuris trichiura*. *Trans. Roy. Soc. Trop. Med. Hyg.*, **84**, 272–6.

Gompels, M. M., Todd, J., Peters, B. S. *et al.* (1991) Disseminated strongyloides in AIDS: uncommon but important. *AIDS*, **5**, 329–32.

Guyatt, H. L. and Bundy, D. A. P. (1991) Estimating prevalence of community morbidity due to intestinal helminths: prevalence of infection as an indicator of the prevalence of disease. *Trans. Roy. Soc. Trop. Med. Hyg.*, **85**, 778–82.

Guyatt, H. L., Bundy, D. A. P., Medley, G. F. and Grenfell, B. T. (1990) The relationship between the frequency distribution of *Ascaris lumbricoides* and the prevalence and intensity of infection in human communities. *Parasitology*, **101**, 139–43.

Hagan, P., Blumenthal, U. J., Dunn, D. *et al.* (1991) Human IgE, IgG4 and resistance to reinfection with *Schistosoma haematobium*. *Nature*, **349**, 243–5.

Haswell-Elkins, M. R., Elkins, D. B., Manjula, K. *et al.* (1987) The distribution and abundance of *Enterobius vermicularis* in a South Indian fishing community. *Parasitology*, **95**, 339–54.

Haswell-Elkins, M. R., Elkins, D. B. and Anderson, R. M. (1987) Evidence for predisposition in humans to infection with *Ascaris*, hookworm, *Enterobius* and *Trichuris* in a South Indian fishing community. *Parasitology*, **95**, 323–37.

Haswell-Elkins, M. R., Kennedy, M. W., Maizels, R. M. *et al.* (1989) The antibody recognition profiles of humans naturally infected with *Ascaris lumbricoides*. *Parasite Immun.*, **11**, 615–27.

Hirayama, K., Matsushita, S., Kikuchi, I. *et al.* (1987) HLA-DQ is epistatic to HLA-DR in controlling in the immune response to schistosoma antigen in humans. *Nature*, **327**, 426–30.

Holland, C. V., Asaolu, S. O., Crompton, D. W. T. *et al.* (1989) The epidemiology of *Ascaris lumbricoides* and other soil-transmitted helminths in primary school children from Ile-Ife, Nigeria. *Parasitology*, **99**, 275–85.

Hominick, W. M., Dean, C. G. and Schad, G. A. (1987) Population biology of hookworms in West Bengal: analysis of numbers of infective larvae recovered from damp pads applied to the soil surface at defaecation sites. *Trans. Roy. Soc. Trop. Med. Hyg.*, **81**, 978–86.

Hsieh, H. C. (1970) Studies on endemic hookworm: I. Survey and longitudinal observation in Taiwan. *Jap. J. Parasit.*, **19**, 508–22.

Hussein, R. and Ottesen, E. A. (1986) IgE responses in human filariasis IV. Parallel antigen recognition by IgG and IgG4 subclass antibodies. *J. Immun.*, **136**, 1859.

Iskander, R., Das, P. K. and Aalberse, R. C. (1981) IgG4 antibodies in Egyptian patients with schistosomiasis. *Int. Arch. Allergy Appl. Immun.*, **66**, 200–7.

Jordon, P. and Webbe, G. (1982) *Schistosomiasis: Epidemiology, Treatment and Control*, William Heinemann Medical Books Ltd., London.

Kennedy, M. W., Qureshi, F., Haswell-Elkins, M. and Elkins, D. B. (1987) Homology and heterology between the secreted antigens of the parasitic larval stages of *Ascaris lumbricoides* and *Ascaris suum*. *Clin. Exp. Immun.*, **67**, 20–30.

Keusch, G. T. (1982) Summary and recommendations, in *The Biology of Parasitic Infections: Workshop on Interactions of Nutrition and Parasitic Diseases. Reviews of Infectious Diseases* **4** (4), 901–7.

Keymer, A. and Pagel, M. (1989) Predisposition to hookworm infection, in *Hookworm Infection: Current Status and New Directions* (eds G. A. Schad and K. S. Warren), Taylor and Francis, London.

Keymer, A. E. and Slater, A. F. G. (1987) Helminth fecundity: Density dependence or statistical illusion? *Parasit. Today*, **3** (2), 56–8.

Lillywhite, J. E., Bundy, D. A. P., Didier, J. M. *et al.* (1991) Humoral responses in human infection with the whipworm *Trichuris trichiura*. *Parasite Immun.*, **13**, 491–507.

Lwambo, N., Bundy, D. A. P. and Medley, G. F. (1991) A new approach to morbidity risk assessment in hookworm endemic communities. *Epidemiology and Infection*, **108**, 469–81.

Martinez-Torres, C., Ojeda, A., Roche, M. and Laryisse, M. (1967) Hookworm infestation and intestinal blood loss. *Trans. Roy. Soc. Trop. Med. Hyg.*, **61**, 373–83.

McCallum, H. I. (1990) Covariance in parasite burdens: the effect of predisposition to infection. *Parasitology*, **100**, 153–9.

Morera, P. (1987) Abdominal angiostrongyloidiasis, in *Intestinal Helminthic Infections* (ed. Z. S. Pawlowski), *Baillière's Clinical Tropical Medicine and Communicable Diseases*, **2**, 747–53.

Mott, K. E. (1989) Selective population chemotherapy in *Schistosoma haemotobium* infection: pros and cons, in *Parasitic Diseases: Treatment and Control* (eds M. J. Miller, and E. J. Love), CRC Press, Florida.

Nakada, K., Kohakura, M., Komoda, H. and Hinuma, Y. (1984) High incidence of HTLV antibody in carriers of *Strongyloides stercoralis*. *Lancet*, **i**, 633.

Nokes, C., Cooper, E. S., Robinson, B. A. and Bundy, D. A. P. (1991a) Geohelminth infection and academic assessment in Jamaican children. *Trans. Roy. Soc. Trop. Med. Hyg.*, **85**, 272–3.

Nokes, C., Grantham-McGregor, S. M., Sawyer, A. W. *et al.* (1991b) Moderate to high infections of *Trichuris trichiura* and cognitive function in Jamaican school children. *Proc. Roy. Soc.*, **247**, 77–81.

Ogilvie, B. M., Bartlett, A., Godfrey, R. C. *et al.* (1978) Antibody responses in self-infections with *Necator americanus*. *Trans. Roy. Soc. Trop. Med. Hyg.*, **72**, 66–71.

Pawlowski, Z. S. and Davis, A. (1989) Morbidity and mortality in ascariasis, in *Ascariasis and its Prevention and Control* (eds D. W. T. Crompton, M. C. Nesheim and Z. S. Pawlowski), Taylor and Francis, London, pp. 71–86

Pawlowski, Z. S. (1989) Epidemiology, prevention and control, in *Strongyloidiasis, a Major Roundworm Infection of Man* (ed. D. I. Grove), Taylor and Francis, London, pp. 233–49.

Pritchard, D. I., Quinell, R. J., Slater, A. F. G. *et al.* (1990) Epidemiology and immunology of *Necator americanus* infection in a community in Papua New Guinea: humoral responses to excretory-secretory and cuticular collagen antigens. *Parasitology*, **100**, 317–26.

Sadun, E. H. and Maiphoom, C. (1953) Studies on the epidemiology of the human intestinal fluke

Fasciolopis buski (Lankester) in Central Thailand. *Am. J. Trop. Med. Hyg.*, **2**, 1070.

Sahba, G. H., Arfaa, F. and Bijan, H. (1967) Intestinal helminthiasis in the rural area of Khuzestan, south-west Iran. *Ann. Trop. Med. Parasit.*, **61**, 352–7.

Sasazuki, T., Ohta, N., Kaneoka, R. and Kojima, S. (1980) Association between an HLA haplotype and low responsiveness to schistosomal worm antigen in man. *J. Exp. Med.*, **152**, 314–18.

Sato, Y. (1986) Epidemiology of strongyloidiasis in Okinawa, in *Collected Papers on the Control of Soil- transmitted Helminthiases* (eds M. Yokogawa *et al.*), The Asian Parasite Control Organization, Tokyo, **Vol. III**, pp. 20–31.

Schad, G. A. and Anderson, R. M. (1985) Predisposition to hookworm infection in humans. *Science*, **228**, 1537–40.

Schad, G. A., Nawalinski, T. A. and Kochar, V. K. (1983) Human ecology and distribution and abundance of hookworm populations, in *Human Ecology and Infectious Disease* (ed. N. A. Croll and J. Cross), Academic Press, New York, pp. 187–223.

Seo, B. S., Cho, S. Y. and Chai, J. Y. (1979) Frequency distribution of *Ascaris lumbricoides* in rural Korea with special reference on the effect of changing endemicity. *Korean J. Parasit.*, **17**, 105–13.

Singhi, S., Singhi, P. and Adwani, G. B. (1981) Role of psychosocial stress in the cause of pica. *Clin. Paed.*, **20**, 783–5.

Soroczan, W. (1976) *Strongyloides stercoralis* in eastern and south-eastern Poland. *Wiadomosci Parazytologiczne*, **22**, 515–16.

Stephenson, L. S. (1987) *The Impact of Helminth Infections on Human Nutrition*. Taylor and Francis, London.

Stephenson, L. S., Latham, M. C., Kruz, K. M., *et al.* (1989) Treatment with a single dose of Albendazole improves physical fitness of Kenyan school boys with hookworm, *T. trichiura* and *A. lumbricoides* infections. *Am. J. Trop. Med.*, **41**, 78–87.

Suskind, R. M. (1980) Malnutrition and the immune response, in *The Impact of Malnutrition on Immune Defence in Parasitic Infection* (eds H. Isliker and B. Schurch), Hans Huber Publishers, Vienna.

Thein-Hlaing, Than-San and Myat-Lay-Kyin (1991) The impact of three-monthly age-targeted chemotherapy on *Ascaris lumbricoides* infection. *Trans. Roy. Soc. Trop. Med. Hyg.*, **85**, 519–22.

Wakelin, D. and Blackwell, J. M. (1988) *Genetics of Resistance to Bacterial and Parasitic Infection*. Taylor and Francis, London.

Wakelin, D. and Lee, T. D. G. (1987) Immunobiology of *Trichuris* and *Capillaria* infections, in *Immune Responses in Parasitic Infections: Immunology, Immunopathology, and Immunoprophylaxis*. Vol I: Nematodes (ed. E. J. L. Soulsby), CRC Press, Florida, pp. 61–88.

Walsh, J. A. (1984) Estimating the burden of illness in the tropics, in *Tropical and Geographical Medicine* (eds K. S. Warren and A. A. F. Mahmoud), McGraw-Hill Book Company, New York, pp. 1073–85.

Warren, K. S., Bundy, D. A. P., Anderson, R. M. *et al.* (1993) Helminth infections, in *Disease and Disease Control in Developing Countries* (eds D. T. Jamison and W. H. Mosley), OUP, World Bank, Washington DC, Chapter 17, pp. 131–60.

Wassom, D. L., Krco, C. J. and David, C. S. (1987) I-E expression and susceptibility to parasite infection. *Immun. Today*, **8**, 39–43.

Wassom, D. L., Wakelin, D., Brooks, B. O. *et al.* (1984) Genetic control of immunity to *Trichinella spiralis* infections of mice. Hypothesis to explain the role of H-2 genes in primary and challenge infections. *Immunology*, **51**, 625–31.

Wilkins, H. A., Blumenthal, U. J., Hagan, P. *et al.* (1987) Resistance to reinfection after treatment of urinary schistosomiasis. *Trans. Roy. Soc. Trop. Med. Hyg.*, **81**, 29–35.

Wong, M. S. and Bundy, D. A. P. (1990) Quantitative assessment of contamination of soil by the eggs of *Ascaris lumbricoides* and *Trichuris trichiura*. *Trans. Roy. Soc. Trop. Med. Hyg.*, **84**, 567–70.

Wong, M. S., Bundy, D. A. P. and Golden, M. H. N. (1988) Quantitative assessment of geophagous behaviour as a potential source of exposure to geohelminth infection. *Trans. Roy. Soc. Trop. Med. Hyg.*, **82**, 621–5.

Wong, M. S., Bundy, D. A. P. and Golden, M. H. N. (1991) The rate of ingestion of *Ascaris lumbricoides* and *Trichuris trichiura* eggs in soil and its relationship to infection in two children's homes in Jamaica. *Trans. Roy. Soc. Trop. Med. Hyg.*, **85**, 89–91.

THREE

Molecular aspects of colonization and helminth pathogenicity

J. W. Kazura

Enteric helminthic infections are among the most prevalent parasitoses of humans and other mammalian hosts. One-quarter of the world's population has been estimated to be infected by the nematode *Ascaris lumbricoides* and iron deficiency anemia secondary to hookworm infection is an important cause of morbidity in children living in developing countries. Several gastrointestinal nematodes also have an adverse impact on economic aspects of the meat industry, especially those related to raising cattle and sheep. Despite the global importance of these infectious diseases, there is relatively little knowledge of the molecular mechanisms by which these helminths establish themselves within the gut and how colonization in this site is maintained. This is in contrast with the case of many enteric bacteria and protozoan parasites, such as *Entamoeba histolytica* and *Giardia lamblia* (Tse and Chadee, 1991).

Several reasons account for this difference. Firstly, relative to unicelullar protozoa and bacteria, intestinal helminths are multicellular and biochemically complex. In the case of nematodes, with which this chapter is primarily concerned, these organisms have five distinct developmental stages that include first- to fourth-stage larvae (L1 through L4) and sexually mature adult male and female worms. Each of these parasite stages has distinct antigenic and biochemical characteristics which are adapted to their unique environments within or outside the host. With respect to gastrointestinal nematodes, there is a great deal of heterogeneity in terms of the specific developmental stages that interact with this organ system. In the simplest case such as pinworms or *Oxyuridae,* all of the developmental stages are limited to the gut. In some cases, only adult worms are present in the gut (e.g. *Ancylostoma* and *Necator* species), whereas in others in addition to adult and larval stages in the gut, a second generation of L1 develops parenterally (e.g. *Trichinella spiralis*). With some exceptions, such as *Strongyloides stercoralis,* the intensity of infection in the gut is directly related to the inoculum of infective stage parasite acquired outside the body (i.e. through ingestion or skin penetration). *Strongyloides* also has an autoinfective life cycle in which infective larvae are produced in the gastrointestinal tract and re-initiate their life cycle from this location.

These diverse biologic features suggest that observations made in one host–parasite system may not be generalized to other nematode infections. Another reason for

Enteric Infection 2. Intestinal helminths. Edited by M.J.G. Farthing, G.T. Keusch and D. Wakelin. Published in 1995 by Chapman and Hall, London. ISBN 0 412 39140 6

slow progress in this area of investigation is related to the lack of axenic systems for production of sufficient numbers of cloned parasite populations to isolate and characterize molecules involved in attachment of nematodes to mucins or gastrointestinal epithelia. There are currently no widely used *in vitro* methods which enable harvest of large numbers of each developmental stage of *Nippostrongylus brasiliensis*, *Trichinella spiralis* or *Heligmosomoides polygyrus*, nematode parasites which are the most commonly employed for experimental work. Finally, and most importantly, there are at present few *in vitro* models which reliably mimic the complex interaction of enteric nematodes with the gastrointestinal tract, whether it be limited to the small intestine or colon. Explants of mammalian gastrointestinal tract generally do not survive for more than several days, which is often shorter than the period of time adult nematode parasites live in the gut of the intact host.

Despite the difficulties of the experimental systems, there has been progress in understanding the environmental cues which result in development of nematodes in the gastrointestinal tract. In addition, recent studies of *Trichinella spiralis* have provided insight into the possible contributions of nematode–mucus interactions in establishing the niche of adult worms in the gut. Although the host immune response clearly plays a major role in expulsion of nematodes from the gut (see Chapter 5) and the attendant local pathology (see Chapter 4), it is also likely that select host-derived effector molecules interact with the parasite enzymes in a manner that promotes survival of the invading organism. These aspects of nematode interaction with the gastrointestinal tract will be discussed in this chapter.

3.1 ORAL INFECTION PROCESS AND TRIGGERS FOR NEMATODE DEVELOPMENT

A complex process of moulting (i.e. shedding of the surface cuticle) and somatic development is initiated when infective eggs or L3 are ingested by the mammalian host. Prior to their introduction into the host, these infective stages may have undergone periods of dormancy or hypobiosis in the external environment, allowing them to survive adverse conditions. In moulting, the organisms rapidly lose their cuticle and undergo developmental processes morphologically characterized by an increase in size and changes in the neural system. The precise parasite molecules which initiate this moulting event have not been identified. However, several lines of evidence support the notion that ecdysteroids are involved. The biologic function of these sterols is best characterized in insects, where they have been shown to be critical in moulting not only of immature larval stages but also in regulation of reproductive activities of adult insects (Barker and Rees, 1990). There is indirect evidence that ecdysteroids are synthesized by nematodes (Bottjer, Whisenton and Weinstein, 1984). Moreover, addition of exogenous ecdysteroids to *Ascaris suum* larvae increases the rate of moulting *in vitro*. Finally, diminution of the bioavailability of ecdysteroids by immunization of the host with these sterols conjugated to protein prior to infection with the nematode *Dirofilaria immitis* diminishes the intensity of microfilaremia (Koolman, Walter and Zahman, 1984). Since nematodes are incapable of *de novo* cholesterol synthesis, the requisite precursor of ecdysone and related ecdysteroids, the availability of cholesterol in the gut is likely to be important in initiating development of the organisms.

Studies of strongyloid enteric nematodes (Rogers and Somerville, 1968) and *Haemon-*

chus contortus (Rogers, 1960) indicate that changes in carbon dioxide content in the gastrointestinal tract at temperatures within the physiologic range of the normal host are additional important factors which 'trigger' moulting. The precise molecular basis by which carbon dioxide induces these alterations is not known. However, it has been proposed that a decrease in the internal pH of the worm results in activation of a mitochondrial calcium–hydrogen ion exchanger. These events ultimately result in increased levels of free intracellular calcium ions (Petronijevic and Rogers, 1987a). Ex-sheathment is thought to be calcium-dependent (Petronijevic and Rogers, 1987b). Verification of this hypothetical series of events will require identification of the putative mitochondrial ion pump and examination of its functional state at various times during the moulting process. Examination of similar events using more tractable models in which tissue L3 behaviour can be easily manipulated by exposure to serum or its active components should provide additional insight into this problem (Hawdon and Schad, 1990).

3.2 HABITAT SELECTION

The molecular basis by which enteric nematodes select the gut or specific locations within it as their niche have not been determined. As is described in several chapters in this volume, many nematodes remain localized to the small intestine (hookworms) while others are maintained in the colon (pinworms). The process of habitat selection is a general biologic phenomenon of parasitism and there is little understanding of the chemical or physical cues and the corresponding sensors in helminths that guide the organisms to the appropriate tissue site. In cestodes such as *Fasciola hepatica*, carbon dioxide and glycocholic acid present in bile appear to be involved in regulating the migratory path of this liver fluke (Sukhdeo, 1990). Similar regulatory pathways and the means by which the nervous system of intestinal nematodes sense them, have not been described.

3.3 NEMATODE INTERACTIONS WITH MUCUS AND GASTROINTESTINAL EPITHELIA

Mucus in the gastrointestinal tract is a complex biomaterial consisting of mucus glycoproteins, lipids, peptides, several host immune proteins including IgA, endogenous bacterial microflora and debris from enterocytes and other gut cells. There are at least two forms of mucus in the gut. The first is a thin layer of water-insoluble material covering the mucosal surface and the second a more viscous material containing a relatively greater amount of non-mucin glycoproteins in the gut lumen (Allen and Carroll, 1985). The source of mucus glycoproteins, the most important constituent of mucus from the perspective of invading parasites, are goblet cells (Neutra and Forstner, 1987).

Mucus glycoproteins or mucins consist of polymers of glycoprotein subunits linked by disulphide bonds through their protein cores (Neutra and Forstner, 1987). The proteinaceous component of mucus generally constitutes 20% of the total mass of these macromolecules, which have Mr in the range of 1 to 2 million. The major region of the protein has a high content of serine, threonine and proline, to which the carbohydrate moieties are linked. The oligosaccharide side chains, which consist of approximately 80% of the molecular mass, are joined to the peptide backbone of the major region via hydroxyl groups of serine and threonine. Five sugars are generally found in mammalian mucus glycoproteins: galactose, fucose, N-acetylgalactosamine, N-acetylglucosamine and sialic acid. There is marked heterogeneity in the carbohydrate composition and sequences of peptide backbones of mucins produced by goblet cells located in different segments of the small and large intestine. This variability in chemical structure may contribute to the success of a specific nematode species in colonizing discrete portions of the gut.

The critical role of mucins in colonization of the gut is at present best illustrated by studies of pathogenic protozoa and bacteria (Tse and Chadee, 1991). In the case of the protozoan *Entamoeba histolytica*, trophozoites adhere to mammalian cells by the heavy subunit of a 260 kDa surface lectin which binds to galactose/N-acetylgalactosamine (Petri *et al.*, 1987). Inhibition of this binding by appropriate competitive sugars results in decreased binding to mucin-bearing target cells *in vitro*. Similarly, mucus receptors have been identified for several strains of bacteria, such as *Escherichia coli*, *Shigella flexneri* and *Campylobacter jejuni* (Tse and Chadee, 1991). Specific mucus receptors have not been identified to date in nematodes. Nevertheless, work done by several groups has provided evidence suggesting that mucins may be involved in the colonization and maintenance of some enteric nematodes in the gut niche.

With the use of models in which newborn rats suckling immune or *T. spiralis*-infected dams expel more than 99% of orally inoculated infective larvae – a process referred to as rapid expulsion (Appleton and McGregor, 1984) – or adult rats experience abbreviated infections in the gut (Bell *et al.*, 1984), the contribution of intestinal mucus to this process and the specific parasite molecules mediating this interaction have been investigated. Earlier studies had implicated intestinal mucus in the expulsion of *Nippostrongylus brasiliensis* from the gut of immunized rats (Miller *et al.*, 1981). When challenged orally with muscle-stage or infective larvae of *T. spiralis*, the helminths rapidly become entrapped in mucus, a process markedly enhanced by antibodies directed against the surface of the organisms (Carlisle, McGregor and Appleton, 1991a). Although in some cases there is a correlation between the degree of mucus entrapment mediated by monoclonal antibodies *in vitro* and rapid expulsion *in vivo*, this is not true for several other monoclonal antibodies, allowing the two phenomena to be dissociated. Taken together with related studies in which F(ab')2 fragments of several monoclonal antibodies were found to mediate increased adherence to mucus without effecting expulsion, the investigators concluded that entrapment of *T. spiralis* in mucus is not the primary event in rapid expulsion mediated by antibody. The data suggest that antibody directly interferes with a function of a nematode molecule(s) required for maintenance in the epithelial niche of the gastrointestinal tract (Carlisle, McGregor and Appleton, 1991b). To identify the targets of such molecules, Appleton and Usack (1993) employed immunoprecipitation and Western blot studies to characterize their size and surface disposition on the parasite. Protective antibodies bound most prominently to glycoproteins of approximately 45 kDa and 105/55 kDa, although antigens of other apparent mobilities were noted. Detailed biochemical characterization of these antigens, especially with regard to their carbohydrate composition and homology with other 'receptor' proteins for other gastrointestinal microbes, are needed to extend our knowledge of the molecular mechanisms by which nematodes colonize the gut.

3.4 MOLECULAR BASIS FOR PATHOGENICITY IN THE GASTROINTESTINAL TRACT

Enteric nematodes cause a wide variety of disease manifestations in the gut. In many cases, infections of low intensity are associated with little or no clinically significant disease manifestations. This is the case with many *Ascaris lumbricoides* and *Trichuris trichiura* infections, although in the setting of concurrent malnutrition or other infections of the gut these helminthiases may contribute to morbidity (see relevant chapters in this volume). Other nematodes may cause diarrhea and fluid loss from the bowel, such as Arctic strains of *Trichinella spiralis* and *Strongyloides stercoralis*, or anemia secondary to bleeding in the cases of *Ancylostoma* and *Necator* infections. For the most part, the specific parasite molecules which mediate these pathologic responses in the gut have not been identified or characterized in great detail. This section will thus summarize details only of those molecules which are known to be involved in these aspects of the host–parasite relationship and suggest some approaches to investigate the mechanisms underlying gut-associated pathologic responses.

As is the case with pathogenic bacteria and protozoa, host effector mechanisms against helminthic parasites may in part be dependent upon generation of reduced oxygen products such as hydrogen peroxide and hydroxyl radicals. These labile highly toxic molecules result in lipid peroxidation and damage to DNA of nearby targets, such as invading helminthic parasites surrounded by local inflammatory cells (e.g. eosinophils, neutrophils and monocytes) in the gut. Studies of *T. spiralis* and other nematodes have shown that there is an inverse relationship between the endogenous content of scavenging enzymes which destroy these toxic molecules, such as glutathione peroxidase and catalase, and susceptibility to killing by reactive oxygen species (Brophy and Pritchard, 1992). During this process, it is likely that surrounding host tissues such as the gastrointestinal mucosa are damaged, with a consequent increase in epithelial cell turnover. The observation that some forms of these parasite scavenger enzymes, such as superoxide dismutase, are actively secreted suggest that lipid peroxidation and other types of oxidative damage may be diverted from the gut-invasive helminth and directed against nearby host tissues. Confirmation of the *in vivo* role of these enzymes will require development of nematode parasites that lack functional scavenging enzymes, such as by genetic disruption, and assessment of the effects of neutralizing antibodies to the parasite enzymes on the pathologic outcome and intensity of infection.

Perhaps the most well-defined basis of pathogenicity in a gastrointestinal helminthiasis is the case of hookworm infection. These organisms attach to the small intestinal mucosa by a series of hooks and secrete proteolytic enzymes which have potent anticoagulant effects (Hotez, LeTrang and McKerrow, 1985 and see Chapter 10). The continual bleeding, which provides the nutritional protein source for the adult parasites, results in iron-deficiency anemia, a disease manifestation which is proportional to the number of parasites in the gut and the oral intake of iron by the host (Schad and Banwell, 1991).

Finally, it is important to emphasize that much of the tissue damage and physiologic alterations associated with enteric nematode infections are not a direct result of interaction with parasite molecules with mucus or gut epithelium but due to the immune response to secreted or surface antigens. For example, the early response to oral infection with *Heligmosomoides polygyrus* (within 12 hours of inoculation) includes marked elevations of cytokines such as IL-3, IL-5 and IL-9 produced by mast cells or other non-T, non-B cells (Svetic *et al.*, 1993). These cytokines are not only involved in commitment and expansion of local CD4+ T-helper cells to produce cytokines characteristic of the Th2 functional phenotype (IL-4, IL-5, IL-10) (Urban *et al.*, 1992) but may also have direct effects on epithelial cell functions such as electrolyte and water transport, mast cell expansion and release of biologically active lipids which include leukotriene D4 (see Chapter 5). Th2-type responses and corresponding production of nematode-specific IgE antibodies may then, in conjunction with local mast cells, result in net chloride ion and water loss from the gut (Harari and Castro, 1991 and see Chapter 4).

REFERENCES

Appleton, J. A. and McGregor, D. D. (1984) Rapid expulsion of *Trichinella spiralis* in suckling rats. *Science*, **226**, 70–72.

Barker, G. C. and Rees, H. H. (1990) Ecdysteroids in nematodes. *Parasit. Today*, **6**, 384–7.

Bottjer, K. P., Whisenton, L. R. and Weinstein, P. P. (1984) Ecdysteroid-like substances in *Nippostrongylus brasiliensis*. *J. Parasit.*, **70**, 986–7.

Brophy, P. M. and Pritchard, D. I. (1992) Immunity to helminths: ready to tip the biochemical balance. *Parasit. Today*, **8**, 419–22.

Carlisle, M. S., McGregor, D. D. and Appleton, J. A. (1991a) Intestinal mucus entrapment of *Trichinella spiralis* larvae induced by specific antibodies. *Immunology*, **74**, 546–51.

Carlisle, M. S., McGregor, D. D. and Appleton, J. A. (1991b) The role of the antibody Fc region in rapid expulsion of *Trichinella spiralis* in suckling rats. *Immunology*, **74**, 552–8.

Harari, Y. and Castro, G. A. (1991) Reconstruction of immune-mediated ion secretion in gut mucosa of the athymic rat. *Parasit. Immunol.*, **13**, 313–28.

Hawdon, J. M. and Schad, G. M. (1990) Serum-stimulated feeding *in vitro* by third-stage infective larvae of the canine hookworm *Ancylostoma caninum*. *J. Parasit.*, **76**, 394–8.

Hotez, P. I., LeTrang, N. and McKerrow, J. H. (1985) Isolation and characterization of a proteolytic enzyme from the adult hookworm *Ancylostoma caninum*. *J. Biol. Chem.*, **260**, 7343–8.

Koolman, J., Walter, J. and Zahman, H. (1984) Metabolism and mode of action of invertebrate hormones, in *Biosynthesis* (eds J. Hoffman and M. Porchet), Springer–Verlag, Amsterdam, pp. 323–30.

Neutra, M. R. and Forstner, J. F. (1987) In *Physiology of the Gastrointestinal Tract* (ed. L. R. Johnson), Raven Press, New York, pp. 975–1008.

Petri, W., Smith, R. D., Schlesinger, P. H. *et al.* (1987) Isolation of the galactose-binding lectin that mediates the *in vitro* adherence of *Entamoeba histolytica*. *J. Clin. Inv.*, **80**, 1238–44.

Petronijevic, T. and Rogers, W. P. (1987a) Undissociated bases as the stimulus for the development of early parasitic stages of nematodes. *Int. J. Parasit.*, **17**, 911–15.

Petronijevic, T. and Rogers, W. P. (1987b) The physiology of infection with nematodes: the role of intracellular pH in the development of the early parasitic stage. *Compar. Biochem. Physiol.*, **88A**, 207–12.

Rogers, W. P. (1960) The physiology of infective processes of nematode parasites; the stimulus from the animal host. *Proc. Roy. Soc. London*, **152B**, 367–86.

Rogers, W. P. and Sommerville, R. I. (1968) The infectious process, and its relation to the development of early parasitic stages of nematodes. *Adv. Parasit.*, **6**, 327–48.

Schad, G. and Banwell, J. (1991) Hookworm, in *Tropical and Geographic Medicine* (eds K. S. Warren and A. A. F. Mahmoud), McGraw-Hill, New York, pp. 379–93.

Smith, A. C. and Podolsky, D. K. (1987) Biosynthesis and secretion of human colonic mucin glycoproteins. *J. Clin. Inv.*, **80**, 300–7.

Sukhdeo, M. (1990) Habitat selection by helminths: a hypothesis. *Parasit. Today*, **7**, 234–7.

Svetic, A., Madden, K. B., Xia, Z. *et al.* (1993) A primary intestinal helminthic infection rapidly induces a gut-associated elevation of Th2-associated cytokines and IL-3. *J. Immun.*, **150**, 3434–41.

Tse, S. -K. and Chadee, K. (1991) The interaction between intestinal mucus glycoproteins and enteric infections. *Parasit. Today*, **7**, 163–72.

Urban, J. F. Jr, Madden, K. B., Svetic, A. *et al.* (1992) The importance of Th2 cytokines in protective immunity to nematodes. *Immun. Rev.*, **127**, 205–20.

FOUR

Mechanisms of injury

Sui Zhang
and
G. A. Castro

Nematodes, trematodes, cestodes and acanthocephalans are helminths that inhabit the gastrointestinal (GI) tract of humans and lower mammals. Naturally occurring helminthiases can be modeled in many cases through infection of experimental animals. The aim of this review is to draw on descriptions of diseases from natural and laboratory-induced infections to demonstrate how helminths interact with their hosts to cause injury.

The format that will be followed is a simple one, being based on the pathological principle that if an injurious stimulus is applied to a tissue, the injury will be reflected over time in biochemical, functional and morphological changes (Figure 4.1). Generally biochemical and functional changes precede morphological alterations, the latter being more easily detectable. Thus, the parasite will be viewed as a stimulus which, through various means, induces subcellular, cellular and organ malfunctions.

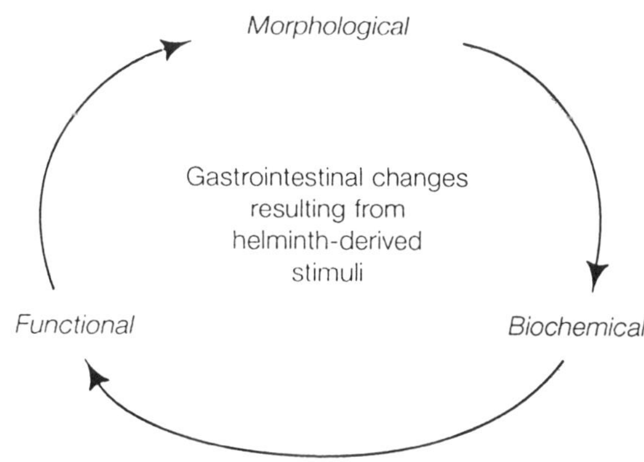

Figure 4.1 Inseparable relationships between biochemical, functional and morphological changes during helminth infection. Biochemical and functional changes generally precede morphological alterations.

4.1 PARASITE FACTORS CONTRIBUTING TO INJURY

4.1.1 MORPHOLOGY

To understand host–parasite interactions it is pertinent to recognize structures of parasites that impinge directly on host tissues, or which produce chemical substances that do so. These structures include body coverings, organs of attachment and organs involved in excretory or secretory processes. Resulting excretions or secretions may influence the parasite's feeding or other behavioral patterns. The general structural aspects of roundworms and variations among sexes and species have been described in detail (Chitwood and Chitwood, 1950). Extensive accounts of functions related to structure in

Enteric Infection 2. Intestinal helminths. Edited by M.J.G. Farthing, G.T. Keusch and D. Wakelin. Published in 1995 by Chapman and Hall, London. ISBN 0 412 39140 6

the giant intestinal roundworm *Ascaris lumbricoides* have come to serve as the basis for generalization. The cylindrical body of nematodes is covered with a chemically complex cuticle, which is also antigenic (Despommier, Kajima and Wostmann, 1967; MacKenzie, Preston and Ogilvie, 1978; Phillip, Parkhouse and Ogilvie, 1981). Surface antigens of nematodes are recognized by antibodies and ensuing reactions are potentially significant in the host–parasite interaction (Ogilvie *et al.*, 1980). The buccal cavity of some nematodes (e.g. hookworms) may contain hooks or cutting plates for attachment to host tissue.

Flukes or trematodes are covered with a tegument and also possess an alimentary canal. Substances are emitted into the parasite's environment from various body orifices. In flukes, such as schistosomes (blood flukes), the reproductive system represents an important component in the host–parasite relationship, since disease is caused by host reactions to the eggs deposited in tissues.

Tapeworms and acanthocephalans are devoid of an alimentary system. Therefore, the tegument is the site of active absorptive processes. The hold-fast organs, such as suckers and hooks on the 'head' of these helminths may damage tissue resulting in inflammation. Acanthocephalans have unique thorny heads which enable the parasites to penetrate the intestinal wall.

4.1.2 BIOCHEMISTRY

Biochemical processes in parasites result in metabolites that are secreted or excreted into or onto host tissues. Although the role of excretory–secretory (ES) products in the host–parasite interaction is vague, these substances must be considered as factors of potential importance in pathologic processes.

ES products of parasites include fermentation acids, ammonia, urea, amines, amino acids and various, mostly uncharacterized macromolecules (Weinstein, 1960; 1967). Macromolecular secretory products may affect structure–function relationships in host tissue through their actions as enzymes, antienzymes, or antigens. Adult enteric helminths may secrete enzymes that function in extracorporeal digestion (Thorson, 1956).

Vast amounts of acetylcholinesterase (AChE) (Lee and Martin, 1977; Yeates and Ogilvie, 1976) are secreted by some nematodes, such as *Nematodirus battus*, a parasite of lambs, *Nippostrongylus brasiliensis* and *Necator americanus*. It has been speculated that AChE may function as a depressant of motor activity. Furthermore, it has been postulated that a depressant of intestinal motor activity might be advantageous to the parasite in preventing expulsion. However, objections to this hypothesis concern observations that not all roundworms secrete AChE, and considerable contractile activity occurs in the gut of parasitized hosts without expulsion being effected (Castro *et al.*, 1976; Schanbacher *et al.*, 1978).

Effects on host digestive functions follow parasite-induced insults on mucosal tissue. Several studies indicate that the physical presence of intestinal tapeworms affects the activity of secreted enzymes. Trypsin and α- and β-chymotrypsin become inactivated in the presence of *Proteocephalus longicollis* (a fish tapeworm) and *Hymenolepis diminuta* (Pappas and Read, 1972a; Pappas and Read, 1972b; Reichenbach-Klinke and Reichenbach-Klinke, 1970; Uglem and Just, 1983). Pappas and Read (1972a) suggested that the trypsin inactivation was associated with the tapeworm glycocalyx, the outermost structural component of the tapeworm tegument. Pancreatic lipase has been shown also to be inactivated by intact *H. diminuta* (Ruff, Uglem and Read, 1973). In contrast, *H. diminuta* enhances the activity of pancreatic amylase (Taylor and Thomas, 1968). Antitryptic and antipeptic factors have been isolated in extracts of *Ascaris* somatic tissues (Collier,

1941). Although it has been postulated that such factors prevent digestion of worms by host enzymes, this has not been supported by experimental evidence.

Reactions to antigenic metabolites, including enzymes, are important in explaining serologic and physiological alterations in the host. The host may produce antibodies in response to ES antigens (Kagan, 1970), and these may be involved in immune (Prosser and Brown, 1961; Soulsby, 1962) or allergic (Murray, 1972; Olson and Schultz, 1963) reactions. Inflammatory lesions in the GI mucosa may be immune-mediated. The linkage of inflammation to mucosal structural and functional changes in these infections (Castro and Fairbairn, 1969; Russell and Castro, 1979; Smith and Castro, 1978; Symons and Fairbairn, 1962) suggests that host responses to parasite antigens may lead to intestinal disorders. The mediation of tissue damage by immediate and delayed hypersensitivity reactions during parasite infections is well known. An intriguing sidelight to the potential importance of homocytotropic antibodies in mediating pathology, i.e. the importance of type I hypersensitivity, is that tissues of parasitic nematodes contain antigens that characteristically induce high levels of such antibodies. Such an antigen has been purified from tissue extracts of *A. lumbricoides* (Hussain, Bradbury and Strejan, 1973), and indications are that it sensitizes the host during the larval migration phase of infection.

Infection with the nematode *N. brasiliensis* in rats stimulates high titers of reaginic antibodies not only against the parasite but against other antigens to which the host's immune system is already primed (Orr and Blair, 1969). An elevated immunoglobulin E (IgE) response to injected ovalbumin also follows infection with the trematode *Fasciola hepatica* (Jarrett, 1972), and suggests that the potentiation of IgE production may be a characteristic of many helminths.

4.2 EVIDENCE OF INJURY

4.2.1 SYMPTOMS

Lumen-dwelling parasites interact superficially with the host, generally inducing only mild responses. On the other hand, tissue invaders induce more severe reactions which, teleologically, are aimed at confining or eliminating the stress on the host. Unlike many micro-organisms, intestinal helminths are not known to produce potent toxins. Pathogenesis of disease is related directly to traumatic damage or lysis of tissue. Indirectly, pathology may be related to cellular influxes associated with either the acute inflammatory response to parasite-induced trauma or the cellular proliferative response stimulated by immunologic reactions.

The vast majority of helminth infections are asymptomatic. However, clinical cases may present with symptoms referable to the intestine, such as abdominal pain, nausea, vomiting, diarrhea or steatorrhea. Conditions such as enteritis, mechanical blockage and intestinal perforation have been noted and judged, because of the association, to be the cause of such signs. Systemic signs of helminth infection may include anorexia, weight loss, dizziness, headaches, convulsive seizures and various hematologic changes (Conrad, 1971). Most controlled studies of weight loss have been in experimental animals. Poor growth rate has been attributed to changes in basal metabolism and to intestinal malabsorption. The relative importance of malabsorption to weight loss is difficult to determine in helminth infections because weight reduction is often associated with anorexia (Castro, 1990a). However, the majority of evidence suggests that decreased food intake is more important than malabsorption in causing weight loss. Also, because various physiological functions vary with the feeding-state (Castro, 1981), changes that are physiologically associated with helminthiases may be a consequence of reduced feeding.

Hematologic changes that characterize many helminth infections include eosinophilia and anemia. Eosinophilia is often associated with immediate hypersensitivity states (Mahmoud, Stone and Kellermeyer, 1977; Zucker–Franklin, 1974) and is the hallmark of infections such as strongyloidiasis and trichinosis. *Ascaris* and *Trichuris* infections are also frequently associated with a lesser rise in circulating eosinophils. Although worms with extraintestinal stages in their life cycle are notorious for their ability to elicit the eosinophilic response, it has been shown in the case of trichinosis that the intestinal stages are causal (Despommier, Weisbroth and Fass, 1974).

Anemia is frequently associated with hookworm infection. The severity is directly related to the intensity and duration of infection in experimental animals (Behnke, 1990). In humans, however, this relationship is complicated by iron content of the diet, iron stores of the patient (Gilles, Williams and Ball, 1964), and by infections with other parasites. Macrocytic anemia occurs in about 1% of human infections with the fish tapeworm, *Diphyllobothrium latum* (von Bonsdorff, 1956), which is due to competitive absorption of free vitamin B_{12} by the parasite (Nyberg, 1963). The parasite is also able to break the B_{12}-intrinsic factor complex and absorb free vitamin B_{12}. This is the only confirmed evidence that host nutrient is depleted by parasite through competitive absorption.

4.2.2 STRUCTURAL CHANGES IN THE INTESTINE – INFLAMMATION

(a) Non-specific

Inflammation is the response of normal tissue to local damage. In the case of intestinal helminthiases, inflammation is evoked by direct tissue-damaging activity of the parasite and/or by parasite-derived metabolites or antigens. Thus, the type and intensity of inflammation is dependent, not only on the tissue-damaging behavior of the parasite, the worm burden and the duration of infection, but also on the immune status of the host. This is supported by the interesting finding of Shelhamer, Neva and Finn (1982). In an immunodeficient patient heavily infected with *Strongyloides stercoralis*, the intestinal biopsies were fairly normal, and the patient had no GI symptoms.

Inflammation is associated with both structural and functional changes in the GI tract. Although helminth-evoked inflammatory changes may play a role in the pathogenesis of infection, inflammation may be beneficial in contributing to the removal of the worms from the intestine (Kennedy, 1980), i.e. inflammation may be involved in acquired resistance or immunity.

Changes caused by inflammation in the intestine may include mucosal edema, increased permeability of the overlying epithelium, submucosal vascular hyperemia, villus atrophy, crypt hyperplasia, epithelial cell abnormalities and sometimes interstitial hemorrhages (Moqbel and MacDonald, 1990). Intestinal smooth muscle may also be affected by inflammation. An increase in smooth muscle mass occurs in rats infected with *Nippostrongylus brasiliensis*, in rats and guineapigs infected with *Trichinella spiralis* (Lin and Olson, 1970; Castro *et al.*, 1976), in rats infected with acanthocephalans (Crompton and Singhi, 1982), and in pigs infected with *Ascaris suum* (Stephenson *et al.*, 1980). Changes in smooth muscle during inflammation are caused directly by inflammatory cells or by the chemical byproducts of these cells. The role of inflammatory mediators in pathological changes during helminth-induced inflammation is summarized in Table 4.1.

Changes in the chemical composition of epithelial cells occur in the brush border. Isolated brush border membranes (BBM) from rats infected with *Trichinella* show a

Table 4.1 Important mediators involved in helminth-induced intestinal inflammation

Mediators	*Role in inflammation*	*Cell source*
Leukotriene B_4	Chemotactic for neutrophil and eosinophil	Eosinophil, mast cell, neutrophil, macrophage
Platelet activating factor (PAF)	Chemotactic for eosinophil; ulcerogenic agent, edema and mucus secretion	Mast cell, platelet, endothelial cell, neutrophil, macrophage, eosinophil
Histamine	Chemotactic for granulocyte; edema, mucus secretion; immunoregulation; neurotransmitter	Mast cell, basophil
Serotonin (5-HT)	Edema; immunoregulation; neurotransmitter, mastocytosis	Mast cell, platelet, enterochromaffin cell
Eosinophil chemotactic factor of anaphylaxis	Chemotactic for eosinophil	Mast cell
Neutrophil chemotactic activity	Chemotactic for neutrophil	Mast cell, mononuclear cell, T cell
Leukotrienes C_4, D_4 (LTC_4, LTD_4, SRS-A)	Mucosal edema; mucus hypersecretion	Mast cell, eosinophil
Prostaglandins	Mucosal edema	Macrophage, platelet, mast cell
Proteolytic enzymes (RMCPII)	Epithelial damage; increased mucosal permeability	Mucosal mast cell
Hydrogen peroxide	Epithelial damage	Neutrophil, macrophage
Major basic protein	Epithelial damage	Eosinophil

reduced capacity to bind the lectin wheat-germ agglutinin (WGA; Harari and Castro, 1988a). The reduction is maximally expressed two weeks after infection and lasts for at least 12 weeks. A decrease in sialic acid residues is the cause of the reduced binding of BBM to WGA (Harari and Castro, 1983). The significance of these changes to host immunity or to the pathogenesis of infection is not clear.

The cell types involved in inflammatory infiltration during intestinal helminth infection include neutrophils, small and large lymphocytes, macrophages, eosinophils and mast cells (Moqbel and MacDonald, 1990). Inflammation caused by *T. spiralis*, a tissue-invading nematode has been used as a prototype of helminth-evoked inflammation. In randomly outbred Swiss mice with a moderate-level infection, only minimal cellular infiltration occurs during the first four days of infection. Intensive inflammation starts at six days after infection (Race *et al.*, 1978), peaking at about eight to ten days. Inflammation is a panmucosal phenomenon, rather than a reaction limited to the region of the parasite attachment. At day 38, the intestinal tissue returns to normal.

(b) Immune-mediated

It has been proposed that in late primary infection and in secondary infection the immune system plays a central role in helminth-evoked intestinal inflammation. The term immunophysiology (Castro, 1982) embraces the concept of co-ordination of systems. It draws attention to the dynamic relationships among cells and tissues as they become functionally enmeshed as a result of immunological reactions (Castro, 1976). The realization that physiological responses to enteric helminths are conditioned by the immune state of the host developed from several observations. These include the findings that:

- many enteric helminths incite local inflammation;
- inflammation has an earlier onset following secondary infection than it does after primary infection (Taliaferro and Sarles, 1939; Larsh, 1963);
- the anamnestic nature of the inflammatory response has an immunological basis (Taliaferro and Sarles, 1939; Larsh, 1963);
- inflammation regardless of etiology, influences gastrointestinal physiology in specific ways (Castro, 1976; Sprinz, 1962).

An understanding of how antigenic signals are transduced into physiological changes should lead to the development of working models to guide attempts at preventing or regulating immunopathological responses to parasites, and at simulating favorable responses, e.g. functional immunity, by extrinsic intervention.

Immunologically mediated inflammation is best described under the heading of hypersensitivity. Coombs and Gell (1975) categorized hypersensitivities into four types. Type I hypersensitivity is dependent on the interaction of antigen with anaphylactic antibody (IgE or IgG subclasses) on the surface of amine-containing cells, such as mast cells and basophils. Type II is antibody-dependent cellular cytotoxicity (ADCC) which results in lysis of target cells in the presence of complement. Type III is the Arthus reaction characterized by inflammation due to the formation of antigen–antibody complexes that activate complement and attract neutrophils. Type IV involves antigen-activated T cells that release lymphokines that cause local proliferation of lymphocytes and attract myeloid cells. Because of the delayed expression of inflammation in the type IV response, it is referred to as delayed hypersensitivity. The more rapid onset of types I–III reactions labels them as immediate hypersensitivity responses.

Inasmuch as these hypersensitivity reactions occur in the lamina propria, epithelium and smooth muscle are influenced by elements of immune-mediated inflammation. Cellular elements of the immune system may induce structural and functional changes in these tissues directly through paracrine secretions or, more indirectly, through intrinsic neural pathways.

Type I hypersensitivity has been suggested to play a role in both pathological changes occurring in helminth infection (Castro, 1990) and in host defense against the parasites (Zhang and Castro, 1990). The hallmarks of helminth infection, namely mastocytosis, eosinophilia and increased IgE synthesis are all related to type I hypersensitivity. Mast cells have surface receptors for IgE (high affinity receptors, FcεRI receptors; Metzger, 1983). Depending on the species, other isotypes can also bind to mast cells with low affinities (Haig and Miller, 1990). Cross-linking of IgE molecules on the surface of mast cells by helminth antigens or by other multivalent ligands leads to mast cell degranulation. Other mast cell activators include complement components, $C3_a$ and $C5_a$ (Befus *et al.*, 1988), vasoactive intestinal peptide, somatostatin, bradykinin (Shanahan *et al.*, 1984), substance P (Denburg and Bienenstock, 1983) and interleukin 1 (Subramanian and Bray, 1987).

In helminth infection, mast cell degranulation can occur shortly after the arrival of worms in the intestine without preimmunization of the host, presumably through mediation by a worm-derived factor (Block, Cygan and Waltin, 1972). Preformed inflammatory mediators, such as histamine, mast cell protease and serotonin are released during degranulation. The degranulation process is also associated with the *de novo* synthesis of mediators such as prostaglandins, leukotrienes and platelet-activating factor (PAF). These inflammatory mediators are able to cause structural damage and disturbance of physiological functions of the intestine. In rats, for example, mast cell protease II (RMCPII) is able to digest type IV collagen in the epithelial basal lamina (Patrick *et al.*, 1988). Other mediators such as leukotrienes, PAF, oxygen-free radicals (Schwartz and Austen, 1984) and cytokines (Gordon, Burd and Galli, 1990) may alter blood flow. Furthermore, mast cells can release chemotactic factors for neutrophils and eosinophils, recruiting these cells to an area of inflammation.

Eosinophils in both peripheral blood and tissue are increased in number by helminth infection, especially by infections with tissue-invading parasites (Befus and Bienenstock, 1982). Besides T-cell-mediated eosinophilopoiesis, certain chemotactic factors, such as eosinophil chemotactic factor of anaphylaxis (ECF-A), PAF and leukotriene B_4 (LTB_4) which are released from mast cells as a result of IgE-antigen interaction, can cause local accumulation of eosinophils. Like mast cells, eosinophils also have granules containing preformed mediators. The mechanisms of mediator release from eosinophils is not completely understood. Eosinophils bear surface receptors such as FCτR for IgG, complement (CR1 and C3) receptors (Kay, 1985) and low-affinity FcεRII (Capron *et al.*, 1981). The interaction between antigen and IgE molecules stimulates mediator release (Wardlaw and Kay, 1987).

Preformed mediators from eosinophils that are released following activation include:

- major basic protein which is a tissue-damaging protein and highly toxic to parasites *in vitro*;
- eosinophil cationic protein which is able to damage tissue and worms and promote histamine release from mast cells;
- eosinophil granule peroxidase which can also induce histamine release from mast cells.

Activation of eosinophils also leads to release of membrane associated mediators such as leukotriene C_4 and PAF which are proinflammatory and are able to mediate the release of mucus.

Mastocytosis, eosinophilia and the development of IgE response appear to be induced by cytokines from TH2 subset of CD4+ T cells (Finkelman *et al.*, 1991). In mouse, CD4+ T cells are required for intestinal mastocytosis and IgE response during primary infection with *N. brasiliensis* (Katona, Urban and Finkelman, 1988). In *T. spiralis*-infected rats, mastocytosis is induced by OX22+ subset of CD4+ T-helper cells and an increase of eosinophils is mediated by OX22− subset (Wang *et al.*, 1990). Cytokines that are able to induce mucosal mastocytosis include IL-3, IL-4, IL-9 and IL-10 (cytokine synthesis inhibitory factor, CSIF). IL-3 and IL-4 appear to be the major cytokines that induce intestinal mastocytosis (Finkelman *et al.*, 1991). D'Inca *et al.* (1992) demonstrated that the number of mast cells was increased in the intestine of nude rats infected with *N. brasiliensis*. Although there is a possibility that T-cell-like activity exists in the intestine of nude rats, other mechanisms may also contribute to the mastocytosis in nude rats. There is evidence that mastocytosis could be induced by mast cell degranulation products (Marshall *et al.*, 1990) which include IL-3 (Gordon *et al.*, 1990). On the other hand, serotonin, another mast cell mediator, may play a role in intestinal mastocytosis. Parmentier *et al.* (1987) demonstrated that mastocytosis induced by *T. spiralis* infection was significantly inhibited by methysergide and ketanserin, antagonists of the serotonin 5-HT_2 receptor.

T cells, through their regulatory effects on other types of cells, and through more direct effects cause structural changes in tissues. MacDonald and Spencer (1988) demonstrated that activated T cells can rapidly cause epithelial cell hyperplasia and villous atrophy. T-cell-depleted rats do not show villous atrophy and crypt cell hyperplasia which are caused by *N. brasiliensis* in normal rats (Ferguson and Jarrett, 1975).

Overwhelming evidence indicates that T cells play a major role in changes caused by helminth-induced granulomas. Granulomas occur in infections with a variety of helminths, such as tapeworms, filarial worms and hookworms. Granuloma formation has been extensively studied in infections with *Schistosoma* spp. In schistosomiasis, antigens released from the miracidium within the egg can induce a T-cell-mediated hypersensitivity reaction, or type IV hypersensitivity (Phillips *et al.*, 1980; Cheever *et al.*, 1985). The cells involved include macrophages, lymphocytes and eosinophils, which may contribute to the tissue damage, and fibroblasts which are responsible for fibrosis of the lesion (Grimaud *et al.*, 1987). One interesting feature of granuloma development is that the size of the granuloma decreases as the infection progresses. The underlying mechanism is not clear, although T-suppressor cells and IgG_1 anti-idiotypic antibodies are postulated to be modulatory factors (Stavitsky, 1987).

Overall, the involvement of type I and type IV hypersensitivities in helminth-evoked tissue damage has been well documented. The role of ADCC (type II reaction) and complement in villus cell damage was discussed by Kniker (1987). Type III reactions have been related to celiac disease, enteritis, and malabsorption. The evidence of involvement of type II and type III in helminth-evoked intestinal inflammation is scarce, although their involvement is likely because during inflammation different types of hypersensitivity are considered to act synergistically, one type being regulated by another. The different types may be expressed sequentially or in parallel.

The immediate (type I) hypersensitivity may play a role in the induction of the delayed (type IV) hypersensitivity (Castro, 1990b). Recent findings (Ptak, Geba and Askenase, 1991) in studies of skin delayed-type hypersensitivity (DTH) induced by contact with certain chemicals, provide insight into the interaction between types I and IV hypersensitivities. It is necessary that CD4+ cells are recruited to the specific site and activated before manifestation of DTH. Lymphokines released from these CD4+ cells then promote inflammatory changes through recruiting other effector cells. Therefore, the recruitment of CD4+ cells from the circulation to the site of DTH is called initiation. IgE, participating in a type I reaction, is able to initiate DTH by recruiting DTH effector T cells to mediate the manifestation of DTH. The recruiting effect is mediated by 5-hydroxytryptamine (5-HT) through 5-HT_2 receptors (Ameisen, Meade and Askenase, 1989). The initiation effect of IgE can be inhibited by histamine through H_2 receptors.

4.2.3 FUNCTIONAL CHANGES IN THE INTESTINE

The primary function of the GI tract is to assimilate dietary nutrients. In this regard secretory, digestive, absorptive and motor activities are of primary importance. GI hormones are important regulators of these processes. Changes in assimilation, that often associate with helminth infections, pose a threat to optimal host nutrition and to fluid and electrolyte balance. Alterations in specific physiological processes induced by helminths and their influence on food assimilation are discussed below.

(a) Gastric and pancreatic secretion – maldigestion

Secretory activities are under intricate control by GI hormones. In several helminthiases, endocrine regulatory systems involving these hormones are impaired. This is clearly demonstrated in altered gastric and pancreatic secretion.

There are a multitude of points of potential parasitic interaction in stimulus-coupled gastric secretory events. Acetylcholine, histamine and gastrin are the principal physiological regulators of gastric acid secretion, acting on the parietal cell after release from postganglionic nerves, gastric mucosal cells and antral G cells, respectively. Most stimuli that increase the secretion of acid also increase the secretion of pepsinogen. Secretion of pepsinogen from chief cells is dependent in part on an acid-activated local cholinergic reflex. Once secreted, pepsinogen is converted by acid to the active proteolytic enzyme.

Inflammation in the gastric mucosa of sheep (Anderson, Hansky and Titchen, 1976) and intestinal mucosa of pigs (Titchen, 1982) and rats (Yeates and Ogilvie, 1976) infected with nematodes, has been associated with hypergastrinemia. Also, gastrin levels 20-fold higher than normal were reported in rats harboring hepatic stages of the tapeworm, *Taenia taeniaeformis* (Cook, Williams and Lichtenberger, 1981). It was assumed that the elevated gastrin level was responsible for the enormous hyperplastic changes in the gastric and intestinal mucosae associated with this tapeworm infection. However, subsequent findings (Cook, Williams and Lichtenberger, 1981) showed that there was no cause–effect relationship, since gastric hyperplasia occurred in antrectomized rats in the absence of elevated gastrin levels.

Secretion of HCl and pepsin in the canine host is stimulated by the hormone gastrin, and this output is suppressed by secretin when released from duodenal mucosa by the presence of H^+. The regulation of gastric acid and enzyme output by secretin is altered in dogs infected with the enteric stages of the nematode *T. spiralis* due to impaired synthesis or release of secretin from the gut (Dembinski, Johnson and Castro, 1979a). A major function of secretin in addition to regulating gastric secretion, is to cause water and bicarbonate secretion by duct cells of the exocrine pancreas. It also stimulates the acinar cells to secrete enzymes, but is less effective in this regard than the hormone cholecystokinin (CCK). In dogs infected with enteric stages of *T. spiralis* the release of endogenous secretin and CCK is reduced, imparing both gastric and pancreatic responses to physiological secretagogues (Dembinski, Johnson and Castro 1979a,b). Impaired hormone release may be due to local inflammation which reduces endocrine cell number, decreases the number or avidity of receptors for secretagogues or impairs hormone synthesis and release.

Ovington, Bacarese-Hamilton and Bloom (1985), in an examination of nippostrongylosis in rats, observed altered plasma levels of several GI hormones. CCK and insulin levels were reduced, whereas secretin, enteroglucagon and pancreatic glucagon were elevated, and gastrin and pancreatic polypeptide were unchanged as compared with weight-matched, pair-fed, uninfected hosts.

(b) Intestinal secretion

Although intestinal helminths are relatively less likely to cause diarrhea than protozoa, bacteria or viruses, this symptom of infection is still frequently observed (Wolfe, 1986). An increase in intestinal solute/water secretion or decrease in solute/water absorption, which contribute to the volume and fluidity of the stool, are important causes of diarrhea. Diarrhea can be a result of the osmotic retention of water in the gut lumen, exudative protein loss, increased intestinal secretion or decreased contact time between fluid in the gut lumen and the absorptive surface. The latter involves changes in intestinal motility. All the above mechanisms have been implicated in diarrhea caused by intestinal helminths (Castro, 1990a), and it is possible in a single infection that more than one mechanism may be operating.

Retention of water in the intestinal lumen is dependent on the porosity or the hydraulic conductivity of the mucous membrane and the hydrostatic pressure difference between the interstitial fluid compartment and the luminal compartment. The transmembrane pressure difference which is due to asymmetrical distribution of osmotically active solutes is equivalent to hydrostatic pressure in causing volume flow. Porosity or hydraulic conductivity of mucous membranes can be affected by changes in capillary filtration and by leakiness of epithelial tight junctions.

Increased water movement between the interstitial compartment and the luminal compartment may result from the porosity changes of mucous membrane but occurs only when a pressure difference is present between the two compartments. Osmotic diarrhea is caused by accumulation of osmotically active molecules in the intestinal lumen. Reduced absorption of Na^+, Cl^-, glucose and amino acids has been observed in rats infected with *Moniliformis dubius* (Mettrick, Budziakowski and Podesta, 1979) and *N. brasiliensis* (Symons, 1969; Scofield, 1977). Diarrhea could result from the osmotic effects of these solutes. The detailed mechanism and affected cellular pathways responsible for reduction of Na^+/Cl^- absorption is not well understood. Mediators released during inflammation undoubtedly play a role (Sartor and Powell, 1991).

Leakage of proteins and other macromolecules often results from an increase in mucosal permeability associated with intestinal parasitism (Bloch *et al.*, 1979; Cobden, Rothwell and Axon, 1979; Murray, 1969). Leakage of serum proteins occurs through capillary endothelium and mucosal tight junctions during nippostrongylosis, and is associated temporally with the development of mucosal inflammation marked by mast cell hyperplasia. Protein-losing enteropathy occurs in sheep infected with *Ostertagia circumcincta* (Halliday and Mulligan, 1968). Diarrhea may develop due to the osmotic effect of excess protein in the intestinal lumen. Intraluminal antigenic molecules, on the other hand, may diffuse through the leaky mucosa driven by a local lumen-to-tissue concentration gradient. Contact of these antigenic molecules with mucosal immune system may lead to the release of mediators that stimulate ion and water secretion.

Secretory diarrhea is typically induced by bacterial enterotoxins in Asiatic cholera, staphylococcal and clostridial food poisoning and infections with various strains of *Escherichia coli*. These enterotoxins are believed to induce secretion by increasing intracellular cAMP, or in the case of *E. coli*, heat-stable toxin, cGMP which act as second messengers to mediate active Cl^- secretion.

The active serosal-to-mucosal movement of Cl is accompanied by passive movement of Na^+, which provide the driving force for water movement. Agents such as GI hormones, mediators released in inflammation, luminally derived long-chain fatty acids and hydroxy bile acids can increase intracellular cAMP and cause Cl^-/fluid secretion by direct action on enterocytes or indirectly through stimulation of the enteric nervous system.

Some hormones, neurotransmitters or inflammatory mediators may cause Cl^-/fluid secretion through other second messengers such as protein kinase C and/or Ca^{++}. Table 4.2 summarizes Cl^- secretagogues and their second messengers. Although secretory diarrhea caused by parasites is not recognized by a WHO scientific work group (World Health Organization, 1980), evidence is accumulating suggesting that parasites may evoke this type of diarrhea. Infection with *Strongyloides stercoralis* is associated with secretion of water, Na^+ and Cl^- into the lumen of the jejunum in humans (Kane, Luby and Krejs, 1984). Watery diarrhea has been seen in human infections with *Capillaria philippinensis*. Although the mechanism of diarrhea in this infection is not clear, it has been postulated as an analog of that in cholera patients (Whalen *et al.*, 1969).

A gut perfusion technique involving the dilution or concentration of a radioactive, non-absorbable marker was used to estimate net fluid movement in *T. spiralis*-infected rats (Castro, Hessel and Whalen, 1979). A decrease in net fluid absorption and increase in secretion was detected several days after

Table 4.2 Mediators released in inflammation that cause Cl^- secretion in the intestine

Secretagogues	*Intracellular mediator*	*Possible cell origin*
Histamine	cAMP Ca^{++}?	Mast cell, basophil
Serotonin (5-HT)	Protein kinase C/Ca^{++}	Mast cell, platelet, enterochromaffin cell
Prostaglandins	cAMP, protein kinase C/Ca^{++}	Macrophage, platelet, mast cell, cells in subepithelial tissues
Bradykinin	cAMP and protein kinase C/Ca^{++}	Plasma precursor produced in liver, activated in mast cell-mediated inflammation
Adenosin	cAMP, protein kinase C/Ca^{++}?	Stimulated mast cell
Platelet-activating factor (PAF)	cAMP	Phagocyte, platelet, mast cell, vascular endothelium
Vasoactive intestinal peptide	cAMP	Enteric neurons
Substance P	Protein kinase C/Ca^{++}	Enteric neurons
Acetylcholine	Protein kinase C/Ca^{++}	Enteric neurons
IL-1, IL-3	cAMP, protein kinase C and Ca^{++}	Macrophage, T cell, fibroblast
Reactive oxygen metabolites	cAMP, Protein kinase C and Ca^{++}	Phagocytes

Summarized from reviews by Hinterleitner and Powell (1991); and by Chang and Rao (1991).

primary infection. The same changes in fluid flux occurred within minutes after a secondary infection implicating involvement of the local immune response.

The physiological changes that account for the altered fluid flux have been studied in an *in vitro* system. Jejunal segments from rats infected (immunized) with *T. spiralis* were mounted in Ussing chambers and ion transport properties of the tissue were monitored by changes in net transmural short circuit current (I_{SC}). Challenge of the tissue with *Trichinella*-derived antigen induced a net Cl^- secretion within seconds after stimulation (Russell and Castro, 1987). The biphasic Cl^- secretory response induced by antigenic challenge could be mimicked by a combination of mast cell-derived mediators such as histamine, 5-HT and prostaglandin E_2, and inhibited by antagonists or inhibitors of these mediators (Castro, Harari and Russell, 1987; Figure 4.2). Further experiments demonstrated that antigen-induced Cl^- secretory response was mediated by intestinal anaphylaxis (Harari, Russell and Castro, 1987). Antigen-induced intestinal Cl^- secretion is also evident in rats infected with *N. brasiliensis* (Harari and Castro, 1988b).

The hypothesis that antigen-induced Cl^- secretion is the major driving force for intestinal fluid secretion was tested and confirmed in a series of *in vivo* experiments in which the volume of fluid in the small intestine was measured directly (Zhang, Myers and Castro, 1991). Reinfection of rats immunized to *T. spiralis* caused a 10-fold increase in the volume of fluid accumulated in the small intestine within 30 min. Like the antigen-evoked Cl^- secretion, the worm-induced fluid accumulation is mediated by intestinal anaphylaxis and inhibited by simultaneous administration of indomethacin (cyclooxygenase inhibitor) and diphenhydramine (histamine H_1 receptor blocker). Therefore, the secretory response induced by mediators released in inflammation or specific immune reactions could play a role in diarrhea caused by helminth infections.

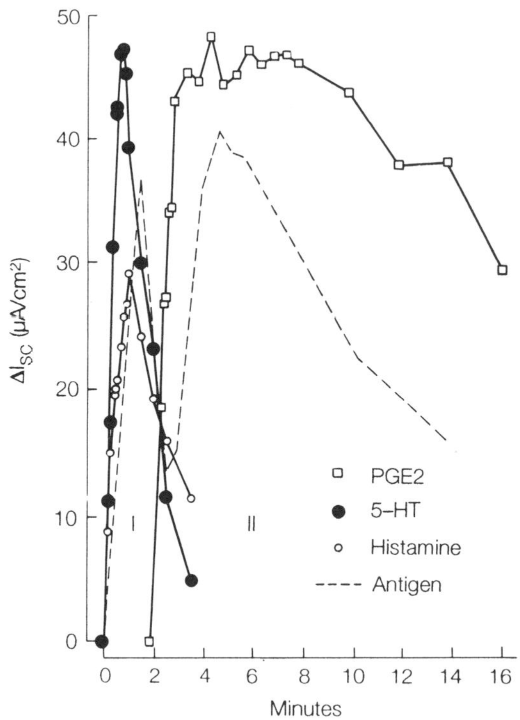

Figure 4.2 Changes in transmural short-circuit current (ΔI_{SC}) induced in rat jejunum by homologous challenge with antigen (25 μg protein/ml), 5-hydroxytryptamine (5-HT; 10^{-4} M), histamine (10^{-4} M), and prostaglandin E_2 (10^{-5} M). I and II = first and second phases of antigenic response respectively. All agents added to serosal solution of Ussing chamber. (Source: Castro, 1990b, with permission.)

(c) Intestinal motility

Intestinal helminths can cause both anatomical and functional changes in smooth muscle layers of the gut wall. An early report of structural alterations was that of a marked thickening of the muscularis externa in the small intestine of rats infected with *Nippostrongylus brasiliensis*. Analogous observations have been reported in rats and guineapigs infected with *T. spiralis*, rats with *Moniliformis dubius*, horses with *Parascaris equorum* and pigs with *Ascaris suum* (Castro, 1988).

The cause of increased muscle mass in these infections is unknown but may involve physical effects of parasites, parasite-derived substances, or chemical mediators of inflammation. The induction of hypertrophic changes in intestinal smooth muscle of rats and guineapigs by surgically produced stenosis (Gabella, 1975) implies that smooth muscle 'hypertrophy' in ascarid and acanthocephalan infections could involve adaptive changes resulting from moving contents through an intestine undergoing stenosis due to the presence of large worms. In guineapigs with secondary trichinosis, an accelerated onset of inflammation is associated with an increase in intestinal smooth muscle mass (Lin and Olson, 1970). Since immune elements mediate inflammation in secondary infection, they may be responsible for the increased mass of smooth muscle. The suggestion that the immunological system regulates smooth muscle cell proliferation or growth remains problematic.

A variety of parameters, such as intraluminal pressure, gastric emptying, intestinal transit, myoelectric activity, contraction of smooth muscle and fluid propulsion have been measured and used as indices of GI motor functions (Castro, 1988). A correlation between morphological changes and responsiveness to stimulation is evident in the rat-*N. brasiliensis* system. The increase in muscle mass seen in primary nippostrongylosis (Miller, 1987) is associated with hyper-responsiveness to chemical (5-HT) and electrical stimulation (Farmer and Laniyonu, 1984). Similarly, intestinal muscle in rats with trichinosis is hyper-responsive to acetylcholine (Vermillion and Collins, 1986). Despite the doubts about the influence of the immune system on smooth muscle structure, immune reactions clearly cause functional changes (Castro, 1988). Historically, the impact of an immune reaction on smooth muscle function was first demonstrated in the Schultz–Dale reaction (Coulson, 1953). That reaction, which is based on type I hypersensitivity, is characterized by the contraction of isolated segments of intestine in response to antigenic challenge. The Schultz–Dale response has been used to study the allergenicity of a number of helminths (Olson and Schultz, 1963). Guineapigs infected with *Toxocara canis, A. lumbricoides* and *T. spiralis* show a marked hypersensitivity to antigens derived from those worms (Sharp and Olson, 1962).

Variations in the methods used to study the Schultz–Dale phenomenon have supported the notion that the immune system regulates smooth muscle function in the gut. Fluid-filled segments of small intestine from guineapigs infected with *T. spiralis* challenged with *T. spiralis* antigen *in vitro* undergo immediate changes in fluid-propelling behavior. The antigen-induced changes in propulsion can be mimicked by histamine and blocked by a histamine H_1 antagonist, but not by a 5-HT antagonist (Alizadeh, Weems and Castro, 1988). The probability that the Schultz–Dale reaction has an *in vivo* equivalent was demonstrated by measurements of small bowel myoelectric activity. This correlate of motility was quickly altered in conscious rats sensitized by primary infection with *T. spiralis* and challenged by reinfection (Palmer and Castro, 1986). The myoelectric changes were not inducible in *T. spiralis*-sensitized rats infected with another enteric parasite, *Eimeria nieschulzi*, illustrating the immunological specificity of the response.

Profoundly important observations relating to the immune regulation of smooth muscle function are those that implicate the activity of the enteric nervous system in some of the pathways through which antigens induce effector responses. The electrical activity of myenteric neurons, measured with intracellular microelectrodes, was altered by an immune reaction. Challenge of the myenteric plexus from *T. spiralis*-infected guineapigs with parasite-derived antigen led to changes in transmembrane potential and resistance in the impaled neurons (Palmer, Tamura and Wood, 1988). The transduction of the antigenic signal to elicit the neuronal changes presumably involved a response initiated by mast cells. This experiment

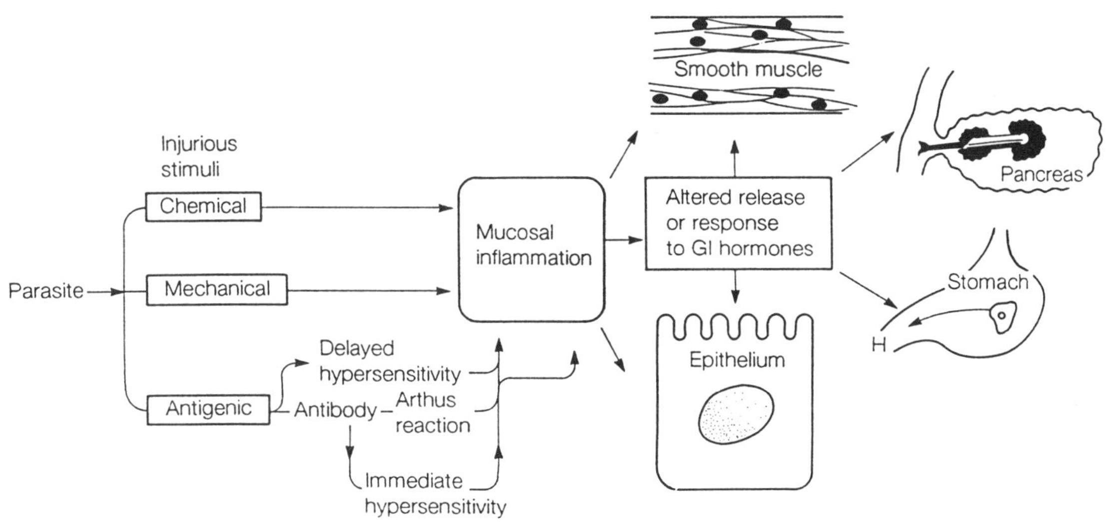

Figure 4.3 Summary of structural and functional inter-relationships during enteric infection with helminths. Emphasis is on various components and forms of inflammation as a bridge between morphologic and physiologic alterations. (Source: Russell and Castro, 1987, with permission.)

provides direct evidence that enteric neurons in sensitized gut tissue respond physiologically to antigenic stimulation. The capacity of the host to modulate smooth muscle function through immune reactions coupled to the enteric nervous system has significant implications in the ways that enteric helminths cause injury.

4.3 CONCLUSIONS

This review summarizes factors that underlie intestinal injuries caused by helminths. The host response is often a sum of injuries caused by multiple factors (Figure 4.3). The observations that similar pathological changes are induced by different parasites imply that specific actions of parasites are less important than host responses in causing injury. Inflammation, which is either non-specifically induced or immunologically mediated, plays a key role in transducing parasite stimuli into morphological and functional changes. Despite a growing knowledge of GI alterations induced by helminths, a major challenge remains in interpreting available information to decide whether the effect of a helminth on the host is adaptive or maladaptive in nature, i.e. whether observed changes are harmful, beneficial or without effect on the host.

REFERENCES

Alizadeh, H., Weems, W. A. and Castro, G. A. (1988) Histamine-regulated intestinal propulsion in guinea pigs infected with *Trichinella spiralis*. *FASEB J.*, **2**, A325.

Ameisen, J.-C., Meade, R. and Askenase, P. W. (1989) A new interpretation of the involvement of serotonin in delayed-type hypersensitivity. Serotonin-2 receptor antagonists inhibit contact sensitivity by an effect on T cells. *J. Immunol.*, **142**, 3171–3179.

Anderson, N., Hansky, J. and Titchen, D. A. (1976) Hypergastrinemia during parasitic gastritis in sheep. *J. Physiol. (Lond.)*, **256**, 51P-52P.

Befus, A. D., and Bienenstock, J. (1982) Factors involved in symbiosis and host resistance at the mucosa-parasite interface. *Prog. Allergy*, **31**, 76–177.

Befus, A. D., Fujimaki, H., Lee, T. D. C. and Swieter, M. (1988) Mast cell polymorphisms – present concepts, future directions. *Dig. Dis. Sci.*, **33** (Supplement), 165–245.

Behnke, J. M. (1990) Laboratory animal models, in *Hookworm Disease: Current Status and New Directions* (eds G. A. Schad and K. S. Warren), Taylor and Francis, London, pp. 105–28.

Bloch, K. J., Bloch, D. B., Stearns, M. and Walker, W. A. (1979) Intestinal uptake of macromolecules. VI. Uptake of protein antigen *in vivo* in normal rats and in rats infected with *Nippostrongylus brasiliensis* or subjected to mild systemic anaphylaxis. *Gastroenterology*, **77**, 1039–44.

Block, K. J., Cygan, R. W. and Waltin, J. (1972) The IgE system and parasitism: role of mast cells, IgE, and other antibodies in host response to primary infection with *Nippostrongylus brasiliensis*, in *The Biological Role of the Immunoglobulin E System* (eds K. Ishizaka and J. Dayton), US Government printing, Washington, pp. 119.

Capron, M., Capron, A., Dessaint, J. P. *et al.* (1981) Fc receptors for IgE on human and rat eosinophils. *J. Immunol.*, **126**, 2087.

Castro, G. A. (1976) Spatial and temporal integration of host responses to intestinal stages of *Trichinella spiralis*: Retro- and prospective views, in *Biochemistry of Parasites and Host–Parasite Relationship* (ed. H. Van den Bossche), North Holland Publishing Company, Amsterdam, pp. 343–58.

Castro, G. A. (1981) Physiology of the gastrointestinal tract in the parasitized hosts, in *Physiology of the Gastrointestinal Tract*. Vol. 1 (ed. L. R. Johnson), Raven Press, New York, pp. 1381–406.

Castro, G. A. (1982) Immunological regulation of epithelial function. *Am. J. Physiol.*, **243**, G321–9.

Castro, G. A. (1988) Parasitic infections and gastrointestinal motility, in *Handbook of Physiology: Gastrointestinal System*, Section 6, Vol. 1 (ed. J. D. Wood), The American Physiological Society, Bethesda, pp. 1133–52.

Castro, G. A. (1990a) Intestinal pathology, in *Parasites: Immunity and Pathology: the Consequences of Parasitic Infection in Mammals* (ed. J. M. Behnke), Taylor and Francis, London, pp. 283–316.

Castro, G. A. (1990b) Immunological regulation of electrolyte transport, in *Textbook of Secretory Diarrhea* (eds E. Lebenthal and M. Duffey), Raven Press, New York, pp. 31–45.

Castro, G. A. and Fairbairn, D. (1969) Comparison of cuticular and intestinal absorption of glucose by adult *Ascaris lumbricoides*. *J. Parasit.*, **55**, 13–16.

Castro, G. A., Harari, Y. and Russell, D. A. (1987) Mediators of anaphylaxis-induced ion transport changes in small intestine. *Am. J. Physiol.*, **253**, G540–8.

Castro, G. A., Hessel, J. J. and Whalen, G. (1979) Altered intestinal fluid movement in response to *Trichinella spiralis* in immunized rats. *Parasite Immun.*, **1**, 259–66.

Castro, G. A., Badial-Aceves, F., Smith, J. W. *et al.* (1976) Altered small bowel propulsion associated with parasitism. *Gastroenterology*, **71**, 620–5.

Chang, E. B. and Rao, M. C. (1991) Intracellular mediators of intestinal electrolyte transport, in *Current Topics in Gastroenterology. Diarrheal Diseases* (ed. M. Field), Elsevier Science Publishing Co., New York, pp. 49–72.

Cheever, A. W., Byram, J. E. and von Lichtenberg, F. (1985) Immunopathology of *Schistosoma japonicum* infection in athymic mice. *Parasite Immun.*, **7**, 387–98.

Chitwood, B. C. and Chitwood, M. B. H. (1950) *An Introduction to Nematology. Section I, Anatomy.* Catholic University of America Press, Washington, DC.

Cobden, I., Rothwell, J. and Axon, A. T. R. (1979) Intestinal permeability in rats infected by *Nippostrongylus brasiliensis*. *Gut*, **20**, 716–21.

Collier, H. B. (1941) Trypsin-inhibiting fraction of *Ascaris*. *Can. J. Res.*, **819**, 90–8.

Conrad, M. W. (1971) Hematologic manifestations of parasitic infections. *Semin. Hematol.*, **8**, 267–303.

Cook, R. W., Williams, J. F. and Lichtenberger, L. (1981) Hyperplastic gastropathy in the rat due to *Taenia taeniaeformis* infection: Parabiotic transfer and hypergastrinemia. *Gastroenterology*, **80**, 728–34.

Coombs, R. R. A. and Gell, P. G. H. (1975) Classification of allergic reactions responsible for clinical hypersensitivity and disease, in *Clinical Aspects of Immunology*, 3rd edn (eds P. G. H. Gell, R. R. A. Coombs and P. J. Lackman), Blackwell Publications, Oxford, England, pp. 761–81.

Coulson, E. J. (1953) The Schultz–Dale technique. *J. Allergy*, **24**, 458–73.

Crompton, D. W. T. and Singhi, A. (1982) Intestinal responses of rats to *Moniliformis* (Acanthocephala), *Parasitology*, **84**: 1XX (abstract).

Dembinski, A. B., Johnson, L. R. and Castro, G. A. (1979a) Influence of parasitism on secretin-inhibited gastric secretion. *Am. J. Trop. Med. Hyg.*, **28**, 854–9.

Dembinski, A. B., Johnson, L. R. and Castro, G. A. (1979b) Influence of enteric parasitism on hormone-regulated pancreatic secretion in dogs. *Am. J. Physiol.*, **237**, R232–8.

Denburg, J. A. and Bienenstock, J. (1983) Mast cell subpopulations and their response to substance P, in *Substance P* (eds P. Skrabanek and D. Powell), Dublin Book Press, pp. 145–6.

Despommier, D. D., Kajima, M. and Wostmann, B. S. (1967) Ferritin-conjugated antibody studies on the larvae of *Trichinella spiralis*. *J. Parasit.*, **53**, 618–24.

Despommier, D., Weisbroth, S. and Fass, C. (1974) Circulating eosinophils and trichinosis in the rat: the parasitic stage responsible for induction during infection. *J. Parasit.*, **60**, 280–4.

D'Inca, R., Ernst, P., Hunt, R. H. and Perdue, M. H. (1992) Role of T lymphocytes in intestinal mucosal injury: inflammatory changes in athymic nude rats. *Dig. Dis. Sci.*, **37**, 33–9.

Farmer, S. G. and Laniyonu, A. A. (1984) Effects of p-chlorophenylalanine on the sensitivity of rat intestine to agonists and on intestinal 5-hydroxytryptamine levels during *Nippostronglylus brasiliensis* infection. *Br. J. Pharmac.*, **82**, 883–9.

Ferguson, A. and Jarrett, E. E. E. (1975) Hypersensitivity reactions in the small intestine. 1. Thymus dependence of experimental 'partial villous atrophy'. *Gut*, **16**, 114–17.

Finkelman, F. D., Pearce, E. J., Urban, J. F. Jr. and Sher, A. (1991) Regulation and biological function of helminth-induced cytokine responses. *Immun. Today.*, **12**, A62–6.

Gabella, G. (1975) Hypertrophy of intestinal smooth muscle. *Cell Tiss. Res.*, **163**, 199–214.

Gilles, H. M., Williams, E. J. W. and Ball, P. A. J. (1964) Hookworm infection and anemia. *Q. J. Med.*, **33**, 1–24.

Gordon, J. R., Burd, P. R. and Galli, S. J. (1990) Mast cells as a source of multifunctional cytokines. *Immun. Today*, **11**, 458–64.

Grimaud, J. A., Boros, D. L., Takiya, C. *et al.* (1987) Collagen isotypes, laminin, and fibronectin in granulomas of the liver and intestines of *Schistosoma mansoni*-infected mice. *Am. J. Trop. Med. Hyg.*, **37**, 335–44.

Haig, D. M. and Miller, H. R. P. (1990) Differentiation of bone marrow cells into effector cells, in *Parasites: Immunity and Pathology: the Consequences of Parasitic Infection in Mammals* (ed J. M. Behnke), Taylor and Francis, London, pp. 42–62.

Halliday, G. J. and Mulligan, W. (1968) Parasitic hypoalbuminemia: studies on type II ostertagiasis in cattle. *Res. Vet. Sci.*, **9**, 224–30.

Harari, Y. and Castro, G. A. (1983) Sialic acid deficiency in lectin-resistant intestinal brush border membranes from rats following the intestinal phase of trichinellosis. *Molec. Biochem. Parasit.*, **9**, 73–81.

Harari, Y. and Castro, G. A. (1988a) Evaluation of a possible functional relationship between chemical structure of intestinal brush border and immunity to *Trichinella spiralis* in the rat. *J. Parasit.*, **74**, 244–8.

Harari, Y. and Castro, G. A. (1988b) Simulation of parasite-induced gut hypersensitivity: implications for vaccination. *Immunology*, **66**, 302–7.

Harari, Y., Russell, D. A. and Castro, G. A. (1987) Anaphylaxis mediated Cl^- secretion and parasite rejection in rat intestine. *J. Immun.*, **138**, 1250–5.

Hinterleitner, T. A. and Powell, D. W. (1991) Immune system control of intestinal ion transport. *Proc. Soc. Exp. Biol. Med.*, **197**, 249–60.

Hussain, R., Bradbury, S. M. and Strejan, G. (1973) Hypersensitivity to *Ascaris* antigens. VIII. Characterization of a highly purified allergen. *J. Immun.*, **111**, 260–8.

Jarrett, E. E. E. (1972) Potentiation of reaginic (IgE) antibody to ovalbumin in the rat following sequential trematode and nematode infections. *Immunology*, **22**, 1099–101.

Kagan, I. G. (1970) Evaluation of the immune state by immunologic techniques, in *Immunity to Parasitic Animals* (eds G. J. Jackson, R. Hermann and I. Singer), Appleton-Century-Crofts, New York, pp. 137–63.

Kane, M. G., Luby, J. P. and Krejs, G. J. (1984) Intestinal secretion as a cause of hypokalemia and cardiac arrest in a patient with strongyloidiasis. *Dig. Dis. Sci.*, **29**, 768–72.

Katona, I. M., Urban, J. F., Jr. and Finkelman, F. D. (1988) The role of L3T4+ and Lyt-2+ T cells in the IgE response and immunity to *Nippostrongylus brasiliensis*. *J. Immun.*, **140**, 3206–11.

Kay, A. B. (1985) Eosinophils as effector cells in immunity and hypersensitivity disorders. *Clin. Exp. Immun.*, **38**, 294.

Kennedy, M. W. (1980) Immunologically mediated, non-specific interactions between the intestinal phases of *Trichinella spiralis* and *Nippostrongylus brasiliensis* in the mouse. *Parasitology*, **80**, 61–72.

Kniker, W. T. (1987) Immunologically mediated reactions to food: state of the art. *Ann. Allergy*, **59** (2), 60–70.

Larsh, J. E., Jr. (1963) Experimental trichinosis, in *Advances in Parasitology* (ed. B. Dawes), Academic Press, New York, pp. 213–86.

Lee, D. L. and Martin, J. (1977) Changes in *Nematodirus battus* associated with the development of immunity to this nematode in lambs, in *Biochemistry of Parasites and Host–Parasite Relationships* (ed. H. Van der Bossche), North–Holland Publishing Co., Amsterdam, pp. 311–18.

Lin, T. M. and Olson, L. J. (1970) Pathophysiology of reinfection with *Trichinella spiralis* in guinea pigs during the intestinal phase. *J. Parasit.*, **56**, 529–39.

MacDonald, T. T. and Spencer, J. (1988) Evidence that activated mucosal T cells play a role in the pathogenesis of enteropathy in human small intestine. *J. Exp. Med.*, **167**, 1341–9.

MacKenzie, C. D., Preston, P. M. and Ogilvie, B. M. (1978) Immunological properties of the surface of parasitic nematodes. *Nature*, **276**, 826–8.

Mahmoud, A. A. F., Stone, M. K. and Kellermeyer, R. W. (1977) Eosinophilopoietin. *J. Clin. Invest.*, **60**, 675–82.

Marshall, J. S., Stead, R. H., McSharry, C. *et al.* (1990) The role of mast cell degranulation products in mast cell hyperplasia. *J. Immun.*, **144**, 1886–92.

Mettrick, D. F., Budziakowski, M. E. and Podesta, R. B. (1979) Net fluxes of electrolytes in the rat intestine infected with *Moniliformis dubius* (Acanthocephala). *Can. J. Physiol. Pharmac.*, **57**, 882–6.

Metzger, H. (1983) The receptor on mast cells and related cells with high affinity for IgE. *Contemp. Topics Molec. Immun.*, **9**, 115.

Miller, H. R. P. (1987) Immunopathology of nematode infestation and expulsion, in *Immunopathology of the Small Intestine* (ed. M. N. Marsh), John Wiley Sons, Chichester, pp. 177–208.

Moqbel, R. and MacDonald, A. J. (1990) Immunological and inflammatory responses in the small intestine associated with helminthic infections, in *Parasites: Immunity and Pathology: the Consequences of Parasitic Infection in Mammals* (ed. J. M. Behnke), Taylor and Francis, London, pp. 249–82.

Murray, M. (1969) Structural changes in bovine ostertagiasis associated with increased permeability of the bowel wall to macromolecules. *Gastroenterology*, **56**, 763–72.

Murray, M. (1972) Immediate hypersensitivity effector mechanisms, in *Immunity to Animal Parasites* (ed. E. J. L. Soulsby), Academic Press, New York, pp. 115–90.

Nyberg, W. (1963) *Diphyllobothrium latum* and human nutrition with particular reference to vitamin B_{12} deficiency. *Proc. Nutr. Soc.*, **22**, 8–14.

Ogilvie, B. M., Philipp, M., Jungery, M. *et al.* (1980) The surface of nematodes and the immune response of the host, in *The Host Invader Interplay* (ed. H. Van der Bossche), Elsevier/North-Holland Biomedical Press, Amsterdam, pp. 99–104.

Olson, L. J. and Schultz, C. W. (1963) Nematode induced hypersensitivity reactions in guinea pigs: Onset of eosinophilia and positive Schultz–Dale reactions following graded infections with *Toxocara canis*. *Ann. NY Acad. Sci.*, **113**, 440–55.

Orr, T. S. C. and Blair, A. M. J. N. (1969) Potentiated reagin response to egg albumin and conalbumin in *Nippostrongylus brasiliensis* infected rats. *Life Sci.*, **8** (Part 2), 1073–7.

Ovington, K. S., Bacarese-Hamilton, A. J. and Bloom, S. R. (1985) *Nippostrongylus brasiliensis*: Changes in plasma levels of gastrointestinal hormones in the infected rat. *Exp. Parasit.*, **60**, 276–84.

Palmer, J. M. and Castro, G. A. (1986) Anamnestic stimulus-specific myoelectric responses associated with intestinal immunity in the rat. *Am. J. Physiol.*, **250**, G266–73.

Palmer, J. M., Tamura, K. and Wood, J. D. (1988) Electrical and synaptic properties of myenteric plexus neurons from guinea-pig small intestine during infection with *Trichinella spiralis*. *FASEB J.*, **2**, A325.

Pappas, P. W. and Read, C. P. (1972a) Trypsin inactivation by intact *Hymenolepis diminuta*. *J. Parasit.*, **58**, 864–71.

Pappas, P. W. and Read, C. P. (1972b) Inactivation of α- and β-chymotrypsin by intact *Hymenolepis diminuta* (Cestoda). *Biol. Bull.*, **143**, 605–16.

Parmentier, H. K., de Vries, C., Ruitenberg, E. J. and Van Loveren, H. (1987) Involvement of serotonin in intestinal mastocytopoiesis and inflammation during a *Trichinella spiralis* infection in mice. *Int. Archs. Allergy Appl. Immun.*, **83**, 31–8.

Patrick, M. K., Dunn, I. J., Buret, A. *et al.* (1988) Mast cell protease release and mucosal ultrastructure during intestinal anaphylaxis in the rat. *Gastroenterology*, **94**, 1–9.

Philipp, M., Parkhouse, R. M. E. and Ogilvie, B. M. (1981) The molecular basis for stage specificity of the primary antibody response to the surface of *Trichinella spiralis*, in *Trichinellosis* (eds C. W. Kim, E. J. Ruitenberg and J. S. Teppema), Reedbooks, Chertseg, UK, pp. 59–64.

Phillips, S. M., Reid, W. A., Doughty, B. L. and Bentley, A. G. (1980) The immunologic modulation of morbidity in schistosomiasis. Studies in athymic mice and *in vitro* granuloma formation. *Am. J. Trop. Med. Hyg.*, **29**, 820–31.

Prosser, C. L. and Brown, F. A. (1961) *Comparative Animal Physiology*, W. B. Saunders Co., Philadelphia, pp. 1–5.

Ptak, W., Geba, G. P. and Askenase, P. W. (1991) Initiation of delayed-type hypersensitivity by low doses of monoclonal IgE antibody. Mediation by serotonin and inhibition by histamine. *J. Immun.*, **146**, 3929–36.

Race, G. J., Larsh, J. E., Martin, J. H. *et al.* (1978) Histopathologic observations of mice after expulsion of *Trichinella spiralis*, in *Trichinellosis, Proceedings of the Fourth International Conference on Trichinellosis* (eds C. W. Kim and Z. S. Pawlowski), University Press of New England, Hanover, New Hampshire, pp. 239–61.

Reichenbach-Klinke, H.H. and Reichenbach-Klinke, K.E. (1970) (Translated title) Enzyme studies in fishes. II. Inhibitors of trypsin and α-amylase. *Arch. Fischereiwiss.*, **21**, 67–72.

Ruff, M. D., Uglem, G. L. and Read, C. P. (1973) Interactions of *Moniliformis dubius* with pancreatic enzymes. *J. Parasit.*, **59**, 839–43.

Russell, D. A. and Castro, G. A. (1979) Physiological characterization of a biphasic immune response to *Trichinella spiralis* in the rat. *J. Infect. Dis.*, **139**, 304–12.

Russell D. A. and Castro G. A. (1987) Physiology of the gastrointestinal tract in the parasitized host, in *Physiology of Gastrointestinal Tract*, 2nd edn (ed. L. R. Johnson), Raven Press, New York, pp. 1749–80.

Sartor, B. R. and Powell, D. W. (1991) Mechanisms of diarrhea in intestinal inflammation and hypersensitivity: Immune system modulation of intestinal transport, in *Current Topics in Gastroenterology, Diarrheal Diseases* (ed. M. Field), Elsevier Science Publishing Co., New York, pp. 75–114.

Schanbacher, L. M., Nations, J. K., Weisbrodt, N. W. and Castro, G. A. (1978) Intestinal myoelectric activity in parasitized dogs. *Am. J. Physiol.*, **234**, R188–95.

Schwartz, L. B. and Austen, K. F. (1984) Structure and function of the chemical mediators of mast cells. *Prog. Allergy*, **34**, 271–321.

Scofield, A. M. (1977) Intestinal absorption of hexose in rats infected with *Nippostrongylus brasiliensis*. *Int. J. Parasit.*, **7**, 159–65.

Shanahan, F., Denburg, J. A., Bienenstock, J. and Befus, A. D. (1984) Mast cell heterogeneity. *Can. J. Physiol. Pharmac.*, **62**, 734–7.

Sharp, A. P. and Olson, L. J. (1962) Hypersensitivity responses in *Toxocara-*, *Ascaris-*, and

Trichinella-infected guinea pigs to homologous and heterologous challenge. *J. Parasit.*, **48**, 362–7.

Shelhamer, J. H., Neva, F. A. and Finn, D. R. (1982) Persistent strongyloidiasis in an immunodeficient patient. *Am. J. Trop. Med. Hyg.*, **31**, 746–751.

Smith, J. W. and Castro, G. A. (1978) Relation of peroxidase activity in gut mucosa to inflammation. *Am. J. Physiol.*, **234**, R72–9.

Soulsby, E. J. L. (1962) Antigen-antibody reactions in helminth infections. *Adv. Immun.*, **2**, 265–308.

Sprinz, H. (1962) Morphological response of intestinal mucosa to enteric bacteria and its implication for sprue and Asiatic cholera. *Fed. Proc.*, **21**, 57–64.

Stavitsky, A. B. (1987) Immune regulation in *Schistosomiasis japonica*. *Immun. Today*, **8**, 228–33.

Stephenson, L. S., Pond, W. G., Nesheim, M. C. *et al.* (1980) *Ascaris suum*: Nutrient absorption, growth and intestinal pathology in young pigs experimentally infected with 15-day old larvae. *Exp. Parasit.*, **49**, 15–25.

Subramanian, N. and Bray, M. A. (1987) Interleukin-1 releases histamine from human basophils and mast cells *in vitro*. *J. Immun.*, **138**, 271–5.

Symons, L. E. A. (1969) Pathology of gastrointestinal helminthiases. *Int. Rev. Trop. Med.*, **3**, 49–100.

Symons, L. E. A. and Fairbairn, D. (1962) Pathology, absorption, transport, and activity of digestive enzymes in rat jejunum parasitized by the nematode *Nippostrongylus brasiliensis*. *Fed. Proc.*, **21**, 913–18.

Taliaferro, W. H. and Sarles, M. P. (1939) The cellular reactions in the skin, lungs and intestine of normal and immune rats after infection with *Nippostrongylus muris*. *J. Infect. Dis.*, **64**, 157–92.

Taylor, E. W. and Thomas, J. N. (1968) Membrane (contact) digestion in the three species of tapeworm *Hymenolepis diminuta, Hymenolepis microstoma* and *Moniezia expansa*. *Parasitology*, **58**, 535–46.

Thorson, R. E. (1956) The stimulation of acquired immunity in dogs by injection of extracts of the esophagus of adult hookworms. *J. Parasitol.*, **42**, 501–4.

Titchen, D. A. (1982) The role of hormones in the reactions of the host to enteric parasites, in *Parasites – Their World and Ours* (eds D. F. Mettrick and S. S. Dresser), Elsevier Biomedical Press, Amsterdam, pp. 245–7.

Uglem, G. L. and Just, J. J. (1983) Trypsin inhibition of tapeworms: Antienzyme secretion or pH adjustment. *Science*, **220**, 79–81.

Vermillion, D. L. and Collins, S. M. (1986) Differential responses of longitudinal and circular muscle to inflammation induced in the rat by *Trichinella spiralis*. *Gastroenterology*, **90**, 1680.

von Bonsdorff, B. (1956) Parasitological review: *Diphyllobothrium latum* as a cause of pernicious anemia. *Exp. Parasit.*, **5**, 207–30.

Wang, C. H., Korenaga, M., Greenwood, A. and Bell, R. G. (1990) T-helper subset function in the gut of rats: differential stimulation of eosinophils, mucosal mast cells and antibody-forming cells by OX8-OX22 and OX8-OX22+ cells. *Immunology*, **71**, 166–75.

Wardlaw, A. J. and Kay, A. B. (1987) The role of the eosinophil in the pathogenesis of asthma. *Allergy*, **42**, 321.

Weinstein, P. P. (1960) Excretory mechanisms and excretory products of nematodes, in *Host Influence on Parasite Physiology* (ed. L. A. Stauber), Rutgers University Press, New Brunswick, NJ, pp. 65–92.

Weinstein, P. P. (1967) Immunologic aspects of parasitic infections, in *Immunologic Aspects of Parasitic Infections*, Pan American Health Organization Sci. Publication No. 150, Washington, DC, pp. 91–106.

Whalen, G. E., Strickland, G. T., Cross, J. H. *et al.* (1969) Intestinal capillariasis: a new disease in man. *Lancet*, **i**, 13–16.

Wolfe, M. S. (1986) Parasites, in *Infectious Diarrhea* (ed. S. L. Gorbach), Blackwell Scientific Publications, Boston, pp. 141–55.

World Health Organization (1980) Parasite-related diarrheas. Bull. WHO, **58**, 819–30.

Yeates, R. A. and Ogilvie, B. M. (1976) Nematode acetylcholinesterases, in *Biochemistry of Parasites and Host–Parasite Relationships* (ed. H. Van den Bossche), North-Holland Publishing Co. Amsterdam, pp. 307–10.

Zhang, S. and Castro, G. A. (1990) Involvement of type I hypersensitivity in rapid rejection of *Trichinella spiralis* from adult rats. *Int. Arch. Allergy Appl. Immun.*, **93**, 272–9.

Zhang, S., Myers, S. and Castro, G. A. (1991) Inhibition of anaphylaxis-evoked intestinal fluid secretion by the dual application of an H1 antagonist and cyclooxygenase inhibitor. *Gastroenterology*, **100**, 922–8.

Zucker-Franklin, D. (1974) Eosinophil function and disorders. *Adv. Intern. Med.*, **19**, 1–25.

FIVE

Immune responses: protective immunity, adaptation and pathogenesis

A. D. Befus

5.1 BACKGROUND

This volume seeks to emphasize that intestinal helminth infections are important causes of disease in humans (WHO Expert Committee, 1987) and in domestic animals (e.g. Urban and Gamble, 1989) and of significant social and economic losses. Accordingly, in order to seek for innovative therapeutic interventions for these infections, researchers have studied host immune responses throughout much of the present century (Chandler, 1953). Although a great deal of information has been generated, including a wealth of knowledge about aspects of the immune system not readily forthcoming from studies of other infections or immunologic diseases (such as IgE, mast cells and eosinophils), we do not understand the precise mechanisms of host resistance in any helminth infection. Moreover, which effector cells or molecules are important is not clear. Even empirical studies of vaccination, a strategy that has been effective for the development of vaccines in many viral and bacterial infections, has been unproductive for helminths of the gastrointestinal (GI) tract, and with the exclusion of cattle lungworm, worms living elsewhere in the body.

Over the last two decades a number of approaches have been widely employed to help elucidate the nature of the host immune and inflammatory responses to intestinal helminths. These can be summarized as follows:

- time course analyses of parasite establishment, development, fecundity and survival in naive and previously infected hosts of differing genotypes;
- correlation between these analyses and histopathologic responses at site of infection;
- vaccination with attenuated parasites or their products;
- cellular and/or serum transfer of immunity to naive or immunocompromised hosts;
- manipulation of cells or mediators postulated to be important in host defense using agonistic or antagonistic drugs or antibodies;
- definition of local microenvironmental components of antigen-specific and non-specific responses to parasites or their antigens (Befus *et al.*, 1986). These investigations have been extensively reviewed by many authors (e.g. Befus and Bienenstock, 1984; Befus, 1986; Castro, 1989; Miller, 1987a,b; Moqbel, 1986; Russell and Castro,

Enteric Infection 2. Intestinal helminths. Edited by M.J.G. Farthing, G.T. Keusch and D. Wakelin. Published in 1995 by Chapman and Hall, London. ISBN 0 412 39140 6

1987; Rothwell, 1989; Smith, 1989; Wakelin, 1986; and Wassom and Kelly, 1990).

Because of numerous logistic difficulties and the expense of studies in humans or large domestic animals, most of the studies of immune responses to intestinal helminths have employed nematode models in mice, rats or guineapigs, notably with *Nippostrongylus brasiliensis, Strongyloides ratti, Trichinella spiralis, Trichostrongylus colubriformis and Trichuris muris*. Perhaps with the exception of *Trichuris*, each of these infections induces a pronounced inflammatory infiltration in the GI tract with some neutrophils and mononuclear cells, but also with striking local mastocytosis and eosinophilia. Not surprisingly, these inflammatory cells have been a focus for the study of mechanisms of resistance and pathogenesis.

Although in comparison with nematode infections the immunology of cestode infections of the GI tract has received relatively little investigation, future studies with these flatworms may be enlightening, because immunologic resistance is generated in the absence of major inflammatory infiltrates. For example, primary infections with the tapeworm *Hymenolepis diminuta* are expelled from the intestine of mice, and mice are resistant to secondary challenge infections through unknown mechanisms not involving obvious inflammatory responses. It may be that even in nematode infections with pronounced inflammatory infiltrates, mechanisms of protective immunity are not necessarily directly associated with the inflammation, but with mechanisms similar to those with cestode infections, albeit masked by the more obvious, and thus compelling, inflammatory changes.

Immune responses to trematode or acanthocephalan infections of the GI tract have received less study than for nematodes and cestodes, although recently it has been proposed that IgA antibody responses, perhaps generated in the intestinal mucosa, to human infections with *Schistosoma mansoni*, may be highly relevant in protective immunity in at least some individuals (Capron *et al.*, 1992; Dessein *et al.*, 1992). Given the paucity of information on immune responses to intestinal trematode and acanthocephalan infections, this review will draw heavily from concepts developed with nematode and cestode models.

It is critical to appreciate the limitations of the literature evolving from these models, because natural infections do not always follow the course predicted by these models and future vaccine development for humans or domestic animals may require considerable modification from protocols developed in experimental systems. Experimental models are rigorously defined to be highly reproducible through efforts to employ genotypically and phenotypically homogeneous hosts and parasites. Not only are genetic variations selected against, but nutrition, other infections and numerous environmental conditions such as light, temperature, humidity, etc. are stringently controlled. Furthermore, relatively large numbers of worms are employed in infections, almost always given as a single bolus to hosts of highly selected ages, with or without a subsequent secondary infection. As highlighted by Schweitzer and Anderson (1991), the emphasis is on statistically significant responses in relatively homogeneous populations, rather than on the mechanisms underlying the heterogeneity of outcomes exhibited among individuals in natural populations.

Moreover, despite considerable evidence that repeated low level infections can induce differing inflammatory and immune responses (e.g. Ferens, Arai and Befus, 1992) than these bolus infections, repeated low-level infection protocols are seldom used, largely because of the highly repetitive technical demands and financial constraints, including the time required for such studies.

Experimental systems are also designed to

isolate a low number of variables and often employ strategies to enhance or ablate a single mediator or cell type. Unfortunately, it is seldom that a deficiency, such as in CD4+ cells or mast cells is absolute, or that a single cell type or mediator can be isolated from all others, or that worm expulsion or the lack thereof is complete. Yet conclusions are generated on the basis of partial worm loss or cell depletion, or marked cell enrichment. It is not necessary to dwell on these deficiencies of our experimental tools, although it is essential that they be recognized and that an appropriate caution is employed in generating conclusions and in their generalization.

It is disturbing that our understanding is limited such that in a comprehensive review of 1989, Rothwell concluded that despite the volume of literature, we are unable to answer clearly general but fundamental questions such as: 'does an individual host have the option of a variety of expulsion processes', or 'do different host species use the same or different processes to expel a particular parasite'? One interpretation of the literature suggests that the answers to these questions are yes; this would certainly help explain some of the potential confusion that exists. In this chapter, an up-to-date summary is presented of the mucosal immune apparatus of the GI tract and an overview of present concepts of host defenses in the intestinal mucosa (see McGhee *et al.*, 1989; Husband and Dunkley, 1990; Targan and Shanahan, 1990; Cerf-Bensussan and Guy-Grand 1991). Finally some focused studies are identified which may provide important new comprehension of immunity and pathogenesis of GI helminthiasis.

5.2 ANTIGEN UPTAKE, PROCESSING AND PRESENTATION AT MUCOSAL SURFACES

Despite significant advances in our understanding of antigen uptake, processing and presentation (e.g. Golub and Green, 1991), knowledge of these mechanisms in the GI tract or other mucosal surfaces is limited (Bland, 1988; Mayer, 1990). In the immune system in general, B cells are thought to interact directly with antigen through their specific surface immunoglobulin receptors. By contrast, T cell activation by antigen requires the participation of antigen-presenting cells (APC) of the same major histocompatibility complex (MHC) haplotype. Many cells can act as APC, including B cells, fibroblasts, various tissue-specific macrophage populations, dendritic cells and even epithelial and endothelial cells.

Processing of antigen for presentation to CD4+ T helper cells (T_H) requires uptake of exogenous antigen into endosomal vesicles and cleavage into fragments which bind to MHC class II molecules subsequently expressed at the cell surface for presentation to the T cell receptor (TCR). The TCR complex can be of two major types, namely TCR γ/δ and TCR α/β, (see below) and together with CD3 includes at least seven distinct polypeptide chains (Golub and Green, 1991). MHC class II-antigen recognition by TCR involves the CD4 molecule itself as a coreceptor.

For presentation of antigens to CD8+ cells, antigen must be in the cytoplasm of the APC, often an endogenous viral or tumour antigen, where it is cleaved into fragments, subsequently complexed to class I MHC molecules and finally expressed at the cell surface for interaction with the CD8 coreceptor and TCR. This model of antigen presentation explains MHC restriction as a process where the TCR together with the CD4 or CD8 coreceptor recognizes the antigen fragment bound in a groove on the corresponding MHC molecule.

For many years a major concern for students of GI immune responses was the mechanism of uptake of lumenal antigen. The epithelium and its mucus is a prominent barrier to antigen uptake (Russell and Walker, 1990)

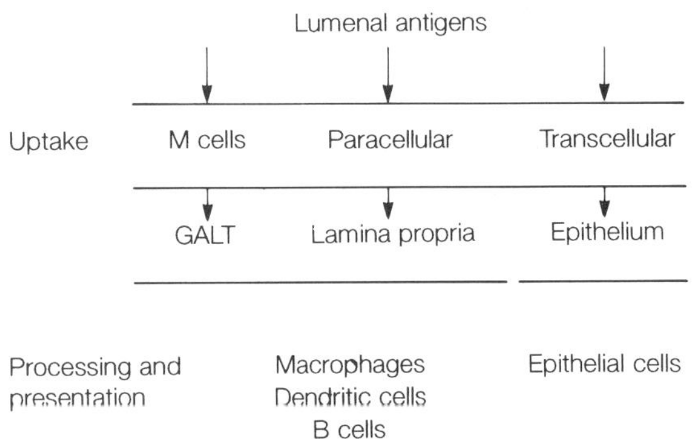

Figure 5.1 Antigen uptake, processing and presentation in the gastrointestinal tract.

and it was thought that unless there was disruption of this barrier through injury by an infectious agent or other inflammatory events, antigen uptake was minimal. However as summarized by Mayer (1990), three pathways are thought to be important for antigen uptake from the GI tract, namely:

- uptake by microfold (M) cells in the lymphoepithelium overlying the Peyer's patches and other gut-associated lymphoid tissues (GALT);
- paracellular;
- transcellular pathways through epithelial cells (Figure 5.1).

Following the careful observations by Owen and Jones (1974), M cells were identified as specialized epithelial cells derived from the base of the crypts and capable of rapid uptake and transport of antigens to cells within the Peyer's patches. Paradoxically, a number of bacteria and viruses appear to utilize M cells for colonization or to gain access to the body from the intestinal lumen (Befus and Bienenstock, 1984), but to date no relationship between these cells and any intestinal helminth has been noted. Perhaps M cells provide some physical or chemical signals which helminths utilize for site selection or as other microenvironmental clues for survival. Interestingly, M cells do not appear to express MHC II molecules and thus may not be directly involved in antigen processing or presentation. Dendritic cells, macrophages or B cells in the Peyer's patches may be most relevant for these functions.

In attempts to dissect the mechanisms which dictate pathway selection in immune responses, such as the classical dichotomy of antibody versus delayed hypersensitivity responses, or isotype restriction, APC have become a favoured target. The predilection for IgA responses by GALT appears at least partially to involve the ability of Peyer's patch-derived dendritic cells selectively to promote polyclonal IgA responses *in vitro*, regardless of whether the T cell help was derived from Peyer's patches or spleen cells (Spalding and Green, 1986).

Unfortunately, the role of paracellular pathways through the epithelium in antigen uptake, processing and presentation in the intestine is unknown. It is assumed that this pathway is most important when the epithelial barrier is breached by some injury, thereby exposing APC of the lamina propria to lumen antigens. These APC have received little study because of difficulties in their *in situ* visualization, isolation and purification. Thus, we may not appreciate the abundance or relative importance of these cells. They may form an interdigitating network below the intestinal epithelium similar to that recently identified for the remarkable network of MHC class II-positive dendritic cells underlying the respiratory epithelium (Holt *et al.*, 1990), reminiscent of the Langerhan cell latticework in the skin (Dezutter-Dambuant, 1988). Whether they exhibit some selectivity in the nature of the immune responses that they induce remains to be determined, but given the abundance of local IgG responses in inflammatory diseases such as inflammatory bowel disease (IBD; MacDermott and Stenson, 1990) and trichinosis (Zettel *et al.*, 1992), they may promote IgG responses.

The transcellular pathway through the intestinal epithelium is also relatively poorly known, but *in vitro* studies by Bland (e.g. Bland, 1988) and Mayer (Mayer, 1990) have established that isolated rat and human intestinal epithelial cells present antigens to CD8+ T cells. Interestingly, this activation of CD8+ cells was inhibitable by antibodies to MHC II molecules, suggesting a novel form of presentation rather than the anticipated MHC class I restriction normally involved in CD8+ cell activation. Mayer (1990) postulated that a hitherto unknown ligand for CD8 exists on intestinal epithelial cells. The molecular and functional definition of such a ligand would open new areas of investigation of GI immune responses, especially given the predominance of CD8+ lymphoid cells in the epithelium, largely expressing the homodimeric CD8 α/α complex in conjunction with TCR γ/δ+ or in the absence of CD3 and TCR (CD3-, TCR-; Cerf-Bensussan and Guy-Grand, 1991 and see discussion below). Given the phenotypic heterogeneity of CD8+ cells in the intestinal epithelium, the specific functions of this pathway of antigen uptake and presentation are likely to be diverse. Whether or not this pathway exhibits some selectivity in the generation of immune responses is unknown, but the CD8+ phenotype suggests that it may be important in oral tolerance (McGhee *et al.*, 1989) or contrasuppression (Fujihashi *et al.*, 1990).

There have been no studies of uptake, processing or presentation of helminth antigens in the GI tract or elsewhere. It remains to be determined which antigens are relevant, the pathway(s) of their uptake, types of APC utilized and nature of processing and presentation. Whether or not the remarkable predominance of IgE, mast cell and eosinophil responses in GI helminth infections can be directly attributed to the pathways of uptake, processing and presentation of worm antigens, or to other characteristics of the host–parasite relationship remains to be established.

5.3 GENERATION OF MUCOSAL IMMUNE AND INFLAMMATORY RESPONSES

In addition to highly specialized lymphoid aggregates such as Peyer's patches in the GI mucosa, there is an abundance of lymphoid and myeloid cells in the lamina propria and epithelium of the intestine. Major efforts have been made to investigate the specialization and unique compartmentalization of portions of the immune system in these sites, and significant advances have been made in the last few years. The cellular and molecular mechanisms of the local production and transport of secretory IgA (IgA) have become increasingly clear, although the complexity of regulatory mechanisms appears to be baffling (McGhee *et al.*, 1989). The nature of the heterogeneous leucocyte population in the intestinal epithelium has been more fully described and recent information about the abundance of cells bearing TCR γ/δ and/or the homodimeric form (α/α) of CD8 (Cerf-Bensussan and Guy-Grand, 1991) promises to stimulate innovative investigations. The excitement generated in the entire field of immunology by the recent categorization of T_H subsets (Mosmann and Coffman, 1989) has stimulated a focus on the distribution, abundance and function of these cells in the intestinal mucosa. The activation or preferential enhancement or survival of one of these two T_H subsets appears to be highly relevant in host defenses and pathogenesis of parasitic infections in the intestine and elsewhere (Finkelman *et al.*, 1991; King and Nutman, 1991; Locksley and Scott, 1991).

5.3.1 COMPARTMENTALIZATION OF THE IMMUNE SYSTEM IN THE GASTROINTESTINAL MUCOSA

(a) Gut-associated lymphoid tissues (GALT)

GALT include Peyer's patches and solitary lymphoid nodules, the appendix and sacculus rotundus in some species, and in birds, the bursa of Fabricius. Apart from the avian bursa and mammalian Peyer's patches, little is known about distinct functions of these various forms of GALT. However, studies in sheep have demonstrated that in this species at least there are two types of Peyer's patch one in the terminal ileum arising prenatally, apparently independent of exogenous antigenic stimulation, and another found largely in the jejunum which develops later in a relatively antigen-dependent manner (Reynolds and Kirk, 1989). The ileal Peyer's patch appears to be analogous to the avian bursa in its production of B lymphocytes, whereas jejunal Peyer's patch appears to function as a reactive lymphoid tissue. In rodents and perhaps in humans, Peyer's patches appear to function in a manner analogous to that in the jejunum of sheep. It is these that will be described in greater detail below. Similar lymphoid aggregates are found at other mucosal surfaces, such as the respiratory tract where they are known as bronchus-associated lymphoid tissue (BALT; Bienenstock, Johnston and Perey, 1973).

The lumenal surfaces of Peyer's patches are covered by a lymphoepithelium containing large numbers of CD4+ and CD8+ T lymphocytes, B lymphocytes and M cells specialized for antigen uptake. Below this lymphoepithelium, there is a follicle, referred to as an IgA 'inductive' environment, a site of rapid B cell proliferation and selective cell death. This programmed cell death, called apoptosis, appears to be analogous to a similar process in the thymus where T cell specificities for antigens are determined, and it has been postulated that in the Peyer's patch this selective death or survival determines the repertoire of B cell antigen specificities in the individual (Motyka and Reynolds, 1992). Adjacent to the B cell-rich follicles with their smaller populations of T subsets, macrophages and dendritic cells, there are T cell-rich interfollicular zones. These zones also contain high endothelial venules, sites highly active in the emigration of lymphocytes from the circulation.

(b) Lamina propria

In contrast to the IgA 'inductive' environment of the Peyer's patch, the lamina propria is referred to as an 'effector' site (IgA and other). It contains large numbers of IgA-producing plasma cells, as well as T cells, macrophages, mast cells, eosinophils and neutrophils interspersed among the connective tissue framework, portions of the enteric nervous system and blood vessels. As outlined below, the immigration of lymphoid and myeloid cells into this compartment often involves specialized endothelial receptor–ligand systems and multiple other cellular communication systems. Details of some of the regulatory components of the cell populations in the lamina propria, as well as their effector functions will be outlined below.

(c) Intraepithelial leucocytes (IEL)

The population of leucocytes in the intestinal epithelium (probably epithelial sites elsewhere also) is heterogeneous and consists of some novel cell types (reviewed by Cerf-Bensussan and Guy-Grand, 1991). The majority of IEL are lymphocyte-like in morphology; 20 to 70% possess cytoplasmic granules containing mucopolysaccharides and, at least in mice, the markers of cytotoxic cells, perforin and granzymes (Guy-Grand *et al.*, 1991a). In an elegant and enlightening study, Guy-Grand *et al.* (1991b) described the heterogeneity of surface phenotype of IEL in the mouse intestine (Table 5.1), and confirmed unequivocally the presence of two distinct populations of CD8+ cells, one bearing homodimeric CD8+ alpha chains (Lyt2+, α/α) and the other with heterodimeric CD8+ alpha and beta (Lyt3+) chains (α/β).

In the normal mouse small intestine, about 95% of all IEL are CD3+, 90% are CD8+ and

Table 5.1 Abundance of intraepithelial leucocyte populations in the murine intestine

		Phenotype						
				CD_8			*TCR*	
Mice	*Cell number* (× 10^6)	*Thy1*	*CD_4*	α/α	α/β	*CD_3*	α/β	γβ
Normal adult								
Total	7.5	50	10	56	33	95	72	27
Thy1	–*	<0.1	<0.1	92	<0.1	93	56	–*
Nu/Nu	1	6	<1	84	<1	37	0	53
SCID	0.3	9	1	46	4	3	0	–*
Suckling	1.5	11	2	74	5	89	12	81
Germ-free	0.6	25	4	63	2	82	14	–*
GVHR	5	<99	5	1	94	>99	>99	0

* Where data is absent from Table, none is available.
Abbreviations: Nu/Nu, athymic nude; SCID, severe combined immmunodeficient; GVHR, graft versus host reaction.
Adapted from Guy-Grand *et al.*, 1991b.

about 10% are CD4+ (Table 1). Only 50% express what was previously considered to be a murine pan T cell marker, Thy1 and of the Thy1− cells, >90% are CD3+ and CD8+. About 70% of IEL from normal mice are TCR α/β+ and 27% are TCR γ/δ+. Of the CD8+ IEL in normal mice, about 63% are homodimeric CD8 α/α and 37% are heterodimeric CD8 α/β. Of the Thy1-IEL of normal mice, 100% are CD8 α/α.

The proportions of various subpopulations of IEL are modified in mice with selected immune deficiencies or in suckling, germ-free mice or mice with graft-versus-host reactions (GVHR). For example, thymus-deficient nude mice lack Thy1+, CD4+ and TCR α/β+ cells. Nevertheless, IEL from nude mice have a high proportion of CD8+ (84%), CD3+ (37%) and TCR γ/δ+ (53%) cells. Thus, many CD8+, TCR γ/δ+ IEL appear to be capable of development in a thymus-independent manner. Mice with severe combined immune deficiency (SCID) have low numbers of Thy1+, CD4+, CD3+ and TCR α/δ+ cells, but maintain a CD8+ (50%) population of IEL. This indicates that many of the CD8+ cells in IEL are independent of the expression of genetic rearrangements which define classical T and B lymphocyte lineages.

In mice with limited antigenic exposure (e.g. suckling or germ-free mice), the numbers and proportions of Thy1+ cells are low (11 to 25%) and the CD4+ cells are few (2 to 4%), but the proportions of CD3+ and CD8+ cells are near normal. The proportion of TCR α/β+ cells is reduced from normal, but the proportion of TCR γ/δ+, at least as studied in the suckling mice, appears to be elevated. From this information, the authors suggested that antigenic stimulation is important in the expression of Thy1+, CD4+ and α/β+ cells, but the expression of CD8+, CD3+ and TCR γ/δ+ cells is relatively antigen-independent. By contrast, in mice with a strong T cell-dependent reaction, namely GVHR, 99% of the IEL are Thy1+, CD3+ and TCR α/β+. About 95% of these cells are CD8+ (Table 5.1).

Guy-Grand *et al.* (1991b) concluded that IEL consist of two major populations, one which is Thy1+, TCR α/β+ and heterodimeric CD8 α/β+. It is derived from antigen-driven proliferating T cells in the Peyer's patches. The second major population is largely Thy1−, TCR γ/δ+ and homodimeric CD8 α/α+; it can develop independently of the thymus and of antigenic stimulation. Klein and coworkers (Mosley, Styre and Klein, 1990) also provided strong evidence for the presence of thymic-independent IEL using athymic chimeras, a conclusion initially reached by Mayrhofer (1980). In addition, both Rocha's and Whetsell's work established that for many IEL, gene rearrangements in TCR involve a major extrathymic pathway of T cell differentiation (Rocha, Vassalli and Guy-Grand, 1991; Whetsell *et al.*, 1992). Rocha *et al.* (1991) established that the homodimeric CD8 α/α is the major population in this pathway and proposed that CD8 α/α IEL may contribute to a first line of defense against exogenous superantigens.

Evidence suggests that IEL in the normal adult human small intestine also possess populations analogous to the murine thymic-independent and thymic-dependent cells, as well as a small (>20%) population of T cell precursors (CD7+, CD3−, CD2−, TCR−) (see Cerf-Bensussan and Guy-Grand, 1991).

From these observations, Guy-Grand *et al.* (1991b) postulated that 'the gut epithelium (an endoderm derivative, as the thymic epithelium) has an inductive property, attracting progenitors of bone marrow origin, and triggering their TCR rearrangement and α/α CD8 chains expression, thus giving rise to a T-cell population that appears to belong to the same lineage as γ/δ thymocytes and to recognize an antigenic repertoire different from that of α/β CD8+ IEL'.

Functional investigations of IEL have established that many of the populations, including TCR α/β+, TCR γ/δ+ and cells negative for T-cell markers, express cytotoxic activity (reviewed by Cerf-Bensussan and Guy-Grand, 1991). Moreover, mast cell, natural killer and T-cell precursors are present in IEL. IEL can secrete large amounts of γ interferon (γIFN) and tumor necrosis factor alpha (TNFα), but smaller amounts of IL-2 (Cerf-Bensussan and Guy-Grand, 1991); they also produce IL-5 (Taguchi *et al.*, 1990).

A critical question to be answered is the nature of antigen recognition and MHC involvement in TCR γ/δ IEL. It has been calculated that TCR γ/δ have a potentially diverse repertoire for antigen recognition and, given the localization of TCR γ/δ at epithelial surfaces, they may interact with superantigens of some microbes, or heat-shock antigens common to a number of organisms which inhabit these sites (Janeway, Jones and Hayday, 1988). The role of MHC is unknown and the significance of CD8 α/α remains unknown. Perhaps there are novel interactions with ligands on the surface of epithelial cells. As described below in greater detail, it appears that IEL produce factors that play important physiological roles in their microenvironment, including epithelial cell development and turnover.

Despite the heterogeneity, functional repertoire and recent excitement generated by study of IEL, there is little information about their role in helminthic infections. Although the numbers of IEL increase in giardiasis and in celiac disease, no such increases have been found in helminth infections. Whether alterations in selected sub-populations occur in helminth infections, as in celiac disease (Halstensen, Scott and Brandtzaeg, 1989), remains to be determined. Although changes in the numbers of IEL have not been noted, it seems probable that IEL are important in host defenses, pathogenesis or adaptation in helminth infections.

5.3.2 SYNTHESIS AND SECRETION OF IGA

A high proportion of B cells in Peyer's patches that survive the selection of apoptosis, become IgA-producing plasma cells, although the mechanisms underlying this isotype restriction are incompletely understood. It appears that this cannot be explained by the selective recruitment to Peyer's patches of precursors committed to IgA production from sites such as bone marrow, but local mechanisms are involved for rearrangements of the Ig genes which select for α heavy chain expression. To date this cannot be attributed to any known cytokine or combination of cytokines from T cells, dendritic cells (Spalding and Griffin, 1986) or other sources, although Kawanishi, Saltzman and Strober (1983) isolated T-cell clones from Peyer's patches which appear to act early in the pathway of IgA production, because they induced a commitment of surface IgM+ B cells to IgA production (switch to surface IgA positive). These T-switch cells could be activated by autologous lymphoreticular cells, Thy 1+, Lyt-1+ (CD5+) and Ia+, but neither they, nor their supernatants, would augment Ig secretion by B cells (reviewed by McGhee *et al.*, 1989).

Many other cells, including both classical T_H and T suppressor (T_S) cells are involved in the regulation of IgA synthesis and secretion. Some, but not all of these cells produce IgA binding factors involved in isotype-specific regulation. Once commitment of the B cell to IgA has occurred, the mitogen LPS, and the cytokine IL-4, can activate the precursor to begin its maturation into an IgA-secreting plasma cell (McGhee *et al.*, 1989). After IL-4 activation, IL-5 can induce the activated B cells to proceed through the cell cycle and clonally expand. Subsequently, IL-6, perhaps together with IL-5, induces final differentiation into plasma cells secreting IgA (McGhee *et al.*, 1989). Many other factors influence this induction, proliferative and differentiation pathway of IgA B cells, including IgA binding factors, many neuropeptides (Stanisz, Befus and Bienenstock, 1986), and the seemingly ubiquitous growth factor, transforming growth factor β (TGFβ). TGFβ has been identified as a costimulator of IgA production, perhaps by potentiation of switch to IgA by a timely inhibition of cell proliferation (Kim and Kagnoff, 1990).

Maturation of IgA cells to plasma cells does not occur in the Peyer's patches, but involves migration in lymph efferent from the Peyer's patches to the mesenteric lymph nodes (MLN), followed by migration in the lymph to the thoracic duct and into the circulation (Figure 5.2). A high proportion of these cells home specifically to the intestinal lamina propria through specialized venules in the basal area of the villus or in the crypt, or in other mucosal surfaces where they become fully functional plasma cells secreting IgA antibody. The mechanisms of this highly selective localization are incompletely understood, but involve exquisite endothelial and B cell ligand–receptor systems and unknown adhesion and activation mechanisms for local cell retention and proliferation (e.g. Ottaway, 1990).

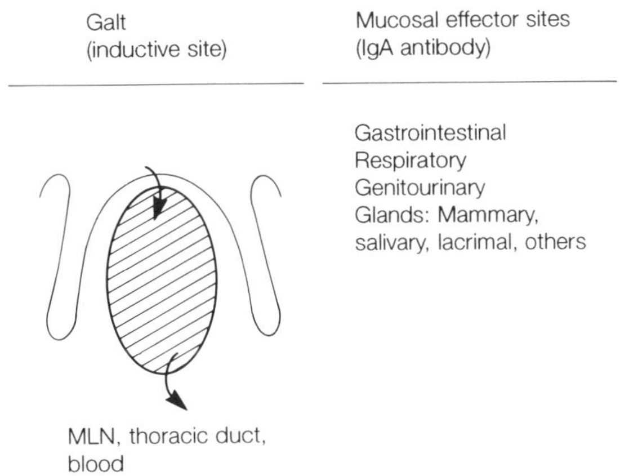

Figure 5.2 Development and migration of IgA-producing cells.

5.3.3 T-HELPER SUBSETS IN THE INTESTINAL MUCOSA

(a) Overview

The identification of two populations of CD4+ T_H cells, T_{H1} and T_{H2}, promises to enhance our understanding of how the immune system generates a particular effector pathway (Mosmann and Moore, 1991). Through studies of the patterns of cytokine secretion by murine T-cell clones, Mosmann and Coffman (1989) defined two prominent profiles. T_{H1} cells produce large amounts of IL-2, γIFN and lymphotoxin, whereas T_{H2} cells produce IL-4, IL-5, IL-6 and IL-10 (Table 5.2). CD8+ cells produce cytokines as well,

Table 5.2 Cytokine secretion profiles of murine T lymphocytes

	Cell type				
Cytokine	T_{H1}	T_{H2}	$CD8^+$	T_{HP}	T_{HO}
IL-2	++	−	+/−	++	++
γIFN	++	−	++	−	++
Lymphotoxin	++	−	+		
IL-4	−	++		−	++
IL-5	−	++	+	−	++
IL-6	−	++			
IL-10	−	++		−	++
GM-CSF	++	+	+	−	++
TNFα	++	+	+		
IL-3	++	++	+	−	++

Modified and extended from Mosmann and Moore (1991).

but do not necessarily fall into either T_{H1} or T_{H2} patterns (e.g. Mosmann and Moore, 1991; Taguchi *et al.*, 1990).

Subsequent studies on the patterns of cytokine secretion established that not all T_H cells fall into these two discrete categories. Moreover, the nature of the growth and differentiation pathways which yield T_{H1} or T_{H2} cells, or cells with other patterns of cytokine production, is unclear. It is not known if multiple cytokine secretion patterns arise from a single precursor cell after antigen activation, or if a single cytokine pattern is programmed in the precursor before exposure to antigen (Mosmann and Moore, 1991). In an effort to present these ideas clearly and cautiously, Mosmann and Moore (1991) postulated that a T_{HP} (precursor) which appears to make only IL-2, differentiates into a T_{HO} population making a variety of cytokines (Table 5.2). Subsequently, T_{H1} and T_{H2} populations evolve during the course of a particular immune response, their products orchestrating particular effector pathways and inhibiting others. Thus, development proceeds from an initial, predominantly proliferative and inductive signal (T_{HP}), through a diverse maze of chemical messages (T_{HO}), and finally to effector pathways of delayed hypersensitivity/cellular immunity (T_{H1}) or antibody-mediated immunity (T_{H2}). This working model must be rigorously tested in a number of experimental systems in animals, as well as in humans where recent evidence suggests that stable cytokine secretion patterns similar to those of murine T_{H1} and T_{H2} exist (Del Prete *et al.*, 1991).

Given the spectrum of cytokine production by T_{H1} and T_{H2} cells, it is not surprising that their functions differ in the generation of immune responses. T_{H1} cells mediate delayed hypersensitivity and can also help B cells in antibody production. In general, they appear to be effective in responses to intracellular pathogens, whereas T_{H2} may be critical in dealing with extracellular pathogens, such as helminths. T_{H2} are potent in the facilitation of antibody production and in the absence of the inhibitory effects of γIFN, IL-4 markedly enhances IgE responses. Moreover, IL-3 and IL-4 are mast cell growth factors, and IL-5 induces eosinophil proliferation and differentiation. Thus, T_{H2} are strongly associated with immediate hypersensitivity responses involving IgE, mast cells and eosinophils, responses which are the hallmark of so many helminth infections of the intestine and other sites.

(b) T-helper subsets in the GI tract

In the GI tract, the distribution in time and space of what is likely to be a constantly evolving balance among the spectrum of cytokine secretion patterns by T cells has received limited study. Husband and Dunkley (1990) postulated an attractive model of T_{H1} and T_{H2} balance in the distinctive 'inductive' environment of the Peyer's patch and the 'effector' environment of the lamina propria. T_{H1}, characterized by the production of γIFN, IL-2 and lymphotoxin, and derived from the pool of small recirculating T cells, are able to help B cells in their early inductive phases of development. In contrast, T_{H2} cells, which are derived from short-lived non-recirculating T cells, produce IL-4, IL-5 and IL-6, interleukins which can directly induce proliferation and differentiation in large B cells. Thus, in Peyer's patches, where small naive resting B cells undergo induction and commitment to the IgA pathway, T_{H1} may predominate. In the lamina propria where recent immigrants include large B cells committed to IgA production, the actions of T_{H2} in the final phases of IgA synthesis and secretion may be most influential. In a manner consistent with this model, Dunkley and Husband (1989) observed that small recirculating T_H from the thoracic duct of rats, localized selectively to the Peyer's patches, and as predicted by the model, large activated T_H, likely to contain T_{H2}, localized to the intestinal lamina propria within 1 h of injection. These observations are interesting, but not a direct test of cytokine production by cells in specific compartments of the intestinal immune system.

Using ELISPOT assay to detect individual T cells producing γIFN or IL-5, Taguchi *et al.* (1990) determined the production profile of cells from murine Peyer's patches, lamina propria and IEL. IL-5 was produced by a greater proportion of lymphocytes derived from the lamina propria than from Peyer's patches or IEL, although cells from all sites produced both cytokines. This observation is consistent with the postulated dominance of T_{H2} in the lamina propria. In a study with non-human primates, James, Kwan and Sneller (1990) established that, in the 'inductive' environment of the MLN, mRNA levels suggested a low potential for T_{H1} (γIFN, IL-2) and a high potential for T_{H2} (IL-4, IL-5) activity. The lamina propria 'effector' compartment exhibited high levels of mRNA for γIFN, IL-2, IL-4 and IL-5, indicative of an activated or memory state, but apparently not predominantly T_{H1} or T_{H2}. It is clear that additional studies are required to describe the cytokine secretion profiles of the normal intestinal mucosa and the changes induced during the evolution of immune and inflammatory responses in helminth or other infections, or in other diseases of the gut.

(c) Observations with GI helminth infections

Interesting and enlightening results relating to pathogenesis and protective immunity have been generated from studies of T_H subsets and cytokine profiles in leishmaniasis (e.g. Locksley and Scott, 1991) and more recently with human filariasis (King and Nutman, 1991). With gastrointestinal nematode infections, Finkelman *et al.* (1991) suggested that in some infections T_{H2} cytokines appear to contribute to host protection, but in others they appear to contribute to survival of the parasite. Undoubtedly, important information will be forthcoming, as recombinant cytokines, respective nucleic acid probes and monoclonal antibodies are used to map cytokine production and importance in host defenses, pathogenesis and adaptation in helminth infections of the gut. Unfortunately, as the information unravels, it is unlikely to be marked by its simplicity. There is pronounced redundancy in the actions of many cytokines, their time course of synthesis and secretion can be variable, and the competency of other cells to respond varies. Moreover, these cytokines are not made solely by T cells; other cells, including epithelial cells, mast cells and many stromal elements are potent producers of selected cytokines (e.g. Gordon, Burd and Galli, 1990; Shirota *et al.*, 1990; Radema, Van Deventer and Cerami, 1991; Stadnyk and Gauldie, 1991) and hence unsubstantiated emphasis on T_H cells as the sole or predominant source of these chemical messages must be viewed cautiously.

5.3.4 INFLAMMATION IN THE INTESTINAL MUCOSA

(a) Overview

Acute inflammation is a normal physiologic response designed to restrict damage at a site of infection or other injury. As reviewed by Stadnyk and Gauldie (1991), it involves complex local and systemic changes with increased protein catabolism and gluconeogenesis, and a negative nitrogen balance. Local responses include coagulation, kinin generation, phospholipid metabolism, increased blood flow and permeability, and leucocyte infiltration. Systemic responses include fever, leucocytosis, alterations in plasma concentrations of heavy metals and increased plasma levels of hepatocyte-derived proteins important in the cascade of events following the injury. If the source of the injury persists or the appropriate regulation of inflammation is compromised, chronic inflammation with repair and scarring results in loss of normal function.

Inflammatory responses in the intestinal mucosa are often assessed by histologic analysis of mononuclear or granulocytic (neutrophils, eosinophils, mast cells) infiltration, or disruption of the normal integrity of the epithelium, mucosa or muscle layers. Recently emphasis has been placed upon the analysis of specific inflammatory mediators stored in or rapidly generated by the inflamed tissue. For example, especially in conjunction with studies of the pathogenesis of IBD, mediators such as myeloperoxidase, leukotrienes, platelet activating factor (PAF), oxygen radicals, biogenic amines and cytokines, including IL-1 and TNFα, have been measured and where possible their actions agonized or antagonized by drugs or antibodies (e.g. Wallace, 1991). Cellular and molecular mechanisms regulating inflammatory cell influx are being investigated, as are pathologic and adaptive changes in the local physiology. With these approaches the characteristics of intestinal inflammation and its consequences are being defined.

(b) Cellular infiltration

Given our present knowledge, the infiltration of neutrophils and eosinophils into the intestinal mucosa appears to involve mechanisms common to all tissue sites and thus will not be reviewed further here. However, given that mast cell infiltration in the intestinal mucosa in helminthic infections involves a mast cell phenotype expressed predominantly in mucosal surfaces, and thought to be an important element in host defenses (e.g. Befus, 1989; Galli, 1990; Rothwell, 1989; Miller, 1991; and see below), the mechanisms involved will be briefly reviewed.

Mast cell precursors are widely distributed and following helminthic infections their precursor frequency increases in mucosal sites. It appears that in the local environment these precursors are activated by variety of factors, including stem cell factor, IL-3, IL-4 and IL-10. γIFN and TGF_{β} are able to inhibit mast cell development. Bell and coworkers have extended the work of others on T-cell control of intestinal mastocytosis and established that CD4+, OX22+, but not OX22− cells from the thoracic duct lymph of rats infected with *T. spiralis* induced intestinal mastocytosis upon transfer into infected recipients (Wang *et al.*, 1990a). OX22 is a monoclonal antibody which recognizes a high molecular weight moiety of rat leucocyte common antigen (CD45). In general, it can subdivide rat T_H into two subpopulations, OX22+ which mediate cellular alloreactivity, and OX22− which help B cells in secondary immune responses. Interestingly, to induce intestinal eosinophilia, OX22−, but not OX22+, CD4+ lymphocytes were active.

Intestinal mucosal mast cells (IMMC) are biochemically and functionally distinct from mast cells widely distributed in connective tissues elsewhere and their activation and secreted mediators have been extensively investigated. There is no evidence that intestinal eosinophils are distinct from eosinophils elsewhere, although this has not been investigated fully.

Table 5.3 Hepatocyte-derived proteins elevated in plasma during acute inflammatory responses

C-Reactive protein	Fibrinogen
α1 Acid glycoprotein	Haptoglobin
Serum amyloid A	Serum amyloid P
α2 Macroglobulin	Ceruloplasmin
α1 Cysteine protease inhibitor	Complement C3
	Angiotensinogen
α1 Proteinase inhibitor	Fibronectin
α1 Antichymotrypsin	Glycosyltransferases

Modified from Stadnyk and Gauldie (1991).

(c) Acute phase reactions

The production of systemic inflammatory responses, particularly the generation of hepatocyte-derived acute phase proteins, has received little attention in GI inflammation. Attempts have been made to utilize the levels of some of these proteins as diagnostic or prognostic indicators in IBD, but in general this approach has not provided the sensitivity or specificity needed in such tests. In helminthic infections there is little information.

Stadnyk and Gauldie (1991) reviewed the acute phase proteins (Table 5.3) and the cytokines, including IL-1, IL-6 and TNFα, which induce synthesis and release of these proteins by the liver. The precise roles of all the acute phase proteins are unknown; many are antiproteases, others are active in tissue repair and in a variety of metabolic processes. Interestingly, in studies of *T. spiralis* infections in rats no increases in acute phase proteins were detected and, although normal *N. brasiliensis* infections induced acute phase responses, *N. brasiliensis* infections which avoided the lung phase (direct transplantation of 4th stage larvae into the duodenum), were similar to *T. spiralis* in not generating acute phase responses (Stadnyk *et al.*, 1990). Nevertheless, rats infected with *T. spiralis* could generate acute phase protein responses to appropriate stimuli and thus the response was not inhibited by the infection. Why these helminth infections of the intestine do not generate acute phase protein responses remains to be determined. It is clearly a critical question to establish if this unresponsiveness relates to some property of the worms, or to some more general distinction of the intestinal mucosa in the development of systemic inflammatory responses.

(d) Physiologic adaptations

Associated with the generation of immune and inflammatory responses in the GI tract, there are a number of alterations in the normal physiology of the site (Castro, 1989; Befus, 1990). These changes have been most extensively described for the epithelium and smooth muscle, although recently some alterations in the enteric nervous system and vasculature have been described

Thymus-dependent villus atrophy and crypt hyperplasia occurs in helminth infections (Ferguson and Jarrett, 1975). Goblet cell hyperplasia also develops (e.g. Wells, 1963; McKay *et al.*, 1990) and this response can be transferred by sensitized T cells (Miller *et al.*, 1979). Antigen challenge of animals sensitized with nematode infection induces epithelial sloughing, decreased activities of brush border enzymes, local and systemic release of inflammatory mediators and increases in epithelial permeability and ion transport (e.g. Castro, 1989; D'Inca *et al.*, 1990). MHC class II antigen expression on the epithelium is altered as a consequence of the inflammatory responses (Masson and Perdue, 1990). Whether or not there are alterations in the production of cytokines by epithelial cells themselves in response to helminth infection remains to be determined. IL-1 (Radema, Van Deventer and Cerami, 1990), IL-6 (Shirota *et al.*, 1990), TNFα (Keshav *et al.*, 1990) and the defensin-like moiety, cryptdin (Ouellette *et al.*, 1989), are potentially important cytokines, whose synthesis by the intestinal epithelium and local activity could be markedly altered in helminthic infections. Moreover, given that IL-1, TNFα and γIFN (Kvale,

Brandtzaeg and Lovhang, 1988; Kelleher *et al.*, 1991) regulate the expression of genes such as secretory component and MHC class I in epithelial cells, it may be that during helminth infections major changes occur in epithelial cell responsiveness and responses to cytokines and other messages such as neuropeptides and secretagogues which influence the magnitude of the injury and facilitate its repair. Such questions need to be addressed to understand the pathogenic process and recovery.

Fundamentally similar questions can be raised about the mechanisms and significance of the T lymphocyte-dependent alterations in smooth muscle responses following helminth infection (Vermillion *et al.*, 1988; Vermillion, Ernst and Collins, 1991). Until recently the potentially analogous effects of helminth infections on the enteric nervous system were ignored. However, Stead and coworkers established that there was a strong association between the newly developed mast cells and the enteric nerves in the jejunal mucosa of rats infected with *N. brasiliensis* (Stead *et al.*, 1987). Careful time-course analysis of the development of this association established that within 10 days of infection there is dilation and degeneration of enteric nerves, but that subsequently these regenerate (Stead *et al.*, 1992). The authors proposed that even in normal animals there is an ongoing modelling of mucosal nerve fibres. The significance of this plasticity of the nervous system in intestinal infections and the impact that it has on enteric nerve function require study.

Other important, but largely neglected, physiologic targets in the intestinal mucosa in helminth infections have been the vasculature and the stromal elements. Ottaway *et al.* (1980) established that increases in blood flow occur in the intestine during infection of mice with *T. spiralis*, whereas Mathison *et al.* (1990) noted that after the expulsion of *N. brasiliensis* from the rat intestine there was a PAF-dependent depression of intestinal blood flow. There appear to be no studies of the intestinal stromal elements in helminth infections, but presumably significant alterations may occur in cell types such as fibroblasts, which are well known for altering their phenotype and making various cytokines in inflamed tissues (e.g. Stadnyk and Gauldie, 1991).

5.4 EFFECTOR RESPONSES IN THE INTESTINAL MUCOSA

Despite the diversity of information about the generation of immune and inflammatory responses in the intestinal mucosa, investigations of effector mechanisms in intestinal helminth infections have focused in more limited areas, namely on the types of antigen-specific cells which can transfer immunity or selected cellular responses to naive hosts, the IgE-mast cell axis and the role of selected chemical mediators, including mucus. In general the effector mechanisms appear to involve antigen-specific T-cell responses which induce antibody responses and inflammatory changes, in turn releasing a plethora of chemical mediators ultimately responsible for the expulsion of the worms (Figure 5.3). This network of responses is highly integrated, but can be subdivided into cellular, antibody and inflammatory mediator components.

5.4.1 ANTIGEN SPECIFIC T-CELL RESPONSES

Rothwell (1989) reviewed the literature on the transfer of sensitized T cells to dissect the cellular basis of protective immunity to GI helminths. Since this exhaustive review, Bell and associates have provided new information which clarifies the role of some of the T-cell subsets. CD8- (presumably CD4+), OX22− lymphocytes collected from the thoracic duct of rats 3 days after infection with *T. spiralis* transferred immunity (evident within

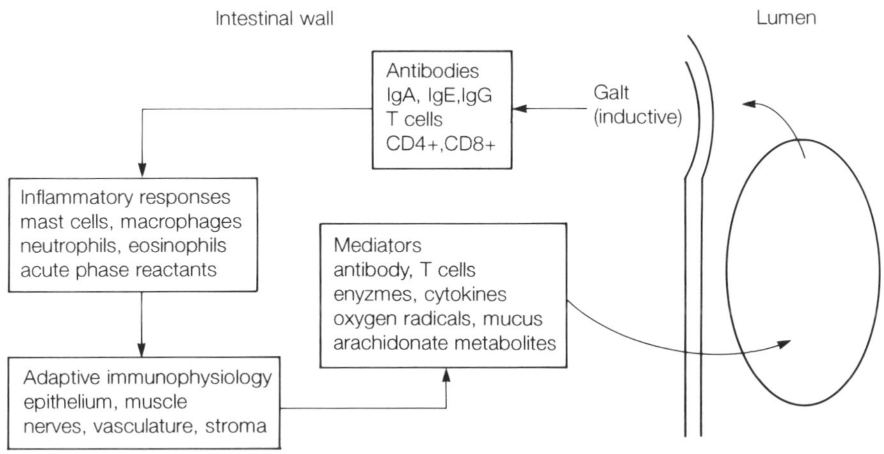

Figure 5.3 Host responses to intestinal infections.

9 days of infection) to adult worms in naive rats (Wang *et al.*, 1990a). This protection correlated with the transfer of eosinophilia by day 9, but not mastocytosis, which by contrast was transferred with CD4+ OX22+ cells. By day 9 increased numbers of antibody-producing cells were also found in the spleens and MLN of recipients of OX22−, but not OX22+ cells. Additionally, within 24 h three to four times as many CD4+, OX22− lymphocytes migrated into the intestinal epithelium as CD4+, OX22+ lymphocytes (Wang *et al.*, 1990b) a distinction not seen with their localization in the intestinal lamina propria. These intraepithelial immigrants were predominantly large dividing cells and required MHC class II compatibility for epithelial localization. Thus, in this model CD4+, OX22− blasts capable of inducing eosinophilia but not mastocytosis, and with a MHC class II-dependent predilection for the intestinal epithelium, transfer protective immunity to adult worms which is expressed within 9 days of infection. The precise mechanisms of protection are unknown.

Cellular transfer of the ability to express *rapid expulsion* (within 1 to 24 h) of 30 to 80% of *T. spiralis* larvae was also achieved with CD8−, OX22−, OX38+ (T_H) dividing cells from the thoracic duct, in combination with immune serum (Ahmad *et al.*, 1991a). Neither cells or serum alone transferred rapid expulsion; the cellular component was long-lived and the serum component was transient (< 1 week) following transfer; mucus trapping did not appear to be involved (Ahmad *et al.*, 1990).

Analysis of the component in immune serum which collaborated with the T_H in the transfer of rapid expulsion to larval infection established that purified IgE was responsible, but that when the serum levels of antiworm IgE had decreased, non-IgE fractions also contained protective activity (Ahmad *et al.*, 1991b). Thus, transfer of rapid expulsion required CD4+, OX22− T_H cells which localize in the intestinal epithelium within 24 h and could induce eosinophilia, but not mastocytosis within 9 days. IgE can mediate the T_H-dependent rapid expulsion, but in its absence, non-IgE fractions from immune serum can also be active. How these dividing T_H, many of which localize in the epithelium, act together with IgE or other components of immune serum to express rapid expulsion (1 to 24 h) in otherwise naive hosts without obviously expanded populations of IgE receptor-bearing (or other) cells, is unknown.

It may be that T_H which migrate into the epithelium produce an essential cytokine or profile of cytokines which activates other IEL (e.g. TCR γ/δ, CD8 α/α) to produce factors (e.g. TNFα, perforin or granzymes) which directly influence the parasite, or act indirectly through epithelial or other cells to prevent the larvae from maintaining their position in the intestine. This does not appear to involve mucus secretion (Ahmad *et al.*, 1990), but may involve Cl− (Castro, 1989), cytokine (e.g. IL-1, IL-6, TNFα or cryptdin), or other mediator production by epithelial cells. IgE likely sensitizes resident populations of high (mast cells or basophils) or low (eosinophils, IEL, lymphocytes, macrophages, neutrophils, platelets) affinity receptor-bearing cells, activated by locally produced cytokines. Whether smooth muscle, nervous, vascular or stromal responses are also involved in the rapid expulsion generated in the transfer model is unknown. However, in expulsion of primary infections or in accelerated or rapid expulsion generated against challenge infections in actively sensitized animals, where inflammatory cell infiltration and numerous adaptive responses have occurred, all of these responses are likely to be activated and integrated in some manner.

In mice, expulsion of adult *N. brasiliensis* in primary, but not in secondary infections, was inhibited by infusion of antibodies to CD4 (Katona, Urban and Finkelman, 1988). These antibodies also inhibited the development of mastocytosis in primary infections and IgE responses in both primary and secondary infections. Although antibodies to IL-5 inhibited eosinophilia, they failed to enhance worm survival. Similarly antibodies to IL-4 inhibited IgE responses and antibodies to IL-3 and IL-4 inhibited mastocytosis, but these treatments did not block worm expulsion (Finkelman *et al.*, 1991). These results confirm T_H involvement, but do not clarify the roles of IgE, eosinophils and mast cells in worm expulsion.

5.4.2 ANTIBODY-DEPENDENT RESPONSES

IgE, IgA and IgG are considered to be the most relevant antibodies in intestinal defenses and pathogenesis. Although IgG responses are well documented, most studies of intestinal helminthiasis have focused on IgE and IgA antibodies and the present state of knowledge for these will be outlined below.

(a) IgA

Although IgA is the most prominent immunoglobulin in intestinal secretions, possesses multiple effector functions (Kilian, Mestecky and Russell, 1988) and knowledge of its synthesis and secretion has increased dramatically in the last decade (see above), it is disappointing that there have been no significant advances in the study of this class of antibody in helminth infections in the same period (see Befus and Bienenstock, 1982). Perhaps postulates by Capron *et al.* (1992) and Butterworth *et al.* (1992) that in human schistosomiasis (*S. mansoni*), IgA antibodies are relevant in protective immunity, might stimulate additional studies of this isotype of immunoglobulin.

IgA receptors on IEL (Tagliabue *et al.*, 1984) may be critical in novel activation and effector pathways presently unknown in TCR γ/δ+, CD8 α/α+ or other IEL. IgA induction of eosinophil degranulation (Abu-Ghazaleh *et al.*, 1989) may be an important helminthocidal pathway. Alternately, or perhaps synergistically, oligosaccharides on secretory IgA which have been shown to interact with mannose-specific lectins on certain microbes (Wold *et al.*, 1990), may be important in helminthiasis by depression of helminth metabolic activities or modulation of host immune responses. It may be that within the next few years these types of investigations of intestinal helminth infections will be initiated.

(b) IgE

Despite the apparently ubiquitous nature of IgE responses in GI helminth infections and evidence that IgE can be involved in protective immunity, its mode of action is unclear. Evidence strongly suggests that mast cells with their high affinity IgE receptors are important, but many experimental models have shown that markedly elevated numbers of mast cells are not required. Whether or not small resident or infiltrating populations of these cells are sufficiently active remains to be investigated; these may be all that is necessary given the common suggestion that <5% of the total lung histamine (mast cell-derived) must be released to generate a severe asthmatic attack. Unfortunately, it is difficult to study small populations of cells, especially when their potential importance is shrouded by pronounced cellular infiltrations.

Cells bearing low affinity receptors for IgE, especially eosinophils, are potent *in vitro* mediators of IgE-dependent helminthotoxicity (e.g. Capron *et al.*, 1992; Butterworth *et al.*, 1992), but their role is unclear in GI helminthiasis. It is intriguing that the transfer of CD4+, OX22− cells produces protective immunity and a correlated eosinophilia (Wang *et al.*, 1990a) and that eosinophils produce a plethora of helminthocidal molecules such as major basic protein. Unfortunately, it will be particularly challenging to establish that IgE-mediated activation of any of the cells bearing low affinity IgE receptors will be important in immunity, because these cells also possess receptors for the much more abundant immunoglobulin, IgG. Nevertheless, given recent evidence that IgE can mediate protective immunity in intestinal helminth infections (Ahmad *et al.*, 1991b) and in human schistosomiasis (Hagan *et al.*, 1991; Dessein *et al.*, 1992) the challenge must be met.

5.4.3 INFLAMMATORY MEDIATORS

The list of inflammatory mediators thought to be involved in immunity and pathogenesis of intestinal helminth infections is growing rapidly (see above). Some of these are derived from a single cell type, e.g. RMCP II, major basic protein, whereas others can be produced by many different cell types, e.g. IL-1, TNFα, oxygen radicals. For some mediators, selective antagonists or agonists are available, but for others such experimental tools are unavailable. However, despite the wealth of information and wide acceptance that inflammatory mediators are important, there is no unequivocal evidence that a particular mediator is essential for worm expulsion. Perhaps this state is best explained by the postulate of multiple pathways for host defenses and a marked redundancy in the actions of the mediators involved (see Section 5.1).

Rothwell (1989) and Miller (1991) reviewed the spectrum of mast cell mediators that may be involved, notably histamine, arachidonic acid metabolites and the serine proteases. Other mediators such as TNFα which can be produced by mast cells (Gordon, Burd and Galli, 1990) have received little study. Nevertheless, there is no doubt that following infection, mast cell numbers increase and mediator secretion occurs. Significant amounts of mast cell-derived mediators may be released during the period of worm loss, even when this is not necessarily the period of most pronounced mast cell hyperplasia. Thus despite experiments where worm loss occurs in the absence of mast cell hyperplasia, it remains to be established that mediators derived solely from mast cells, albeit present at relatively low levels, are not involved.

Certain observations require additional study, as for example those of Douch *et al.*

(1983) who showed that a component of mucus from infected sheep, probably a leukotriene, had paralytic activity against nematodes. Following observations of Moqbel *et al.* (1985) on arachidonic acid metabolites in the intestine in *N. brasiliensis* infections of rats, further studies of these mediators are relevant.

Recent observations on their biological activities and production by a variety of cell types suggest that studies of cytokines such as TNFα, IL-1, IL-6 and γIFN may be helpful in elucidating integrated cascades of immune and inflammatory responses in intestinal helminthiasis. Novel mediators such as cryptdin or other Paneth cell-derived factors must be explored for their expression and role during intestinal infections. Emphasis on oxygen radicals is also well justified (Smith, 1989). Perhaps at this stage in our understanding it is unrealistic to expect that a single mediator will prove to be solely responsible for host defenses, especially in genetically heterogeneous populations of hosts and parasites. A model of host resistance which incorporates multiple interacting pathways with considerable overlap and redundancy in cell and mediator function is attractive. All cells in the local microenvironment should be considered potentially relevant as sources of important mediators, not just those that increase dramatically in number or exhibit obvious markers of activation. Such an approach provides a solid basis for future studies.

5.5 DIRECTIONS FOR FUTURE STUDY

Many important directions for future investigations of host–parasite relationships in intestinal helminth infections are evident. Antigens relevant to protective immunity of pathogenic responses must be defined. The uptake, processing and presentation of these antigens must be dissected and the T_{H1}/T_{H2} activation pathways established. This information will help elucidate the mechanisms underlying the selection of specific immune responses, notably IgE/mast cell/eosinophil pathways. Major attempts must be made to evaluate the importance of IgA production in helminth infections, as well as the activation and function of selected subsets of IEL, particularly those which have only recently been defined (e.g. TCR γ/δ+, CD8 α/α+, Thy1−). What is the nature of antigen recognition by these cells, the role of MHC and the cytokines or other mediators produced?

Mediators produced by cells throughout the intestinal mucosa during the course of infection must be mapped and their functions evaluated in reductionist experiments *in vitro*, as well as in *in vivo* experiments with agonists or antagonists, including monoclonal antibodies and gene depletions. Undoubtedly, mediators such as TNFα, γIFN, cryptdin, TGF and many others will be the subject of such studies very soon.

Immunophysiologic investigations are in their infancy, but their importance is obvious, especially as it is becoming increasingly recognized that classical boundaries of immune and inflammatory responses and the cell types involved are challenged. Perhaps of greatest value will be experiments to explore the bidirectional interactions between the immune and nervous system in the intestine and elsewhere. It is disappointing that more progress has not been made in characterizing alterations in worm metabolism caused by components of the host response. This type of immunophysiologic information about the parasite would provide an important tool to dissect the effects of individual elements of the immune response.

Although the types of studies outlined above will contribute much to our knowledge base, it will be essential to have concurrent investigations in the challenging areas of human infections, low level repeated infections and infections with more heterogeneous hosts and parasites. The question posed by Schweitzer and Anderson (1991) about the fundamental mechanisms of the heterogeneity of parasite survival and host pathogenesis patterns in natural populations should serve as the ultimate objective for our studies.

REFERENCES

Abu-Ghazaleh, R. I. *et al.* (1989) IgA-induced eosinophil degranulation. *J. Immunol.*, **142**, 2393–400.

Ahmad, A. *et al.* (1990) Synergistic interaction between immune serum and thoracic duct cells in the adoptive transfer of rapid expulsion of *Trichinella spiralis* in adult rats. *Exp. Parasit.*, **71**, 90–9.

Ahmad, A. *et al.* (1991a) Characterization of the thoracic duct T-helper cells that co-mediate, with antibody, the rapid expulsion of *Trichinella spiralis* in adult rats. *Parasite Immun.*, **13** (in press).

Ahmad, A. *et al.* (1991b) A role for IgE in intestinal immunity. Expression of rapid expulsion of *Trichinella spiralis* in rats transfused with IgE and thoracic duct lymphocytes. *J. Immun.*, **146**, 3563–70.

Befus, D. (1986) Immunity in intestinal helminth infections: present concepts, future directions. *Trans. Roy. Soc. Trop. Med. Hyg.*, **80**, 735–41.

Befus, D. (1989) Mast cells are that polymorphic! *Reg. Immun.*, **2**, 176–87.

Befus, A. D. (1990) Immunophysiology: influence of the mucosal immune system on intestinal function, in *Immunology and Immunopathology of the Liver and Gastrointestinal Tract* (eds S. R. Targan and F. Shanahan), Igaku-Shoin, New York, pp. 205–29.

Befus, A. D. and Bienenstock, J. (1982) Factors involved in symbiosis and host resistance at the mucosa–parasite interface. *Prog. Allergy*, **31**, 76–7.

Befus, A. D. and Bienenstock, J. (1984) Induction and expression of mucosal immune responses and inflammation to parasitic infections, in *Contemporary Topics in Immunobiology: Immunobiology of Parasites and Parasitic Infections* (ed. J. J. Marchalonis), Plenum Press, New York, pp. 71–108.

Befus, D. *et al.* (1986) Unique characteristics of local responses in host resistance to mucosal parasitic infections. *Vet. Parasit.*, **20**, 175–94.

Bienenstock, J., Johnston, N. and Perey, D. Y. E. (1973) Bronchial lymphoid tissue. I. Morphological characteristics. *Lab. Invest.*, **28**, 686–92.

Bland, P. (1988) MHC class II expression by the gut epithelium. *Immun. Today*, **9**, 174–8.

Butterworth, A. *et al.* (1992) Human immunity to *Schistosoma mansoni*: observations on mechanisms, and implications for control (in press).

Capron, A. *et al.* (1992) Schistosomiasis: from effector and regulation mechanisms in rodents to vaccine strategies in man (in press).

Castro, G. A. (1989) Immunophysiology of enteric parasitism. *Parasit. Today*, **5**, 11–19.

Cerf-Bensussan, N. and Guy-Grand, D. (1991) Intestinal intraepithelial lymphocytes. *Gastro. Clin. N. Amer.* (in press).

Chandler, A. C. (1953) Immunity in parasitic diseases. *J. Egypt. Med. Assoc.*, **36**, 811–35.

Del Prete, G. F. *et al.* (1991) Purified protein derivative of *Mycobacterium tuberculosis* and excretory secretory antigen(s) of *Toxocara canis* expand *in vitro* human T cells with stable and opposite (type 1 T helper or type 2 T helper) profile of cytokine production. *J. Clin. Invest.*, **88**, 346–50.

Dessein, A. *et al.* (1992) Environmental, genetic and immunological factors in human resistance to *Schistosoma mansoni* (in press).

Dezutter-Dambuant, C. (1988) Role of Langerhans cells in cutaneous immunologic processes. *Semin. Dermat.*, **7**, 163–70.

D'Inca, R. *et al.* (1990) Antigen-induced mucosal damage and restitution in the small intestine of the immunized rat. *Int. Arch. Allergy Appl. Immun.*, **91**, 270–7.

Douch, P. G. C. *et al.* (1983) *In vitro* bioassay of sheep gastrointestinal mucus for nematode paralysing activity mediated by a substance with some properties characteristic of SRS-A. *Int. J. Parasit.*, **13**, 207–12.

Dunkley, M. L. and Husband, A. J. (1989) Role of antigen in migration patterns of T cell subsets arising from gut-associated lymphoid tissue. *Reg. Immun.*, **2**, 213–24.

Ferens, W. A., Arai, H. P. and Befus, D. (1992) Trickle infections with *Nippostrongylus brasiliensis* in rats: broncho-alveolar leucocyte responses. *J. Parasit.* (in press).

Ferguson, A. and Jarrett, E. E. E. (1975) Hypersensitivity reactions in the small intestine. I. Thymus dependence of experimental 'partial villous atrophy'. *Gut*, **16**, 114–17.

Finkelman, F. D. *et al.* (1991) Regulation and biological function of helminth-induced cytokine responses. *Immun. Today*, **12**, A62–6.

Fujihashi, K. *et al.* (1990) Regulatory function for murine intraepithelial lymphocytes. Two subsets of CD3+, T cell receptor-1+ intraepithelial lymphocyte T cells abrogate oral tolerance. *J. Immun.*, **145**, 2010–19.

Galli, S. J. (1990) New insights into 'the riddle of the mast cells': microenvironmental regulation of mast cell development and phenotypic heterogeneity. *Lab. Invest.*, **62**, 5–33.

Golub, E. S. and Green, D. R. (1991) *Immunology: A Synthesis*, 2nd edn, Sinauer Associates, Inc., Sunderland, MA.

Gordon, J., Burd, P. R. and Galli, S. J. (1990) Mast cells as a source of multifunctional cytokines. *Immun. Today*, **11**, 458–64.

Guy-Grand, D. *et al.* (1991a) Cytotoxic differentiation of mouse gut thymodependent and independent intraepithelial T lymphocytes is induced locally. Correlation between functional assays, presence of perforin and granzyme transcripts, and cytoplasmic granules. *J. Exp. Med.* (in press).

Guy-Grand, D. *et al.* (1991b) Two gut intraepithelial CD8+ lymphocyte populations with different T cell receptors: a role for the gut epithelium in T cell differentiation. *J. Exp. Med.*, **173**, 471–81.

Hagan, P. *et al.* (1991) Human IgE, IgG4 and resistance to reinfection with *Schistosoma haematobium*. *Nature*, **349**, 243–5.

Halstensen, T. S., Scott, J. and Brandtzaeg, P. (1989) Intraepithelial T cells of the TCR γ/δ+ CD8− and V δ1/J δ+ phenotypes are increased in coeliac disease. *Scand. J. Immun.*, **30**, 665–72.

Holt, P. G. *et al.* (1990) A contiguous network of dendritic antigen-presenting cells within the respiratory epithelium. *Int. Archs. Allergy Appl. Immun.*, **91**, 155–9.

Husband, A. J. and Dunkley, M. (1990) Helper T cell control of mucosal immune responses. *Today's Life Sci.*, **2**, 22–31.

James, S. P., Kwan, W. C. and Sneller, M. C. (1990) T cells in inductive and effector compartments of the intestinal mucosal immune system of nonhuman primates differ in lymphokine mRNA expression, lymphokine utilization, and regulatory function. *J. Immun.*, **144**, 1251–6.

Janeway, C. A., Jones, B. and Hayday, A. (1988) Specificity and function of T cells bearing γ/δ receptors. *Immun. Today*, **9**, 73–6.

Katona, I. M., Urban, J. F. Jr and Finkelman, F. D. (1988) The role of L3T4+ and LYT2+ T cells in the IgE response and immunity to *Nippostrongylus brasiliensis*. *J. Immun.*, **140**, 3206–11.

Kawanishi, H., Saltzman, L. E. and Strober, W. (1983) Mechanisms regulating IgA class-specific immunoglobulin production in murine gut-associated lymphoid tissues. I. T cells derived from Peyer's patches that switch Sigm B cells to Siga B cells *in vitro*. *J. Exp. Med.*, **157**, 433–50.

Kelleher, R. S. *et al.* (1991) Endocrine, neural, and immune control of secretory component output by lacrimal gland acinar cells. *J. Immun.*, **146**, 3405–12.

Keshav, S. *et al.* (1990) Tumor necrosis factor mRNA localized to Paneth cells of normal murine intestinal epithelium by in situ hybridization. *J. Exp. Med.*, **171**, 327–32.

Kilian, M., Mestecky, J. and Russell, M. W. (1988) Defense mechanisms involving Fc-dependent functions of immunoglobulin A and their subversion by bacterial immunoglobulin A proteases. *Microbiol. Rev.*, **52**, 296–303.

Kim, P. H. and Kagnoff, M. F. (1990) Transforming growth factor β1 increases IgA isotype switching at the clonal level. *J. Immun.*, **145**, 3773–8.

King, C. L. and Nutman, T. B. (1991) Regulation of the immune response in lymphatic filariasis and onchocerciasis. *Immun. Today*, **12**, A54–8.

Kvale, D., Brandtzaeg, P. and Lovhaug, D. (1988) Up-regulation of the expression of secretory component and HLA molecules in a human colonic cell line by tumour necrosis factor-α and gamma interferon. *Scand. J. Immun.*, **28**, 351–7.

Locksley, R. M. and Scott, P. (1991) Helper T-cell subsets in mouse leishmaniasis: induction, expansion and effector function. *Immun. Today*, **12**, A58–61.

MacDermott, R. P. and Stenson, W. F. (1990) Inflammatory bowel disease, in *Immunology and Immunopathology of the Liver and Gastrointestinal Tract* (eds S. R. Targan and F. Shanahan), Igaku-Shoin, New York, pp. 459–86.

Masson, S. D. and Perdue, M. H. (1990) Changes in distribution of Ia antigen on epithelium of the jejunum and ileum in rats infected with *Nippostrongylus brasiliensis*. *Clin. Immun. Immunopath.*, **57**, 83–95.

Mathison, R. *et al.* (1990) Alterations in regional blood flow in rats following sensitization to the nematode *Nippostrongylus brasiliensis*: effects of PAF antagonists. *Br. J. Pharmac.*, **101**, 93–6.

Mayer, L. (1990) Antigen presentation in the intestine, in *Immunology and Immunopathology of the Liver and Gastrointestinal Tract* (eds S. R. Targan and F. Shanahan), Igaku–Shoin, New York, pp. 33–48.

Mayrhofer, G. (1980) Thymus-dependent and thymus-independent subpopulations of intestinal intraepithelial lymphocytes: a granular subpopulation of probable bone marrow origin and relationship to mucosal mast cells. *Blood*, **55**, 532–5.

McGhee, J. R. *et al.* (1989) Regulation of IgA synthesis and immune response by T cells and interleukins. *J. Clin. Immun.*, **9**, 175–99.

McKay, D. M. *et al.* (1990) *Hymenolepis diminuta*: intestinal goblet cell response to infection in male C57 mice. *Exp. Parasit.*, **71**, 9–20.

Miller, H. R. P. (1987a) Gastrointestinal mucus, a medium for survival and for elimination of parasitic nematodes and protozoa. *Parasitology*, **94**, S77–100.

Miller, H. R. P. (1987b) Immunopathology of nematode infestation and expulsion, in *Immunopathology of the Small Intestine* (ed. M. N. Marsh), John Wiley & Sons, Ltd, London, pp. 177–208.

Miller, H. R. P. (1991) Mast cells: their function and heterogeneity, in *Parasites and Allergy* (ed. R. Moqbel), Taylor and Francis, UK (in press).

Miller, H. R. P., Nawa, Y. and Parish, C. R. (1979) Intestinal goblet cell differentiation in *Nippostrongylus brasiliensis*-infected rats after transfer of fractionated thoracic duct lymphocytes. *Int. Archs. Allergy Appl. Immun.*, **59**, 281–5.

Moqbel, R. (1986) Helminth-induced intestinal inflammation. *Trans. Roy. Soc. Trop. Med. Hyg.*, **80**, 719–27.

Moqbel, R. *et al.* (1986) Enteral and systemic release of leukotrienes during anaphylaxis of *Nippostrongylus brasiliensis* primed rats. *J. Immun.*, **137**, 296–301.

Mosley, R. L., Styre, D. and Klein, J. R. (1990) Differentiation and functional maturation of bone marrow-derived intestinal epithelial T cells expressing membrane T cell receptor in athymic radiation chimeras. *J. Immun.*, **145**, 1369–75.

Mosmann, T. R. and Coffman, R. L. (1989) T_{H1} and T_{H2} cells: different patterns of lymphokine secretion lead to different functional properties. *Ann. Rev. Immun.*, **7**, 145–73.

Mosmann, T. R. and Moore, K. W. (1991) The role of IL-10 in crossregulation of T_{H1} and T_{H2} responses. *Immun. Today*, **12**, A49–53.

Motyka, B. and Reynolds, J. R. (1991) Apoptosis is associated with the extensive B cell death in the sheep ileal Peyer's patch and the chicken bursa of Fabricius: a possible role in B cell selection. *Eur. J. Immun.*, **21**, 1951–8.

Ottaway, C. A. (1990) Migration of lymphocytes within the mucosal immune system, in *Immunology and Immunopathology of the Liver and Gastrointestinal Tract* (eds. S. R. Targan and F. Shanahan), Igaku–Shoin, New York, pp. 49–69.

Ottaway. C. A. *et al.* (1980) Regional blood flow and localization of lymphoblasts in small intestine of the mouse II. The effects of a primary infection with *Trichinella spiralis*. *Immunology*, **41**, 963–71.

Ouellette, A. J. *et al.* (1989) Developmental regulation of cryptdin, a corticostatin/defensin precursor mRNA in mouse small intestinal crypt epithelium. *J. Cell. Biol.*, **108**, 1687–95.

Owen, R. L. and Jones, A. L. (1974) Epithelial cell specialization within human Peyer's patches: an ultrastructural study of intestinal lymphoid follicles. *Gastroenterology*, **66**, 189–203.

Radema, S. A., Van Deventer, S. J. H. and Cerami, A. (1991) Interleukin 1β is expressed predominantly by enterocytes in experimental colitis. *Gastroenterology*, **100**, 1180–6.

Reynolds, J. R. and Kirk, D. (1989) Two types of sheep Peyer's patches: location along gut does not influence involution. *Immunology*, **66**, 308–11.

Rocha, B., Vassalli, P. and Guy-Grand, D. (1991) The Vβ repertoire of mouse gut homodimeric α CD8+ intraepithelial T cell receptor α/β+ lymphocytes reveals a major extrathymic pathway of T cell differentiation. *J. Exp. Med.*, **173**, 483–6.

Rothwell, T. L. W. (1989) Immune expulsion of parasitic nematodes from the alimentary tract. *Int. J. Parasit.*, **19**, 139–68.

Russell, D. A. and Castro, G. A. (1987) Physiology of the gastrointestinal tract in the parasitized host, in *Physiology of the Gastrointestinal Tract* (ed. L. R. Johnson), Raven Press, New York, pp. 1749–80.

Russell, G. A. and Walker, W. A. (1990) Role of the intestinal mucosal barrier and antigen uptake, in *Immunology and Immunopathology of the Liver and Gastrointestinal Tract* (eds S. R. Targan and F. Shanahan), Igaku-Shoin, New York, pp. 15–31.

Schweitzer, N. and Anderson, R. (1991) Helminths, immunology and equations. *Immun. Today*, **12**, A76–81.

Shirota, K. *et al.* (1990) Interleukin-6 and its receptor are expressed in human intestinal epithelial cells. *Virchows Archiv. B Cell Pathol.*, **58**, 303–8.

Smith, N. C. (1989) The role of free oxygen radicals in the expulsion of primary infections of *Nippostrongylus brasiliensis*. *Parasit. Res.*, **75**, 423–38.

Spalding, D. M. and Griffin, J. A. (1986) Different pathways of differentiation of pre-B cell lines are induced by dendritic cells and T cells from different lymphoid tissues. *Cell*, **44**, 507–15.

Stadnyk, A. W. and Gauldie, J. (1991) The acute phase protein response during parasitic infection. *Immun. Today*, **12**, A7–12.

Stadnyk, A. W., Baumann, H. and Gauldie, J. (1990) The acute-phase protein response in parasite infection. *Nippostrongylus brasiliensis* and *Trichinella spiralis* in the rat. *Immunology*, **69**, 588–95.

Stanisz, A., Befus, A. D. and Bienenstock, J. (1986) Differential effects of vasoactive intestinal peptide, substance P, and somatostatin on immunoglobulin synthesis and proliferation by lymphocytes from Peyer's patches, mesenteric lymph nodes, and spleen. *J. Immun.*, **136**, 152–6.

Stead, R. H. *et al.* (1987) Intestinal mucosal mast cells in normal and nematode-infected rat intestines are in intimate contact with peptidergic nerves. *Proc. Natl. Acad. Sci. USA.*, **84**, 2975–9.

Stead, R. H. *et al.* (1992) Remodelling of B-50 (GAP-43) – and NSE-immunoreactive mucosal nerves in the intestines of rats infected with *Nippostrongylus brasiliensis* (in press).

Tagliabue, A. *et al.* (1984) IgA-dependent cell-mediated activity against enteropathogenic bacteria: distribution, specificity and characterization of the effector cells. *J. Immun.*, **133**, 988–92.

Taguchi, T. *et al.* (1990) Analysis of Th1 and Th2 cells in murine gut-associated tissues: frequencies of CD4+ and CD8+ T cells that secrete IFNγ and IL-5. *J. Immun.*, **145**, 68–77.

Targan, S. R. and Shanahan, F. (1990) *Immunology and Immunopathology of the Liver and Gastrointestinal Tract*, Igaku–Shoin, New York.

Urban, J. F. and Gamble, H. R. (1989) Intestinal immune responses of mammals to nematode parasites. *Amer. Zool.*, **29**, 469–78.

Vermillion, D. L., Ernst, P. B. and Collins, S. M. (1991) T-lymphocyte modulation of intestinal muscle function in the *Trichinella*-infected rat. *Gastroenterology*, **101**, 31–8.

Vermillion, D. L. *et al.* (1988) Antigen-induced contraction of jejunal smooth muscle in the sensitized rat. *Am. J. Physiol.*, **255**, G701–8.

Wakelin, D. (1986) Genetic and other constraints on resistance to infection with gastrointestinal nematodes. *Trans. Roy. Soc. Trop. Med. Hyg.*, **80**, 742–7.

Wallace, J. L. (1991) Strategies for therapeutic modulation of colitis, in *Inflammatory Bowel Diseases: Progress in Basic Research and Clinical Implications* (eds H. Goebell, B. M. Peskar and H. Malchow), M.T.P. Press Ltd., Lancaster, UK, pp. 179–89.

Wang, C. H. *et al.* (1990a) T-helper subset function in the gut of rats: differential stimulation of eosinophils, mucosal mast cells and antibody-forming cells by OX8− OX22− and OX8− OX22+ cells. *Immunology*, **71**, 166–75.

Wang, C. H. *et al.* (1990b) Intraintestinal migration to the epithelium of protective, dividing, anti-*Trichinella spiralis* CD4+ OX22− cells requires MHC class II compatibility. *J. Immun.*, **145**, 1021–8.

Wassom, D. L. and Kelly, D. A. B. (1990) The role of the major histocompatibility complex in resistance to parasite infections. *Crit. Rev. Immun.*, **10**, 31–52.

Wells, P. D. (1963) Mucin-secreting cells in rats infected with *Nippostrongylus brasiliensis*. *Exp. Parasit.*, **14**, 15–22.

Whetsell, M. *et al.* (1992) Rearrangement and diversity of T cell receptor gamma genes in intestinal intraepithelial lymphocytes in murine athymic chimeras (in press).

Wold, A. E. *et al.* (1990) Secretory immunoglobulin A carries oligosaccharide receptors for *Escherichia coli* type 1 fimbrial lectin. *Infect. Immun.*, **58**, 3073–7.

World Health Organization Expert Committee (1987) Public health significance of intestinal parasitic infections. *Bull. WHO*, **65**, 575–88.

Zettel, L. A. *et al.* (1992) Perturbation of isotype regulation in mice with intestinal inflammation induced by *Trichinella spiralis* (in press).

SIX

Geohelminth infections and nutritional status

J. S. Edirisinghe
and
A. M. Tomkins

Nearly 13 million children die each year in developing countries and in the majority of cases infections, especially parasitic diseases, are responsible for these deaths. Many of these children die malnourished (Tomkins and Watson, 1989). The magnitude or the precise role of malnutrition contributing to these deaths are not known. It is established, however, that all children, from the time of birth, are caught up in a cycle of malnutrition and infection (Figure 6.1 and Figures 6.2 and 6.4 (colour plate section)) which many do not survive (Rivera and Mortorell, 1988). A considerable proportion of childhood infections are due to parasites, particularly those associated with poor hygiene, sanitation and poverty. Current global estimates indicate that the soil-transmitted helminthiases are among the most common of all parasitic infections (Stephenson, 1987). According to Pawlowski (1984), three major geohelminth infections, ascariasis, hookworm disease and trichuriasis, are among the 11 most common infections of the developing world. The actual prevalence of strongyloidiasis is not known and difficult to estimate. The prevalence of protein energy malnutrition and iron deficiency anaemia, two most common forms of malnutrition, is high and estimated at 500 million (mostly children) and 350 million (women of reproductive age) respectively. A major nutritional deficiency disorder associated with geohelminth infections in Asia, Africa and Latin America is vitamin A deficiency. Apart from visual complications such as partial or total blindness (Figure 6.3, colour plate section), vitamin A deficiency causes high mortality in children and lowers resistance to a range of infections.

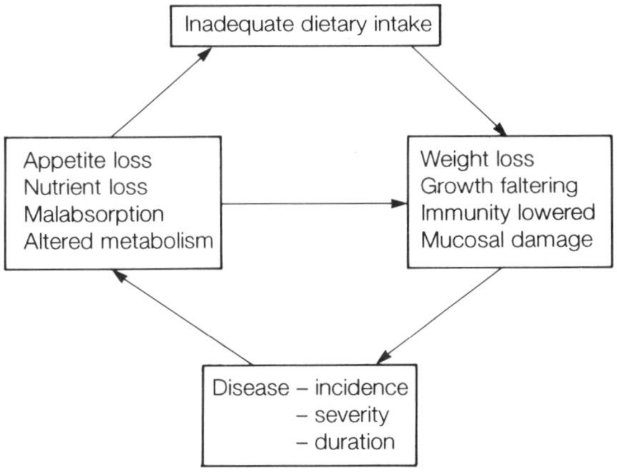

Figure 6.1 Malnutrition/infection cycle. (Source: Tomkins and Watkins, 1989.)

Parasitic intestinal helminths are in a good physiological position to interfere with host nutrition (Stephenson, 1987) (Figures 6.5(a) and (b), colour plate section). *Ascaris lumbri-*

Enteric Infection 2. Intestinal helminths. Edited by M.J.G. Farthing, G.T. Keusch and D. Wakelin. Published in 1995 by Chapman and Hall, London. ISBN 0 412 39140 6

coides, *Necator americanus*, *Ancylostoma duodenale* and *Strongyloides stercoralis* spend the greater part of their lives in the small intestine where a major part of digestion and absorption of nutrients take place. The larvae of *Strongyloides stercoralis* cause damage to the mucosa of the large intestine during internal autoinfection while the adult *Trichuris trichiura* worms live with part of their bodies buried in the mucosa of the large intestine.

6.1 MECHANISMS OF MALNUTRITION IN INTESTINAL HELMINTH INFECTIONS

Several nutritional deficiencies occur as a result of intestinal helminth infections. These include weight loss as a result of losses of body protein or fat stores. On other occasions it may include deficiencies of micronutrients and vitamins, even in the presence of relatively satisfactory body stores of proteins and fat. Intestinal helminth parasites may affect the nutritional status by causing:

- decrease in food intake
- increase in nutrient loss
- decrease in nutrient absorption and utilization.

6.1.1 FOOD INTAKE

Inadequate dietry intake is a frequent cause of malnutrition in many infections. In certain circumstances there may be cultural factors such as the avoidance of certain foods that are thought to be deleterious in the presence of intestinal infections. Sometimes the patient has severe anorexia as a result of abdominal pain, diarrhoea, febrile episodes or even the passage of helminths through respiratory tissues. Recent evidence suggests that appetite is under the control of cytokines which are released during systemic infections (Klasing, 1988). When parasitic infections occur in immunocompromised hosts, the secondary infection of the buccal cavity by monilia may produce painful lesions which make eating difficult.

6.1.2 MALABSORPTION

Gut infections may damage the intestinal mucosa with resulting decrease in surface area for absorption of micronutrients. Disturbances of motility in the upper intestine as a result of intestinal helminths may encourage the proliferation of bacterial numbers such that a 'blind loop' syndrome occurs. The bacterial deconjugation of bile acids accounts for some of the steatorrhoea in giardiasis. Vitamin A deficiency is particularly likely to occur when steatorrhoea is present.

6.1.3 INCREASED REQUIREMENTS

Requirements for energy are increased by about 10% for every 1° rise in body temperature (Tomkins and Watson, 1989). This may be a significant feature in the development of weight loss during infections associated with febrile responses. Systemic infections are also known to increase requirements for protein as a result of increased rates of synthesis and breakdown of proteins, particularly in muscle. Such phenomena may well account for marked wasting in parasitic diseases. The magnitude of the increases in requirements are especially great when infections affect children, during periods of fast growth and development, and women during pregnancy and lactation when the demands are increased; also requirements increase following increased catabolism and losses due to other paths mentioned earlier.

6.1.4 INTESTINAL LOSSES

In health, large numbers of intestinal cells are exfoliated and broken down and their constituent amino acids are reabsorbed. In certain gut parasitic infections this mechanism is impaired with resulting loss of endogenous proteins. The loss of blood from the small intestinal mucosa in hookworm infection is considerable and may precipitate protein energy malnutrition and severe iron deficiency anaemia. In addition the losses of blood and mucus in association with certain colonic parasites may profoundly influence the nutritional status of the host. As well as the losses of protein there may be heavy losses of body stores of iron, zinc and potassium.

The nutritional effects and their mechanisms are caused by four major geohelminths: *A. lumbricoides*, hookworms, *S. stercoralis* and *T. trichiura*, are discussed in this chapter.

6.2 *ASCARIS LUMBRICOIDES* (LINNAEUS 1758)

Ascaris lumbricoides is the largest intestinal helminth parasite of man and ascariasis is the commonest parasitic infection in the world (Davis, 1985). It has a cosmopolitan distribution and occurs in temperate, tropical and subtropical environments, but is more common in warm, humid countries where poverty, illiteracy, overcrowding and poor sanitation coexist.

Ascariasis is particularly common in children and is associated with malnutrition (Stephenson, 1987). Increasing evidence suggest that ascariasis affects health (Pawlowski and Davis, 1989), growth (Stephenson, 1987; Stephenson *et al.*, 1989a), and physical fitness of infected children (Stephenson *et al.*, 1988). The impact of these deleterious effects of ascariasis on other developmental factors such as scholastic attainment is not known.

6.2.1 EPIDEMIOLOGY

Current estimates suggest a global prevalence of 0.8 to 1.3 billion infected persons or about one quarter of the world's population (Stephenson, 1987). Infection is known to occur in 153 of the 218 recognized countries of the world (Crompton, 1988). These countries are also the poorest nations where minimal or no facilities are available for safe disposal of faeces, where sanitation is substandard, and where health education on disease prevention is generally non-existent. It is often the rule rather than the exception to find helminthic infections coexisting with malnutrition, where poverty forms the major common factor. It is in these areas where parents find it difficult to provide sufficient food for their children or lack the knowledge that small children need frequent feeding to prevent the development of protein energy malnutrition and need to consume green and yellow vegetables to avoid vitamin A deficiency (Stephenson, 1987).

The prevalence of infection with *Ascaris* increases sharply during the second and third years of life rising to a maximum between 4 and 14 years of age, finally declining or remaining at a slightly lower level during adulthood. The intensity of infection is greatest in the 2–10-year age group (Bundy *et al.*, 1987c; Haswell-Elkins, Elkins and Anderson, 1989; Haswell–Elkins *et al.*, 1989). Predisposition of individuals and families to heavy infection with *A. lumbricoides* is known to occur (Forrester *et al.*, 1988; Holland *et al.*, 1989; Forrester *et al.*, 1990). The frequency distribution of *A. lumbricoides* in cross-sectional community studies show a highly overdispersed pattern with a large number of persons with small worm burdens and small number of persons with heavy infections (Bundy *et al.*, 1987; Forrester *et al.*, 1988). However, when the same population is studied during a period when several treatments and opportunities for reinfection are included, it appears that the proportion of individuals who are heavily infected at one time or other may be considerably greater than that estimated from single cross-sectional studies (Hall *et al.*, 1992). The maximum prevalence and the greatest intensity of infection occur in the age group in which rapid growth and development are seen under normal circumstances.

6.2.2 PATHOGENESIS OF MALNUTRITION

The extent and severity of malnutrition in ascariasis is related to its effect on host food intake, digestion of nutrients and absorption of nutrients within the body of the host (Schultz, 1982; Stephenson, 1980).

(a) Reduced food intake

Reduced food intake during a range of infections is a common phenomenon in man and animals (Mata, 1978; Martorell and Yarborough, 1983; Crompton, 1984). Low food consumption is an important feature of *A. suum* infection in pigs (McCance, 1960; Forsum, Nesheim and Crompton, 1981; Stephenson, 1987). The decrease in the rate of weight gain of the infected pigs correlates well with the worm burden (Forsum, Nesheim and Crompton, 1981). The physiological mechanisms responsible for reduced food intake are not clear but a range of cytokines are likely to be important. Anorexia may accompany the pulmonary manifestations of ascariasis during the acute stage of the infection associated with larval migration.

(b) Altered nutriet digestion and absorption

Architectural alterations of the small intestine in human ascariasis include thickening and irregular folding of the mucosa (Tripathy *et al.*, 1972; Legundoye, 1972). A range of changes in the microvilli, from fusion of adjacent villi to total loss, has been demonstrated in pigs infected with *A. suum* (Martin *et al.*, 1985). Hypertrophy of the tunica muscularis leading to an increase in the wet weight of the small intestine occurs in pig ascariasis. The degree of changes in the intestine is related to the worm load (Stephenson *et al.*, 1980a; Forsum, Nesheim and Crompton, 1981). Alterations of small intestinal morphology may be responsible for the defective digestion that occurs in human ascariasis. Low lactase activity with associated lactose maldigestion is a feature of *A. suum* infection in pigs. These findings have been confirmed in children infected with *A. lumbricoides* (Carrera, Nesheim and Crompton, 1984; Taren *et al.*, 1987). It is not clear whether *A. lumbricoides* has a significant effect on the hydrolysis of macronutrients although they are able to produce substances which inhibit activity of trypsin and chymotrypsin *in vitro* (Chappel, 1980). The effects of the pancreatic protease inhibitors isolated from adult worms are not known (Green, 1957; Homanberg and Peanasky, 1976).

(c) Alteration of nutrient absorption

Disturbances of the absorptive capacity of the intestinal mucosa may result in nutrient loss. The physical presence of a large number of worms and their habit of remaining close to the intestinal mucosa may reduce the available absorptive area. Although adult *Ascaris* worms are known to have a glycogen consumption rate of around 1.3 g/100 g of body weight/24 h, competition for nutrients with the host is probably negligible as many gut parasites have relatively low energy needs compared with their hosts (Crompton *et al.*, 1981).

Nitrogen absorption may be reduced in children infected with *A. lumbricoides* and improves after deworming (Tripathy *et al.*, 1972; Brown *et al.*, 1980; Northrop *et al.*, 1987). Some studies suggest an improvement in the absorption of D-xylose following deworming (Tripathy *et al.*, 1972) while others dispute it (Brown *et al.*, 1980). Several studies fail to demonstrate any effect of ascariasis on intestinal absorption (Teotia *et al.*, 1969; Freij *et al.*, 1979). Mouth-to-caecum transit time is reduced in children with ascariasis and is related to the worm burden (Taren *et al.*, 1987). Rapid passage of food through the intestinal tract could contribute to the decreased nutrient absorption. In areas where year-round transmission is the rule, the respiratory symptoms associated with fever may contribute to increased nutritional requirements and thus to increased urinary nitrogen loss aggravating the already compromised nutritional status.

(d) Alterations of micronutrient absorption

Ascariasis lowers vitamin A absorption (Sivakumar and Reddy, 1975; Mahalanabis *et al.*, 1976; 1979). Impaired absorption of fat-soluble vitamins may be related to the histological changes in the small intestine in ascariasis. Effects of ascariasis on iron utilization have also been documented (Pollitt, 1990). Ascariasis and iron deficiency often coexist but the contribution of deworming to improvement of iron status has not been investigated.

(e) Growth and development

There are several reasons why ascariasis may cause growth faltering. The common abdominal clinical manifestations such as abdominal pain, nausea, vomiting, diarrhoea and anorexia may be related to allergic reactions to 'toxins' produced by the worms, to a peptide causing histamine release or to other allergens resulting in immunopathology or a combination of these factors (Coles, 1985). Anti-ascaris IgE may release histamine from mast cells which may be responsible for the allergic manifestations in these patients (Coles, 1985). Such reactions may impair appetite. Improvement of growth has been demonstrated following deworming (Gupta *et al.*, 1977; Gupta, 1985; Willett, Kilama and Kihamia, 1979; Stephenson *et al.*, 1980b; 1989a). Ascariasis together with other intestinal parasites can also impair physical fitness of infected children which could be improved by deworming (Stephenson *et al.*, 1990). It is claimed that *Ascaris* also contributes to the development of the syndrome of severe protein energy malnutrition (Stephenson, 1987). *Ascaris* can also lead to deterioration in aptitude, time-on-task, perseverance and educational achievement (Pollitt, 1990). This effect may be partially mediated through an effect on protein energy malnutrition (Pollitt, 1990).

6.3 *NECATOR AMERICANUS* (STILES 1902; STILES 1906) AND *ANCYLOSTOMA DUODENALE* (DUBINI 1843)

Two hookworm species infect man: *Necator americanus* (the New World hookworm) and *Ancylostoma duodenale* (the Old World hookworm). *Ancylostoma ceylanicum*, a hookworm of dog, is a potential parasite of minor importance (Gilman, 1982). *N. americanus* and *A. duodenale* parasitize the small intestine. The adult worms remain attached to the intestinal mucosa with teeth or cutting plates found in the buccal capsule. The global distribution of the two species overlap although at one time it was thought to be discrete. There are no animal reservoirs. Distinct morphological features identify each species. With the possible exception of the degree of clinical effects and the mode of entry into the human body, the parasitology, pathology, clinical manifestations, diagnosis and the management of the infection are similar for the two species. Hookworm disease denotes the disease condition that follows infection.

6.3.1 PATHOGENESIS OF MALNUTRITION

The pathogenesis of hookworm disease is intimately related to the attachment of worms to the intestinal mucosa. Blood is sucked into and passed through the worms as well as being spilt around the feeding worms. This leads to blood loss, iron deficiency anaemia and clinical features of hookworm disease. The area of mucosal destruction increases as successive plugs of mucosa are digested by individual worms. In less than two hours inflammatory exudate with polymorphs develops around the worms. The injury is limited to the muscularis mucosa. The amount of bleeding depends on the worm load. Once the worms are detached the changes seen in the mucosa are minimal and consist of a generalized increase of crypt mitotic activity with immature cells travelling up the villi (Symons and Fairbairn, 1962). Small haemorrhagic erosive lesions in the mucosa with engorged capillaries and tissue oedema is seen in experimental animals and human biopsies.

Chronic blood loss is responsible for the anaemia of hookworm disease. The loss is estimated at 0.03 ml of blood/day/worm for *N. americanus* and 0.26 ml/day/worm for *A. duodenale* (Roche and Layrisse, 1966). The major proportion of blood loss occurs in the upper small intestine but some of the iron lost in the haemoglobin is re-absorbed lower down in the intestinal tract. The amount reabsorbed is variable.

(a) Impaired intestinal absorption

The association between hookworm disease and impaired absorption is complicated by concurrent features of malnutrition, hypoproteinaemia and enteropathy endemic to tropical areas (Variyan and Banwell, 1982). Hence it is difficult to define exactly the role of mucosal injury in causing impaired absorption. Careful balance studies in Uganda have shown impaired nitrogen balance in severe hookworm disease (Darke, 1959). Later studies in the same area (where tropical malabsorption syndromes are usually absent) showed that the altered nitrogen balance was due to increased loss of protein into the intestine rather than a reduced absorptive capacity (Banwell *et al.*, 1967; Tandon *et al.*, 1969a). Features of a malabsorption syndrome with impaired absorption of fat, carbohydrate and vitamin A, have been reported in hookworm disease (Sheehy *et al.*, 1962; Abdalla *et al.*, 1963; Layrisse *et al.*, 1964; Chuttani, Puri and Misra, 1967; Banwell *et al.*, 1967; Aziz and Siddiqui, 1968). Histological changes range from relatively minor abnormalities to the presence of short, broader villi (Sheehy *et al.*, 1962; Layrisse *et al.*, 1964). Although the serum vitamin B_{12} levels may be low in some patients with hookworm disease (Saraya, Tandon and Ramachandran, 1971; Layrisse *et al.*, 1964) there is little evidence to suggest that it is due to malabsorption (Holland, 1987a). Impaired absorption of folic acid and low serum folate levels have been found in hookworm disease (Layrisse *et al.*, 1959; 1964) but they did not correlate with worm burdens (Saraya, Tandon and Ramachandran, 1971).

(b) Hypoproteinaemia

Hypoproteinaemia of severe hookworm disease may be related to poor intake, impaired absorption, increased loss or a combination of these factors. Low serum albumin levels, lowered fat and D-xylose absorption associated with villus atrophy are features of severe hookworm disease (Tandon *et al.*, 1969b; Saraya, Tandon and Ramachandran, 1971; Mayoral *et al.*, 1967; Falaiye, Oladapo and Wali, 1974). The hookworms are directly responsible for blood loss leading to iron deficiency anaemia while hypoalbuminaemia is, to a great extent, a result of anorexia and gastrointestinal protein loss (Banwell *et al.*, 1967) rather than due to a malabsorption syndrome.

Anorexia is known to accompany hookworm infection (Koshy *et al.*, 1978; Cline *et al.*, 1984), but it is not clear whether the anorexia is 'self imposed' in fear of precipitating abdominal pain or is physiological in nature. Abdominal pain is a common symptom in hookworm disease (Koshy *et al.*, 1978; Cline *et al.*, 1984; Ovartlarnporn *et al.*, 1990). Nausea and vomiting are common with all intestinal helminth parasites and can reduce appetite and interfere with food intake.

Increased protein loss into the intestine may occur as a result of blood loss due to hookworms or due to an accompanying protein-losing enteropathy. Both mechanisms operate in *A. braziliense* infection in dog (Miller, 1971; 1979). It is not clear whether similar mechanisms operate in human hookworm disease. A relationship between the degree of protein or albumin loss and the worm load or faecal egg counts has been established in experimental animals (Darke, 1959; Blackman *et al.*, 1965; Areekul *et al.*, 1971; Gupta, Basu and Tandon, 1974).

(c) Altered small bowel motility

Increased peristaltic activity and segmentation have been described in the small intestine of patients with hookworm infection (Hodes and Keefer, 1948). Rapid passage of food down the small intestine may impair the absorption of nutrients and contribute to malnutrition.

(d) Growth stunting, impaired development and productivity

Impairment of nutrient absorption, intestinal protein loss and lowered food intake contribute to growth faltering in children. However, the precise role of hookworms in growth stunting is not known. Improved growth of children with concurrent infections due to *Schistosoma haematobium* and hookworm following treatment with the drugs metrifonate or praziquantel has been reported from Kenya (Stephenson *et al.*, 1985; 1989b). Low body weight is a frequent accompaniment of chronic anaemia, reversible with correction of the anaemic state (Judisch, Naiman and Oski, 1966). Micronutrient and mineral deficiencies have important effects on linear growth.

The severity of anaemia and the accompanying signs and symptoms depend on the worm load, iron intake, the iron stores and requirements of the host (e.g. during active growth or pregnancy), and the bioavailability of iron in the diet (Holland, 1987a). It is clear that individuals with high dietary intakes of utilizable iron and good iron stores can harbour high worm loads for a long time before developing anaemia (Holland, 1987a).

Children with chronic hookworm disease with associated malnutrition show growth faltering, low scholastic attainment and poor physical fitness (Stephenson *et al.*, 1985; 1989b; 1990, Pollitt, 1990). Adults with chronic hookworm disease may suffer from diminished capacity to perform physical activity leading to poor productivity.

Iron deficiency anaemia can cause impairment of mental and motor development during infancy (Walter, 1989; Lozoff, 1989) and poor scholastic attainment during childhood (Pollitt *et al.*, 1989; Soewondo, Hu Saini and Pollitt, 1989; Seshadri and Gopaldas, 1989; Soemantri, 1989). Because hookworm disease is a major cause of iron deficiency anaemia, it may have profound effects on developmental increments in children via its influence on micronutrient status.

6.4 *TRICHURIS TRICHIURA* (LINNAEUS 1771; STILES 1901)

Trichuris trichiura is a geohelminth which has received renewed attention during the past decade because of the increasing recognition that it has important effects on growth (Bundy and Cooper, 1989). That the parasite, causes loss of blood and mucous diarrhoea, has been known for a long time but it was only in the last decade that gastrointestinal nematodiases, including trichuriasis, received global recognition as major causes of poor health and impaired growth. The infection is often referred to as one of the 'neglected infections' (Holland, 1987b). Evidence for much more profound effects of the infection, apart from growth faltering, (e.g. impairment of cognitive and mental development) has been recently presented (Nokes *et al.*, 1991; Callender *et al.*, 1992; Nokes *et al.*, 1992).

6.4.1 PATHOGENESIS OF MALNUTRITION, ANAEMIA AND GROWTH STUNTING

(a) Malnutrition

Trichuriasis and malnutrition co-exist in poor communities of warm tropical climates. Polyparasitism makes it difficult to ascribe a causal relationship between trichuriasis and malnutrition. However, in trichuriasis there is a strong correlation between intensity of infection and the pattern of symptoms such as diarrhoea, dysentery, rectal prolapse and vomiting (Gilman *et al.*, 1983; Holland, 1987b). The trichuris dysentery syndrome is generally associated with burdens over 500 worms (Bundy, 1986). The severity of symptoms in the syndrome can lead to reduced food intake and increased nutrient loss or both resulting in malnutrition. A causal relationship between trichuriasis and malnutrition in heavy infections has been proposed by some (Gilman *et al.*, 1983).

(b) Anaemia

This has been reported in heavy *Trichuris* infection (Wong and Tan, 1961; Layrisse *et al.*, 1967; Bundy, 1985; Cooper and Bundy, 1988). The anaemia in trichuriasis is hypochromic and microcytic, suggesting iron deficiency (Wong and Tan, 1961). The main causes for anaemia are blood loss from the mucosal surface and/or ingestion by worms. Macroscopic blood loss in stools is obvious in trichuris dysentery syndrome. Although large bleeding ulcers such as occur in amoebiasis are not seen in the colonic mucosa, bleeding can be easily provoked from the congested mucosa, particularly from the prolapsed rectum (Bundy and Cooper, 1989). The daily blood loss in trichuriasis has been estimated at 0.005 ml per worm (Layrisse *et al.*, 1967). Blood leaks from the focal area where the worms have burrowed into the mucosa (MacDonald *et al.*, 1991). The damage to the mucosa may be such that complete red cells cross the large bowel epithelium as has been demonstrated by electron microscopy in disorders such as ulcerative colitis (Donellan, 1966). A similar phenomenon is possible in trichuriasis (MacDonald *et al.*, 1991). It is still not clear whether *Trichuris trichiura* is a 'blood sucker'. The issue remains controversial but it is highly probable that the worms do suck blood (Bundy and Cooper, 1989). As symptomatic trichuriasis is generally chronic, the continuing blood loss together with the compromised iron status prevailing in endemic areas may contribute to the anaemic state.

(c) Growth stunting

This has been demonstrated in trichuriasis (Bundy and Cooper, 1989; Cooper *et al.*, 1990), even in moderately severe infections (Bundy and Cooper, 1989). The mechanisms responsible for growth stunting are poorly understood but reduced food intake, nutrient loss due to vomiting and diarrhoea are contributory. It has been postulated that losses of zinc and potassium may contribute to the metabolic causes of stunting.

6.4.2 SEVERE TRICHURIASIS OR TRICHURIS DYSENTERY SYNDROME (TDS)

TDS was first described by Ramsey in 1962. The clinical manifestations are insidious and chronic, and resemble those of ulcerative colitis and Crohn's disease which are also associated with growth stunting. Diarrhoea with blood and mucus, finger clubbing, iron-deficiency anaemia and stunting are the main features. Chronicity of the manifestations, previous history of frequent loose mucus stools and sometimes a history of dirt eating or pica are notable features.

6.4.3 GROWTH, PHYSICAL FITNESS AND COGNITIVE FUNCTIONS

Trichuriasis may contribute to the impairment of cognitive function of schoolchildren (Nokes *et al.*, 1991; 1992). Improvement in growth and physical fitness of infected children following deworming is known to occur (Stephenson *et al.*, 1989a; Cooper *et al.*, 1990; Stephenson *et al.*, 1990). The possibility that *Trichuris* has a 'toxic effect', independent of its effect on nutrition, is an intriguing possibility but unproven.

6.5 *STRONGYLOIDES STERCORALIS* (BAVAY 1876)

Strongyloides stercoralis is an intestinal nematode parasite with a world-wide distribution, but is more common in tropical and subtropical regions of the world. It is a pathogen of major importance because of its ability to remain as a low grade infection in the human host for long periods and to cause overwhelming infections in immunocompromised patients which is often fatal. Non-human primates and dogs may act as reservoir hosts. Biologically *Strongyloides stercoralis* occupies a unique position among the geohelminths. It is the only parasitic intestinal worm which can multiply within the host while being capable of going through generations of free-living cycles outside the host body. The unusual relationship between the host and the parasite came to light with the descriptions of the persistent disease in former prisoners of World War II who had acquired the infection while in captivity in endemic areas (Gill and Bell, 1979; Grove, 1980; Oliver *et al.*, 1989; Suzuki *et al.*, 1989).

Strongyloides fulleborni, a closely related species, is primarily a parasite of Asian and African non-human primates that can infect man (Wallace, Moorey and Sanders, 1948; Pampiglione and Ricciardi, 1972; Hira and Patel, 1980; Barnish and Ashford, 1989).

6.5.1 PATHOGENESIS OF MALNUTRITION IN STRONGYLOIDIASIS

A definite causal relationship between strongyloidiasis and malnutrition is difficult to establish but severe nutritional deficiencies have been described in previously well nourished subjects. The infection produces malabsorption syndrome in expatriates (Milner *et al.*, 1965; O'Brien, 1975; Tomkins, 1979). Malnutrition in turn predisposes individuals to severe hyperinfection (Purtilo and Connor, 1975; Garcia *et al.*, 1977; Rosenberg and Bowman, 1984). The mechanisms underlying the development of malnutrition include decreased food intake, impaired nutrient absorption and increased nutrient loss.

(a) Decreased food intake

Anorexia is a notable feature of strongyloidiasis (Burke, 1978; Tomkins, 1979; Pelletier, 1984; Onile, Komolafe and Oladiran, 1985). It is not clear whether the anorexia is centrally induced or self-imposed. Abdominal pain, often mimicking peptic ulcer pain and abdominal discomfort can lead to voluntary rejection of food (Burke, 1978; Carvalho Filho, 1978).

(b) Increased nutrient loss

Diarrhoea and vomiting are two of the most common manifestations of chronic and severe infection. Vomiting results from the invasion of the stomach by larvae, together with the accompanying oedematous inflammation and hypotonia of the duodenum (Carvalho Filho, 1978). Frequent vomiting causes loss of fluid, nutrients and electrolytes and may lead to severe dehydration. The brunt of the intestinal pathology is borne by the duodenum and the proximal jejunum, the areas involved in the absorption of a major proportion of fats and carbohydrates (Carvalho Filho, 1978).

(c) Impaired nutrient absorption

Chronic strongyloidiasis may cause a malabsorption syndrome (Bras *et al.*, 1964; Milner *et al.*, 1965; Willis and Nwokolo, 1966; O'Brien and England, 1971; Fraga, Subral and Arnates, 1974; O'Brien, 1975). Inflammation of the small intestine, particularly the duodenum and the proximal jejunum, is associated with blunting of villi, with malabsorption of D-xylose, vitamin B_{12}, folic acid, iron and steatorrhoea. Mesenteric adenitis with lymphangiectasia of the intestinal villi and resulting malabsorption have been described (de Paola, Dias and da Siva, 1962; Amit-Ahmadi *et al.*, 1968). There have been other studies which failed to demonstrate the presence of a malabsorption syndrome in chronic strongyloidiasis (Kotcher *et al.*, 1966; Garcia *et al.*, 1977). Garcia *et al.* (1977) failed to demonstrate a malabsorption syndrome in their patients even when radiological evidence of loss of normal mucosal patterns was present. The evidence suggest that the malabsorption accompanying strongyloidiasis may be due to concurrent protein energy malnutrition resulting from dietary causes, anorexia, increased nutrient loss due to vomiting and diarrhoea or parasite-induced jejunitis (Holland, 1987b).

Intestinal mucosal cell loss has been established in patients with strongyloidiasis (da Costa, 1971). A case report of a patient showing intestinal protein loss and malabsorption has been published (Laudana *et al.*, 1973). The pathological changes in the intestine in strongyloidiasis suggest that many of them are immunologically mediated and that a large component involves immediate hypersensitivity (Neva, 1986).

(d) Severe strongyloidiasis

Severe strongyloidiasis, often ending fatally has been described in association with neoplastic diseases such as lymphomas (Genta, Miles and Fields, 1989; Suzuki *et al.*, 1989); T-cell leukaemia virus infections (Sato and Shiroma, 1989; Dixon *et al.*, 1989); malnutrition (Bras *et al.*, 1964; Poltera, 1974) and immunosuppressive and corticosteroid therapy (Scowdden, Schaffner and Stone, 1978; Willis and Nwokolo, 1966, Suzuki *et al.*, 1989). The balance established between the host and parasite in uncomplicated chronic infection appears to be controlled, at least to a considerable degree, by cell-mediated immunity (Purtilo and Connor, 1975; Dwork, Jaffe and Lieberman, 1975; Ingra-Siegman *et al.*, 1981; Genta *et al.*, 1983). Malnutrition associated with strongyloidiasis may account for the depressed cell-mediated immunity (Purtilo and Connor, 1975). The experience with ex-POWs from World War II, however, shows that these individuals with persistent infection have had no apparent immune defects to account for this phenomenon. High mortality rates have been described in patients immunocompromised by therapy (Ingra-Siegman *et al.*, 1981). In the majority of these cases bacterial sepsis contributed to the fatal outcome.

(e) Disseminated strongyloidiasis and AIDS

Disseminated strongyloidiasis is widely believed to be precipitated by impairment of cell-mediated immunity (Ingra-Siegman *et al.*, 1981; Genta, 1986). The AIDS pandemic was expected to be accompanied by disseminated strongyloidiasis as one of the major opportunistic infections (Murray *et al.*, 1987). However, only a few cases have been reported in AIDS patients (Mayaan *et al.*,

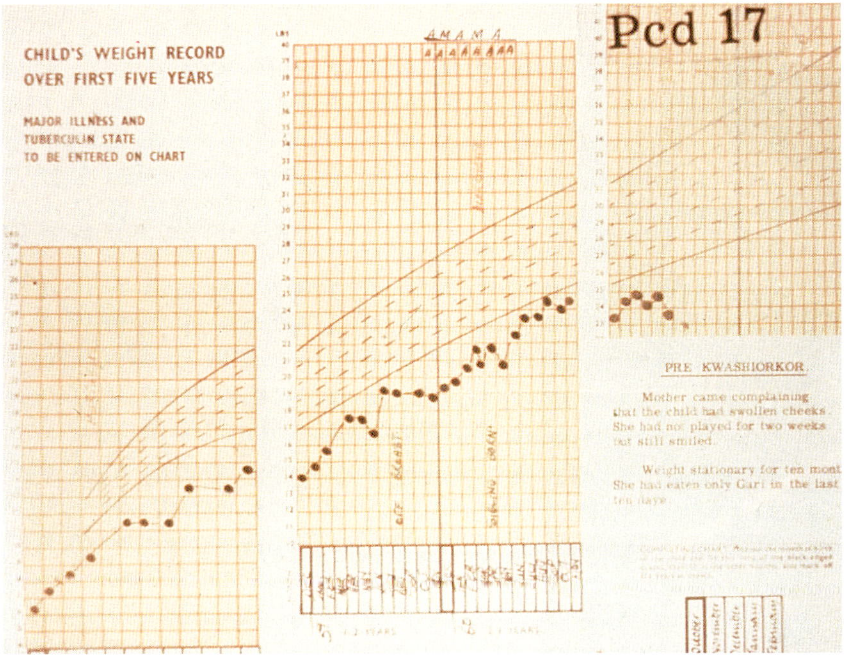

Figure 6.2 Child's weight chart showing longstanding poor weight gain below the 3rd centile.

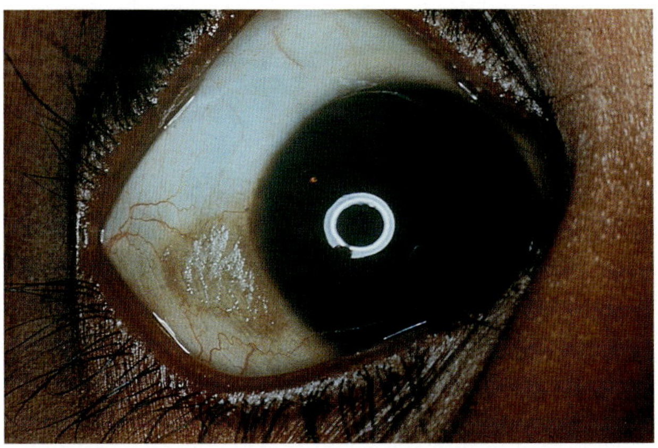

Figure 6.3 Bitot spot in severe vitamin A deficiency.

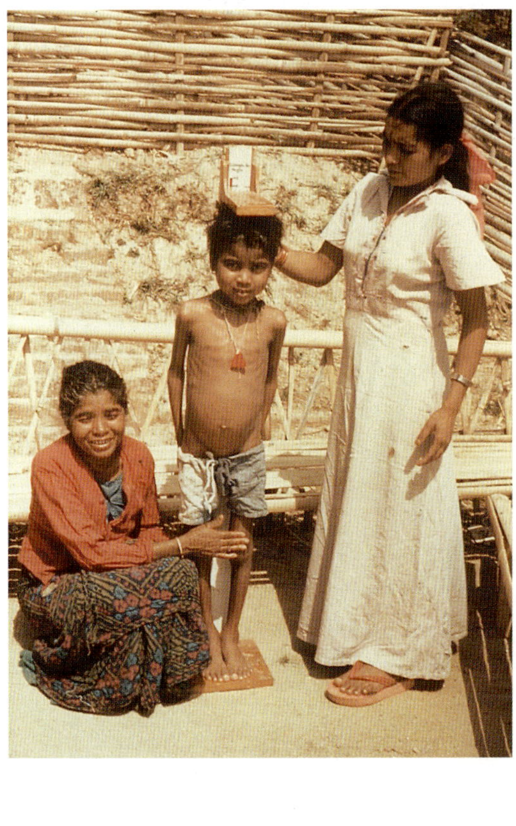

Figure 6.4 Growth stunting due to infection and undernutrition.

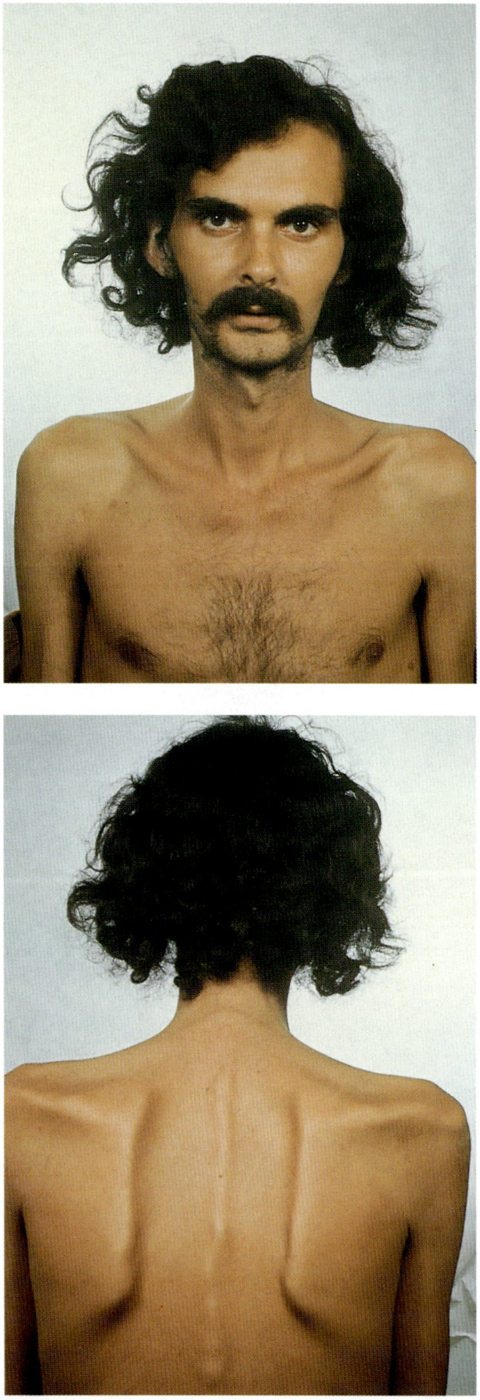

Figure 6.5 a and b Undernutrition due to intestinal malabsorption.

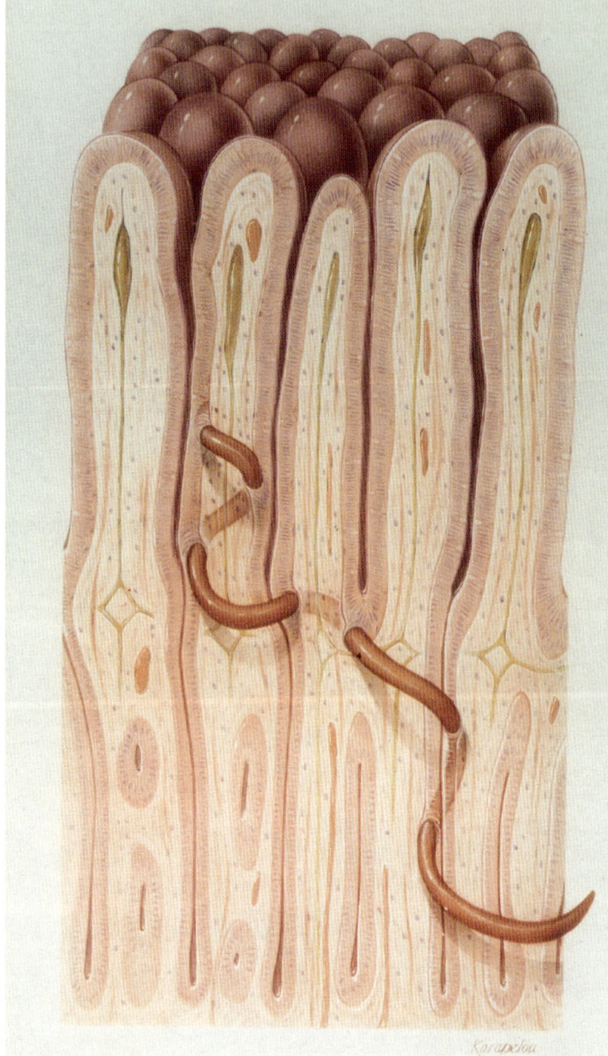

Figure 8.1 Schematic representation of the enteral niche and the adult stage of *Trichinella spiralis in situ*. The parasite is approximately 3 mm in length.

1987) even in areas where epidemiologic overlap of the two conditions occur, as in sub-Saharan Africa, Haiti and Brazil (Genta, 1989).

ACKNOWLEDGEMENTS

Dr Edirisinghe was in receipt of a fellowship from the Association of Commonwealth Universities. The authors wish to thank Madeleine Green for assistance in word processing.

REFERENCES

Abdella, A., Gad-El-Mawla, N., Shaker, E. M. and Galil, N. (1963) Studies on the malabsorption syndrome among Egyptians. 1. Fecal fat and D-xylose absorption tests in pellagra and ancylostomiasis. *J. Egypt. Med. Assoc.*, **46**, 544–52.

Amit-Ahmadi, H., Braun, F., Neva, F. A. *et al.* (1968) Strongyloidiasis at the Boston City Hospital. Emphasis on gastrointestinal pathophysiology and successful therapy with thiabendazole. *Am. J. Dig. Dis.*, **13**, 959–73.

Areekul, S., Devakul, K., Chantachun, Y. *et al.* (1971) Gastrointestinal protein loss in patients with hookworm infection. *J. Med. Assoc. Thailand*, **54**, 28–33.

Aziz, M. A. and Siddiqui, A. R. (1968) Morphological and absorption studies of small intestine in hookworm disease in West Pakistan. *Gastroenterology*, **55**, 242–50.

Banwell, J. G., Marsden, P. D., Blackman, V. *et al.* (1967) Hookworm infection and intestinal absorption amongst Africans in Uganda. *Am. J. Trop. Med. Hyg.*, **16**, 304–8.

Barnish, G. and Ashford, R. W. (1989) *Strongyloides fulleborni* in Papua New Guinea: epidemiology in an isolated community and results of an intervention study. *Ann. Trop. Parasit.*, **83**, 499–506.

Blackman, V., Marsden, P., Banwell, J. and Hall-Craggs, M. (1965) Albumin metabolism in hookworm anaemia. *Trans. Roy. Soc. Trop. Med. Hyg.*, **59**, 472–82.

Bras, G., Irvine, R. A., Richards, R. C. *et al.* (1964) Infection with *Strongyloides stercoralis* in Jamaica. *Lancet*, **ii**, 1257–60.

Brown, K. H., Gilman, R. H., Khatun, M. and Ahmed, M. G. (1980) Absorption of macronutrients from a rice vegetable diet before and after treatment of ascariasis in children. *Am. J. Clin. Nutr.* **33**, 1975–82.

Bundy, D. A. P. (1985) Parasitic worms in the aetiology of iron deficiency anaemia in the Caribbean region. *Q. J. Carib. Food Nutr. Inst. (PAHO/WHO)*, **18**, 197–215.

Bundy, D. A. P. (1986) Epidemiological aspects of *Trichuris* and Trichuriasis in Caribbean communities. *Trans. Roy. Soc. Trop. Med. Hyg.*, **80**, 706–18.

Bundy, D. A. P. and Cooper, E. S. (1989) *Trichuris* and trichuriasis in humans. *Adv. Parasit.*, **28**, 107–73.

Bundy, D. A., Cooper, E. S., Thompson, D. E. *et al.* (1987) Epidemiology and population dynamics of *Ascaris lumbricoides* and *Trichuris trichiura* infection in the same community. *Trans. Roy. Soc. Trop. Med. Hyg.*, **81**, 987–93.

Burke, J. A. (1978) Strongyloidiasis in childhood. *Am. J. Dis. Child.*, **132**, 1130–6.

Callender, J. E. M., Grantham-McGregor, S., Walker, S. and Cooper, E. S. (1992) Trichuris infection and mental development in children. *Lancet*, **339**, 181.

Carrera, E., Nesheim, S. C. and Crompton, D. W. T. (1984) Lactose maldigestion in ascaris-infected preschool children. *Am. J. Clin. Nutr.*, **39**, 255–64.

Carvalho Filho, E. (1978) Strongyloidiasis. *Clinics Gastroent.*, **7**, 179–202.

Chappel, L. H. (1980) *Physiology of Parasites*. Blackie, Glasgow and London.

Cline, B. L., Little, M. D., Bartholomew, R. K. and Halsey, N. A. (1984) Larvicidal activity of albendazole against *Necator americanus* larvae in human volunteers. *Am. J. Trop. Med. Hyg.*, **33**, 387–94.

Chuttani, H. K., Puri, S. K. and Misra, R. C. (1967) Small intestine in hookworm disease. *Gastroenterology*, **53**, 381–8.

Coles, G. C. (1985) Allergy and immunopathology of ascariasis, in *Ascariasis and its Public Health Significance* (eds D. W. T. Crompton, M. C. Nesheim and Z. S. Pawlowski), Taylor and Francis, London, pp. 167–84.

Cooper, E. S. and Bundy, D. A. P. (1988) *Trichuris* is not trivial. *Parasit. Today*, **4**, 301–6.

Cooper, E. S., Bundy, D. A. P., MacDonald, T. T. and Golden, M. H. N. (1990) Growth suppression in the *Trichuris* dysentery syndrome. *Eur. J. Clin. Nutr.*, **44**, 285–91.

Crompton, D. W. T., (1984) Influence of parasitic infections on food intake. *Fed. Proc.*, **43**, 239–45.

Crompton, D. W. T., (1988) The prevalence of ascariasis. *Parasit. Today*, **4**, 162–9.

Crompton, D. W. T., Singhvi, A., Nesheim, M. C. and Walter, D. E. (1981) Competition for dietary fructose between Moniliformis (Acanthocephala) and growing rats. *Int. J. Parasit.*, **11**, 457–61.

da Costa, L. R., (1971) Small intestinal cell turnover in patients with parasitic infections. *Brit. Med. J.*, **3**, 281–3.

Darke, S. J. (1959) Malnutrition in African adults. 5. Effects of hookworm infestation on absorption of foodstuffs. *Brit. J. Nutr.*, **13**, 278–82.

Davis, A. (1985) in *Ascaris and its Public Health Significance* (eds D. W. T. Crompton, M. C. Nesheim and Z. S. Pawlowski), Taylor and Francis, London, pp. 1, 239–44.

de Paola, D., Dias, L. B. and da Silva, J. R. (1962) Enteritis due to *Strongyloides stercoralis*. A report of 5 fatal cases. *Am. J. Dig. Dis.*, **7**, 1086–98.

Dixon, A. C., Yanagihara, E. T., Kwock, D. W. and Nakamura, J. M. (1989) Strongyloidiasis associated with human T-cell lymphotropic virus type i infection in a non endemic area. *West. J. Med.*, **151**, 410–13.

Donellan, W. L. (1966) Early histological changes in ulcerative colitis: a light and electron microscopic study. *Gastroenterology*, **50**, 519–40.

Dwork, K. G., Jaffe, J. R. and Lieberman, H. D. (1975) Strongyloidiasis with massive hyperinfection. *N. Y. State J. Med.*, **75**, 1230–4.

Falaiye, J. M., Oladapo, J. M. and Wali, S. C. (1974) Hookworm enteropathy. *J. Trop. Med. Hyg.*, **77**, 211–14.

Forrester, J. E., Scott, M. E., Bundy, D. A. and Golden, M. H. (1988) Clustering of *Ascaris lumbricoides* and *Trichuris trichiura* infections within households. *Trans. Roy. Soc. Trop. Med. Hyg.*, **82**, 282–8.

Forrester, J. E., Scott, M. E., Bundy, D. A. and Golden, M. H. (1990) Predisposition of individuals and families in Mexico to heavy infection with *Ascaris lumbricoides* and *Trichuris trichiura*. *Trans. Roy. Soc. Trop. Med. Hyg.*, **84**, 272–6.

Forsum, E., Nesheim, M. C. and Crompton, D. W. T. (1981) Nutritional aspects of ascaris infection in young protein deficient pigs. *Parasitology*, **83**, 497–512.

Fraga, C. F., Subral, D. T. and Arnates, M. R. (1974) Disturbios da absorcão intestinal na estrongiloidese. *Rev. Soc. Brasiliera Med. Trop.*, **8**, 209–16.

Freij, L., Meeuwisse, G. W., Berg, N. O. *et al.* (1979) Ascariasis and malnutrition. A study in urban Ethiopian children. *Am. J. Clin. Nutr.*, **3**, 1545–53.

Garcia, F. T., Sessions, J. T., Strum, W. B. *et al.* (1977) Intestinal function and morphology in strongyloidiasis. *Am. J. Trop. Med. Hyg.*, **26**, 859–65.

Genta, R. M. (1986) *Strongyloides stercoralis*: immunobiological considerations on an unusual worm. *Parasit. Today*, **2**, 141–6.

Genta, R. M. (1989) Global prevalence of strongyloidiasis: critical review with epidemiologic insights into the prevention of disseminated disease. *Rev. Infect. Dis.*, **11**, 755–67.

Genta, R. M., Miles, P. and Fields, K. (1989) Opportunistic *Strongyloides stercoralis* infection in lymphoma patients. Report of a case and review of the literature. *Cancer*, **63**, 1407–11.

Genta, R. M., Ottesen, E. A., Neva, F. A. *et al.* (1983) Cellular responses in human strongyloidiasis. *Am. J. Trop. Med. Hyg.*, **32**, 990–4.

Gill, G. V. and Bell, D. R. (1979) *Strongyloides stercoralis* infection in former Far East prisoners of war. *Brit. Med. J.*, **2**, 572–4.

Gilman, R. H. (1982) Hookworm disease: Host–pathogen biology. *Rev. Infect. Dis.*, **4**, 824–9.

Gilman, R. H., Chong, Y. H., Davis, C. *et al.* (1983) The adverse consequences of heavy *Trichuris* infection. *Trans. Roy. Soc. Trop. Med. Hyg.*, **77**, 432–8.

Green, N. M. (1957) Protease inhibitors from *Ascaris lumbricoides*. *Biochem. J.*, **66**, 416–30.

Grove, D. I. (1980) Strongyloidiasis in allied exprisoners of war in South-East Asia. *Brit. Med. J.*, **280**, 598–601.

Gupta, M. C. (1985) Ascariasis and malnutrition in children: studies in India and Guatemala, in *Ascariasis and its Public Health Significance* (eds D. W. T. Crompton, M. C. Nesheim and Z. S. Pawlowski), Taylor and Francis, London, pp. 203–12.

Gupta, M. C., Basu, A. K. and Tandon, B. N. (1974) Gastrointestinal protein loss in hookworm and roundworm infections. *Am. J. Clin. Nutr.*, **27**, 1386–9.

Gupta, M. C., Mithal, S., Arora, K. L. and Tandon, B. N. (1977) Effect of periodic deworming on nutritional status of *Ascaris* infected preschool children. *Lancet*, **ii**, 108–10.

Hall, A., Bundy, D. A. P., Anderson, R. M. and Tomkins, A. M. (1992) Predisposition and ascaris infection. *Lancet*, **340**, 113–14.

Haswell-Elkins, M., Elkins, D. and Anderson, R. M. (1989) The influence of individual, social group and household factors on the distribution of *Ascaris lumbricoides* within a community and implications for control strategies. *Parasitology*, **98**, 125–33.

Haswell-Elkins, M. R., Kennedy, M. W., Maizels, R. M., Elkins, D. B. and Anderson, R. M. (1989b) The antibody recognition profiles of human naturally infected with *Ascaris lumbricoides*. *Parasite Immunol.* **11**, 615–27.

Hira, R. R. and Patel, B. G. (1980) Human strongyloidiasis due to the primate species *Strongyloides fulleborni*. *Trop. Geog. Med.*, **32**, 23–9.

Hodes, P. J. and Keefer, G. P. (1948) Hookworm disease: a small intestine study. *Am. J. Roentgen. Radium Ther. Nuc. Med.*, **54**, 728–42.

Holland, C. (1987a) Hookworm infection, in *Impact of Helminth Infections on Human Nutrition* (ed. L. S. Stephenson), Taylor and Francis, London, New York and Philadelphia, pp. 128–60.

Holland, C. (1987b) Neglected infections – trichuriasis and strongyloidiasis, in *Impact of Helminth Infections on Human Nutrition* (ed. L. S. Stephenson), Taylor and Francis, London, New York and Philadelphia, pp. 161–201.

Holland, C. V., Assolu, S. O., Crompton, D. W. *et al.* (1989) The epidemiology of *Ascaris lumbricoides* and other soil transmitted helminths in primary school children from IleIfe, Nigeria. *Parasitology*, **99**, 275–85.

Homanberg, G. A. and Peanasky, R. J. (1976) Characterisation of proteins *Ascaris lumbricoides* which bind specifically to carboxyl peptidase. *J. Biol. Chem.*, **251**, 2226–33.

Ingra-Siegman, Y., Kapila, R., Sen, P. *et al.* (1981) Syndrome of hyperinfection with *Strongyloides stercoralis*. *Rev. Infect. Dis.*, **3**, 397–407.

Judisch, J. M., Naiman, J. L. and Oski, F. A. (1966) The fallacy of the fat iron-deficient child. *Pediatrics*, **37**, 987–90.

Klasing, K. C. (1988) Nutritional aspects of leucocytic cytokines. *J. Nutr.*, **118**, 1436–46.

Koshy, A., Raina, V., Sharma, M. P. *et al.* (1978) An unusual outbreak of hookworm disease in North India. *Am. J. Trop. Med. Hyg.*, **27**, 42–5.

Kotcher, E., Miranda, M. G., Esquivel, R. R. *et al.* (1966) Intestinal malabsorption and helminthic and protozoan infections of the small intestine. *Gastroenterology*, **50**, 366–71.

Laudanna, A. A., Polack, M., Betarello, A. and Kieffer, J. (1973) Evidence of protein losing enteropathy in strongyloidiasis. *Rev. Inst. Med. Trop. São Paulo*, **15**, 222–6.

Layrisse, M., Blumenfeld, N., Dugarte, I. and Roche, M. (1959) Vitamin B_{12} and folic acid metabolism in hookworm infected people. *Blood*, **12**, 1269–79.

Layrisse, M., Blumenfeld, N., Carbonell, L. *et al.* (1964) Intestinal absorption tests and biopsy of the jejunum in subjects with heavy hookworm infection. *Am. J. Trop. Med. Hyg.*, **13**, 297–305.

Layrisse, M., Aparcedo, L., Martinez-Torres, C. and Roche, M. (1967) Blood loss due to infection with *Trichuris trichiura*. *Am. J. Trop. Med. Hyg.*, **16**, 613–18.

Legundoye, S. B. (1972) Disordered small bowel pattern in ascariasis. *Trop. Geog. Med.*, **24**, 226–31.

Lozoff, B. (1989) Methodologic issues in studying behavioral effects of infant iron-deficiency anaemia. *Am. J. Clin. Nutr.*, **50**, 641–54.

MacDonald, T. T., Choy, M. Y., Spencer, J. *et al.*, (1991) Histopathology and immunochemistry of the caecum in children with the Trichuris dysentery syndrome. *J. Clin. Path.*, **44**, 194–9.

McCance, R. A. (1960) Severe undernutrition in growing and adult animals. 1. Production and general effects. *Brit. J. Nutr.*, **14**, 59–73.

Mahalanabis, D., Jalan, K. N., Maitra, T. K. and Agarwal, S. K. (1976) Vitamin A absorption in ascariasis. *J. Clin. Nutr.*, **29**, 1372–5.

Mahalanabis, D., Simpson, T. W., Chakraboty, M. L. *et al.* (1979) Malabsorption of water miscible vitamin A in children with giardiasis and ascarisis. *Am. J. Clin. Nutr.*, **32**, 313–18.

Martin, J., Crompton, D. W. T., Carrera, E. and Nesheim, M. C. (1985) Mucosal surface lesions in young protein deficient pigs infected with *Ascaris suum* (Nematoda). *Parasitology*, **88**, 333–40.

Martorell, R. and Yarborough, C. (1983) The energy cost of diarrhoeal disease and other common illnesses in children, in *Diarrhoea and Malnutrition* (eds L. C. Chen and N. S. Scrimshaw), Plenum, New York, pp. 125–41.

Mata, L. J. (1978) The children of Santa Maria Canque: a prospective field study of health and growth, MIT Press, Cambridge, Massachusetts.

Mayan, S., Wormser, G. P., Widerhorn, J., Sy, E. R., Kim, Y. H. and Ernst, J. A. (1987) *Strongyloides stercoralis* hyperinfection in a patient with acquired immunodeficiency syndrome. An update. *Am. Rev. Respir. Dis.* **135**, 504–9.

Mayoral, L. G., Tripathy, K., Garcia, F. T. *et al.* (1967) Malabsorption in the tropics. A second look. 1. The role of protein malnutrition. *Am. J. Clin. Nutr.*, **20**, 866–83.

Miller, T. A. (1971) Vaccination against canine hookworm diseases. *Adv. Parasit.*, **9**, 153–83.

Miller, T. A. (1979) Hookworm infection in man. *Adv. Parasit.*, **17**, 315–83.

Milner, P. F., Irvine, R. A., Barton, C. J. *et al.* (1965) Intestinal malabsorption in *Strongyloides stercoralis* infestation. *Gut*, **6**, 574–81.

Murray, J. F., Garay, S. M., Hopewell, P. C. *et al.* (1987) NHLBI workshop summary: pulmonary complications of acquired immunodeficiency syndrome. An update. *Am. Rev. Respir. Dis.*, **135**, 504–9.

Neva, F. A. (1986) Pathology and immunology of human strongyloidiasis. *J. Infect. Dis.*, **153**, 397–406.

Nokes, C., Cooper, E. S., Robinson, B. A. and Bundy, D. A. P. (1991) Geohelminth infection and academic assessment in Jamaican children. *Trans. Roy. Soc. Trop. Med. Hyg.*, **85**, 272–3.

Nokes, C., Grantham-McGregor, S. M., Sawyer, A. W. *et al.* (1992) Parasitic helminth infection and cognitive function in school children. *Proc. Roy. Soc. Lond.*, **247**, 77–81.

Northrop, C. A., Lunn, P. G., Wainwright, M. and Evans, J. (1987) Plasma albumin concentrations and intestinal permeability in Bangladeshi children infected with *Ascaris lumbricoides*. *Trans. Roy. Soc. Trop. Med. Hyg.*, **81**, 811–15.

O'Brien, W. (1975) Intestinal malabsorption in acute infection with *Strongyloides stercoralis*. *Trans. Roy. Soc. Trop. Med. Hyg.*, **69**, 69–77.

O'Brien, W. and England, M. W. J. (1971) *Tropical Sprue and Megaloblastic Anaemia*. Wellcome Trust Collaborative Study, Churchill Livingstone, Edinburgh and London, p. 25.

Onile, B., Komolafe, F. and Oladiran, B. (1985) Severe strongyloidiasis presenting as occult gastrointestinal tract malignancy. *Ann. Trop. Med. Parasit.*, **79**, 301–4.

Oliver, N. W., Rowbottom, D. J., Sexton, P. *et al.* (1989) Chronic strongyloidiasis in Tasmanian veterans – clinical diagnosis by the use of a screening index. *Aust. N. Z. J. Med.*, **19**, 458–62.

Ovartlarnporn, B., Chamroonkul, N., Sirithanaratanakul, N. and Kosolbharn, P. (1990) Gastrointestinal lesions in patients over 40 years of age with iron deficiency anaemia and hookworm infection. *SE Asian J. Trop. Med. Public Hlth.*, **21**, 594–7.

Pampiglione, S. and Ricciardi, M. L. (1972) Experimental infestation with human strain *Strongyloides fulleborni* in man. *Lancet*, **i**, 663–5.

Pawlowski, Z. S. (1984a) Ascariasis. *Ann. Soc. Belge. Med. Trop.*, **64**, 125–34.

Pawlowski, Z. S. and Davis, A. (1989) Morbidity and mortality in ascariasis, in *Ascariasis and its Prevention and Control* (eds D. W. T. Crompton, M. C. Nesheim and Z. S. Pawlowski), Taylor and Francis, London, pp. 71–86.

Pelletier, L. L., Jr. (1984) Chronic strongyloidiasis in World War II Far East ex-prisoners of war. *Am. J. Trop. Med. Hyg.*, **33**, 55–61.

Pollitt, E. (1990) *Malnutrition and Infection in the Class Room*. UNESCO, Paris, pp. 137–49.

Pollitt, E., Hathirat, P., Kotchabhakdi, N. J. *et al.* (1989) Iron deficiency and educational achievement in Thailand. *Am. J. Clin. Nutr.*, **50**, 687–97.

Poltera, A. A. (1974) Fatal strongyloidiasis in Uganda. *Ann. Trop. Med. Parasit.*, **68**, 81–90.

Purtilo, D. and Connor, D. H. (1975) Fatal infections in protein-calorie malnourished children with thymolymphatic atrophy. *Archs Dis. Child.*, **50**, 149–52.

Rivera, J. and Martorell, R. (1988) Nutrition, infection and growth. Part 1. Effects of infection on growth. *Clin. Nutr.*, **1**, 156–62.

Roche, M. and Layrisse, M. (1966) The nature and causes of 'hookworm anaemia'. *Am. J. Trop. Med. Hyg.*, **15**, 1030–100.

Rosenburg, I. H. and Bowman, B. B. (1984) Impact of intestinal parasites on digestive function in humans. *Fed. Proc.*, **43**, 246–50.

Saraya, A. K., Tandon, B. N. and Ramachandran, K. (1971) Study of vitamin B_{12} and folic acid deficiency in hookworm disease. *Am. J. Clin. Nutr.*, **24**, 3–6.

Sato, Y. and Shiroma, Y. (1989) Concurrent infections with strongyloidiasis and T-cell leukemia virus and their possible effect on immune responses of host. *Clin. Immun. Immunopath.*, **52**, 214–24.

Schultz, M. G. (1982) Ascariasis: nutritional implications. *Rev. Infect. Dis.*, **4**, 815–19.

Scowden, E., Schaffner, W. and Stone, W. (1978) Overwhelming strongyloidiasis. An unappreciated opportunistic infection. *Analyt. Rev. Int. Med. Dermatol. Neurol. Pediat. Psych.*, **57**, 527–44.

Seshadri, S. and Gopaldas, T. (1989) Impact of iron supplementation on cognitive functions in preschool and school aged children: the Indian experience. *Am. J. Clin. Nutr.*, **50**, 675–84.

Sheehy, T. W., Meroney, M. H., Cox, R. S. and Soler, J. E. (1962) Hookworm disease and malabsorption. *Gastroenterology*, **42**, 148–56.

Sivakumar, B. and Reddy, V. (1975) Absorption of vitamin A in children with ascariasis. *J. Trop. Med. Hyg.*, **78**, 114–15.

Soemantri, A. G. (1989) Preliminary findings on iron supplementation and learning achievement of rural Indonesian children. *Am. J. Clin. Nutr.*, **50**, 698–701.

Soewondo, S., Husaini, M. and Pollitt, E. (1989) Effects of iron deficiency on attention and learning processes in preschool children: Bandung, Indonesia. *Am. J. Clin. Nutr.*, **50**, 667–73.

Stephenson, L. (1980) Contribution of *Ascaris lumbricoides* to malnutrition in children. *Parasitology*, **81**, 221–33.

Stephenson, L. S. (1987) *Impact of Helminth Infections on Human Nutrition*, Taylor and Francis, London, New York, Philadelphia, pp. 1–20.

Stephenson, L. S., Pond, W. G., Nesheim, M. C., Karook, L. P. and Crompton, D. W. T. (1980a)

Ascaris suum: nutrient absorption, growth and intestinal pathology in young pigs experimentally infected with 15 day old larvae. *Expl. Parasitol.* **49**, 15–25.

Stephenson, L. S., Crompton, D. W. T., Latham, M. C. *et al.* (1980b) Relationship between *Ascaris* infection and growth of malnourished preschool children in Kenya. *Am. J. Clin. Nutr.*, **33**, 1165–72.

Stephenson, L. S., Latham, M. C., Kurz, K. M. *et al.* (1985) Relationship of *Schistosoma haematobium*, hookworm and malarial infections and metrifonate treatment to growth of Kenyan school children. *Am. J. Trop. Med. Hyg.*, **34**, 519–28.

Stephenson, L. S., Latham, M. C., Kurz, K. M. *et al.* (1988) Albendazole treatment improves physical fitness of Kenyan school children with hookworm, *Trichuris trichiura* and *Ascaris lumbricoides* infections. (Abstract), in *Proc. XIIth International Congress of Tropical Medicine and Malaria* (eds P. A. Kager and A. M. Polderman), Excerpta Medica, Amsterdam, New York and Oxford, p. 14.

Stephenson, L. S., Latham, M. C., Kurz, K. M. and Kinoti, S. N. (1989a) Single dose of metrifonate or praziquantel treatment in Kenyan children. ii. Effects on growth in relation to *Schistosoma haematobium* and hookworm egg counts. *Am. J. Trop. Med. Hyg.*, **41**, 445–53.

Stephenson, L. S., Latham, M. C., Kurz, K. M. *et al.* (1989b) Treatment with a single dose of albendazole improves growth of Kenyan school children with hookworm, *Trichuris trichiura* and *Ascaris lumbricoides* infections. *Am. J. Trop. Med. Hyg.*, **41**, 78–87.

Stephenson, L. S., Latham, M. C., Kinoti, S. N. *et al.* (1990) Improvements in physical fitness of Kenyan schoolboys infected with hookworm, *Trichuris trichiura* and *Ascaris lumbricoides* following a single dose of albendazole. *Trans. Roy. Soc. Trop. Med. Hyg.*, **84**, 277–82.

Suzuki, T., Nara, N., Miyake, S. *et al.* (1989) Fatal strongyloidiasis latent over 42 years in the antineoplastic chemotherapy of a case with malignant lymphoma. *Jap. J. Med.*, **28**, 96–9.

Symons, L. E. A. and Fairbairn, D. (1962) Pathology, absorption, transport and activity of digestive enzymes in rat jejunum parasitized by the nematode *Nippostrongylus brasiliensis*. *Fed. Proc.*, **21**, 913–18.

Tandon, B. W., Kohle, R. K., Saraya, A. K. *et al.* (1969a) Role of parasites in the pathogenesis of intestinal malabsorption in hookworm disease. *Gut*, **10**, 293–8.

Tandon, B. N., Saraya, A. K., Ramachandran, K. and Sama, S. K. (1969b) Relationship of anaemia and hypoproteinaemia to functional and structural changes in the small bowel in hookworm disease. *Gut*, **10**, 360–5.

Taren, D. L., Nesheim, M. C., Crompton, D. W. T. *et al.* (1987) Contribution of ascariasis to poor nutritional status of children from Chiriqui Province, Republic of Panama. *Parasitology*, **95**, 603–13.

Teotia, S. P. S., Teotia, M., Kunwar, K. B. and Misra, S. S. (1969) Fat malabsorption in intestinal parasitic infections. *J. Indian Med. Assoc.*, **53**, 577–82.

Tomkins, A. (1979) The role of intestinal parasites in diarrhoea and malnutrition. *Trop. Doc.*, **9**, 21–4.

Tomkins, A., Watson, F. (1989) Malnutrition and infection. A review, United Nations Administrative Committee on Coordination/Subcommittee on Nutrition. State of the art series. Nutrition policy discussion paper No. 5. p. 1, London.

Tripathy, K., Duque, E., Bolanos, O. *et al.* (1972) Malabsorption syndrome in ascariasis. *Am. J. Clin. Nutr.*, **25**, 1276–87.

Variyan, E. P. and Banwell, J. G. (1982) Nutrition implications of hookworm infection. *Rev. Infect. Dis.*, **4**, 830–5.

Wallace, F. G., Mooney, R. D. and Sanders, A. (1948) *Strongloides fulleborni* infection in man. *Am. J. Trop. Med.*, **2**, 299–302.

Walter, T. (1989) Infancy: mental and motor development. *Am. J. Clin. Nutr.*, **50**, 655–64.

Willet, W. C., Kilama, W. L. and Kihamia, C. M. (1979) *Ascaris* and growth rates: a randomized trial of treatment. *Am. J. Public Hlth*, **69**, 987–91.

Willis, A. J. P. and Nwokolo, C. (1966) Steroid therapy and strongyloidiasis. *Lancet*, **i**, 1396–8.

Wong, M. S. and Tan, K. (1961) Severe whipworm infestation in children. *Singapore Med. J.*, **2**, 34–7.

SEVEN

Strongyloides stercoralis

F. Neva

Strongyloides stercoralis is an intestinal nematode of humans which can produce serious, even fatal disease in an immunocompromised host because of certain unusual biological characteristics of the parasite. This tiny worm normally resides in the upper small intestine and produces relatively few symptoms in the majority of infected individuals. In this situation diagnosis is difficult because excretion of the parasite is scanty and sporadic. However, the parasite can persist in the human host for long periods of time, perhaps indefinitely, and then reinvade or autoinfect its host under conditions of immunosuppression. When this happens the parasite actually multiplies in the host, a state referred to as hyperinfection syndrome, with invasion of other tissues and organ systems. Therefore, this parasite deserves special recognition as a unique infectious agent with potential for causing serious human disease.

7.1 HISTORICAL ASPECTS

The parasite and the disease caused by it were first discovered and described by a French naval physician, Louis Normand, in 1876, during investigation of diarrheal disease in troops returning from Cochin, China (present day Vietnam). Hence, the synonym, Cochin diarrhea. Although *S. stercoralis* has a world-wide distribution, the generally high prevalence of strongyloides infection in inhabitants of the south-east Asian region suggest that this may be the ancestral home of the parasite. French investigators initially named the parasite, and many French-speaking parasitologists still refer to it as *Anguillula stercoralis* (meaning 'dung eel' in Latin). Several years were required for European parasitologists to differentiate *S. stercoralis* from hookworm larvae, and to work out the complicated *Strongyloides* life cycle. The parasite can either develop directly to an infective lava (homogonic cycle) after it is excreted, or it may undergo a free-living generation before development to an infective larva (heterogonic or indirect cycle). In either event, the parasite was found to be biologically similar to hookworm by the fact that infection is initiated by penetration of intact skin. *Strongyloides stercoralis* was officially accepted as the name of the parasite by the International Commission on Zoologic Nomenclature in 1915. There was another period of confusion and controversy about details of the life cycle before it was realized that *S. stercoralis* is parthenogenetic, and no convincing evidence for the existence of a parasitic adult male worm has been found. With a related species, *S. ratti*, patent infection can be initiated by a single infective larva. This early history of the subject is presented in greater detail by Grove (1989a).

From observations in infected dogs and in

Enteric Infection 2. Intestinal helminths. Edited by M.J.G. Farthing, G.T. Keutch and D. Wakelin. Published in 1995 by Chapman and Hall, London. ISBN 0 412 39140 6 patients with urticarial skin lesions over the buttocks and perianal area, Fullerborn (1926) suggested that *S. stercoralis* was capable of developing to infective filariform larvae and reinvading the same host, i.e. autoinfection. This concept of autoinfection was supported by autopsy studies which showed filariform larvae in the wall of the colon of patients whose sputum during life contained filariform larvae (Gage, 1911). Thus, it seemed that in some cases with heavy strongyloides infections, many of the parasites were reinfecting, or multiplying in the host to produce a syndrome of hyperinfection.

The association of very severe, often fatal, hyperinfection syndrome with various forms of immunosuppression can be considered a historic milestone in our understanding of strongyloidiasis. This realization came from multiple reports between 1964 and 1978 (Bras *et al.*, 1964; Cruz, Reboucas and Rocha, 1966; Purtilo, Meyers and Connor, 1974; Scowden, Schaffner and Stone, 1978) which linked administration of steroids, and other immunosuppressive states, with a fatal outcome of strongyloides infection.

The latest finding of historical proportions, because of its epidemiological significance, is the evidence that untreated strongyloides infections may persist indefinitely. The first convincing report was that of Gill and Bell (1979) who found 12% of 443 British former prisoners of Second World War (POWs) from Burma were infected with the parasite after living for 23 to 33 years without presumed re-exposure to *S. stercoralis*. Up to 27% infection rates with the parasite were found in Australian (Grove, 1980) and American (Pelletier, 1984) ex-POWs from the same region. Thus, it is difficult to escape the conclusion that, at least with certain strains of *S. stercoralis*, infections may persist essentially for life, even in presumably normal hosts. This suggests, furthermore, that some degree of internal autoinfection occurs very commonly with this parasite.

7.2 MICROBIOLOGY

Strongyloides stercoralis is a nematode belonging to the Order Rhabditoidea. Other members of the genus *Strongyloides* include *S. fulleborni*, a parasite of Old World primates, as well as of humans; *S. cebus*, which occurs in New World monkeys; *S. ransomi* of pigs and *S. papillosus* of sheep. *S. ratti*, as indicated by the name, is found naturally in rats, and can be adapted for passage in certain strains of mice as well. At least 40 other species have been described, but different species have a fairly high degree of host specificity.

S. stercoralis is the only human pathogen within the Rhabditoidea. Other genera in this group are free-living in the soil and include the worm *Caenorhabditis elegans*, upon which so much attention has been lavished recently by developmental and molecular geneticists. The primitive nature of *S. stercoralis*, in comparison to other parasitic nematodes, is evidenced by the fact that it still retains capacity for a free-living, or indirect, mode of reproduction and development, the heterogonic cycle referred to above. In addition, *S. stercoralis* undergoes the more conventional direct or homogonic cycle of development, in which infective larvae develop directly from the first stage rhabditiform larva.

The adult parasitic female worm, which is barely visible to the naked eye because of its transparent appearance and small size, up to 2.5 mm long and 40–45 μm in diameter, lives deep between the villi or threaded just under the mucosa of the upper small intestine. A long esophagus extending about one fourth the length of the worm, and paired uteri which contain up to a dozen eggs arranged in single file, are the most prominent internal structures. The female adult worm would easily be overlooked at autopsy or surgery because it is so small and is embedded in the mucosa (Figure 7.1).

The adult free-living male is smaller than the free-living female (0.7 mm × 45 μm), and

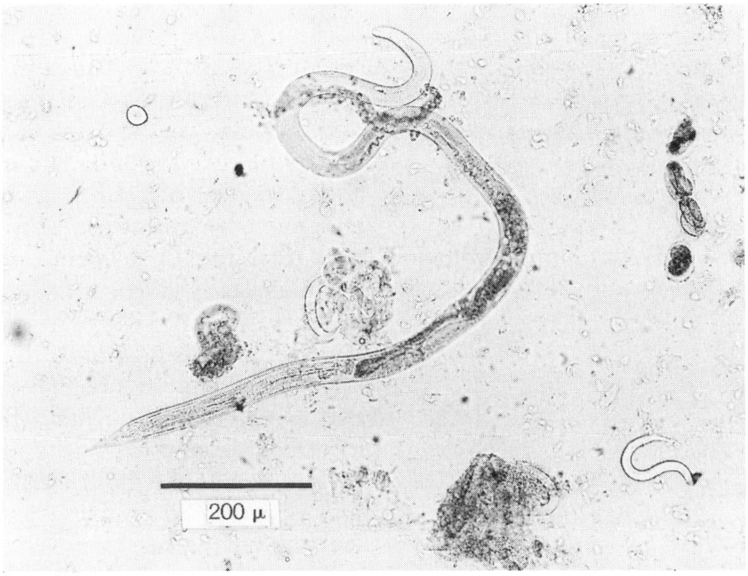

Figure 7.1 Parasitic female *S. stercoralis* from small intestinal contents of a patient with hyperinfection; it is slightly immature since there are no eggs in the uterus. A rhabditiform larva is present on the lower right.

has a characteristic hooked or J-shape at the pointed posterior end. Paired copulatory spicules, chitinous structures utilized by the male worm to immobilize the female during copulation, are also prominent at the posterior end. Both the free-living male and female worms require low-power microscopic magnification to be seen and identified. They exhibit sluggish and jerky movements when observed (Figure 7.2).

First-stage rhabditiform larvae (L1), which hatch from eggs laid by the free-living, as well as by the parasitic female, are morphologically identical. They are approximately 250 μm in length and 15 μm in width, but the length can vary considerably depending upon the duration of time after hatching. The rhabditiform larvae display a prominent esophagus and esophageal bulb and an elongated tapered tail. The L1 is usually actively motile, but often will remain still for a few seconds before resuming a graceful snake-like movement. Not before the end of the second larval stage (L2) can it be determined

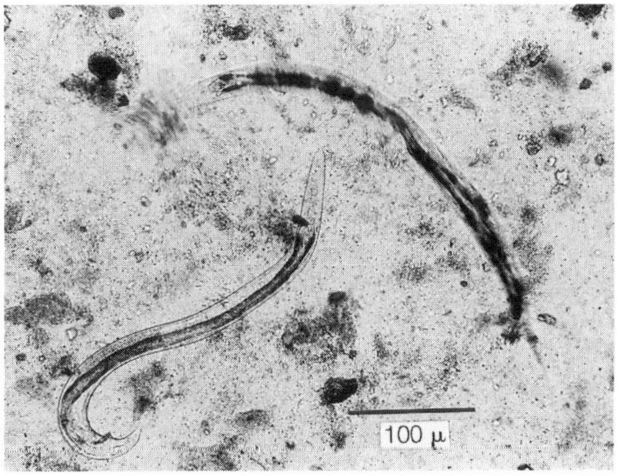

Figure 7.2 Free-living adult male (with sharply curved and pointed posterior end) and female *S. stercoralis* in a fecal culture; the gut of both is darkly outlined by ingested material.

morphologically as to the type of future development either direct or indirect, to which the larva is committed. If destined for the free-living (indirect) stage there is general growth and development of male or female reproductive systems. If the larva is to

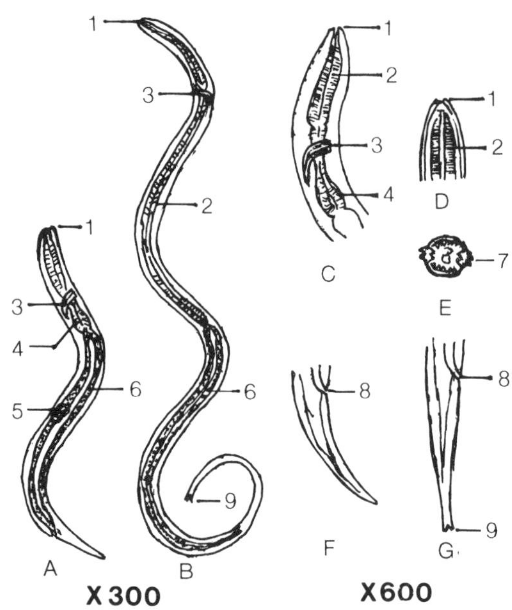

Figure 7.3 Larvae of S. stercoralis. (A) = rhabditiform larva; (B) = filariform larva; (C) and (D) = anterior end of rhabditiform and filariform larva, respectively; (E) = cross-section of filariform larva; (F) and (G) = posterior end of rhabditiform and filariform larva, respectively. 1 = mouth; 2 = esophagus; 3 = nerve ring; 4 = esophageal bulb; 5 = genital primordium; 6 = intestine; 7 = lateral alae; 8 = anus; 9 = notched tail. (Redrawn from Belding, 1942.)

become an infective filariform worm via the direct stage of development it becomes long and thin (Figure 7.3).

The third stage (L3) infective, or filariform, larva is 400 to 700 μm long by 12–20 μm in diameter. It exhibits sweeping and rapid directed movement. The mouth is a small pore which is probably impervious even to liquids. The main morphologic features are a long esophagus extending almost half the length of the worm and encircled at its upper third by a nerve ring. Although inconspicuous and visible only in cross-section, parallel ridges, or alae, run the length of the worm and even extend slightly beyond the tip of the tail. These provide the filariform larva with an important morphologic feature of a notched tail that distinguishes it from other filariform larvae, such as that of the hookworm (Figure 7.3). The sense organs in the anterior end of the worm (cervical papillae or deirids), and in the tail end (phasmids) are situated between the lateral alae. The nature and location of glands that produce the enzyme(s) required for skin penetration by the larvae have not been identified.

Strongyloides fulleborni, originally described as a parasite of baboons and chimpanzees in Africa, has been found to be a common infection of humans in many parts of Africa and New Guinea. *S. fulleborni* shares many morphologic and biologic similarities with *S. stercoralis*, but the main differential feature is that eggs of the parasite, instead of larvae, are passed in the feces. Therefore, *S. fulleborni* is considered in this review, along with *S. stercoralis*, as a human pathogen; significant differences between the two species will be noted.

7.3 LIFE CYCLE OF *S. STERCORALIS*

Infection is initiated by penetration of intact skin by infective filariform larvae (L3), regardless of whether they are the product of the direct or indirect cycle of development (Figure 7.4). After access to the blood stream or lymphatics, most larvae are believed to pass through the lungs in the usual migratory route exhibited by hookworm and *Ascaris* larvae. However, in view of recent studies with *S. ratti* (Dawkins, Thomason and Grove, 1982) and with *S. stercoralis* in dogs (Schad, Aikens and Smith, 1989), in which less than 5% of infecting larvae were demonstrated to pass through the lungs, the classical route of larval migration with *Strongyloides* has been questioned. Although differences in parasite strains, and technical difficulties inherent in performing such experiments may account for some of these discrepancies, the issue of larval migratory route for *Strongyloides* species remains open.

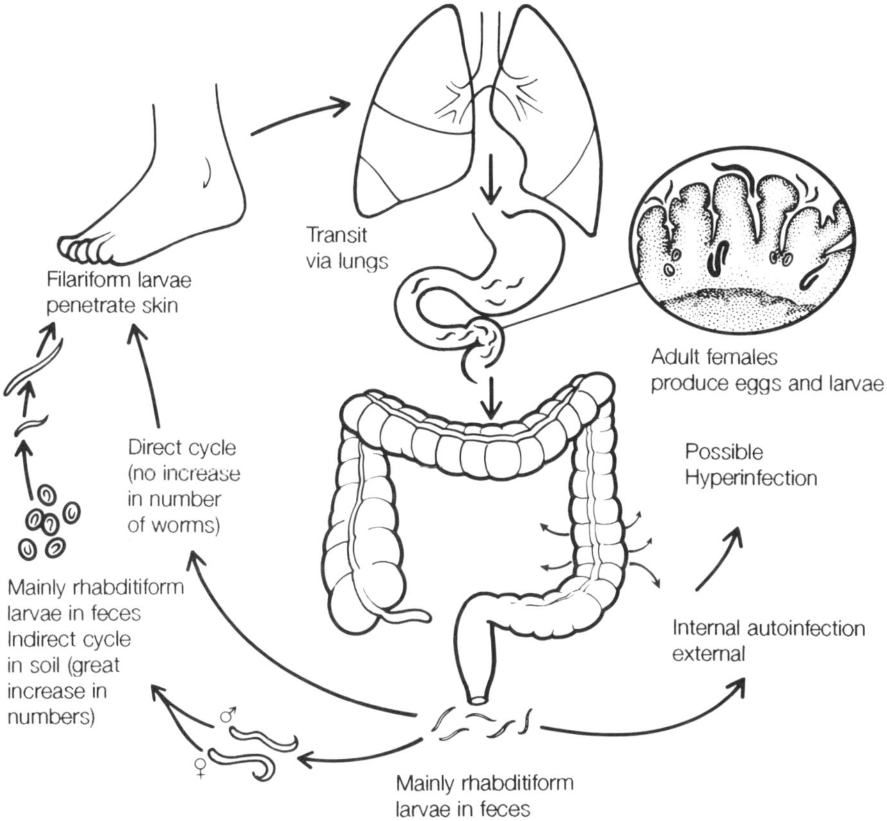

Figure 7.4 Life cycle of *S. stercoralis*. (Source: Neva and Brown, 1994.)

Larvae in transit through the lungs are still morphologically similar to infective L3 forms, but after breaking out of alveoli and migrating up the trachea, several additional molts occur during development to the adult stage. Detection and identification of the type of larvae in sputum has important clinical implications. Finding a rare or occasional filariform larva in the sputum is compatible with internal autoinfection; large numbers of L3 forms suggest hyperinfection, while presence of rhabditiform larvae indicates that adult female worms are present in the lungs.

The larvae which ascend the respiratory tract and are swallowed, or reach the upper gastrointestinal tract by other routes of tissue migration grow rapidly to adult females. They curl up deep in the crypts between intestinal villi, or embed themselves in or just under the mucosal epithelium of the upper small bowel and begin to lay eggs (Figure 7.4). The eggs hatch in or under the mucosa, and the L1 rhabditiform larva migrate out to the intestinal lumen to pass out with the feces. Although larvae in the feces of chronically infected individuals are all or predominantly rhabditiform, some may be larger, indicating development to L2 and L3 stage. Also, it is not unusual to find a few filariform larva present in routine specimens.

Although Kreis (1932) and Faust (1933) described the presence of parasitic male worms in the lungs and for a short period of time in the gut before being expelled, this has not been confirmed by subsequent workers. Their observations involved mainly strains of *S. stercoralis* from Louisiana that were passaged in dogs. The overwhelming evidence and prevailing current view is that *S. stercoralis* and related species have a parasitic female worm that is parthenogenetic. The prepatent period, i.e. the time after infection before larvae appear in the stool, is variable but can be as short as 10 or 11 days up to 3 or 4 weeks. In 26 monkeys (*Erythrocebus patas*) infected with 750 to 2500 larvae of the same serially passaged strain of *S. stercoralis* from south-east Asia, the prepatent period varied from 10 to 27 days.

After passage to the external environment, larvae may develop directly to the infective stage (homogonic type), or undergo a free-living generation (heterogonic or indirect type). In the latter case, some of the passed larvae must first develop into a free-living adult male and female worm. The female worm must be inseminated by male sperm in order to produce eggs, although apparently true fertilization does not occur. The resulting larva will then be a parasitic female worm. The net result of the indirect free-living cycle is that the parasite is amplified in numbers to optimize continued survival, even though only one free-living generation takes place. Whether produced by a direct or indirect cycle of development, the result is a filariform infective larva that initiates a new infection.

Infective larvae can develop from the L1 stage via the direct cycle within a day or two after passage in the feces. Six or seven days are required for development of infective larvae via the indirect cycle. In either case the actively motile L3 larvae crawl on to soil particles, literally standing on their tails, and if present in large numbers, aggregate into bunches, waiting to contact the skin of a potential host.

Many studies have attempted to identify the environmental and physiologic factors that determine direct or indirect larval development. Most investigations have been with non-human species of *Strongyloides*. Some authors have concluded that intrahost factors, such as density and duration of infection, or perhaps immunologic status of the host can affect the type of larval development. This could be very important if, for example, accelerated direct development resulted in production of large numbers of infective larvae and enhanced auto-infection. External environmental conditions, such as pH, temperature, and availability of food, can push the mode of larval development in one direction or another. These issues are discussed in greater detail by Schad (1989).

Parasitic females of *S. fulleborni* are also localized to the mucosa of the upper small bowel, and as noted earlier, discharge eggs rather than larvae, which are excreted. The eggs are about 50 × 30 μm in size, slightly smaller than hookworm eggs. Internal auto-infection presumably is not possible under these circumstances with this species, but the indirect cycle of development can occur. In fact, several authors have reported that multiple free-living generations can take place.

7.4 EPIDEMIOLOGY

Human infection with *S. stercoralis* is worldwide in distribution, but varies greatly in prevalence. Transmission is favored by conditions of poor sanitation, specifically with regard to fecal contamination of the environment, high humidity, and moderate to warm temperatures. Thus, highest levels of infection are found in the American, African and Asian tropics.

Prevalence rates of infection detected with this parasite will obviously depend upon the number and type of stool examinations, as well as the skill and experience of the examiners. Even allowing for such variables, certain regions of the world with very high rates can be identified, and a rough ranking of infection frequencies can be made. In some areas of rural Africa or South America overall infection rates of 10–20% of the population by a single stool examination are not unusual. Among certain urban populations in the developing world, 5–10% infection rates may be found. However, parasitologic surveys which find high infection rates with the common intestinal nematodes, such as *Trichuris, Ascaris* and hookworm, will generally report *Strongyloides* larvae in only 1 or 2%. Locally acquired strongyloidiasis has been reported from virtually all countries of Europe, including England and the southern former USSR. With a few exceptions, such as Ryukyu Island of southern Japan, a known endemic area, strongyloidiasis appears to be scarce or absent in northern regions of the temperate zone, but transmission of the parasite still occurs in the southern and south-eastern USA. In a local rural area of Kentucky, strongyloides infection was found in 3% (Walzer *et al.*, 1982).

Current surveys for prevalence of strongyloidiasis in the USA and northern Europe will be influenced by immigrant populations from endemic areas. For example, 11.5% of 776 newly arrived south-east Asian immigrants to the state of New Mexico were positive for *S. stercoralis* on a single stool exam (Skeels, Nims and Mann, 1982). Strongyloides infection was found to be the most common cause of eosinophilia in recent refugees from south-east Asia attending an out-patient clinic in the Washington DC area (Nutman *et al.*, 1987). A retrospective review of cases diagnosed in Paris concluded that very few were contracted in France, most had probably been acquired abroad while on work or military assignments, but many were Europeans from countries with a higher prevalence of stronglyloidiasis (Junod, 1987). The long duration of infections with *S. stercoralis* has additional implications, in contrast to other intestinal helminth infections of a much shorter life span. However, even Junod's study indicated that there was a progressive decrease in *S. stercoralis* infections detected in North Africans living in France for 20 years or more.

The long-term persistence of strongyloidiasis raises the pertinent question of whether new foci of transmission can be initiated by imported cases, and the likelihood of transmission within families. Where general levels of sanitation are adequate and fecal contamination of the environment does not occur, transmission would not be expected. However, sanitary conditions in some migrants labor camps in the USA might well permit transmission of strongyloidiasis. Outbreaks of strongyloidiasis have been described in mental hospitals and other institutions where adequate levels of personal hygiene are difficult to maintain (Yoeli *et al.*, 1972). Contributing factors include the possible presence of a few infective larvae in freshly passed stools, and the fact that a shorter time and less demanding physical conditions are required for larval development of *S. stercoralis* than for hookworm, for example. Grove (1982) found no serologic evidence of infection in any of 24 wives of ex-POWs who had been infected with *S. stercoralis* for 30 years or more – unusual but convincing evidence that even with intimate person-to-person contact transmission did not occur. Even transmission to homosexual partners does not appear to be common (Junod, 1987).

Although the evidence is anecdotal or circumstantial, infection with *S. stercoralis* seems more likely to involve certain occupational groups. Miners working underground in confined spaces cannot avoid contact with unplanned fecal deposits of fellow workers, where conditions of darkness, temperature and humidity are ideal for larval survival. The variety of *Strongyloides* found in dogs (Jaskoski, Barr and Borges, 1982) and in monkeys is indistinguishable from the human variety; indeed, in some instances it may have been acquired from humans. Yet, human infections presumably acquired from dogs appear to be rare (Georgi and Sprinkle, 1974). Sometimes outbreaks of strongyloidiasis occur in monkeys used for biomedical research (Harper *et al.*, 1982). In any event, animal caretakers, veterinarians, and underground miners may be at increased risk for acquisition of strongyloidiasis.

The epidemiology of *S. fulleborni* in humans has special features. Both in Africa and in New Guinea, infants a few months to a few years old are infected with this species. The predilection for the very young is even more striking in New Guinea where babies show evidence of infection by week 3 of life, and more than half of the population has patent infections by the age of 3 months (Ashford and Barnish, 1989). The rates are nearly 100% by 3 to 5 years of age and then fall off to 15–20% in adults. Since patent infections are not seen in the first two weeks of life, transmission is believed to occur postnatally, rather than congenitally. Infective larvae have been found in a mother's milk in Africa (Brown and Girardeau, 1977), but this has not yet been demonstrated in New Guinea. Nevertheless, the transmammary route is believed to be the major mechanism of transmission of the New Guinea parasite.

7.5 PATHOGENESIS

Penetration of the skin by infective larvae is the first critical event in the pathogenesis of strongyloidiasis. Recently, a metalloprotease was identified in excretions/secretions of infective larvae (McKerrow *et al.*, 1990), and penetration of larvae through rat skin preparations was shown to be blocked by inhibitors of this class of proteases. Elastase activity and ability to degrade an artificial extracellular matrix was demonstrated for the protease, suggesting that it also functioned in tissue migration of filariform larvae. These observations, plus the report by Dresden, Rege and Murrell (1985) of metalloprotease activity in extracts of another species, *S. ransomi*, provide a molecular basis for the earlier general observation of Lewert and Lee (1956) that larval extracts of *S. ratti* had collagenase-like properties. Pruritic, erythematous papules that persist for hours to days have been noted in the skin of subjects experimentally infected by local application of infective larvae. These presumably are a reaction to materials produced by the larvae, and are not a consequence of previous allergic sensitization. Whatever the nature of the enzymes that allow larval movement through the skin, the material has striking biologic activity as evidenced by the rate of larval movement. They have been 'clocked' at speeds of 2–10 cm/h by several different observers (Grove, 1989b). This is the manifestation termed larval currens, produced by larvae as they migrate in the skin of the buttocks after reinvasion from the rectal or perianal area.

On route to their ultimate destination in the intestine, a variable proportion of larvae traverse the lungs where they may produce several types of pathologic changes. A single exposure to large numbers of larvae may be associated with a non-productive, irritative cough lasting a day or two within 4 to 7 days of infection. This is probably due to local tissue damage as larvae break out of pulmonary vessels, undergo growth and molting, and start their journey up the respiratory tract. In some situations, and for unknown reasons, some larvae may remain in the lungs, develop to adult female worms, and produce rhabditiform larvae that can be demonstrated in the sputum. In studies of dogs infected with *Strongyloides* from humans and monkeys, Faust (1935) was impressed with the frequent finding of parasitic female worms in the lungs. Pulmonary strongyloidiasis, as evidenced by larvae in the sputum, seems to be reported commonly in patients with underlying chronic pulmonary disease, such as bronchiectasis or emphysema, suggesting that damaged bronchi provide favored sites for development of adult female worms. However, this association may simply reflect the greater likelihood for such patients to be treated with corticosteroids and to develop hyperinfection syndrome.

Hyperinfection syndrome is frequently associated with pneumonitis or pneumonia, along with systemic signs and symptoms of fever, cough, purulent sputum and pulmonary infiltrates by chest radiograph. Some of this picture is certainly due to large numbers of larvae migrating through the lungs as a consequence of hyperinfection. Cases that come to autopsy show larvae in tissue sections, but not in numbers that would be expected; yet, patchy hemorrhages are a prominent feature. Carriage of gram negative bacteria from the gut by migrating larvae has been postulated as a cause of the pneumonia, but no consistent bacterial flora has been documented in such cases.

Rarely, but dramatically, strongyloidiasis can present clinically as tropical pulmonary eosinophilia, with cough, wheezing and very high peripheral blood eosinophilia (Nwokolo and Imohiosen, 1973). The clinical picture, and probably the basic pathophysiology as well, is similar to that associated with filarial infections in which microfilariae are trapped in the lungs (Neva and Ottesen, 1978). Since patients with hyperinfection syndrome frequently exhibit variable degrees of respiratory symptoms, such as cough and wheezing, an IgE-mediated allergic component may be the basis for some of their pathology and symptomatology.

The major sites of pathologic changes in strongyloidiasis are the upper and lower gastrointestinal tracts. The duodenum and upper jejunum harbor the adult female worms, eggs and larvae, while various levels of the colon may show evidence of invading filariform larvae. Female worms burrow deep in the crypts between intestinal villi, often penetrating the mucosa into the lamina propria, and then lay their eggs. From these sequestered locations, motile rhabditiform larvae work their way to the lumen of the small intestine to be carried along with intestinal contents and excreted. Thus, the relationship between the parasite and cellular elements of the mucosa and submucosa are intimate enough to ensure immunologic recognition by the host. Yet, there is great variability in the inflammatory response around the worms and larvae in the gut. Alterations in the small bowel mucosa are generally proportional to the severity of symptoms. With increased numbers of worms the intestinal villi show a cellular infiltrate of lymphocytes and eosinophils, and there is edema of the underlying lamina propria. The villous structure may show some flattening, and dilatation of lymphatic lacteals.

The most severe small bowel changes are associated with hyperinfection syndrome. A prominent inflammatory exudate, including parasites, fills the lamina propria, completely disrupting the normal villous pattern, and producing mucosal erosions (Figure 7.5a). But these severely affected areas may be patchy, with adjacent relatively normal areas. Malabsorption and/or diarrhea is often present. Damage to ganglion cells of the myenteric plexus may contribute to paralytic ileus which is frequently seen in patients with hyperinfection due to *S. stercoralis*. Striking enlargement of mesenteric lymph nodes is seen in some cases. In patients with achlorhydria and long-standing infections, parasites may be found in the gastric mucosa and gastric contents. Similarly, the mucosa as far down as the ileum may contain parasitic females.

Pathologic changes in the colon indicate that rhabditiform larvae have already molted to become infective filariform larvae, and are invading. This can occur as proximal as the cecum. Filariform larvae can penetrate into the muscular layer of the colon; their presence is frequently associated with prominent edema in the lamina propria, but they often have no surrounding inflammatory reaction. Other tissue sections in the same patient may show prominent granulomas around degenerating larvae. The colonic mucosa may be sufficiently damaged to result in significant lower intestinal bleeding (Figure 7.5b).

Larvae may be found in virtually any organ

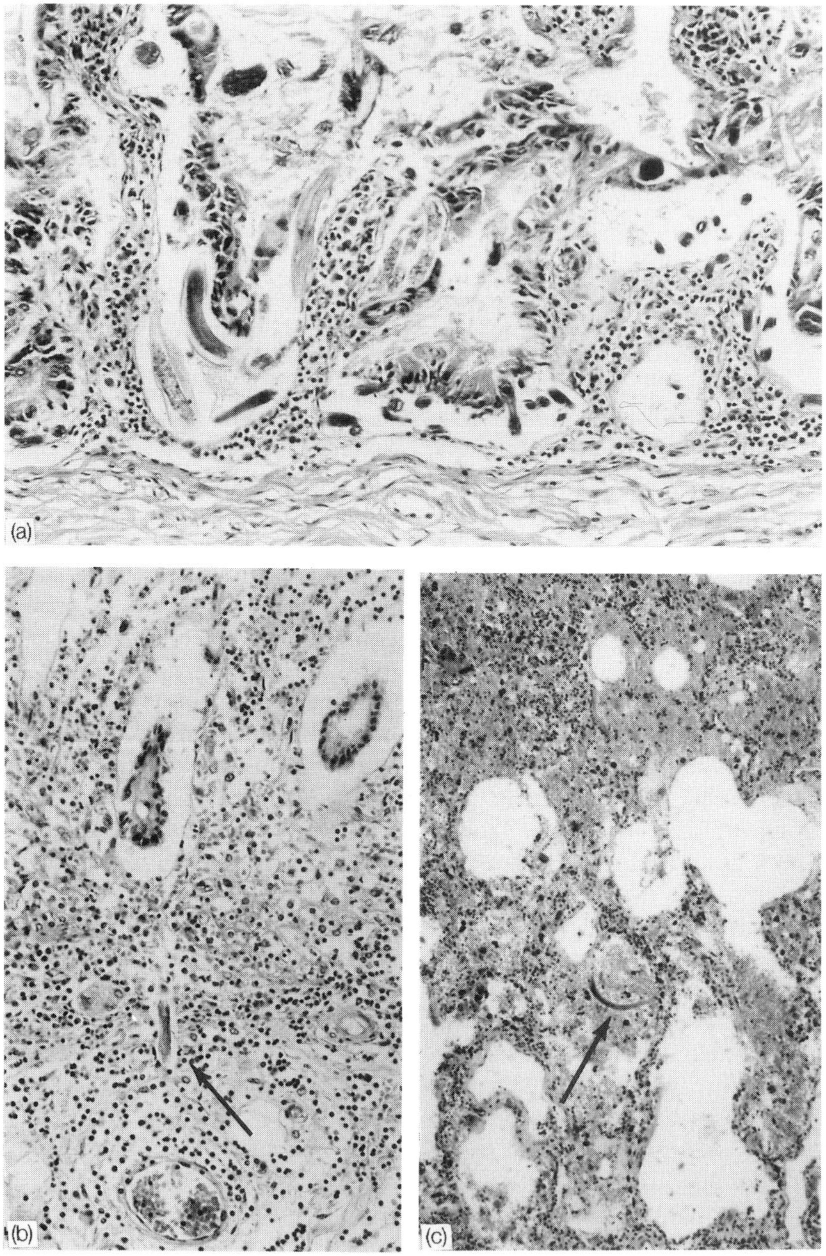

Figure 7.5 (a) Section of small intestine from case of fatal hyperinfection with *S. stercoralis*. Portions of adult worms, larvae, and eggs are seen with disruption of normal villous structure, but inflammation is confined to the lamina propria. (× 200.) (b) Section through colon showing intense inflammation and edema. The arrow points to an invading filariform larva (× 200.) (c) Section of lung from same case showing hemorrhagic pneumonia, with larva in alveolus indicated by arrow (× 100.)

or tissue when hyperinfection occurs. They have frequently been demonstrated in the liver, both in portal tracts and in the hepatic parenchyma. Frequent involvement of the lungs by *S. stercoralis* has already been described (Figure 7.5c). Their presence in the myocardium, urinary tract, spleen and endocrine organs has been reported, but is rare and has not been associated with clinical manifestations. One instance of joint involvement with arthritis has been reported.

Central nervous system invasion by *S. stercoralis* larvae, however, is not unusual, and purulent meningitis caused by gram negative bacteria is quite common. More than 25% of cases of hyperinfection syndrome collected from the literature were reported to have meningitis, and in nearly half of these cases the organism was a gram negative rod (Igra-Siegman *et al.*, 1981). The purulent meningitis is probably secondary to gram negative bacteremia that frequently accompanies the meningitis, rather than caused by bacteria transported on or in migrating larvae.

7.6 EXPERIMENTAL ANIMAL MODELS

Strongyloides ratti infection in the rat or mouse is a convenient animal model for investigation of certain aspects of strongyloidiasis, but it is not suitable to study causative factors of hyperinfection syndrome because autoinfection cannot be induced. The model is well suited, for example, to study events during and soon after skin penetration by infective larvae, such as loss of the external cuticle (Grove *et al.*, 1987) and the fate of larvae in the skin (Dawkins, Thomason and Grove, 1982). Some insights into immune response from an initial infection can be obtained (Genta *et al.*, 1983b), but the phenomenon of spontaneous expulsion of worms from the gut that occurs with *S. ratti* is not a feature of human strongyloidiasis. Although increased duration of *S. ratti* infection is seen after administration of steroids, autoinfection and hyperinfection have never been observed with this parasite in the rat (Olson and Schiller, 1978; Moqbel and Denham, 1978).

Certain primate species and dogs, however, can be infected with human *S. stercoralis* and, in addition, they resemble the human host by developing hyperinfection when steroids are given. This has been well documented in *Erythrocebus patas* (Harper *et al.*, 1984) and in dogs (Grove, Heenan and Northern, 1983) (Genta, Schad and Hellman, 1986). Published and unpublished observations (Neva and Gam, 1992), always using the same south-east Asian human strain of *S. stercoralis*, have given consistent results in *Patas* monkeys. With inocula of 800–1200 larvae, fatal infections developed in several monkeys (3 of 26), but in most animals infections became chronic and administration of prednisone was required to activate a chronic infection. Continued administration of corticosteroid led to fatal hyperinfection, with pulmonary hemorrhage as the most consistent finding at autopsy. Although the experience is small, gibbons appear to be unusually susceptible to infection with *S. stercoralis* (DePaoli and Johnson, 1978). Cumulative experience with experimental infections, especially of dogs, with human *S. stercoralis*, suggest that inconsistent results may be due to geographically different parasite strains, with variable pathogenicity. In addition, conclusions about resistance to infection may have been erroneous due to failure to examine specimens for small numbers of larvae.

7.7 CLINICAL FEATURES

The literature on clinical strongyloidiasis is distorted by its emphasis upon the immunosuppressed patient with hyperinfection syndrome and unusual clinical manifestations. The majority of individuals infected with *S. stercoralis* are asymptomatic and do not generally seek medical care. Yet, if those incidentally found to be infected by *S. stercoralis* by routine surveys are questioned more closely about specific symptoms, many will comment upon various degrees of epigastric discomfort, intermittent loose stools, poor appetite and abdominal bloating after eating. Also, history of intermittent urticarial skin rashes over the buttocks, lower back or upper thighs can often be elicited. The skin rashes may either be linear and migratory, or patchy and non-specific. Larva currens move more rapidly than creeping eruption due to dog and cat hookworm larvae.

A history of gastrointestinal complaints, necessitating use of antacids, or previous upper gastrointestinal surgery tends to be associated with strongyloidiasis. Whether gastric anacidity or impaired motility of the gut or post-surgical blind loops predispose to infection with the parasite, or simply favor its survival is not clear. The diarrhea associated with strongyloides infection is usually not severe and does not contain frank blood, but enough bleeding to produce guaiac-positive stools is common. Small bowel malabsorption due to *S. stercoralis* when the disease process is limited to the gastrointestinal tract may occur (Amir–Ahmadi *et al.*, 1968), but it is more likely to be related to malnutrition rather than to a direct effect of the parasite (Garcia *et al.*, 1977).

In patients with hyperinfection syndrome, gastrointestinal and pulmonary manifestations become more prominent. Instead of diarrhea the patient may present with abdominal distention and ileus, simulating obstruction of the bowel or peritonitis. Cough, production of sputum and evidence of pneumonia often develops, with fever and a septic state progressing to shock. Signs of meningitis or more focal neurologic deficits can occur. Blood or spinal fluid cultures are likely to grow gram negative enteric organisms. This is the type of clinical picture that has been associated with patients with chronic pulmonary disease, lupus erythematosus or rheumatoid arthritis treated with steroids. A large series has been reported by De Vault *et al.* (1990) in patients immunosuppressed for renal transplantation. Interestingly, this report commented upon the absence of reports of strongyloides hyperinfection in renal allograft recipients receiving cyclosporin A.

7.8 HOST DEFENSE

Host defense in strongyloidiasis can be considered in terms of non-specific or poorly defined factors that prevent normal development of the parasite, as well as on the basis of specific humoral and cell-mediated immunologic responses to parasite antigens. The fact that successful infection with various species of *Strongyloides* is restricted to certain hosts is an example of the first category of host defence. Until the specific mechanism to explain accelerated larval development and resultant autoinfection can be defined, the breakdown in host defense associated with hyperinfection also remains in the poorly defined category. The status of humoral, and to a lesser extent, of cell-mediated immune function can be assessed, but up to now these measures have contributed little to understanding host control of strongyloidiasis. Serum IgG antibodies to filariform larval antigens can be demonstrated in 85–95% of infected individuals by ELISA (Neva, Gam and Burke, 1981) or immunofluorescence tests (Dafalla, 1972; Genta and Weil, 1983). IgM responses can be demonstrated in early stages of experimental infections (Grove and Northern, 1982), but are usually negative in human cases, presumably because it is impossible to define when infection was acquired. A test for parasite-specific IgA antibodies has been described (Genta, Frei and Linke, 1987). Severe strongyloidiasis in two patients with hypogammaglobulinemia has been reported (Shelhamer, Neva and Finn, 1982; de Oliveira, Voltarelli and Meneghelli, 1981), but impaired cell-mediated function was also present in one of the cases.

Although elevated total serum IgE levels have been reported in some groups of patients with strongyloidiasis, information on the more significant issue of parasite-specific IgE in such patients is still fragmentary. Using an assay of relative binding of radiolabelled anti-IgE in a few patients, Genta, Douce and Walzer (1986) suggested that hyperinfection may have been due to very low serum levels of parasite-specific IgE. Technical improvements in the assay and a larger experience are needed in further studies correlating clinical status with specific IgE.

The role of direct T lymphocyte function has not provided much insight in evaluating host defenses in strongyloidiasis. However, no published studies are available about possible indirect roles for T cells in terms of cytokine production. Both Genta *et al* (1983a) and Sato and Shiroma (1989) found decreased mitogen responses but neither group found significant responses of T cells to strongyloides antigen in patients. The Japanese results may have been influenced by the high prevalence of HTLV-1 infection in their patients. One problem in interpretation of T cell function in strongyloidiasis is that virtually all patients studied are chronically infected so that cellular responses may be down-regulated.

Although supporting evidence is sketchy, perhaps immediate hypersensitivity responses involving the IgE/mast cell system may be an important host defense system in strongyloidiasis. Expulsion of intestinal nematodes in rodent models is associated with peripheral basophilia and a great increase in blood histamine levels (Roth and Levy, 1980) and delayed expulsion of worms from the gut, was attributed to depletion of intestinal mast cells in rats given cortisone (Olson and Schiller, 1978). Depletion of intestinal mast cell numbers and histamine content was also observed in *S. stercoralis*-infected monkeys after treatment with prednisone (Barrett *et al.*, 1988). We (Neva *et al.*, unpublished data) have been impressed with evidence of impaired reaginic function in certain patients infected with both *S. stercoralis* and the human T cell leukemia retrovirus (HTLV-1). This has been manifested by very low total and specific serum IgE levels, by failure to mount an immediate hypersensitivity skin test response to strongyloides antigens and by only temporary response to treatment with thiabendazole. Failure to cure strongyloidiasis with the drug in strongyloidiasis patients infected with HTLV-1 has also been reported from Jamaica by Terry *et al.* (1989). Interestingly, in a group of HIV-infected patients with strongyloidiasis in Zaire, positive immediate skin test reactions to strongyloides antigens, normal or high IgE levels, and no apparent predisposition to hyperinfection were observed (Neva *et al.*, unpublished).

A number of observations suggest that host defense mechanisms against *S. stercoralis* are only partially and never completely effective. The long persistence of infection in the POWs described earlier, and other instances of prolonged infection, suggest that the infected host usually cannot prevent a continuing low level of internal autoinfection by the parasite. Even though more detailed information to rule out the persistence of a previous infection are lacking, several early workers failed to demonstrate immunity to reinfection in themselves (Freedman, 1991). Similarly, a repeated human self-infection with *S. fulleborni* indicated lack of immunity from a previous infection four months earlier. Evidence both for and against immunity to reinfection with *S. stercoralis* and *S. fulleborni* in dogs has been reported over the years. A convincing example of significant but not total resistance to re-infection with *S. stercoralis* in Patas monkeys is available (Neva, 1986).

7.9 DIAGNOSIS

Direct microscopic visualization of the parasite in the feces, sputum, or other body fluids and tissues is the only definitive method of diagnosis of strongyloidiasis. Since the larvae, the usual form of the parasite observed, are often motile, specimens can be initially scanned with a 2 or 3 × magnification. Unfortunately, excretion of larvae in the stool is frequently scanty and irregular, so that after screening one or two direct smears, concentration methods must be used, such as the formalin-ether or formalin ethylacetate procedure. The formalin will kill motile larvae, so higher magnification (10 ×) is generally required in examining the concentrated sediment, containing a drop or two of iodine solution. The entire sediment must be examined. If these efforts are still negative, and strongyloidiasis must be excluded, examination of additional specimens or more efficient concentration methods are required. A simple technique, although not necessarily more efficient than the formalin concentration, is the Harada–Mori culture. In this procedure, about 0.5 g feces is smeared along the upper three quarters of a strip of filter paper and then inserted, clean end down, into a wide test tube containing about 2 ml of water. The tube is allowed to stand upright in the dark at room temperature, so that larvae can migrate into the water. The water is sampled daily, or after several days for evidence of strongyloides larvae.

The most sensitive methods of fecal examination for *S. stercoralis* are the Baermann concentration procedure or the direct culture technique, which are described in greater detail elsewhere (Neva, 1986). The new technique of agar plate culture, which has received attention recently because of its novel features, involves smearing some of the fecal specimen in the center of an agar plate and examining later for circular streaks of motile larvae (Koga *et al.*, 1990). The most important principle to remember about any method of fecal examination for larvae of *S. stercoralis* is that the likelihood of finding scanty numbers of larvae depends upon the amount of specimen examined. The direct fecal smear generally examines 2 or 3 mg of stool, the formalin concentrate about 0.5 g, while the Baermann concentration can process 10 to 50 g.

Because pulmonary involvement is so common in strongyloidiasis, especially in hyperinfection syndrome, it is useful to remember that larvae can often be demonstrated in sputum, or in bronchial washings (Figure 7.6a, b). Examination of an unfixed specimen will permit spotting motile larvae. In patients with CNS involvement or meningitis, larvae have only rarely been found in the cerebrospinal fluid.

If circumstances and the patient permit, larvae may be sought directly in intestinal contents obtained by duodenal aspiration. The so-called string test can also be used in which an encapsulated string is swallowed, later withdrawn and intestinal mucus stripped for examination. Neither of these procedures is necessarily more efficient than one or more stool examination, but they may yield a positive result at any one time in a given patient when stool examination is negative.

S. stercoralis larvae in the stool must be differentiated from hookworm larvae, which may hatch from hookworm eggs if the stool specimen is held at room temperature for half a day or more. Filariform larvae of *S. stercoralis* are the easiest to identify because they have a notched tail.

Several serologic tests for IgG antibodies to filariform larvae of *S. stercoralis* have been developed and are becoming available in some commercial laboratories. The most commonly used is the ELISA, which will be positive in 85–95% of parasitologically proven cases (Grove, 1989c). The test has been used in the Sudan, Australia, USA and Japan with consistent results. The indirect fluorescent antibody (IFA) test with larval anti-

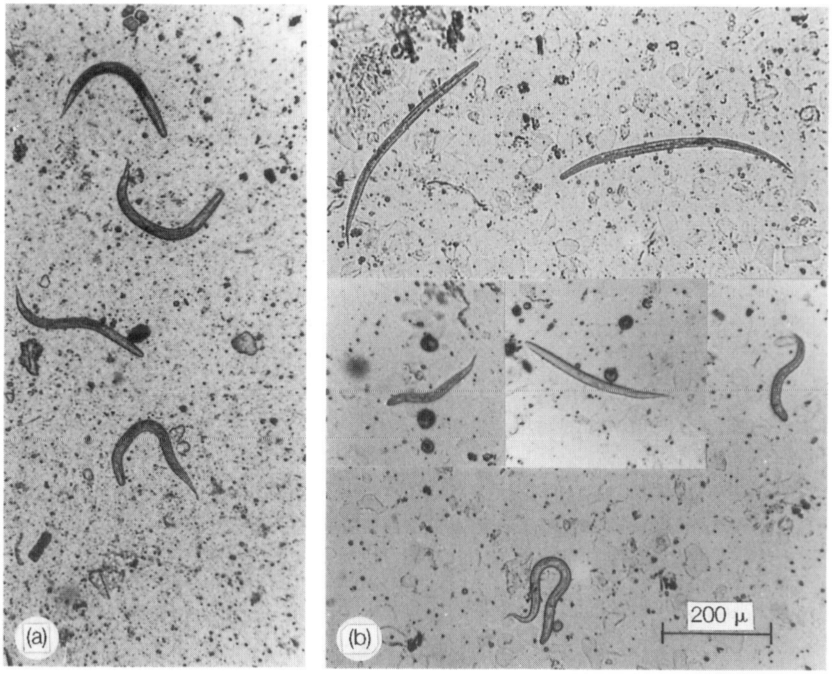

Figure 7.6 *Strongyloides* larvae in the stool (a) and in the sputum (b) of a patient. Note that larvae in the stool are rhabditiform, whereas the sputum contains both filariform and rhabditiform larvae, indicating that adult female worms are present in the lungs. Magnification for (a) is the same as in (b). (Source: Shelhamer, Neva and Finn, 1982.)

gens may be slightly more sensitive, but is also more complicated to use. Sera from some patients with filarial and onchocerca infections, especially those with an exaggerated immune response, will cross-react with *S. stercoralis* larval antigens. A decline in titer or even negative tests for antibody by the ELISA test have been noted within one or two years in many strongyloides patients after therapy. If this can be confirmed and found to be a consistent finding in patients parasitologically negative after treatment, serology would be a convenient way to assess outcome of therapy.

What may be the most rapid, convenient and specific diagnostic test for strongyloidiasis – namely, an immediate hypersensitivity skin test – is available only for research purposes. Encouraging results were obtained by earlier workers using skin test antigens prepared from *S. stercoralis* or *S. fulleborni* filariform larvae. More recently, Sato *et al.* (1986) reported finding positive reactions in 83% of 52 infected patients using a larval extract as antigen. We have found an immediate skin test using excretion/secretion (E/S) antigens of filariform *S. stercoralis* larvae to be more specific and discriminating than somatic antigen (Neva, unpublished data). However, until the antigen(s) can be purified and characterized more fully, such a test will remain investigational.

7.10 TREATMENT

Until thiabendazole was introduced in the early 1960s, the treatment of strongyloidiasis was unsatisfactory. Following a dosage of

25 mg/kg of the drug twice daily for 2 or 3 days, 70% or more of most infections will be temporarily eliminated or cured. However, the experience with immunosuppressed patients who have hyperinfection indicates that treatment should be continued for 5 to 7 days to control the infection. It may also be necessary to use intermittent long-term treatment, such as a 2- or 3-day course every month, or half-doses for a week each month, thereafter. Unfortunately, nausea, anorexia, dizziness and malaise are common side-effects of thiabendazole; it is not an easy drug to tolerate. More serious complications such as erythema multiforme, increased serum transaminase and cholestasis may rarely occur. Critical and long-term evaluation of drug therapy under conditions in which re-infection is unlikely, has seldom been done. This would include multiple Baermann concentrations, since light infections are difficult to detect.

Several subsequent benzimidazole analogues, cambendazole and albendazole, as well as the new antifilarial drug, ivermectin, have been found to be effective in treatment of strongyloidiasis. Cambendazole was withdrawn for human use because of rare fatal reactions in cattle. Albendazole and ivermectin have not yet been approved for treatment of strongyloidiasis in the United States, but both appear to be as effective as thiabendazole and much less toxic. For maximum efficacy, albendazole was given in two separate courses 14 days apart, in a dosage of 16–20 mg/kg daily for 3 days (Mojon and Nielsen, 1987). Ivermectin has been given in a single dose of 200 μg/kg for one or two days. An interrupted course of treatment about two weeks apart, may also be advantageous for ivermectin and thiabendazole, the empirical rationale being that the drugs are more active against the parasite in different stages of development during internal autoinfection. However, experimental studies of drug action against different developmental stages of the parasite are difficult to interpret (Grove and Northern, 1988). Treatment of ill patients with the hyperinfection syndrome should include broad spectrum anti-bacterial medication to avoid septicemia and bacterial meningitis.

7.11 PREVENTION AND CONTROL

Since infection with this parasite is so clearly dependent upon human contact with an environment contaminated with human or animal faeces, measures for prevention and control are straightforward. Educating the population as to how strongyloidiasis and other enteric infectious diseases are transmitted is worthwhile. Provision of latrines or designated sites for defecation is important especially for agricultural and other outdoor workers. People should be encouraged to wear shoes, if they have them, especially when frequenting areas where fecal contamination is likely to be encountered. No special enteric precautions are required for hospital staff and health care workers in caring for a patient with strongyloidiasis. Wet linen soiled with feces should be disposed of appropriately to minimize chances for survival and development of larvae. Health care workers dealing with a patient with hyperinfection should take appropriate precautions, since the patient may be excreting large numbers of larvae in the sputum as well as in feces.

The possible existence of chronic or asymptomatic strongyloidiasis should be considered in patients who are about to undergo organ transplantation or aggressive therapy for malignancy. This is especially pertinent if the patient has lived in areas endemic for the parasite, and if the treatment will include long-term steroid administration. If infection with *S. stercoralis* is suspected, on the basis of a serologic test or presence of eosinophilia, the diagnosis should be pursued further, and kept in mind as a possible future complication.

REFERENCES

Amir-Ahmadi, H., Braun, P., Neva, F. A. *et al.* (1968) Strongyloidiasis at the Boston City Hospital. Emphasis on gastrointestinal pathophysiology and successful therapy with thiabendazole. *Am. J. Digest. Dis.*, **13**, 959–73.

Ashford, R. W. and Barnish, G. (1989) *Strongyloides fulleborni* and similar parasites in animals and man, in *Strongyloidiasis: A Major Roundworm Infection of Man* (ed. D. I. Grove), Taylor and Francis, New York, pp. 271–86.

Barrett, K. E., Neva, F. A., Garn, A. A. *et al.* (1988) The immune response to nematode parasites: modulation of mast cell numbers and function during *Strongyloides stercoralis* infections in non-human primates. *Am. J. Trop. Med. Hyg.*, **38**, 574–81.

Belding, D. L. (1942) *Textbook of Clinical Parasitology*. Appleton–Century Co. Incorp., N. Y. p. 275.

Bras, G., Richards, R. C., Irvine, R. A. *et al.* (1964) Infection with *Strongyloides stercoralis* in Jamaica. *Lancet*, **ii**, 1257–60.

Brown, R. C. and Girardeau, M. H. E. (1977) Transmammary passage of *Strongyloides* sp. larvae in the human host. *Am. J. Trop. Med. Hyg.*, **26**, 215–19.

Cruz, T., Reboucas, G. and Rocha, H. (1966) Fatal strongyloidiasis in patients receiving corticosteroids. *New Eng. J. Med.*, **275**, 1093–6.

Dafalla, A. A. (1972) The indirect fluorescent antibody test for serodiagnosis of strongyloidiasis. *J. Trop. Med. Hyg.*, **75**, 109–11.

Dawkins, H. J. S., Thomason, H. J. and Grove, D. I. (1982) The occurrence of *Strongyloides ratti* in the tissues of mice after percutaneous infection. *J. Helminth.*, **56**, 45–50.

de Oliveira, R. B., Voltarelli, J. C. and Meneghelli, U. G. (1981) Severe strongyloidiasis associated with hypogamma-globulinemia. *Parasite Immun.*, **3**, 165–9.

DePaoli, A. and Johnson, D. O. (1978) Fatal strongyloidiasis in gibbons. *Vet. Parasit.*, **15**, 31–9.

DeVault, G. A., King, J. W., Rohr, M. S. *et al.* (1990) Opportunistic infections with *Strongyloides stercoralis* in renal transplantation. *Rev. Infect. Dis.*, **12**, 653–71.

Dresden, M. H., Rege, A. A. and Murrell, K. D. (1985) *Strongyloides ransomi*: proteolytic enzymes from larvae. *Expl. Parasit.*, **59**, 257–63.

Faust, E. C. (1933), Experimental studies on human and primate species of *Strongyloides*. II The development of *Strongyloides* in the experimental host. *Am. J. Hyg.*, **18**, 114–32.

Faust, E. C. (1935) Experimental studies on human and primate species of *Strongyloides*. IV. The pathology of strongyloides infection. *Archs Path.*, **19**, 769–806.

Freedman, D. O. (1991) Experimental infection of human subjects with *Strongyloides* species. *Rev. Infect. Dis.*, **13**, 1221–6.

Fulleborn, F. (1926) Hautquaddeln und 'Autoinfection' bei *Strongyloides*-stagern, *Arch. Schiffs Trop. Hyg.*, **30**, 721–32.

Gage, J. G. (1911) A case of *Strongyloides intestinalis* with larvae in the sputum. *Archs Int. Med.*, **7**, 55–9.

Garcia, F. T., Sessions, J. T. and Strum, W. B. (1977) Intestinal function and morphology in strongyloidiasis. *Am. J. Trop. Med. Hyg.*, **26**, 859–65.

Genta, R. M. and Weil, G. J. (1983) Antibodies to *Strongyloides stercoralis* larval surface antigens in chronic strongyloidiasis. *Lab. Invest.*, **47**, 87–90.

Genta, R. M., Douce, R. W. and Walzer, P. D. (1986a) Diagnostic implications of parasite-specific immune responses in immunocompromised patients with strongyloidiasis. *J. Clin. Microbiol.*, **23**, 1099–103.

Genta, R. M., Schad, G. A. and Hellman, M. E. (1986b) *Strongyloides stercoralis*: parasitological, immunological and pathological observations in immunosuppressed dogs. *Trans. Royal Soc. Trop. Med. Hyg.*, **80**, 34–41.

Genta, R. M., Frei, D. F. and Linke, M. J. (1987) Demonstration and partial characterization of parasite-specific IgA responses in human strongyloidiasis. *J. Clin. Microbiol.*, **25**, 1505–10.

Genta, R. M., Ottesen, E. A., Neva, F. A. *et al.* (1983a) Cellular responses in human strongyloidiasis. *Am. J. Trop. Med. Hyg.*, **32**, 990–4.

Genta, R. M., Ottesen, E. A., Gam, A. A. and Neva, F. A. (1983b) Immunologic responses to experimental strongyloidiasis in rats. *Z. Parasitenk.*, **69**, 667–75.

Georgi, J. R. and Sprinkle, C. L. (1974) A case of human strongyloidiasis apparently contracted from asymptomatic colony dogs. *Am. J. Trop. Med. Hyg.*, **23**, 899–901.

Gill, G. V. and Bell, D. R. (1979) Strongyloides infection in former Far East prisoners of war. *Br. Med. J.*, **2**, 572–4.

Grove, D. I. (1980) Strongyloidiasis in Allied ex-prisoners of war in southeast Asia. *Br. Med. J.*, **280**, 598–601.

Grove, D. I. (1982) Strongyloidiasis: is it transmitted from husband to wife? *Br. J. Vener. Dis.*, **58**, 271–2.

Grove, D. I. (1989a) Historical introduction, in *Strongyloidiasis: A Major Roundworm Infection of Man* (ed. D. I. Grove), Taylor and Francis, New York, pp. 1–9.

Grove, D. I. (1989b) Clinical manifestations, in *Strongyloidiasis: A Major Roundworm Infection of Man* (ed. D. I. Grove), Taylor and Francis, New York, pp. 155–73.

Grove, D. I. (1989c) Diagnosis, in *Strongyloidiasis: A Major Roundworm Infection of Man*, (ed. D. I. Grove), Taylor and Francis, New York, pp. 175–97.

Grove, D. I. and Northern, C. (1982) Infection and immunity in dogs infected with a human strain of *Strongyloides stercoralis*. *Trans. Roy. Soc. Trop. Med. Hyg.*, **76**, 833–8.

Grove, D. I. and Northern, C. (1988) The effects of thiabendazole, mebendazole and cambendazole in normal and immunosuppressed dogs infected with a human strain of *Strongyloides stercoralis*. *Trans. Roy. Soc. Trop. Med. Hyg.*, **82**, 146–9.

Grove, D. I., Heenan, P. J. and Northern, C. (1983) Persistent and disseminated infections with *Strongyloides stercoralis* in immunosuppressed dogs. *Int. J. Parasit.*, **13**, 483–90.

Grove, D. I., Warton, A., Northern, C. and Papadimitrou, J. M. (1987) Electron microscopical studies of *Strongyloides ratti* larvae: loss of surface coat during skin penetration. *J. Parasit.*, **73**, 1030–4.

Harper, J. S., Rice, J. M., London, W. T. *et al.* (1982) Disseminated strongyloidiasis in *Erythrocebus patas*. *Am. J. Primat.*, **3**, 89–98.

Harper, J. S., Genta, R. M. and Gam, A. *et al.* (1984) Experimental disseminated strongyloidiasis in *Erythrocebus patas* I. Pathology. *Am. J. Trop. Med. Hyg.*, **33**, 431–43.

Igra-Siegman, U., Kapila, R., Sen, P. *et al.* (1981) Syndrome of hyperinfection with *Strongyloides stercoralis*. *Rev. Infect. Dis.*, **3**, 397–407.

Jaskoski, B., Barr, V. and Borges, M. (1982) Intestinal parasites of well-cared-for-dogs: an area revisited. *Am. J. Trop. Med. Hyg.*, **31**, 1107–10.

Junod, C. (1987) Etude retrospective de 1934 cas de strongyloidose diagnostiques à Paris (1970–1986). *Bull. Soc. Path. Exot.*, **80**, 357–69.

Koga, K., Kasuya, S., Khamboonruang, C. *et al.* (1990) An evaluation of the agar plate method for the detection of *Strongyloides stercoralis* in northern Thailand. *J. Trop. Med. Hyg.*, **93**, 183–8.

Kreis, H. (1932) Studies on the genus *Strongyloides* (Nematoda). *Am. J. Hyg.*, **16**, 450–1.

Lewert, R. M. and Lee, C. L. (1956) Quantitative studies of the collagenase-like enzymes of cercariae of *Schistosoma mansoni* and the larvae of *Strongyloides ratti*. *J. Infect. Dis.*, **99**, 1–14.

McKerrow, J. H., Brindley, P., Brown, M. *et al.* (1990) *Strongyloides stercoralis*: identification of a protease that facilitates penetration of skin by the infective larvae. *Exp. Parasit.*, **70**, 134–43.

Mojon, M. and Nielsen, P. B. (1987) Treatment of *Strongyloides stercoralis* with albendazole. A cure rate of 86 percent. *Zentbl. Bakt. Hyg., A.*, **263**, 619–24.

Moqbel, R. and Denham, D. A. (1978) *Strongyloides ratti*: the effect of betamethasone on the course of infection in rats. *Parasitology*, **76**, 289–98.

Neva, F. A. (1986) Biology and immunology of human strongyloidiasis. *J. Infect. Dis.*, **153**, 397–406.

Neva, F. A. and Brown, H. W. (1994) *Basic Clinical Parasitology*. 6th edn, Appleton and Lange, Norwalk, Connecticut.

Neva, F. A. and Gam, A. A. (1992) Unpublished data.

Neva, F. A. (1994) *Basic Clinical Parasitology*, 6th edn, Appleton & Lange, Norwalk, CT (in press).

Neva, F. A. and Ottesen, E. A. (1978) Tropical (filarial) eosinophilia. *New Engl. J. Med.*, **298**, 1129–31.

Neva, F. A., Gam, A. A. and Burke, J. (1981) Comparison of larval antigens in an enzyme-linked immunosorbent assay for strongyloidiasis in humans. *J. Infect. Dis.*, **144**, 427–32.

Nutman, T. B., Ottesen, E. A., Ieng, S. *et al.* (1987) Eosinophilia in Southeast Asian refugees; evaluation at a referral center. *J. Infect. Dis.*, **155**, 309–13.

Nwokolo, C. and Imohiosen, E. A. E. (1973) Strongyloidiasis of respiratory tract presenting as 'asthma'. *Br. Med. J.*, **2**, 153–4.

Olson, C. E. and Schiller, E. L. (1978) *Strongyloides ratti* infections in rats. II. Effects of cortisone treatment. *Am. J. Trop. Med. Hyg.*, **27**, 527–31.

Pelletier, L. L. (1984) Chronic strongyloidiasis in World War II Far East ex-prisoners of war. *Am. J. Trop. Med. Hyg.*, **33**, 55–61.

Purtilo, D. T., Meyers, W. M. and Connor, D. H. (1974) Fatal strongyloidiasis in immunosuppressed patients. *Am. J. Med.*, **56**, 488–93.

Roth, R. L. and Levy, D. A. (1980) *Nippostrongylus brasiliensis*: peripheral leukocyte responses and correlation of basophils with blood histamine concentration during infection in rats. *Exp. Parasit.*, **50**, 331–41.

Sato, Y. and Shiroma, Y. (1989) Peripheral lymphocyte subsets and their responsiveness in human strongyloidiasis. *Clin. Immun. Immunopath.*, **53**, 430–8.

Sato, Y., Otsura, M., Takara, M. and Shiroma, Y. *et al.* (1986) Intradermal reactions in strongyloidiasis. *Int. J. Parasit.*, **16**, 87–91.

Schad, G. A. (1989) Morphology and life history of *Strongyloides stercoralis*, in *Strongyloidiasis: A*

Major Roundworm Infection of Man (ed. D. I. Grove), Taylor and Francis, New York, pp. 85–104.

Schad, G. A., Aikens, L. M. and Smith, G. (1989) *Strongyloides stercoralis*: is there a canonical migratory route through the host? *J. Parasit.*, **75**, 740–9.

Scowden, E. B., Schaffner, W. and Stone, W. J. (1978) Overwhelming strongyloidiasis; an unappreciated opportunistic infection. *Medicine (Baltimore)*, **57**, 527–44.

Shelhamer, J. H., Neva, F. A. and Finn, D. R. (1982) Persistent strongyloidiasis in an immunodeficient patient. *Am. J. Trop. Med. Hyg.*, **31**, 746–51.

Skeels, M. R., Nims, L. J. and Mann, J. M. (1982) Intestinal parasitoses among Southeast Asian immigrants in New Mexico. *Am. J. Publ Health*, **72**, 57–9.

Terry, S. I., Blattner, W., Neva, F. A. *et al.* (1989) Coincidental HTLV-1 infection influences outcome of treatment of strongyloidiasis. *W. Ind. Med. J.*, **38**, 36 (Suppl.1).

Walzer, P. D., Milder, J. E., Banwell, J. G. *et al.* (1982) Epidemiologic features of *Strongyloides stercoralis* infection in an endemic area of the United States. *Am. J. Trop. Med. Hyg.*, **31**, 313–19.

Yoeli, M., Most, H., Hammond, J. and Scheinesson, G. P. *et al.* (1972) Parasitic infections in a closed community. *Trans. Roy. Soc. Trop. Med. Hyg.*, **66**, 764–76.

EIGHT

Trichinella spiralis

D. Despommier

The nematode parasite, *Trichinella spiralis*, infects a wide variety of mammalian hosts and, in each, occupies several diverse stage-specific niches. The ecological niche consists of the physical site of infection and trophic and hypervolume aspects of that site (Odum, 1983; Despommier, 1993). The infectious 1st stage larva (L1) lives inside a modified striated muscle cell, the Nurse cell (Purkerson and Despommier, 1974). This niche is highly altered and unique to the genus *Trichinella*. The adult worm and developing larval stages (i.e. L1–L4) leading up to that stage also live in a specialized niche, namely within a common cytoplasm derived from a row of enterocytes in the small intestine (Wright, 1979). Thus, the stages of *T. spiralis* in the small intestine live as intramulticellular parasites. While in this site, the worms induce many functional changes in the small intestine frequently resulting in diarrheal disease. Other nematodes also occupy this niche: *Capillaria* spp., *Trichosomides* spp., *Trichuris* spp. and *Strongyloides* spp. being the most common ones. The latter two intestinal helminths are agents of diarrheal disease as well, especially if infection is severe enough (Katz, Despommier and Gwadz, 1989). *Trichuris trichiura* and *S. stercoralis* are soil-transmitted pathogens of humans found primarily throughout the tropical and subtropical world, while, as mentioned. *T. spiralis* infects nearly all mammalian species and is found in all climates and microhabitats (Campbell, 1983). Its transmission depends upon the habit of eating raw or undercooked meat.

This chapter will largely focus on the biology of *T. spiralis* in its enteral niche. Clinical aspects of enteral infection will also be described as they relate to the development of the parasite in this site. However, despite a large number of clinical obsevations (Pawlowoski, 1983), much of what we know about the enteral phase is derived from animal experiments. The gut-associated changes that the enteral stages induce throughout the infection have been well documented and several excellent reviews have been published dealing with this important aspect (Castro, 1988; 1990, Chapter 4). A review of the overall biology and many other aspects of infection with *T. spiralis* can be found in Campbell (1983).

8.1 NICHE SELECTION BEHAVIOR

Infection begins with the ingestion of infected muscle tissue containing nurse cells harboring infectious L1 larvae. The parasite is digested away from the tissue meal in the stomach and is passively carried to the small intestine by peristalsis. Within minutes (Stewart *et al.*, 1987) the freed larvae are activated within the lumen of the small intestine, probably as the result of partial

Enteric Infection 2. Intestinal helminths. Edited by M.J.G. Farthing, G.T. Keusch and D. Wakelin. Published in 1995 by Chapman and Hall, London. ISBN 0 412 39140 6

removal of their epicuticle, an outer bilayer of protein–lipid composite material (Lee, Wright and Shivers, 1984; Wright and Hong, 1988). The partial disruption of this layer is thought to be an essential first step, allowing the worm to receive information regarding its hypervolume niche (i.e. pH, Eh, temperature, the concentration of ions, amino acids, peptides, proteins, fats, carbohydrates, vitamins, etc.). This layer also contains antigenic determinants (Despommier and Kajima, 1967) which elicit responses that protect against reinfection (Silberstein and Despommier, 1986; Ortega-Pierres *et al.*, 1989). The partial removal of the epicuticle is accomplished by the combined action of trypsin, chymotrypsin and bile (Despommier, 1983). This process can be reproduced *in vitro* and worms treated in this fashion exhibit a shift in their behavior, namely from that of a slow coiling–uncoiling motion to that of a thrashing, rapid serpentine movement (Stewart *et al.*, 1987). In addition, the removal of a portion of the epicuticle enables the larvae to take up free glucose and begin the conversion to aerobic metabolism (Ferguson and Castro, 1973). These events are temperature-dependent, occurring at 37°C, but not at 20°C.

Once activated, larvae rapidly penetrate epithelial cells, occupying a row of them throughout the coming weeks of their life (Figure 8.1, see colour plate section). Worms do not disrupt the cell membranes of the epithelia; rather they stretch them to their limits, thus remaining within their intramulticellular niche. The mean diameter of the worm does not change at any time during its development, but its length does, and that is presumably why it is able to maintain its position in this unusual site. The adult female of *Strongyloides* spp. is approximately the same diameter as that of *T. spiralis*. The slender anterior half of *Trichuris* spp. (i.e. the 'whip' end) is serpiginously embedded in a parasite-induced syncytium derived from epithelial cells of the large intestine (Lee and Wright, 1978). The number of contiguous epithelial cells occupied by *Trichinella* varies throughout its life, since the worm grows in length during its morphogenesis to an adult. Hence, the entering L1 worm is approximately 1 mm in length and infects about 30–50 cells, while the 3 mm long adult female occupies some 120 cells.

Larvae do not infect the extreme upper region of small intestine, rather they prefer the area of small intestine below which the pH has changed from acidic to basic, namely the middle and lower duodenum and jejunum (Sukhdeo and Croll, 1981). Thus, *T. spiralis* responds to multiple environmental cues (Despommier, 1982) in order to initiate infection in the gut.

No clinical signs or symptoms have been associated with this early phase of the infection. However, the next few days to weeks uring the enteral infection is the time during which clinical disease characterized by diarrhea, headache, nausea and anorexia develops.

8.2 NICHE MODIFICATION

Life in the intramulticellular niche is anything but static, as uninfected cells are constantly being produced and migrating up and out of the crypts. Peristalsis of the gut represents additional movement of the physical environment. Since each enterocyte normally leaves the villus tip within a two to three day span of time (Cheng and Leblond, 1974), the fate of the infected enterocytes and the worms in them is a subject of some interest. However, only limited data are available suggesting that *T. spiralis* causes the eventual death of each infected enterocyte, with dead cells sloughing off from the mid-portion of the villus surface in some strains of mice, while in others they slough from the tips (Dunn and Wright, 1985; Wright *et al.*, 1987). Nothing was stated in those studies regarding the length of time each enterocyte lives after becoming infected.

Trichinella spiralis is seldom if ever found below the level of the platform at the crypt of Leiberkuhn, regardless of the stage (i.e. L1–L4, adult), while it frequently locates within the cytoplasm of enterocytes of two adjacent villi. Apparently the parasites continually move downward, infecting new cells, while the cells that surround them move upward. Does the infection hasten the migration of cells? Does the mechanism of sloughing of infected cells differ from that of non-infected ones? What is the cause(s) of death of the infected cells? These questions remain to be answered.

Living inside a row of enterocytes also represents a highly specialized niche in terms of nutrition. The parasite lives at a nutrient cross-road where metabolites traverse the outer epithelial membrane, or enter the columnar cells from the circulation within the lamina propria. Presented with these potential pathways, how does *Trichinella* access its nutrients? In attempting to answer this question, Castro and co-workers infected rats with either. *T. spiralis* or *Hymenolepis diminuta*, a lumen-dwelling tapeworm (Castro *et al.*, 1976). After several days of infection, the animals were placed on parenteral nutrition. Adult cestodes were dramatically affected, first losing their proglottids, then reacquiring them within a week. Ordinarily, tapeworms absorb predigested nutrients from the lumenal side of the small intestine. The mechanism(s) by which tapeworms acquire nutrients in the absence of enteral sources remains unknown. In contrast, *T. spiralis* was able to carry out its developmental cycle in its enteral site niche without interruption. The authors concluded that both kinds of parasites can maintain themselves in the host, regardless of the nutrient source, but that *Trichinella* is more efficient than *Hymenolepis* at doing so. Unfortunately, in the case of *Trichinella*, the experiment was terminated prior to the reproductive phase of its development, so that it is still not known if hyperalimentation is sufficient to accommodate this aspect of its life.

If worms infect the lower end of the small intestine or are transplanted into the upper region of large intestine, they produce fewer offspring and are stunted (Sukhdeo and Croll, 1981), suggesting that lumen-obtained nutrients play a major role in the outcome of the overall biology of the infection. However, hypotheses not related to worm nutrition may also account for the stunted worms in those less than ideal sites, such as pH or temperature effects. Regrettably, nothing is known regarding the nutritional requirements of *Trichinella*, other than the fact that this parasite can make all of its macromolecules from small molecular weight precursors (Stewart, 1983).

8.3 DEVELOPMENTAL BIOLOGY

One of the most striking features of the biology of *T. spiralis* is the rapid, stage-specificity of its development within the enteral site niche (Kozek, 1971). The parasite takes only 30 hours to transform from an L1 larva to the adult, molting four times during the process. This represents one of the fastest developmental programs within the phylum Nematoda. With each molt the worm resembles more and more the adult parasite, although its length remains unchanged. The first stage cuticle is shed *in situ* (Figure 8.2) and remains there for some time after the worm has moved to a different region of villus (Capo, Despommier and Silberstein, 1984). It is unlikely that the worm induces much gut damage during this short period, since clinical symptoms associated with such damage rarely develop before the third day after infection (Pawlowski, 1983).

The stichosome is an organ present in all stages of the parasite except the newborn larva. This organ is located in the anterior portion of the worm and is composed of a row of some fifty stichocyte cells (Chitwood

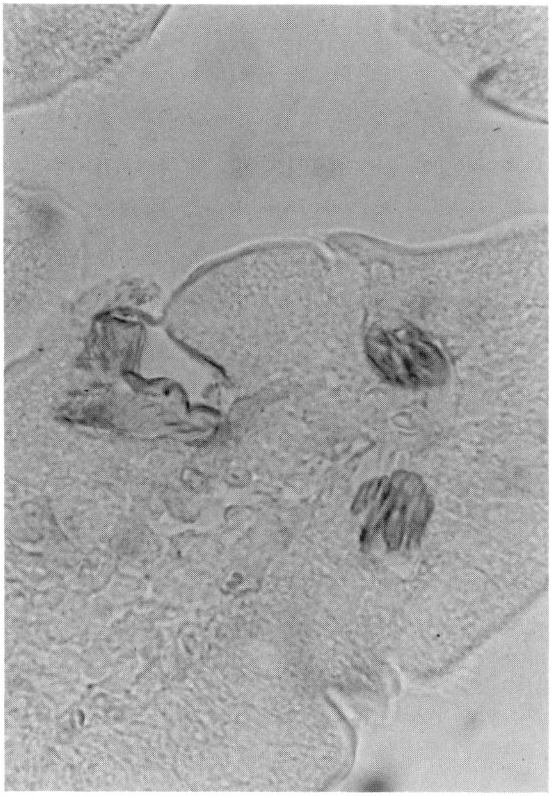

Figure 8.2 A section through a portion of small intestinal villus with portions of shed cuticula (arrows) from first stage larvae of *Trichinella spiralis*. The surface of the cuticle of this larval stage is antigenic and a horseradish peroxidase-labelled antibody directed against these surface epitopes has been used to identify shed cuticula in sections of infected tissue.

and Chitwood, 1950). Each cell contains a unique complement of secretory granules (Despommier and Muller, 1976), while the entire stichosome is made up of five different kinds of stichocyte cells (Takahashi *et al.*, 1989). The majority of the individual proteins (Despommier and Laccetti, 1981) that are contained within each granule type are antigenic. Little is known about the biochemical nature of these proteins except that many of them are glycosylated (Denkers, Wassom and Hayes, 1990), and some elicit strong protective immune responses (Campbell, 1955; Chipman, 1957; Mills and Kent, 1965; Despommier and Laccetti, 1981; Silberstein, 1983; Silberstein and Despommier, 1984; Despommier, 1985; Ortega-Pierres *et al.*, 1989). The stichosome functions by secreting these proteins into the various niches throughout its life cycle (Despommier, 1993).

During the transition from larva to adult – the secreted products of the L1 larva are largely stage-specific (Silberstein, 1983) – the stichocytes undergo redifferentiation (Despommier, 1974) and from then on secrete products largely restricted to the adult stage (Capo, Despommier and Silberstein, 1986; Despommier, 1992). It is reasonable to presume that the presence of these proteins in the intramulticellular environment immediately adjacent to the worm is necessary for the modulation of trophic and hypervolume aspects of that site. However, the precise role of each secreted protein in the overall process of niche modification must first be preceded by the purification of each, and most importantly, the development of an appropriate *in vitro* model for testing its function. Immunocytolocalization data provide some evidence suggesting that these secreted products not only interact with infected enterocytes, but may also affect adjacent enterocytes (Figure 8.3). Thus, the ecological niche of the parasite extends beyond the limits of its immediate intracellular space.

Viewed from the host side of the relationship, the enteral stages induce disease (diarrhea, nausea, vomiting) related to the worm's development and reproduction, but the mechanism(s) remain unknown. It is probable that they are induced by the secretions of the adult stage. However, none of these proteins has been systematically investigated for their pathological effects on the small intestine.

Once the worms have molted for the last time, mating rapidly ensues. The precise anatomic location in the gut where mating occurs is not known. Mating takes place within a very narrow window of time (i.e.

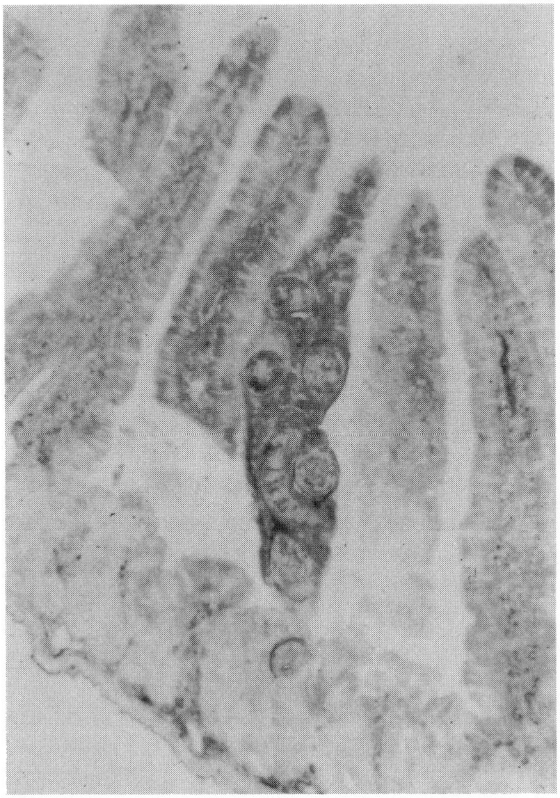

Figure 8.3 Horseradish peroxidase-labelled antibodies directed against secreted proteins of the first stage larva of *Trichinella spiralis* were used to identify the degree to which the worm exerts its biochemical influence on its enteral niche during its early life there (i.e. 0–12 h postoral infection). Note that the distribution of the secreted proteins far exceeds the physical location of the worm, itself. Arrows = sections of larvae.

30–36 hours after infection; Kozek, 1971). As mentioned, it is at this time that clinical symptoms begin. In humans, secretory diarrhea is associated with moderate to heavy infection with *T. spiralis*, but even skilled clinicians often misdiagnose it as food poisoning (Pawlowski, 1983). Intestinal stasis during the first five days of infection (Castro and Bullick, 1983) may facilitate mating, since the parasites apparently communicate with each other through pheromones secreted by both males and females (Bonner and Etges, 1967). Slowing down the gut transit time could allow gradients of these worm attractants to develop unimpaired by normal rates of peristalsis. The nature of the pheromones remains undiscovered. Hypersecretion occurs at the same time as gut stasis and may also be involved in the dispersal of mating signals, supplying the milieu in which worm-specific chemical gradients form. Unfortunately, there are no data to support the above speculation, since precise measurements of gut transit time and peristalsis at this critical time (i.e. 28–34 hours after infection) have not yet been made.

8.4 MORPHOLOGICAL AND FUNCTIONAL CHANGES IN THE INFECTED GUT

Striking physical and biological changes occur in the small intestine during infection with *T. spiralis*, and include flattening of villi, secretory diarrhea and malabsorption of sugars (for reviews see Chapter 4; Castro and Bullick, 1983). In addition, the wheat germ agglutinin receptors along the brush border are reduced (Harari and Castro, 1988), the functional significance of which has yet to be appreciated. Overt pathological changes begin 5–8 days after oral infection. There is evidence that most of these effects of the parasitism are induced by T lymphocytes (Ruitenberg, Leenstra and Elgersma, 1977), since they can be reduced or eliminated by pretreatment of animals with cyclosporin A (Garside, Grencis and Mowat, 1992). Thus, immune complexes may be essential for their development.

Throughout the enteral phase of the infection a progression of lymphoid cells travel through the lamina propria and home in on regions of gut directly adjacent to individual worms (Weatherly, 1983). The majority of cells at any given time consists of plasma cells (Figure 8.4; Race *et al.*, 1974; Capo, Despommier and Silberstern, 1986) mast cells (Castro, 1990) and eosinophils (Larsh, Ottolenghi and

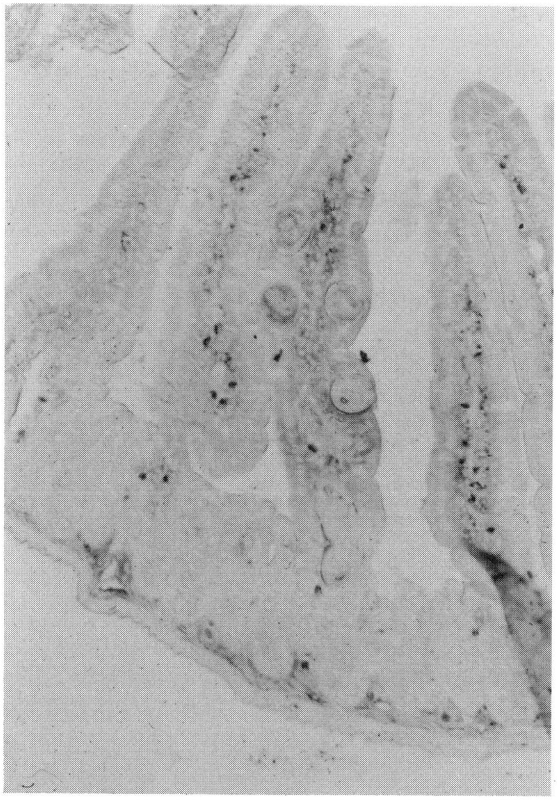

Figure 8.4 Horseradish peroxidase-labelled anti-IgG was used to identify plasma cells in the lamina propria during reinfection with *Trichinella spiralis* larvae. Note the difference in the number of clearly labelled cells in this section compared to the section in Figure 8.3 (i.e. primary infection). Arrows = sections of larvae.

Weatherby, 1974; Wright, Weidman and Hong, 1987). The altered kinetics and site of sloughing of injured epithelial cells (Dunn and Wright, 1985) may be mediated by eosinophils. Eosinophilia in the lamina propria abates when adult worms egress from the host during immune rejection, since it is the adult stage of the worm that elicits the response (Despommier, Weisbroth and Fass, 1974). In rats infected with *T. spiralis*, eosinophilia is induced by a subset of helper T cells that are OX 8(−), OX 22(−) (Wang *et al.*, 1990). The kinetics of tissue and circulating eosinophilia varies according to the immunogenetics of each strain and species of host (Wakelin and Donachie, 1983; Pincus *et al.*, 1986; Wang *et al.*, 1990) but in general it abates over a two-week period following the production of newborn larvae (i.e. weeks 4–6 postinfection).

During the height of the immune responses leading to the expulsion of the parasites, eosinophils degranulate and are thus difficult to identify with common histological stains. However, their presence in tissues can be indirectly assayed by finding increased levels of phospholipase B, an enzyme particularly abundant in eosinophils (Larsh, Ottolenghi and Weatherby, 1974). Immune elimination of adult worms correlates well with increased levels of this enzyme and secretory IgA (DeVos, Danell and Dick, 1992). In special situations, such as rapid expulsion in rats (McCoy, 1940), increased levels of IgE appear to play a role in eliminating larvae during challenge (Amed, Wang and Bell, 1991). In contrast, circulating eosinophilia does not correlate with immunity (Pincus *et al.*, 1986; Wakelin, 1993), and is often markedly elevated in strains of mice that accumulate large numbers of larvae in their musculature.

Worms under immune attack are forced to migrate to the lower part of the small intestine, then into the large intestine (Larsh, Gilchrist and Greenberg, 1952). This latter phase lasts for only several days, and the physiological consequences of the infection in this region of the gut tract are unknown. Within the tissues of the large intestine, the adult worms are stressed beyond their capability to remain there, probably due to a combination of immune damage and a nutrient-poor environment, and they rapidly pass out with the fecal mass; thus infection is terminated.

In summary, *T. spiralis* occupies an unusual ecological niche in the small intestine, living inside the naked cytoplasm of a row of enterocytes. While in this site the parasite induces many changes that favor its reproductive success at the expense of each infected cell. Understanding the linkage of these changes through elucidating the mechanisms employed by this highly evolved nematode to carry out its life in this highly specialized niche has yet to be achieved through scientific inquiry.

8.5 CLINICAL ASPECTS

8.5.1 SYMPTOMS

Symptoms of trichinosis vary during the course of the infection and depend on the location of the parasite within the body. Most descriptions of the clinical course of infection have been obtained from outbreaks, in which the presumed inoculum of muscle cysts has been large. Hence, the impact of light infection is largely unknown, and may be virtually undetectable.

Although the initial interaction of parasite and host is in the upper small bowel and may lead to intestinal symptomatology such as vomiting, cramps, diarrhea or even constipation, in many individuals this phase of illness is asymptomatic. When these symptoms are present, they usually begin approximately 3–10 days following ingestion of tainted meat. It is somewhat surprising that gastrointestinal complaints are so mild considering the major mucosal events and morphological changes occurring after the initial penetration of the infectious larvae. Trichinosis occurring in native Arctic populations is thought to be due to a species called *T. nativa*, although taxonomy is not absolutely clear. This infection is associated with chronic diarrhea as a prominent symptom (MacLean *et al.*, 1989).

The more prominent and hence better known and more characteristic features of trichinosis relate to larval migration. Following mating of the adults, the viviparous birth of larvae (up to several thousand per female) results in invasion of the gut mucosa and dissemination of the parasite via the lymphatic and circulatory systems. This stage of infection can be associated with translocation of bacteria which reach the blood stream, and rare and even fatal cases of systemic sepsis have been described. It is probably fortunate that the upper bowel flora is so sparse, for otherwise this complication of *Trichinella* larval penetration might be more common. The parasites invade a variety of host cells and induce an inflammatory response, but they are able to continue their development only in striated muscle cells, which are modified to support the development of the encysting transmission form of the organism, the Nurse cell–larva complex. The modified muscle cell is termed a 'Nurse cell', suggesting its critical importance in the long-term survival of the young parasite.

Much of the clinical symptomatology of the infection is due to the inflammatory response caused by muscle invasion. Myositis and edema occur approximately 2 weeks after penetration, and result in fever, myalgia, muscle tenderness, edema noted most readily around the eyes, and petechiae often seen in the conjunctivae and in the nail beds ('splinter hemorrhages') as in endocarditis. Heavy infection produces distressing pain and muscle weakness and is associated with fever. These symptoms can at times be so severe as to be confused with the clinical presentation of polymyositis.

However, the clinically most important problems usually result from larval invasion of brain and myocardium. In the brain, the parasite wanders in apparent search for striated muscle in which to continue development, resulting in tissue damage, granulomatous reactions and hemorrhages, headache, and if severe enough, an encephalitic clinical picture with or without seizures (Gay *et al.*, 1982). Myocardial invasion is not usually important because the parasite usually exits the heart muscle quickly; however, on occasion a significant myocarditis can result from the inflammatory response it elicits, with cardiomyopathy-like heart failure. The importance of the inflammatory response in the clinical manifestations of trichinosis is underscored by the relatively mild illness reported in a few immunosuppressed patients (Jacobson and Jacobson, 1977).

8.5.2 DIAGNOSIS

Because initial intestinal symptoms are so non-specific, isolated cases of trichinosis are more difficult to diagnose than those occurring in outbreaks, associated either with ingestion of fresh and undercooked pork or game, such as bear. Symptoms of myositis associated with fever and eosinophilia should prompt a consideration of *T. spiralis*. Once the diagnosis is considered, the two most important diagnostic studies are to measure antibody and/or do a muscle biopsy from a region of muscle tenderness and prepare a fresh crushed sample for direct phase contrast microscopy. If serology is positive, it is not necessary to confirm the diagnosis by biopsy, since this procedure may miss the area of involvement and rather frequently, only one of the two tests is positive.

8.5.3 TREATMENT

In mild to moderate trichinosis, it is not necessary to treat with drugs. Because severe symptoms are associated with the inflammatory reaction induced by larval invasion of cells, patients with myocarditis and heart failure or severe central nervous system involvement may benefit from use of steroids, although controlled studies are not available. Patients with symptomatic myositis may also benefit from a course of thiabendazole or mebendazole, but only very early in the course of the infection prior to encystation in muscle. These drugs do not appear to kill tissue phase larvae very effectively but do seem to alleviate symptoms.

8.5.4 PREVENTION

Cooking infected meat thoroughly will kill encysted larvae. Unfortunately, this does not contribute to the gastronomic virtue of the meal and humans will continue to undercook their meats in spite of the danger of acquisition of a number of zoonotic pathogens. *T. spiralis spiralis* is readily killed by solid freezing of food at −20°C for 3 weeks, however the sylvatic strains appear to be adapted to and more resistant to low temperatures (Eaton, 1979).

ACKNOWLEDGEMENTS

I thank Drs Derek Wakelin, Donald Wassom, Robin Bell, Gilbert Castro and David Denham for the insight and intelligent discussions in which we have engaged throughout my research career. Neither they nor I realized that a distillate of their thoughts would be incorporated into this review; I am nonetheless grateful to each and fortunate for having shared their unpublished data, speculations, suspicions, beliefs and good humor so openly and honestly. I also thank Ms Ramona Polvere and Dr Allen Gold for carefully reviewing the finished manuscript.

REFERENCES

Amed, A., Wang, C. H. and Bell, R. G. (1991) A role for IgE in intestinal immunity. Expression of rapid expulsion of *Trichinella spiralis* in rats transfused with IgE and thoracic duct lymphocytes. *J. Immun.*, **146**, 3563–70.

Bonner, T. P. and Etges, J. F. (1967) Chemically mediated attraction in *Trichinella spiralis*. *Exp. Parasit.*, **21**, 53–60.

Campbell, C. H. (1955) The antigenic role of the excretions and secretions of *Trichinella spiralis* in the production of immunity in mice. *J. Parasit.*, **51**, 185–94.

Campbell, W. C. (ed.) (1983) Trichinella *and Trichinosis*, Plenum Press, New York.

Capo, V., Despommier, D. D. and Silberstein, D. S. (1984) The site of ecdysis of the L1 larva of *Trichinella spiralis*. *J. Parasit.*, **70**, 992–3.

Capo, V., Despommier, D. D. and Silberman, D. S. (1986) Immunocytolocalization of two protection-inducing antigens of *Trichinella spiralis* during its enteral phase in immune and non-immune mice. *J. Parasit.*, **72**, 931–8.

Castro, G. A. (1988) Parasitic infections and gastric motility, in *Handbook of Physiology: Gastrointestinal System*, Section 6, Vol. I. (ed. J. D. Wood), The American Physiological Society, Bethesda, Maryland, pp. 1133–52.

Castro, G. A. (1990) Intestinal pathology, in *Immunity and Pathology: The Consequences of Parasitic Infections in Mammals* (ed. J. M. Behnke), Taylor and Francis, London, pp. 283–316.

Castro, G. A., Johnson, L. R., Copeland, E. M. and Dudrick, S. J. (1976) Course of infection with enteric parasites in hosts shifted from enteral to parenteral nutrition. *J. Parasit.*, **62**, 353–9.

Castro, G. A. and Bullick, G. R. (1983) Pathophysiology of the gastrointestinal phase, in *Trichinella and Trichinosis* (ed. W. C. Campbell), Plenum Press, New York, pp. 209–40.

Cheng, H. and Leblond, C. P. (1974) Origin, differentiation and renewal of the four main epithelial cell types in the mouse small intestine. V. Unitarian theory of the origin of the four epithelial cell types. *Am. J. Anat.*, **141**, 537–62.

Chipman, P. B. (1957) The antigenic role of the excretions and secretions of adult *Trichinella spiralis* in the production of immunity in mice. *J. Parasit.*, **43**, 593–8.

Chitwood, B. G. and Chitwood, M. B. (1950) *An Introduction to Nematology. Section I. Anatomy*. Monumental Printing Company, Baltimore, Maryland, pp. 45–6.

Denkers, E. Y., Wassom, D. L. and Hayes, C. E. (1990) Characterization of *Trichinella spiralis* antigens sharing an immunodominant, carbohydrate-associated determinant distinct from phosphorylcholine. *Molec. Biochem. Parasit.* **41**, 241–50.

Despommier, D. D. (1974) The stichocyte of *Trichinella spiralis* during morphogenesis in the small intestine of the rat, in *Trichinellosis* (ed. C. Kim), Intext Publishers, New York, pp. 239–55.

Despommier, D. D. (1982) Behavioral cues in migration and location of parasitic nematodes, with special emphasis on *Trichinella spiralis*, in *Cues that Influence the Behavior of Internal Parasites* (ed. W. S. Bailey), Agricultural Research Service, US Department of Agriculture, New Orleans, Louisana (May).

Despommier, D. D. (1983) Biology, in Trichinella *and Trichinosis* (ed. W. C. Campbell), Plenum Press, New York, pp. 75–142.

Despommier, D. D. (1985) Antigens, in *Trichinellosis* (ed. C. Kim). The State of New York Press, Albany, New York, pp. 8–16.

Despommier, D. D. (1993) *Trichinella spiralis* and the concept of niches. *J. Parasit.*, **79**, 473–82.

Despommier, D. D. and Kajima, M. (1967) Ferritin-conjugated antibody studies on the larva of *Trichinella spiralis. J. Parasit.*, **53**, 618–24.

Despommier, D. D. and Laccetti, A. (1981) *Trichinella spiralis:* partial characterization of antigens isolated by immuno-affinity chromatography from the large particle fraction of the mature muscle larva. *J. Parasit.*, **67**, 332–9.

Despommier, D. D. and Muller M. (1976) The stichosome and its secretion granules in the mature muscle larva of *Trichinella spiralis. J. Parasit.*, **62**, 775–85.

Despommier, D. D., Weisbroth S. and Fass, C. (1974) Circulating eosinophils and trichinosis in the rat: the parasitic stage responsible for induction during infection. *J. Parasit.*, **60**, 280–4.

DeVos, T., Danell, G. and Dick, T. A. (1992) *Trichinella spiralis:* dose dependence and kinetics of the mucosal immune response in mice. *Exp. Parasit.*, **75**, 95–111.

Dunn, I. J. and Wright, K. A. (1985) Cell injury caused by *Trichinella spiralis* in the mucosal epithelium of B 10A mice. *J. Parasit.*, **71**, 757–66.

Eaton, R. D. P. (1979) Trichinosis in the Arctic. *Can. Med. Ass. J.*, **120**, 22.

Ferguson, J. D. and Castro, G. A. (1973) Metabolism of the intestinal stages of *Trichinella spiralis. Am. J. Physiol.*, **225**, 85–9.

Garside, P., Grencis, R. K. and McI. Mowat, A. (1992) T lymphocyte-dependent enteropathy in murine *Trichinella spiralis* infection. *Parasite Immun.*, **14**, 217–25.

Gay, T., Paukey, G. A., Beckman, E. N. *et al.* (1982) Fatal CNS trichinosis. *J. Am. Med. Ass.*, **247**, 1024–5.

Harari, Y. and Castro, G. A. (1988) Evaluation of a possible functional relationship between chemical structure of the intestinal brush border and immunity to *Trichinella spiralis* in the rat. *J. Parasit.*, **74**, 244–8.

Jacobson, E. S. and Jacobson, H. G. (1977) Trichinosis in an immunosuppressed human host. *Am. J. Clin. Pathol.*, **68**, 791–4.

Katz, M., Despommier, D. D. and Gwadz, R. (1989) *Parasitic Diseases*. 2nd edn, Springer-Verlag, New York and Heidelberg.

Kozek, W. J. (1971) The molting pattern of *Trichinella spiralis*. I. A light microscope study. *J. Parasit.*, **57**, 1015–28.

Larsh, J. E., Jr, Gilchrist, H. B. and Greenberg, B. G. (1952) A study of the distribution and longevity of adult *Trichinella spiralis* in immunized and non-immunized mice. *J. Elisa Mitchell Sci. Soc.*, **68**, 1–11.

Larsh, E. J., Jr., Ottolenghi, A. and Weatherby, N. F. (1987) *Trichinella spiralis*: phospholipase in challenged mice and rats. *Exp. Parasit.*, **36**, 299–306.

Lee, T. D. G. and Wright, K. A. (1978) The morphology of the attachment and probable feeding site of the nematode, *Trichuris muris* (Shrank 1788) Hall 1916. *Can. J. Zool.*, **56**, 1889–905.

Lee, D. L., Wright, K. A. and Shivers, R. R. (1984) A freeze-fracture study of the surface of the infective stage larva of the nematode, *Trichinella spiralis*. *Tiss. Cell*, **16**, 819–28.

MacLean, J. D., Viallet, J., Kaw, C. and Staudt, M. (1989) Trichinosis in the Canadian Arctic: report of five outbreaks and a new clinical syndrome. *J. Infect. Dis.*, **160**, 513–20.

McCoy, O. R. (1940) Rapid loss of *Trichinella spiralis* larvae fed to immune rats and its bearing on the mechanism of immunity. *Am. J. Hyg.*, **32**, 105–16.

Mills, C. K. and Kent, N. H. (1965) Excretions and secretions of *Trichinella spiralis* and their role in immunity. *Exp. Parasit.*, **16**, 300–10.

Odum, E. P. (1983) *Basic Ecology*, Saunders Educational Publishers, Philadelphia and New York, pp. 401–3.

Ortega-Pierres, G., Muniz, E., Coral-Vasquez, R. and Parkhouse, R. M. E. (1989) Protection against *Trichinella spiralis* induced by stage-specific surface antigens of the infective larvae. *Parasit. Res.*, **75**, 563–7.

Pawlowski, Z. S. (1983) Clinical aspects in man, in Trichinella *and Trichinosis* (ed. W. C. Campbell), Plenum Publishers, New York, pp. 367–403.

Pincus, S. H., Cammarrata, P. V., Delima, M. and Despommier, D. D. (1986) Eosinophilia in murine trichinosis. *J. Parasit.*, **72**, 321–4.

Purkerson, M. and Despommier, D. D. (1974) Fine structure of the muscle phase of *Trichinella spiralis* in the mouse, in *Trichinellosis* (ed. C. Kim), Intext Publishers, New York, pp. 7–23.

Race, G. J., Larsh, J. E., Jr, Martin, J. H. and Weatherby, N. F. (1974) Light and electron microscopy of the intestinal tissue of mice parasitized by *Trichinella spiralis*, in *Trichinellosis* (ed. C. Kim), Intext Publishers, New York, pp. 75–100.

Ruitenberg, E. J. and Elgersma, A. (1980) Study of the kinetics of globule leukocytes in the intestinal epithelium of rats after single or double infection with *Trichinella spiralis*. *Br. J. Path.*, **61**, 285–90.

Ruitenberg, E. J., Leenstra, F. and Elgersma, A. (1977) Thymus dependent and independence of intestinal pathology in a *Trichinella spiralis* infection: a study in congenic athymic (nude) mice. *Br. J. Path.*, **58**, 311.

Silberstein, D. S. (1983) Antigens, in Trichinella *and Trichinosis* (ed. W. C. Campbell), Plenum Press, New York, pp. 309–34.

Silberstein, D. S. and Despommier, D. D. (1984) Antigens from *Trichinella spiralis* that induce protection in the mouse. *J. Immun.*, **132**, 898–904.

Stewart, G. L. (1983) Biochemistry, in Trichinella *and Trichinosis* (ed. W. C. Campbell), Plenum Press, New York, pp. 153–72.

Stewart, G. L., Despommier, D. D., Burnham, J. and Reins, K. (1987) *Trichinella spiralis*: behavioral, structural, and biochemical studies on larvae following exposure to components of the host enteric environment. *Exp. Parasit.*, **63**, 195–204.

Sukhdeo, M. V. K. and Croll, N. A. (1981) The location of parasites within their hosts: factors influencing longitudinal distribution of *Trichinella spiralis* in the small intestine. *Int. J. Parasit.*, **11**, 163–8.

Takahashi, Y., Takako, U., Mizuno, N. *et al.* (1989) Ultrastructural localization of antigenic substances in *Trichinella spiralis*. *Parasit. Res.*, **75**, 316–24.

Wakelin, D. (1993) *Trichinella spiralis*: immunity, ecology, and evolution. *J. Parasit.*, **79**, 488–94.

Wakelin, D. and Donachie, A. M. (1983) Genetic control of eosinophilia: mouse strain variation in response to antigens of parasite origin. *Clin. Exp. Immun.*, **51**, 239–46.

Wang, C. H., Korenga, M., Greenwood, A. and Bell, R. G. (1990) T-helper subsets function in the gut of rats infected with *Trichinella spiralis*: deferential stimulation of eosinophils, mucosal mast cells and antibody-forming cells by OX 8 (−), OX 22 (−) and OX 8 (−), OX 22 (+) cells, *Immunology*, **71**, 166–75.

Weatherly, N. F. (1983) Anatomic pathology, in Trichinella *and Trichinosis*, (ed. W. C. Campbell), Plenum Press, New York, pp. 173–208.

Wright, K. A. (1979) *Trichinella spiralis*: an intracellular parasite in the intestinal phase. *J. Parasit.*, **65**, 441–5.

Wright, K. A., Weiden, E. and Hong, H. (1987) The distribution of cells killed by *Trichinella spiralis* in the mucosal epithelium of two strains of mice. *J. Parasit.*, **73**, 935–9.

Wright, K. A. and Hong H. (1988) Characterization of the accessory layer of the cuticle of muscle larvae of *Trichinella spiralis*. *J. Parasit.*, **74**, 440–51.

NINE

Ascariasis

P. O'Hanley
and
T. Pool

Ascariasis is one of the great neglected diseases of mankind since the injurious effects of this most common of all parasitic infections are limited. It is true that the rate of serious complications from ascariasis is low when compared with the number of people that have this disease; however, the enormity of the numbers afflicted by this parasite deserves greater consideration for prevention and control. *Ascaris lumbricoides*, which is the largest nematode causing human disease, afflicts annually an estimated one billion people worldwide (Pawlowski, 1989) and is responsible worldwide for millions of serious complications. They include: pulmonary immunological hypersensitivity reactions, susceptibility to secondary infections due to chronic malnutrition from multiple causes, and gastrointestinal and lung damage. A high adult worm burden may cause intestinal obstruction which is the most common complication of ascariasis. This problem is not unique to developing countries since intestinal obstruction due to intestinal ascariasis occurs even in developed countries. In addition, the annual mortality caused by ascariasis is conservatively estimated worldwide to be 8000 cases, due primarily to intestinal perforation or obstruction in young children (*Lancet* editorial, 1989). Natural infection results from the ingestion of fecally contaminated soil or foods and is strongly correlated with lower socioeconomic living conditions. Other diseases and risk factors associated with lower socioeconomic conditions have made it difficult to quantify specifically the impact of ascariasis. Consequently, national and international health authorities pay little attention to ascariasis.

9.1 EPIDEMIOLOGY

Of the estimated one billion persons infected with ascarids each year, approximately one million will suffer serious complications. Between 8000 and 100 000 people, mostly female children less than 10 years of age, die each year from ascariasis (*Lancet* editorial, 1989). Intestinal obstruction and perforation are responsible for most of the mortality, but very little of the morbidity. While the prevalence of ascariasis is roughly 25 to 30% of the world's population, the prevalence of infection also varies geographically (Crompton, Nesheim and Pawlowski, 1985). The majority of cases occur in the developing world, afflicting up to 70% of the overall population in these regions. The highest prevalence rates for ascariasis are documented in Asia. Children between the ages of 2 and 14 years are most commonly infected in endemic ascaria-

Enteric Infection 2. Intestinal helminths. Edited by M.J.G. Farthing, G.T. Keusch and D. Wakelin. Published in 1995 by Chapman and Hall, London. ISBN 0 412 39140 6

sis areas. It is so common in such regions that the prevalence of ascariasis among children approaches 80% (Martin *et al.*, 1983; Elkins, Haswell-Elkins and Anderson, 1986; Bundy *et al.*, 1981; Bundy, Kan and Rose, 1988; Reinthaler, Mascher and Klem, 1988) and is greater among females than males.

Ascariasis is, however, not confined to developing countries. For example, the prevalence rate of ascariasis in children and young adults from the state of Kentucky in the USA was surprisingly high as recently as 1981 (Jones, 1981). The prevalence was greatest among 3 to 5-year-old preschool children and children 6–12 years old (approximately 32%) followed sequentially by lower rates in adolescents aged 13 to 14 years (20.2%), and 15 to 18 years (15.6%). Jones reviewed medical records in Kentucky over the past 70 years and concluded that the prevalence of ascariasis and *Trichiuris* has remained essentially unchanged during the last 70 years (Jones, 1983). It is clear that ascariasis remains endemic in certain locales both in developing and developed countries.

While the endemic rate of ascariasis is more common in tropical and subtropical climates, the socioeconomic level rather than weather or geology constitutes the critical factor for prevalence. A gram of infected soil from a heavily endemic area may contain several hundred viable *Ascaris* eggs at any time. Local customs can also have a profound impact on transmission kinetics. The use of unprocessed human feces as fertilizer (or 'night soil') has been linked to epidemics of ascariasis (Pawlowski, 1989). Poor sanitation, improper personal hygiene, and eating food by hand from communal vessels have all been associated with increased transmission rates. Children who play on contaminated earth, like night soil-fertilized vegetable gardens, are at considerable risk. Pica, particularly the eating of soil, is not uncommon among children and can also play an important role in the transmission kinetics of ascariasis. In southeastern USA, it is estimated that there are about two obstructions annually due to ascarids per 1000 preschool children who are most likely to eat dirt (Blumenthal and Schultz, 1975). Ascariasis complication rates are much higher in the developing countries than developed countries. For example, 226 (52.3%) of 432 patients presenting as acute abdominal surgical emergencies at a pediatric hospital in Rangoon, Burma, were due to ascariasis (Thein *et al.*, 1990). In this Burmese hospital, ascariasis accounted for 26.3% of all emergency operations and was associated with longer operative times and higher fatality rates than any other emergent surgical condition.

9.2 MORPHOLOGY

The morphological appearances of *Ascaris* adult worms and eggs are the most commonly observed forms of this nematode seen by clinicians and laboratory personnel from clinical specimens. For these reasons, these forms are mentioned here in more detail than other ascarid life-stages. The name *Ascaris lumbricoides* was first used by Linnaeus based on the parasite's remarkable similarity to the earthworm, *Lumbricus terrestrias* (Noble and Noble, 1976). The adult worms are beige in color with females reaching a length of 20–49 cm and a diameter of 3–6 mm. Males are only a little more than half as large. The worms are grossly smooth, rounded and tense since the fluid pressure within the worms may be as high as 225 mm Hg. Three prominent lips guard the gradually tapering anterior tip, while the posterior end is somewhat less tapered in the adult female or hook-shaped in the adult male.

The eggs are broadly oval to almost circular in shape measuring 45–70 μm in length and 35–50 μm in width. Most are bile-stained a yellow-brown color after their passage through the intestines. Each egg is composed of a protein coat, egg shell, pre-vitelline space, and protoplasm. The outer coat is composed of albuminous material with numerous nipple-like projections that acts as a protective barrier and assists in adhesion. This outer coat is absent or incomplete in infertile eggs. The egg proper has a thick, transparent hyaline shell with a thick outer layer for mechanical support and a delicate vitelline inner membrane that is highly impermeable. The eggs are quite resistant to the stresses of cold, desiccation and chemical insult including strong salt solutions and moderate concentrations of hypochlorite and formalin. They are considerably less resistant to heat stress and unfiltered ultraviolet sunlight. In moist temperate soil, the eggs can remain viable for years (5–10 years); in frozen conditions like the Arctic tundra, the eggs can remain viable probably for a century. At oviposition, the shell contains an ovoid mass of unsegmented cytoplasm packed with lecithin granules to be utilized for energy by the developing embryo.

9.3 LIFE CYCLE

Adult roundworms are facultative anaerobes that have a high rate of carbohydrate metabolism. In addition, protein synthesis among adult female worms is especially high in order to sustain their massive egg production. The enormous reproductive potential of the adult female is one of the reasons *Ascaris* species is such a successful human parasite. An adult female may contain over 25 million eggs at any one time and lay almost 250 000 fertilized eggs each day. In contrast to the adults, the eggs and larval stages all depend on aerobic metabolism for their energy needs. Ideal growth conditions for the eggs include: ambient temperatures, moisture, shade from ultraviolet light and oxygen (Blumenthal and Schultz, 1975). Embryonation requires 10 days to 2 weeks under such conditions. Longer periods for embryonation is required when the eggs are exposed to lower temperatures. Infective larvae within the egg shell may remain viable for several years. Desiccation or environmental temperatures that exceed 37°C for short periods of time (i.e. hours) will, however, quickly kill embryonating eggs.

Infective eggs containing L2 larvae must be ingested and hatched in the small intestine for *Ascaris* species to complete their life cycle. Most eggs survive passage through the stomach and are stimulated to hatch by the alkalinity and bile salts present in the small intestine. The L2 larvae penetrate the jejunum and enter capillaries or lymphatics for subsequent migration to the liver. From the hepatic sinusoids, they migrate into the vena cava eventually being translocated from the right side of the heart to the pulmonary capillaries. By this time, three to four days have elapsed since the larvae have penetrated the gastrointestinal mucosa. The larvae develop and molt once or possibly twice over the next two weeks in the pulmonary capillaries. Then, the larvae penetrate the alveolar spaces and begin their migration up the tracheobronchial tree. These 2–3 mm L3 larvae or more mature larval forms are eventually swallowed and pass down the esophagus into the stomach. They are resistant to gastric acid and can survive the passage through the stomach. Once the larvae enter the small intestine, they molt a final fourth-time; thereafter, they will spend the remainder of their lives in the jejunum (Thein *et al.*, 1990). The worms grow rapidly. In about two months, the young females begin passing eggs or fertilized eggs if mating occurs with adult male worms. The entire cycle from egg to adult worm which is capable of reproduction takes about 2.5 to 4 months under normal conditions. The worms do not attach to the luminal surface but 'swim' with strong muscular contractions and feed on the ingesta contained in the jejunum. There is still controversy as to the lifespan of adult worms; however most estimates range from 12 to 24 months. Experimental human infections with *A. suum*, the swine ascarid and closest relative to *A. lumbricoides*, demonstrate that these porcine ascarids fail to molt a final fourth time in the human gut. Because *A. suum* cannot molt a final time and develop into adult forms in the human gastrointestinal lumen, these foreign larval forms are voided with the feces. The life cycles of both ascarid species are otherwise essentially identical except for the strict host specificity.

9.4 CLINICAL FEATURES

The symptomatology of ascariasis has been categorized by Pawlowski as follows: pulmonary ascariasis, intestinal ascariasis, complications of ascariasis and allergy to *Ascaris* species. While the rate of serious complications from ascariasis is low, the absolute number of serious cases is considerable, due to the overall high prevalence of this human parasite. It is for this reason that more emphasis should be placed by health care planners to control and prevent ascariasis.

Most complications are the result of pulmonary hypersensitivity reactions caused by larval antigens which are released during migration or molting. Antigens released by the molting larvae cause inflammation, local and systemic eosinophilia, and elevations of serum IgG. The *Ascaris* allergens are one of the most potent allergens of parasitic origin. For this reason, it is considered appropriate that all members of laboratories working with these worms or their purified products have a common source of medication readily available in the laboratory and be instructed about the guidelines for treating potentially life-threatening anaphylactic reactions among susceptible laboratory personnel or visitors to the laboratory. The intensity of the host response to natural infection is positively correlated with the number of migrating larvae. Light infections are usually clinically inapparent. Following heavy exposure, the patient may suffer intense pneumonitis, hepatic enlargement and generalized toxicity that may last up to two weeks. In classic self-administered experiments performed in 1922 by Shimesu Koino and his younger brother, the clinical effects of the migrating larval load were graphically demonstrated (Noble and Noble, 1976). Shimesu swallowed 2000 infectious *Ascaris lumbricoides* eggs and became seriously ill within four days of ingestion. He remained violently ill for another week. His brother swallowed only 500 infectious eggs and did not experience any severe illness.

The presence of larvae in the liver induces infiltration with eosinophils which may be accompanied by eosinophilic granuloma formation and eventual destruction of the larvae. Eosinophilic infiltration around larvae and peribronchial inflammation causes *Ascaris* pneumonia. This form of pneumonitis may be associated with signs of fever, dyspnea and/or asthma and profound peripheral eosinophilia. The allergens may produce facial edema resembling kwashiorkor. Individuals sensitized by intermittent seasonal exposure usually suffer more intense reactions than chronically infected individuals (Brown and Neva, 1983). Among those intermittently exposed to *Ascaris* antigens, hypersensitivity symptoms may be observed clinically when only a few (6 to 45) eggs have been ingested (Gelpi and Mustapha, 1967). It has been proposed that the acute hypersensitivity reactions to *Ascaris* species antigens are mediated by specific IgE antibodies. In contrast, chronically infected individuals have generally milder symptoms, with severity of symptoms dependent on the migrating larval load. Chronically infected individuals tend to have elevated specific IgG antibodies and not IgE class antibodies.

In general, the host tolerates the intestinal infection with L4 larvae and adult worms without any apparent pathology. A great number of the L4 larvae and the very young mature worms do not survive long in the small intestine probably due to non-specific and immunological activity. The adult worm in the intestines may produce mild abdominal pain and general restlessness, especially if the adult worm load is relatively high (> 20 worms). Most patients first become aware of *Ascaris* infection because of the passage of an adult worm in the stool or regurgitation of a worm during emesis. Symptoms are more severe when the worm burden is high. With a large intestinal adult worm burden (≥ 15 worms within the intestine), the worms may become entangled and form a bolus obstructing the intestinal lumen. Sometimes the intestinal adult worm burden can reach incredible numbers without causing any apparent discomfort or problems to the individual. For example, one asymptomatic patient expelled 667 adult *Ascaris* species worms after taking an anti-helmintic. In another case at autopsy, an individual who died of a non-*Ascaris* related cause had a total of 1488 worms within the intestinal lumen (Noble and Noble, 1976).

In endemic areas, ascariasis is responsible for up to 35% of all intestinal obstructions (Schwartzman, 1991). In chronic intestinal ascariasis, there is usually a coarsening of the mucosal folds of the jejunum. There is also shortened crypt depth, decreased villous length, decreased numbers of goblet cells per number of gastrointestinal epithelial mucosal cells and muscular hypertrophy of the gastrointestinal lamina muscularis. It is presumed that the decreased amounts of intestinal mucosal mucus and the increased intestinal wall muscular tension may contribute to obstruction (Crompton, Nesheim and Pawlowski, 1989); however, there are no empiric data to suggest this cause and effect relationship. Intussusception, infarction, volvulus and intestinal perforation can also be complications of ascariasis. Such cases result frequently in the death of the patient due to the subsequent consequences associated with fatal septicemia.

It has been hypothesized that the spiral swimming motion of the adult worm increases the likelihood of the worm(s) migrating to a gastrointestinal orifice producing obstruction. Factors which have been associated with increased worm migration and correlated with outlet obstruction include: high fever (≥ 40°C), acute and severe diarrhea, peppery foods, anesthesia and other physiological stresses on the host (e.g. induction chemotherapy for leukemia). Worms may migrate through the mouth, out the nares or occlude the Eustachian tube. There have even been cases of asphyxiation caused by worms occluding the trachea.

Biliary ascariasis is a common cause of adult biliary disease and colic in certain areas where the overall endemic rate of ascariasis is high (Khuroo and Zargar, 1985). For example, among 1105 adults randomly selected and screened by ultrasonography from the general population of Kashmir, India, five individuals (0.5%) had *Ascaris* species worms in their biliary tract (Khuroo *et al.*, 1989). This rate of biliary tract ascariasis is apparent only in regions where the prevalence of ascariasis is high among all age groups (e.g. a prevalence rate of ascariasis of 60% among children and 35% among adults in Kashmir). Generally, the elimination of worms or their extraction from the ampullary orifice leads to rapid relief of colic. Even without treatment, most worms in the biliary tract will migrate back into the intestinal lumen in a day or two with resolution of colic. Among 500 patients with hepatobiliary and pancreatic disease due to *Ascaris lumbricoides* infection, only 76 (15.2%) of patients had worm reinvasion of the biliary tree due to *Ascaris* reinfection within a 48-month period (Khuroo, Zargar and Mahajan, 1990). Hepatobiliary ascariasis is difficult to detect by biliary imaging tools (e.g. oral cholecystography or intravenous cholangiography) or surgical explorations. For these reasons documented hepatobiliary ascariasis is rarely diagnosed. There are some investigators who suggest that frequent and early use of endoscopic retrograde cholangiopancreatography might increase the diagnostic yield for hepatobiliary and pancreatic ascariasis. Adult ascarids that invade the bile ducts or the liver parenchyma may result in the formation of granulomatous lesions or liver abscesses. If the worms are trapped in the ducts and die, they form a nidus for the formation of dystrophic calcified stones. Due to the high glucuronidase activity of the *Ascaris* species worm which is responsible for deconjugation of bilirubin, it is also assumed that hepatobiliary ascariasis may be responsible for the genesis of biliary pigment stones (Maki, 1966). Migration of worms into the pancreatic duct can produce severe, life-threatening pancreatitis. There are numerous isolated reports of patients who die with hemorrhagic pancreatitis due to ascarid pancreatic duct obstruction.

The role of *Ascaris* species in causing human nutritional deficiencies is still controversial. The major difficulty is that most malnourished patients suffering with ascariasis often have polyintestinal parasitic infections, notably hookworms and whipworms. Malnutrition in these patients is often exacerbated by coexisting chronic bacterial gastrointestinal infections or other factors related to low socioeconomic living conditions. Although the worms compete with the host for ingested nutrients, the amounts of nutrients required even for the prolific egg laying of the adult females is relatively small. Yet, the impact of a large worm burden on an undernourished child could be significant and hard to measure. Only a few reports on the relation of ascariasis to malnutrition are scientifically based (Pawlowski, 1988). Ascariasis involving heavy worm burden has been shown negatively to affect the absorption of nutrients in children that subsist on a marginal diet (Tripatly Genzale and Lotero, 1971). Adults infected with heavy *Ascaris* species worm loads demonstrate an intestinal loss of 7–9% of dietary fat and abnormal carbohydrate absorption, notably low lactose absorption possibly due to *Ascaris*-induced lactase insufficiency (Carrera, Neisheim and Crompton, 1983). Treatment of ascariasis appears to improve nutrition among patients with heavy intestinal ascariasis infections since there is a dramatic decrease in lactose levels in the stool after curative therapy (Stephenson, 1980). In addition, the result of eradication of intestinal ascarid worms in children produces a significant weight gain relative to placebo controls despite persistent parameters of malnourishment in both groups (Stephenson and Holland, 1987). In another study, 1206 Burmese children aged 2 to 12 years with an overall prevalence of 80% for ascariasis were divided randomly into two groups. One group was treated on a quarterly basis per annum for ascariasis over a 48-month period. Compared with the non-treated placebo control group, acariasis-treated children were 0.65 cm taller and 0.93 kg heavier than the control group (Thein, Thane and Than, 1991). In general, the experimental designs of such studies to assess the effects of ascariasis on human nutrition tend to suffer from difficulties related to confirming the status of *Ascaris* infection. For example, in one study 37% of initially positive individuals for ascariasis treated with placebo became stool negative over a short-time interval based on the absence of *Ascaris* eggs on microscopic observation of isolated stool specimens and 50% of individuals with initially negative stools for *Ascaris* eggs treated with placebo became positive for ascarid eggs in one study (Willett, Kilama and Kihamia, 1979). It is clear that there is a need for more reliable diagnostic tests in order to conduct epidemiological studies and therapeutic trials for ascariasis.

9.5 IMMUNITY

It has been demonstrated that there is increased resistance to *Ascaris* infections in natural hosts and experimental animals by prior ascarid infection with the homologous parasite. The major immune response to *Ascaris* species is thought to be induced by the migrating larval stages and encompasses both humoral and cellular elements (Pawlowski, 1987). Humans are unable to develop a fully protective immunity to reinfection with *Ascaris* species, but immunological and non-specific reactions to *Ascaris* larvae may greatly reduce the final number of parasites eventually infesting humans. In most endemic areas, the prevalence of ascariasis increases sharply after weaning from breast milk during the first 2 to 3 years of life although it is not clear if this is related to passive immunity or reduced exposure to environmental contamination. The prevalence of ascariasis remains consistently at maximum rates for individuals between the ages of 4 and 14 years in most areas and from different races but then declines usually over the subsequent intervening years into adulthood. The prevalence rates of ascariasis even among adults in some endemic areas remains impressive. For example, prevalence rates of 5 to 70% for ascariasis among adults are still not unusual in many Asian, African and Latin American countries. In Jazin, Iran, the overall prevalence of ascariasis in the late 1970s was still 86% among adults and the mean intensity of intestinal ascariasis as evident by the adult worm load was heavy (i.e. average $>$ 8 adult worms per person) (Schwartzman, 1981). Such rates tend to discount the effectiveness of host immunity in protecting the human host from an *Ascaris* infection.

Serum and lymphocytes harvested from previously *Ascaris*-infected guineapigs were able to transfer protective immunity to normal guineapigs to varying degrees in experimental infection models of ascariasis. Most experimental immunization protocols have involved crude lysates of adult worms, eggs and larval stages. It is not surprising that these preparations have resulted in variable findings. During the first days after experimental *Ascaris* infections in small laboratory animals, there is an increase in the numbers and activity of T cells. This activity is expressed by an intense production of lymphokines including those that induce a chemotactic stimulus for eosinophils which are considered a crucial cell type for host protection against invasive ascariasis. Children from an African area endemic for *Ascaris lumbricoides* were found to have specific serum IgG class antibodies to a number of antigens of the parasite. The possibility that this heterogeneity in the immune repertoire has a genetic basis was explored in various strains of inbred mice infected with *Ascaris suum*. No murine strain responded to all of the potential antigens. The investigators determined that it was the major histocompatibility complex (MHC) which controls the response to ascarid antigens in infected humans (Kennedy *et al.*, 1990). Issues of *Ascaris* and its relation to immunopathology and resistance have not been well explored.

9.6 DIAGNOSIS

Intestinal ascariasis is routinely and commonly diagnosed by finding eggs on a fecal smear or after utilizing stool flotation techniques. It is not uncommon for the diagnosis to be made in conjunction with the principal complaint that brought the patient for treatment of ascariasis: passage of an adult worm through the mouth or anus. The worms can so pack a loop of intestine that they are easily palpable through the abdominal wall; sometimes the turgid loop makes a visible impression on the abdomen of an ectomorphic child. X-ray or ultrasound can also reveal the presence of adult worms in the intestine and other extra-intestinal areas.

Larval forms are occasionally identified in biopsies of tissues. L3 and L4 larvae may be recovered from tracheal, oropharyngeal and gastric washings one to two weeks after ingestion of infectious eggs. This is usually an incidental finding, and the search for larvae does not constitute a reliable diagnostic exercise. Eosinophilia as high as 30–50% of peripheral white blood cell counts is common for pulmonary ascariasis when pulmonary larval migration occurs. Eosinophilia remains persistently high for about a month after significant pulmonary ascarid larval infestation. Marked eosinophilia is rare during the intestinal phase of ascariasis which involves only adult worms.

The *Ascaris* eggs produced by newly developed and gastrointestinally located worms will appear in the stool approximately two months following initial ingestion of infectious eggs. A variety of concentrated salt solutions are used to take advantage of the lower density of the eggs to separate them from the fecal debris. Fertile eggs have an oval, coarse appearance caused by the very thick, mammillated shell. Each measures 45–70 μm by 35–50 μm. Infertile eggs are longer, more delicate in appearance, and do not float as well as fertile eggs. Sedimentation techniques or the Kato and Miura thick-smear techniques are considered to be more efficient than flotation techniques in detecting the presence of *Ascaris* eggs. These tests may require slightly more skill on the part of the microscopist. Egg numbers in the stool correlate roughly with the number of adult female worms in the host. Using direct techniques to diagnose a light infection can be challenging. In a study in Korea, false-negative results were found in 15% of ascariasis cases due to the presence of male worms only (52%), old or immature females (33%) or the inadequacy of the examination technique (15%) (Seo, 1981). It is clear, however, that two to three daily stool microscopic examinations for *Ascaris* eggs is the most reliable current method to detect intestinal ascariasis. Failure to detect eggs after such studies does not exclude intestinal ascariasis, as noted above. It is obvious to those who work in the field that there is an urgent need to develop a more sensitive, rapid, cheap but accurate, copradiagnostic test for intestinal ascariasis using a single stool sample. These diagnostic requirements are essential for a better understanding of the epidemiology of ascariasis and the effects of ascariasis on human health, and for more effective therapeutic trials for ascariasis to progress.

Adult worms can also be seen on routine abdominal radiographs in gas-distended loops of intestine. Contrast studies often reveal thin white lines which represent the barium-filled alimentary tracts of the adult worms. Ascarids in the common bile duct or biliary duct radicals may be detected by their smooth cylindrical radiolucent outlines as seen by intravenous, T-tube, or transhepatic cholangiography (Khuroo and Zarqar, 1985).

Indirect methods for diagnosing ascariasis are also available with the use of immunological or biochemical techniques. Sensitivity and specificity of these tests suffer from extreme variations in host response and cross-reactivity of antigens among helminths. It is particularly difficult histologically to distinguish cases of visceral larval migrans caused by migrating larvae of other *Ascaris* species or *Toxocara* (Lloyd, Wijesundera and Soulsby, 1991). Solid-phase radioimmunoassay technique, indirect immunofluorescence and hemagglutination with both larval and adult *Ascaris* antigens have also been utilized but their diagnostic utility remain to be proven.

9.7 TREATMENT

Intestinal ascariasis should always be treated even in the asymptomatic individual since there is no certainty that the individual is not infested with a large number of adult worms (Anon, 1988). It should be stressed and realized by physicians that even one adult worm can potentially cause serious or fatal consequences in an individual. The drugs of choice include pyrantel pamoate and mebendazole. Pyrantel pamoate is preferred over mebendazole because of cost considerations. This is particularly important when considering mass chemotherapy programs in developing countries. Piperazine citrate and levamisole are alternative drugs for the treatment of ascariasis. These agents are probably not as effective after a single attempt for curative treatment of ascariasis; however, due to their relative safety and cheaper cost they are the preferred agents for mass chemotherapy programs in the treatment and control of ascarisis in hyperendemic regions. Most authorities prefer to use levamisole for mass treatment, especially since the use of piperazine has been associated with rare fatal convulsive side-effects among patients with known seizure disorders or inpatients taking chlorpromazine concomitantly. It should be noted by the physician that many of these anti-*Ascaris* drugs have additional curative effects for other intestinal nematodes. This is often ideal since many of the patients with intestinal ascariasis will have polyintestinal parasitic infections, e.g. hookworm and whipworm. The most important consideration for the physician in assessing the effects of therapy is to confirm by repeated (two or three) microscopic examinations of the stool that eggs are no longer being excreted with the feces after two weeks of presumptive curative therapy. Retreatment soon after initiating a first trial of therapy is often required. It should also be realized that repeated quarterly chemotherapy regimens must be utilized for individuals residing in hyperendemic ascariasis regions if a long-term disease-free state is desired. There are really no effective drugs for the treatment of other forms of ascariasis. Some authorities recommend the use of piperazine in cases of intestinal and biliary tract obstruction. When the physician considers extra-intestinal ascariasis, drugs utilized for the treatment of intestinal ascariasis are recommended, as well as other anti-inflammatory agents for the control of secondary inflammation in these sites associated with the killing or clearance of larval or adult worms.

- Pyrantel pamoate: 11 mg/kg (maximum of 1 g) in a single oral dose. This treatment is associated with cure rates of 60–95%. Repeat doses should be given only after assessing the stool for persistent intestinal ascariasis and after two weeks for a maximum of two additional trials. The most common side-effects with this drug include dizziness, vomiting and diarrhea which are all mild.
- Mebendazole: 100 mg twice daily by an oral route for 3 days. Cure rates are in the range of 90–100% after completion of an initial trial. This drug is probably more effective than pyrantel pamoate in terms of producing curative rates for intestinal ascariasis but it is more than double the cost of pyrantel pamoate. This drug causes rare but mild gastrointestinal side-effects.
- Piperazine citrate: 75 mg/kg (maximum 3.5 g) in a single oral dose each day for 2 days. This drug is cheap and is associated with cure rates of >90% when this regimen is taken by infected individuals. There are rare serious and potentially fatal complications associated with this drug. They include seizures and convulsions among patients with epilepsy or those taking chlorpromazine concomitantly.
- Levamisole: 4 mg/kg (maximum of 150 mg) in a single oral dose. After a one-dose administration, cure rates are between 80 and 100%. This drug is safe but can cause (in ~20% patients) a self-limited rash.

9.8 PREVENTION AND CONTROL

The principal goal for control of ascariasis is any intervention that would prevent the ingestion of contaminated soil or foods with infectious ascarid eggs. The use of untreated human feces or night soil as fertilizer is an important source for the transmission of ascariasis. Similarly, defecation by agricultural workers in or about the fields where they work is often a common practice in endemic ascariasis areas. Efforts to alter these behavioral patterns can be expensive and frustrating. Properly composted night soil which can achieve internal temperatures in excess of 50°C for prolonged periods is one measure that appears to decrease the prevalence of ascariasis in endemic regions. This temperature is sufficient to kill embryonated *Ascaris* eggs. This practice is also not prohibitively expensive in terms of labor and in addition improves the quality of the fertilizer which should entice farmers to use this mixture. The additional step to make properly composted night soil requires, however, dedicated and long-term educational efforts if there is any chance of altering the ancient and frugal technique of fertilizing agricultural fields with night soil.

Changing toilet habits of humans has been even more challenging. Even if there are sufficient resources to build and maintain latrines near agricultural fields or living quarters, they often go unused. The odors and lack of available water for washing at the latrines afterwards may greatly minimize their use. It is difficult to argue with people against the apparent good sense of defecating in a clean, private spot near a stream or irrigation waterway. Sometimes the latrines are considered a 'high class' Western innovation and are reserved for village elders or males only. Only the most intensive and long-term educational programs aimed at changing human defecation habits have resulted in success in reducing the rates of ascariasis.

Hand-washing and personal hygiene are of rather less significance in controlling ascariasis, yet still important. Cases often tend to cluster in families even though the members eat the same food and have the same toilet habits as their neighbors. Efforts to sanitize vegetables that are to be eaten raw may succeed in reducing the size of the inoculum as a result of any rinsing. Ascarid eggs can survive sanitizing techniques which most people are willing or able to utilize. Improvements in water and sanitation have been the subject of considerable recent attention as a result of the declaration by the United Nations that the 1980s were to be the International Drinking-Water, Supply and Sanitation Decade. While there have been overall improvements in the health parameters of the recipient populations, reductions in the prevalence of ascariasis due to water-control measures have been modest. Improvements in water availability for domestic hygiene has made more of an impact on ascariasis than improvements in the quality of drinking water (Esrey and Hubicht, 1986).

The cheapest and most effective intervention, at least in the short-term, is chemotherapy. Epidemiologic studies of the target population are preferred to determine the prevalence, intensity and distribution of ascariasis in the community. Yet, logistic and diagnostic problems usually indicate that blanket total population chemotherapy is the most effective course for reducing the prevalence of ascariasis in high endemic areas. It has been calculated for Kenya that the annual cost of mass treatment on a regular basis would amount to only one-fifth of the losses due to human ascariasis (Stephenson, Lathan and Oduori, 1980). This suggests that mass chemotherapy programs for control of ascariasis is cost-effective. Treatments should be repeated at least quarterly per annum and should be maintained for several years due to the remarkable viability of ascarid eggs in benign environments. Unless there are also improvements in water and sanitation, significant rebound epidemics of ascariasis will occur when chemotherapeutic interventions are discontinued (Esrey *et al.*, 1991).

REFERENCES

Anon (1988) Drugs for parasitic infections. *Med. Lett. Drugs. Ther.*, **30**, 15–49.

Blumenthal, D. and Schultz, M. (1975) Incidence of intestinal obstruction in children infected with *Ascaris lumbricoides*. *Am. J. Trop. Med. Hyg.*, **24**, 801–6.

Brown, H. and Neva, F. (1983) *Basic Clinical Parasitology*, 5th edn, Appleton-Century-Crofts, East Norwalk, Connecticut, pp. 99–142.

Bundy, D., Kan, S. and Rose, R. (1988) Age-related prevalence, intensity and frequency distribution of gastrointestinal helminth infection in urban slum children from Kuala Lumpur, Malaysia. *Trans. Roy. Soc. Trop. Med. Hyg.*, **82**, 289–94.

Bundy, D., Cooper, E., Thompson, D. *et al.* (1987) Epidemiology and population dynamics of *Ascaris lumbricoides* and *Trichuris trichiura* infection in the same community. *Trans. Roy. Soc. Trop. Med. Hyg.*, **81**, 987–93.

Carrera, E., Neisheim, M. and Crompton, D. (1983) Lactose maldigestion in Ascaris-infected pre-school children. *Am. J. Clin. Nutr.*, **39**, 255–64.

Crompton, D., Nesheim, M. and Pawloski, A. (eds) (1985) *Ascariasis and its Public Health Significance*. Taylor and Francis, London.

Crompton, D., Nesheim, M. and Pawlowski, A. (eds) (1989) *Ascariasis and its Prevention and Control*, Taylor and Francis, London.

Editorial (1989) Ascariasis. *Lancet*, **i**, 997–8.

Elkins, D., Haswell-Elkins, M. and Anderson, R. (1986) The epidemiology and control of intestinal helminths in the Pulicat Lake region of Southern India. I. Study design and pre- and post-treatment observations on *Ascaris lumbricoides* infection. *Trans. Roy. Soc. Trop. Med. Hyg.*, **80**, 774–92.

Esrey, S. and Habicht, J. (1986) Epidemiologic evidence for health benefits from improved water and sanitation in developing countries. *Epidem. Rev.*, **8**, 117–28.

Esrey, S., Potash, J., Roberts, L. and Shiff, C. (1991) Effects of improved water supply and sanitation on ascariasis, diarrhoea, dracunculiasis, hookworm infection, schistosomiasis, and trachoma. *Bull. WHO*, **69**, 609–21.

Gelpi, A. and Mustapha, A. (1967) Seasonal pneumonitis with eosinophilia: a study of larval ascariasis in Saudi Arabia. *Am. J. Trop. Med. Hyg.*, **16**, 646–57.

Jones, J. (1981) Identification of intestinal parasites using the digital rectal examination. *J. Fam. Pract.*, **12**, 563–5.

Jones, J. (1983) Parasites in Kentucky: the past seven decades. *J. Kentucky Med. Assoc.*, **81**, 621–7.

Kennedy, M., Tomlinson, L., Fraser, E. and Christie, J. L. (1990) The specificity of the antibody response to internal antigens of *Ascaris*: heterogeneity in infected humans and MHC (H-2) control of the repertoire in mice. *Clin. Exp. Immun.*, **80**, 219–24.

Khuroo, M. and Zargar, S. (1985) Biliary ascariasis: a common cause of biliary and pancreatic disease in an endemic area. *Gastroenterology*, **88**, 418–23.

Khuroo, M. S., Zargar, S. and Mahajan, R. (1990) Hepatobiliary and pancreatic ascariasis in India. *Lancet*, **335**, 1503–7.

Khuroo, M., Mahajan R., Zargar, S. *et al.* (1989) Prevalence of biliary tract disease in India: a sonographic study in adult population in Kashmir. *Gut*, **30**, 201–5.

Lloyd, S., Wijesundera, M. and Soulsby, E. (1991) Intestinal changes in puppies infected with *Toxocara canis*. *J. Comp. Pathol.*, **105**, 93–104.

Maki, T. (1966) Pathogenesis of calcium bilirubinate gallstone: role of *Escherichia coli* β-glucuronidase and coagulation by inorganic ions, polyelectolytes, and agitation. *Ann. Surg.*, **164**, 90–100.

Martin, J., Keymer, A., Isherwood, R. and Wainwright, S. (1983) The prevalence and intensity of *Ascaris lumbricoides* infections in Moslem children from northern Bangladesh. *Trans. Roy. Soc. Trop. Med. Hyg.*, **77**, 702–6.

Noble, E. and Noble, G. (1976) *Parasitology*, 4th edn. Lea and Febiger, Philadelphia, Pennsylvania, pp. 304–6.

Pawlowski, Z. (1987) Ascariasis. *Clin. Trop. Med. Comm. Dis.*, **2**, 595–608.

Pawlowski, Z. (1989) Ascariasis, in *Tropical and Geographical Medicine*, 2nd edn (eds K. Warrens and A. Mahmoud), McGraw-Hill Information Services Company, New York, pp. 369–78.

Pawlowski, Z. (1982) Ascariasis: host–pathogen biology. *Rev. Infect. Dis.*, **4**, 806–23.

Reinthaler, F., Mascher, F. and Klem, G. (1988) A survey of gastrointestinal parasites in Ogun State, southwest Nigeria. *Ann. Trop. Med. Parasit.*, **82**, 181–4.

Schwartzman, J. (1991) Intestinal nematodes that migrate through lungs (Ascariasis), in *Hunter's Tropical Medicine* (ed. T. Strickland), Saunders Company, Philadelphia, Pennsylvania, pp. 696–700.

Seo, B. (1981) Ascariasis and its control problems in Korea. *Seoul J. Med.*, **22**, 323–41.

Stephenson, L. (1980) The contribution of *Ascaris lumbricoides* to malnutrition in children. *Parasitology*, **81**, 221–33.

Stephenson, L. and Holland, C. (1987) *The Impact of Helminth Infections on Human Nutrition: Schistosomes and soil-transmitted helminths*, Taylor and Francis, London.

Stephenson, L., Lathan, M. and Oduori, M. (1980) Costs, prevalence, and approaches for control of *Ascaris* infection in Kenya. *J. Trop. Pediatr.*, **26**, 246–63.

Thein, H., Thane, T. and Than, S. (1991) A controlled therapeutic intervention trial on the relationship between *Ascaris lumbricoides* infection and malnutrition in children. *Trans. Roy. Soc. Trop. Med. Hyg.*, **85**, 523–8.

Thein, H., Myat, L., Hlaing, M. and Maung, M. (1990) Role of ascariasis in surgical abdominal emergencies in the Rangoon Children's Hospital, Burma. *Ann. Trop. Paediatr.*, **10**, 53–60.

Tripatly, K., Genzale, F. and Lotero, H. (1971) Effect of ascariasis infection on human nutrition. *Aust. J. Trop. Med. Hyg.*, **20**, 212–18.

Willet, W., Kilama, W. and Kihamia, C. (1979) Ascaris and growth rates: a randomized trial of treatment. *Am. J. Public Health.*, **69**, 987–91.

TEN

Human hookworm infection

P. Hotez

Hookworm infection is one of the most prevalent and clinically significant communicable diseases of humankind, affecting up to one-fifth of the world's population. The hallmark of hookworm disease is iron-deficiency anemia, particularly in developing countries, that occurs when the adult parasite removes blood from the small intestine. Because hookworm anemia is usually insidious and does not present with dramatic symptomatology, its role in human misery and debility is frequently overlooked (Stoll, 1962).

10.1 HISTORICAL ASPECTS

Descriptions of the symptomatology resulting from heavy hookworm infections are recorded from antiquity, but it was not until the nineteenth century that a causal link was made between 'chlorosis' a term used to describe the yellow-green pallor of hookworm anemia, and the presence of intestinal worms (Schad, 1991). Theodore Bilharz implicated hookworms as the etiologic agent of chlorosis and confirmed Dubini's earlier discovery of an adult hookworm recovered from a woman during autopsy. Hookworm disease was largely brought to the attention of the scientific community during an epidemic in 1880 of severe 'miners' anemia' among Italian laborers constructing the Saint Gothard railway tunnel in the Swiss Alps (Peduzzi and Piffaretti, 1983). Twenty years later, Looss (1901), a German scientist working at government medical schools in Egypt, demonstrated percutaneous transmission of hookworm infection and then elucidated the entire life cycle of *Ancylostoma duodenale*, the so-called 'Old World' hookworm.

Working in the 'New World', Charles W. Stiles, discovered a second major hookworm species, *Uncinaria americana* (renamed *Necator americanus*). Carrying out preliminary field studies from his base at the Hygienic Laboratory of the US Public Health Service (the forerunner of the National Institutes of Health), he found it rampant throughout the rural southeastern USA (Stiles, 1902). Stiles' work gained notoriety when a headline appeared in the *New York Sun* announcing his discovery of the 'germ of laziness' (Ettling, 1981). Upon meeting with Stiles, Frederick Gates, a minister and John D. Rockefeller's key advisor for philanthropic endeavors, obtained a pledge for one million dollars to form the Rockefeller Sanitary Commission whose mission was to eradicate hookworm disease from the south (Figure 10.1). In 1913 the International Health Commission was formed to control hookworm overseas. Together the two Rockefeller campaigns helped to produce a generation of scientists studying the biology of hookworms, including William Cort, A. O. Foster, A. C. Chandler, J. Allen Scott and Norman Stoll, who were based at the newly founded Johns Hopkins School of Hygiene and Public Health (Schad, 1991).

Enteric Infection 2. Intestinal helminths. Edited by M.J.G. Farthing, G.T. Keusch and D. Wakelin. Published in 1995 by Chapman and Hall, London. ISBN 0 412 39140 6

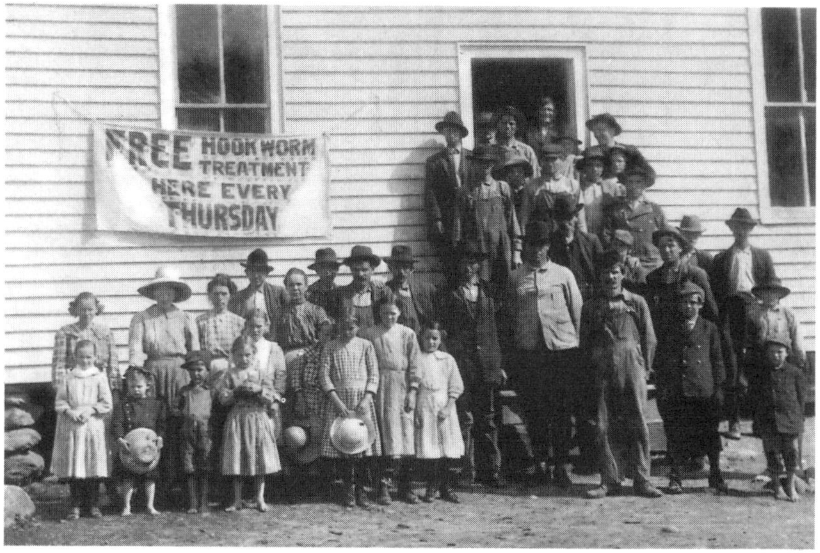

(a)

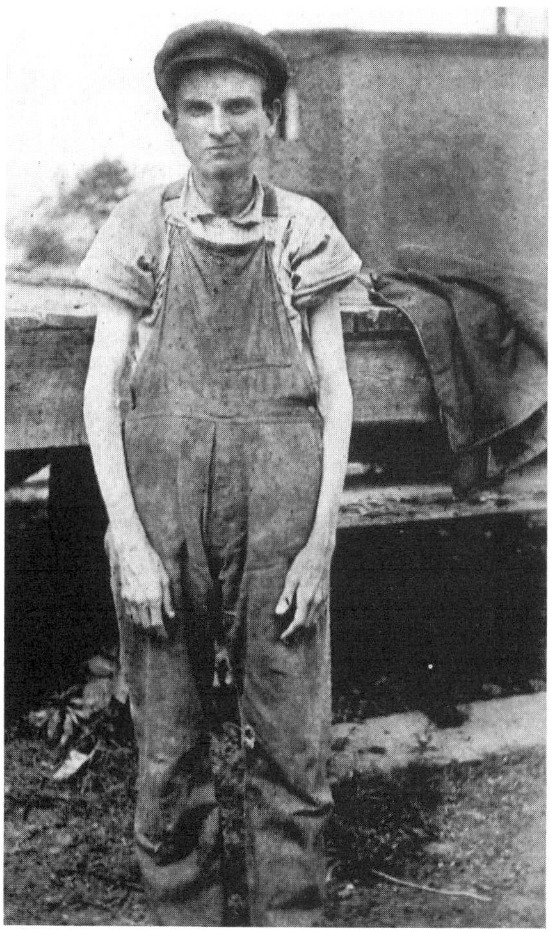

(b)

Figure 10.1 (a) A free clinic for hookworm treatment set up by the Rockefeller Sanitary Commission in the southern USA in the early part of this century. (b) A 29-year-old man with long-standing hookworm infection and consequent physical and intellectual growth delays. (Source: Shaplen, 1964.)

Table 10.1 Differences between *Ancylostoma duodenale* and *Necator americanus**

	Ancylostoma duodenale	*Necator americanus*
Size of adults	8–11 mm (male) 10–13 mm (female)	7–9 mm (male) 9–11 mm (female)
Estimated daily blood loss/worm	0.26 ml	0.03 ml
Daily egg production/worm	10 000–30 000	5000–10 000
Adult natural lifespan	1 year	3–5 years
Prepatent period	53 days	49–56 days
Virulence	++	+
Resistance of eggs to environmental stress	Greater	Less
Oral infectivity	Yes	No
Larval-arrested development	Yes	No

* Source: Hotez (1989) and Hoagland and Schad (1978).

Among the accomplishments resulting from this flurry of investigative activity was the development of quantitative techniques (Stoll, 1923; Cort *et al.*, 1922), strategies for mass chemotherapy and the discovery that resistance to laboratory canine hookworm infection could be elicited by administering repeated small infections with viable larvae (McCoy, 1931; Foster, 1935; Kerr, 1936; Cort and Otto, 1940). These experimental observations laid the foundation for a live canine hookworm vaccine that used attenuated X-irradiated *A. caninum* larvae (Miller, 1971; 1979), but which did not gain commercial acceptance (Miller, 1978). Efforts to reproduce similar resistance in humans have not been successful (Ball and Bartlett, 1969; Ogilve *et al.*, 1978; Miller, 1979; Ottesen, 1990), although they provide much of our current knowledge on the immunobiology of hookworm infection. The current revolution in biotechnology has largely ignored human hookworm infection.

10.2 ETIOLOGY: TAXONOMY, LIFE HISTORY PARAMETERS AND GEOGRAPHY

Hookworms belong to the family Ancylostomatidae, a part of the superfamily Strongyloidea. The two major genera that affect man, *Necator* and *Ancylostoma* are characterized by the presence of oral cutting organs in the adult stage (Faust, Russell and Jung, 1971). *Necator americanus*, whose name literally means the 'American murderer', is the major member of its genus. A second species from badgers, *N. miyazakiensis* has also been described in the Japanese literature (Komiya and Yasuraoka, 1966). The major representative of the genus *Ancylostoma* to infect and complete development in humans is *A. duodenale*.

The major differences between *A. duodenale* and *N. americanus* are summarized in Table 10.1. Unlike *N. americanus* which can complete its life cycle in humans only after skin penetration, *A. duodenale* is also transmitted by oral ingestion of infective larvae. *N. americanus* is smaller than *A. duodenale* and produces fewer eggs, and causes less blood loss. *N. americanus* is also considered less virulent and possibly better accommodated to the human host (Hoagland and Schad, 1978). *A. duodenale*, on the other hand, is considered to be the more 'opportunistic species' based on:

- its greater physiological tolerance when outside the host;
- its ability to infect very young children (discussed below);
- its oral infectivity;
- its greater fecundity;
- its greater virulence (Hoagland and Schad, 1978).

Table 10.2 Etiological agents of human hookworm infection

Organism	*Resevoir host*	*Distribution of human disease*
Ancylostoma duodenale	None	S. Europe, N. Africa, China, N. India
A. ceylanicum	Cats, dogs	India, East Asia
A. caninum	Dogs	Australia
A. malayanum	Bears	Malaysia
Necator americanus	None	Americas, Central Africa, SE Asia

Both major species of human hookworm are distributed widely in the tropics and subtropics, particularly Asia and Africa. In the western hemisphere, *N. americanus* is the predominant species (Martin, 1972) although *A. duodenale* occurs focally in some of the Caribbean Islands and in Central and South America (Banwell and Schad, 1984). *A. duodenale* occurs alone in the Middle East, north Africa, and southern Europe (Banwell and Schad, 1984), and has particularly high prevalence in northern India and China (Wang, 1988).

A. ceylanicum, a parasite of dogs and cats (Garside and Behnke, 1989), is also infective to man both experimentally (Carroll and Grove, 1986) and in naturally exposed individuals living in India (Chowdhury and Schad, 1972), Indonesia (Joe and Siang, 1959), Taiwan (Yoshida, Okamoto and Chiu, 1971), New Guinea (Schad and Banwell, 1984), the Philippines (Velasquez and Cabrera, 1968) and probably elsewhere in Asia (Table 10.2). Recent evidence also suggests that the dog hookworm *A. caninum* may reach adulthood and complete its life cycle in man (Prociv and Croese, 1990; Croese *et al.*, 1990; 1994; Schad, 1994). Beginning in 1988 a clustered number of cases of segmental eosinophilic inflammation of the intestine were diagnosed in northern Queensland, Australia. The patients were previously well and presented with abdominal pain, weight loss, and melena in association with blood eosinophilia and elevated serum IgE. An adult hookworm, identified by scanning electron microscopy as *A. caninum*, was recovered from an inflammatory lesion in the terminal ileum of one patient where there were many discrete, raised, hemorrhagic nodules. *A. malyanum*, the largest member of the genus, is found in bears in India and Malaysia and was reported once from man (Yorke and Maplestone, 1926, quoted by Faust, Russell and Jung, 1971).

Other zoonotic hookworms of the genus *Ancylostoma* penetrate human skin but fail to complete their life cycle and ultimately succumb to the host inflammatory response. For *A. braziliense* this occurs most commonly in the epidermis where serpiginous tunnels in the skin arise to cause the syndrome of cutaneous larva migrans or 'creeping eruption' (Kirby-Smith, Dove and White, 1926; Shelmire, 1928). For others, including *A. caninum*, this can occur in the viscera to cause visceral larva migrans (Little *et al.*, 1983; Beaver, 1956). Overlap of these two syndromes occurs so that pulmonary infiltrates can occur in the setting of creeping eruption (Muhleisen, 1953; Kalmon, 1954).

A schematic representation of the life-history stages of hookworms in humans is presented in Figure 10.2. Descriptions and behaviors of the parasites' external life history stages are provided in section 10.3 and details of the parasitic life history stages are provided in section 10.4.

10.3 EPIDEMIOLOGY

10.3.1 ECOLOGY OF THE EXTERNAL, FREE-LIVING STAGES

Hookworm eggs are discharged from the gravid female adult hookworm and into

Table 10.3 Virulence factors of the parasitic life history stages of hookworms

Virulence factor	*Function*	*Reference*
L3		
Thermotaxis receptor	Host recognition	Croll and Smith (1972)
Chemotaxis receptor	Host recognition	Vetter *et al.* (1985)
Eicosanoids	Immune modulation	Salafsky, Fusco and Siddiqui (1985)
Second-stage cuticle	Immune escape	Pritchard (1990)
Protease (68 kDa)	Tissue invasion Feeding?	Hotez *et al.* (1990b)
Hyaluronidase (49 kDa)	Tissue invasion	Hotez *et al.* (1991)
Protein kinase A and C	Signal transduction	Hawdon and Hotez (unpublished)
L4		
Surface coat	Immune protection	Pritchard (1990)
L5 (Adult)		
Surface coat	Immune protection	Pritchard (1990)
Factor Xa inhibitor	Anticlotting	Cappelio *et al.* (1993)
Platelet aggregating inhibitor	Anticlotting	Spellman and Nossel (1971) Carroll, Howse and Grova (1984)
Proteases (alkaline)	Tissue invasion	Pritchard (1990) Hotez *et al.* (1985) Thorson (1956a)
Proteases (acid)	Hemoglobinase	Pritchard (1990) Oya and Noguchi (1977)
Protease	IgA degradation	Pritchard (1990)
Hemolysin	RBC hemolysis	Foster and Landsberg (1934)
Myelotoxin	Dyserythropoiesis	Foster and Landsberg (1934)
Neurophil inhibitory factor	Immune evasion	Moyle *et al.* (1994)
Hyaluronidase (65 kDa)	Tissue invasion	Hotez *et al.* (1994)

the lumen of the small intestine. The thin-shelled, hyaline, ovoidal eggs, measuring approximately 60 by 40 μm, are generally in the two-cell or four-cell stage when freshly passed (Komiya and Yasuraoka, 1966). The embryos can develop further when fecal retention occurs. Egg development is dependent upon a number of factors including temperature, moisture, sunlight and oxygen content. The lower and upper limits of temperature at which eggs will develop is between 10 and 40°C, with optimal development at 20–30°C (Komiya and Yasuraoka, 1966). These average values neglect information about the precise distribution of development times (Smith and Schad, 1989); mathematical modeling based on laboratory data shows that *A. duodenale* eggs hatch sooner than *N. americanus* but at a marginally slower rate subsequently (Smith and Schad, 1989). Embryos die rapidly in direct sunlight and when the moisture content goes below 9% (Komiya and Yasuraoka, 1966).

Egg hatching and the development of the subsequent external life history stages occur most readily in moist and shady soil where 'decaying vegetation covers a sandy loam' (Faust, Russell and Jung, 1971). Sandy soils usually contain readily visible particles (0.05–2 mm), are well aerated and are non-adhesive (Beaver, 1975) The term 'loam' refers to the additional presence of silt that contains microscopic and barely visible (2–50 μm) soil particles (Beaver, 1975). The first-stage larva (L1) that emerges from eggs is approximately 250–300 μm in length, having a characteristic flask-shaped muscular esophagus that occupies the anterior third of the alimentary canal (Faust, Russell and Jung, 1971). This so-called rhabditiform larva

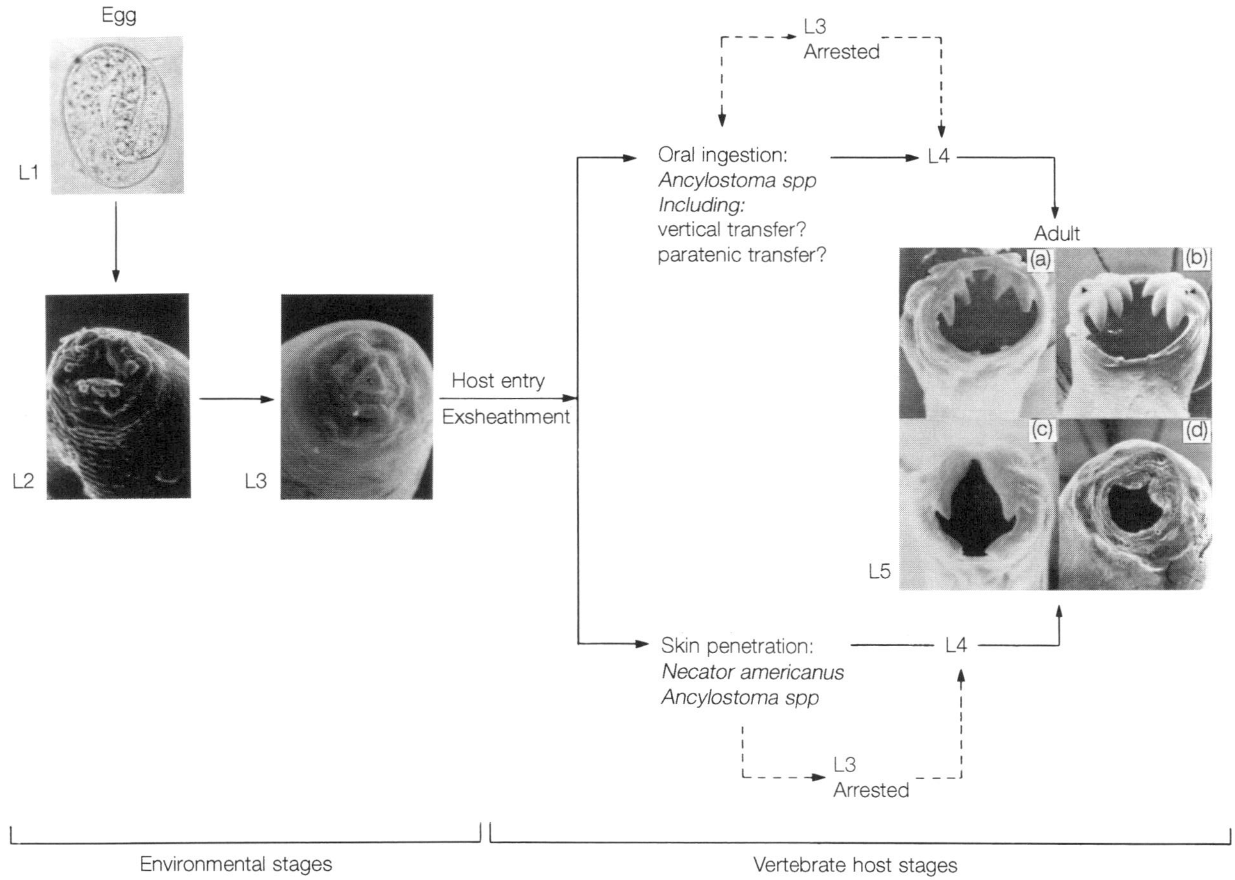

Figure 10.2 The life history stages of human hookworms. L1 = stage one larva; a mature larva of *N. americanus* is coiled within the ova. (Source: Croll and Matthews, 1977.) Scanning electron micrographs are of the L2 and L3 stages of *A duodenale*. (Source: El Naggar, 1987.) Scanning electron micrographs of the L5 or adult stage show four species of hookworm: (1) *A. caninum*, (2) *A. tubaeforme*, (3) *A. ceylanicum*, (4) *N. americanus*. (Source: Croll and Matthews, 1977.) The broken lines refer to facultative growth arrest and resumption of development.

feeds on organic debris and bacteria. After approximately three days of growth the larva undergoes its first ecdysis by paroxysmal movements that facilitate rupture of the cuticle, with the emergence of a second-stage larva or L2 (Komiya and Yasuraoka, 1966). The L2 initially has an open mouth (Figure 10.2) that begins to close by the day 5–8, after hatching. Mouth closure is concurrent with elongation and transformation into the non-feeding third-stage (L3), filariform larva.

The L3 is infective for man, often retaining the cuticle from its previous molt. The ensheathed L3 migrates along films of moisture and will travel vertically in the soil, particularly at night. Around vegetation, larvae will migrate to a height of 30–40 cm in 24–48 h (Komiya and Yasuraoka, 1966), if the film of moisture extends this far. The L3 is highly susceptible to desiccation and will migrate up and down vertically in response to changing moisture conditions (Banwell and Schad, 1984), until the lipid reserves of this non-feeding stage are exhausted (Udonsi, 1984).

10.3.2 HUMAN ECOLOGY

Since survival of the external life-history stages is intimately connected with the soil, it is not surprising that hookworm infection is commonly found in rural and agricultural areas. The association of hookworm infection with agriculture occurs when crops are contaminated with human (and possibly some animal) feces such as when they are applied as fertilizer or deposited onto outdoor defecation grounds. The former situation occurs commonly in rural China where so-called 'night soil' is valued and used widely; the latter situation commonly arises where large plantation-style crops, such as coffee, bananas and cotton, are cultivated (Banwell and Schad, 1984). The scattering actions of rains and the dispersal of feces by dung beetles also enhances the likelihood of transmission (Beaver, 1975). The prevalence of human hookworm infection can reach as high as 90% in rural areas of the moist tropics where sanitation is inadequate (Banwell and Schad, 1984).

Egg and larval viability further depend on soil moisture, and in parts of the tropics where rainfall is seasonal, seasonal variation in human hookworm egg excretion also occurs (Banwell and Schad, 1984). In West Bengal, India, the premonsoon rise in fecal egg counts results from the ability of infective larvae to undergo facultative growth arrest in human tissues during the hot and dry months (see below) and then resume development and mating before the rainy season of the following year (Schad *et al.*, 1973).

Cultural differences profoundly influence the prevalence of hookworm infection. Heavy infections in China, for instance, are often attributed to the wide-spread use of night soil whereas in India, lighter infections often occur partly due to Hindu laws and customs regarding the handling of human feces (Banwell and Schad, 1984). Both Chernin (1954) and Nawalinski, Schad and Chowdhury (1978) found a greater prevalence among Muslims than among Hindus despite the observation that both groups often live in close proximity to one another and that their behavior 'regarding factors determining infection with soil-borne helminths' did not differ.

Gender-associated differences in hookworm prevalence in part reflect occupational exposure, but behavior alone cannot explain a common finding that males are often found more heavily infected than females (Nawalinski, Schad and Chowdhury, 1978). The appearance of gender differences among children emphasizes the possible importance of hormonal, immunological and mechanical factors (Nawalinski, Schad and Chowdhury, 1978). Similar gender differences have been found with animal hookworm infections (Miller, 1965).

10.4 MOLECULAR PATHOGENESIS

10.4.1 LARVAL INVASION AND MIGRATION

The L3 or infective-stage larvae respond to thermal gradients, migrating to the cutaneous surface of mammals by thermotaxis (Croll and Smith, 1972). Larvae actively enter the skin where they separate keratinocytes in the epidermis, penetrate the basement membrane of the epidermal–dermal junction and enter the dermis. Exceptions to this pattern of invasion frequently occur, however. For instance, the zoonotic hookworm *A. braziliense* larva does not usually penetrate the basement membrane, but instead migrates laterally in burrows in the deeper layers of the epidermis and pilosebaceous epithelium (Sulica, Berberian and Kao, 1988) to produce serpiginous tunnels characteristic of cutaneous larva migrans. Lateral migration is facilitated by the release of a hyaluronidase from infective larvae (Hotez *et al.*, 1992), that may hydrolyze the hyaluronic acid adhesion molecules connecting epidermal keratinocytes via CD44 receptors (Miyake *et al.*, 1990; Alho and Underhill, 1989). Moreover, infective hookworm larvae will frequently follow paths of minimal resistance so that increased numbers of larvae can be found beneath breaks in the stratum corneum, including wounds, or at the sites of tears in the epidermis (Hotez *et al.*, 1990b) and within hair follicles (Vetter *et al.*, 1977).

Larvae pass through the basement membrane in order to enter the dermis and the microvasculature (Figure 10.3). Basement membrane dissolution is facilitated by the activity of a larval alkaline protease activity described from *N. americanus* (Matthews, 1982) and a major protease from *Ancylostoma* spp. (Hotez *et al.*, 1990b). The latter protease also has an alkaline pH optimum and is

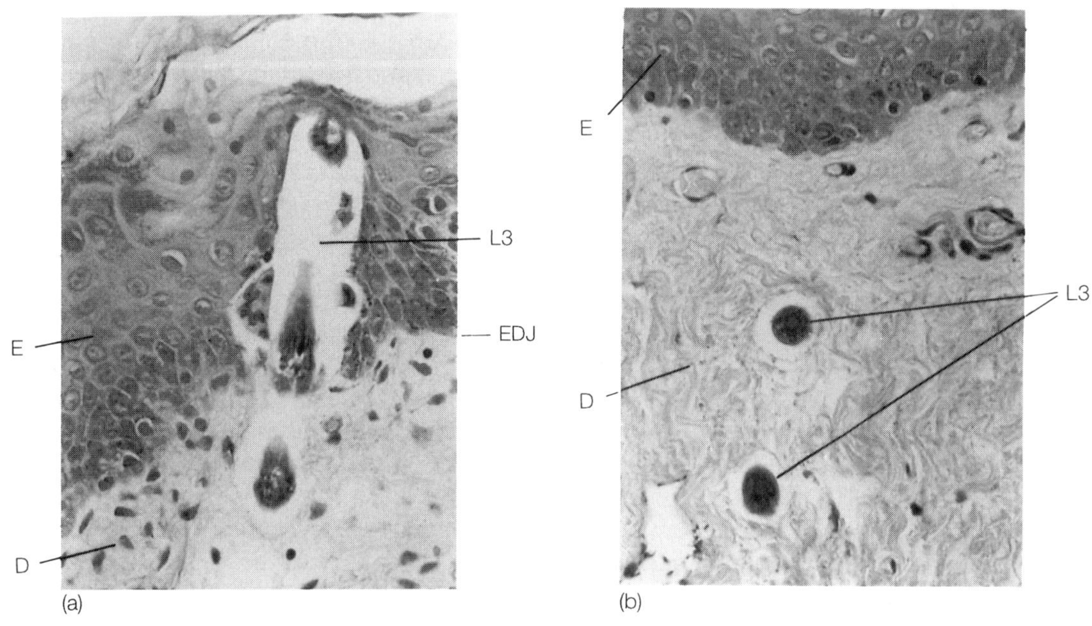

Figure 10.3 Light microscopy of *A. caninum* larvae in skin. Approximately 140 larvae were applied to human neonatal foreskin for 30 min prior to histologic sectioning and staining with periodic acid-Schiff stain. (a) L3 larva traversing the epidermis (E), epidermis–dermis junction (EDJ) and dermis (D). Magnification × 340. (b) L3 larva in the dermis. Magnification × 340. (Source: Hotez *et al.*, 1990b.)

inhibited by *o*-phenanthroline identifying it as a zinc-containing metalloenzyme (Hotez *et al.*, 1990b). Some species, notably *A. tubaeforme*, may also invade via mechanical penetration (Matthews, 1972; 1975). The ground substance of the dermis, which is composed partly of hyaluronic acid, appears to cause little or no hindrance to larval migration (Matthews, 1975) and reflects larval hyaluronidase release (Hotez *et al.*, 1992). Infective larvae shed the cuticle from their previous molt during the early part of invasion by a process known as exsheathment. The location and timing of exsheathment is controversial. Some investigators observe discarded sheaths outside the skin at the site of host entry (Goodey, 1925) and conclude that exsheathment occurs upon host entry, while others observe skin penetration by ensheathed larvae (Matthews, 1975).

As the larvae burrow they elicit a local tissue urticaria ('ground itch'). Skin lipid-induced eicosanoid release by larvae (Salafsky, Fusco and Siddiqui, 1990), in association with cutaneous inflammatory responses resulting from antigen presentation by Langerhans' cells and interleukin production by epidermal keratinocytes, undoubtedly contributes to the immunopathology of 'ground itch'.

From the dermis, larvae enter the microvasculature in response to a 480 dalton host-specific serum chemotactic factor (Vetter *et al.*, 1985). Also in response to a serum factor, larval feeding and development begins (Hawdon and Schad, 1990; 1991; Hawdon *et al.*, 1992). Once in venules and lymphatics the larvae are swept passively to the right atrium, ventricle and pulmonary circulation where they become trapped in pulmonary capillaries. As larvae migrate through the lungs they produce microhemorrhages at the site of ruptured alveolar capillaries, but seldom elicit significant pulmonary hemorrhage and hemoptysis unless large numbers of larvae migrate simultaneously.

Exceptions to the occurrence of this pulmonary phase may occur in humans under two circumstances. First, in the cases of *A. duodenale* (Schad, 1979) and *A. ceylanicum* (Yoshida, Okamotu and Chiu, 1971), infection will occur by the ingestion of L3 larvae. Orally ingested larvae may develop to adulthood directly without requiring a lung migration (Gilman, 1982), although the presence of eosinophilia in patients who ingest larvae (Ottesen, 1990) suggests that tissue invasion occurs. Second, larvae of the genus *Ancylostoma* have been identified in the musculature of humans (Little *et al.*, 1983; Lee, Little and Beaver, 1975) and implicated in the pathogenesis of visceral larva migrans (Beaver, 1956). Thus the possibility exists that larvae can bypass the pulmonary circulation, enter the systemic circulation and disseminate throughout body tissues, including muscle. These tissue-dwelling larvae represent a population of growth-arrested, hypobiotic worms (Nawalinski and Schad, 1974). In the canine host, the 'arrested' or tissue-dwelling larvae migrate from the muscles to the mammary glands of bitches during late pregnancy or parturition and then are transmitted to newborn puppies through the colostrum and milk (Little *et al.*, 1983; Stone and Smith, 1973; Schad, Murrell and Fayer, 1984). This route of migration has also been postulated to occur in humans to produce vertical transmission of hookworm larvae that results in perinatal ancylostomiasis (Hotez, 1989; Wang, 1988). The controlling elements responsible for the induction of hookworm larval arrest as well as the resumption of development from an arrested state are not known. By analogy with an arrested larval stage (named dauer larva) of the free-living nematode *Caenorhabditis elegans*, these phenomena may reflect the presence of worm-derived signal transduction molecules that 'sense' environmental cues (Georgi, Albert and Riddle, 1990; Hotez, Hawdon and Schad, 1993).

10.4.2 INTESTINAL PARASITISM AND ANEMIA

Final development to adulthood occurs in the small intestine. This phase is associated with development of a buccal capsule and attachment and feeding of the adult hookworm onto the mucosa. The average life span for *N. americanus* is calculated to be 3–4 years and that of *A. duodenale* about 1 year (Nawalinski, Schad and Chowdhury, 1978). Adult hookworms will shift positions in the intestine approximately every 4–6 h to search for new feeding sites and sexual partners for mating (Kalkofen, 1970). A correlation exists between hookworm mating behavior and numbers of intestinal lacerations leading to blood loss (Beaver, Yoshida and Ash, 1964). As shown in Figure 10.4, the worms attach by fastening onto the mucosa with their cutting plates and contracting their muscular esophagus to create negative pressure that sucks a plug of intestinal mucosa into their buccal capsule (Kalkofen, 1970; Hotez, 1989). Epithelium dissociates from the lamina propria (Kalkofen, 1970), possibly through the action of a hyaluronidase activity from the adult worm (Hotez *et al.*, 1994). The ingested bolus of host tissue is degraded through the action of proteases (Thorson, 1956a), including the family of proteases released by adult *Ancylostoma* spp. (Hotez *et al.*, 1985; Pritchard, 1990). Hookworm feeding is generally restricted to the mucosa and submucosa; fibers of the muscularis mucosae are seldom incorporated into the feeding bolus (Kalkofen, 1970).

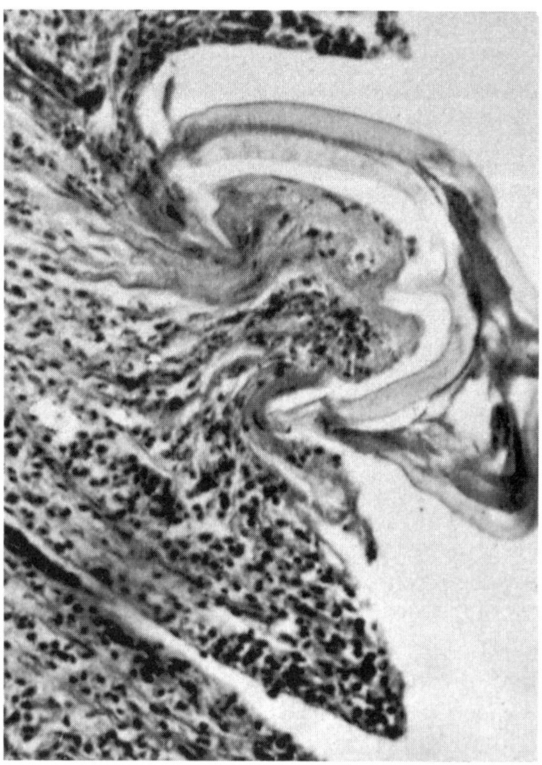

Figure 10.4 Adult *Ancylostoma tubaeforme* hookworm attached to the gut mucosa. (Source: Croll and Matthews, 1977.)

As a general rule, blood loss is incidental to rather than a primary aim of feeding behavior. Blood loss occurs as capillaries in the lamina propria are ruptured within the bolus. Much of the blood is ingested by the worm through efficient esophageal pumping (Roche and Layrisse, 1966), although some of it leaks at the site of attachment (Kalkofen, 1970; 1974). Many of the red blood cells that are ingested by the adult hookworm pass out the anus of the worm still intact. Nevertheless, some red cells are destroyed, in part through the action of cysteinyl hemoglobinases (Oya and Noguchi, 1977; Pritchard, 1990), with the resultant accumulation of iron-containing intestinal pigment granules (Lee, 1970). Blood flow is ensured via the action of parasite-derived anticoagulants secreted from the cephalic glands of the adult worm (Loeb and Smith, 1904; Thorson, 1956b; Eiff, 1966; Spellman and Nossel, 1971). The major anticoagulant from *Ancylostoma* sp. is an kDa peptide that blocks the activity of Xa and VIIa/TF (Capello *et al.*, 1993). Fibrinolytic properties have also been ascribed to the major alkaline protease activity released by adult hookworms (Hotez and Cerami, 1983), analogous to the metalloprotease, hementin, identified from the leech

(Malinconico, Katz and Budzynski, 1984). Adult hookworms of the genus *Ancylostoma* spp. also release antiplatelet-aggregating activities (Spellman and Nossel, 1971; Carroll, Howse and Grove, 1984), that are possibly similar to the apyrase activities described from hematophagous arthropods (Ribeiro, 1987).

Although the early literature describes hemolysins and myelotoxins from adult hookworms that produce a hemolytic anemia and dyserythropoiesis, respectively (Foster and Landsberg, 1934), most of the current literature favors the notion that hookworm anemia occurs directly from mechanical blood withdrawal through the gastrointestinal tract. Blood loss caused by adult hookworms can be measured by labelling circulating erythrocytes with the radioactive isotope chromium-51 and calculating fecal clearance of the isotope relative to the amount in peripheral blood (Roche and Layrisse, 1966). The results show that on average, *A. duodenale* produces a greater order of magnitude of blood loss (0.05–0.3 ml/worm) than does *N. americanus* (0.01–0.04 ml/worm). Measurements for *A. ceylanicum* in a canine host suggest that minimal blood loss occurs during infection with this species (Rep, Van Joost and Vetter, 1971). Some reduction in half-life of circulating erythrocytes has been shown using chromium-51, a phenomenon which has been ascribed to coexisting iron deficiency or protein malnutrition (Miller, 1979).

The development of hypochromic microcytic anemia from intestinal blood loss is highly dependent on the daily iron intake and the iron reserves of the host. In parts of the world where the host is well compensated by high iron intake, a worm load >800 may be required to produce anemia, while in areas where iron intake is poor only 40 worms may be required to precipitate anemia (Gilles, 1985). Similarly, certain populations are particularly vulnerable to blood loss caused by hookworms such as women in their reproductive years in association with menstruation, pregnancy and lactation (Miller, 1979) and growing children who suffer growth failure (Hotez, 1989). Hookworms also injure their host, especially children, through non-hemorrhagic effects of iron deficiency anemia (Pollitt and Leibel, 1976; Oski, 1979; Lozoff and Brittenham, 1987), which produce deficiencies in enzymes with an iron prosthetic group that are essential for the turnover of endogenous neurotransmitters (Mackler *et al.*, 1978; Reeves *et al.*, 1984). Hookworms may cause attention deficits and delay intellectual development by this mechanism.

Plasma protein loss through the intestine also occurs in hookworm infection and leads to hypoalbuminemia which will contribute to kwashiorkor and marasmus in developing countries (Gilles, Watson-Williams and Ball, 1964; Blackman *et al.*, 1965; Gilles, 1990). Mucosal edema and decreased appetite from anorexia and abdominal discomfort also contribute to protein loss (Crompton and Stephenson, 1990). The temporal relationship between the appearance of blood eosinophils and the onset of gastrointestinal symptoms has led to the suggestion that these two processes are related (Ottesen, 1990).

Controversy surrounds the notion of whether intestinal malabsorption occurs in association with hookworm infection, particularly in areas of the world where tropical sprue is endemic (Miller, 1979). Tropical sprue itself appears to exacerbate the morbidity of hookworm infection, particularly in Puerto Rico (Crosby, 1987a). Reductions in gastric acidity and in the secretion and activities of host digestive enzymes caused by hookworm infection have been reported, as have alterations in peristalsis and motility (Miller, 1979; Castro, Behnke and Weisbrodt, 1990).

An association between hookworm infection and Mooren's ulcer of the cornea has been suggested (Kuriakose, 1963). The mechanism by which hookworms may cause corneal ulceration is unknown, although both direct toxin and autoimmune mechanisms have been proposed (Van der gaag *et al.*, 1983).

10.5 IMMUNITY

In many endemic areas the number of hookworms that parasitize the intestine increases in individuals during the first decade of life and then remains relatively constant throughout most of adulthood (Miller, 1979). The contribution of host immunity to this apparent age resistance is unclear, and there is currently no direct evidence that humans develop protective immunity to hookworm infection (Ottesen, 1990). Instead, the development of protective immunity has been postulated from indirect evidence based on the following experimental observations (Ottesen, 1990):

- Resistance to canine hookworm infection can be obtained in laboratory animal models by administering repeated doses of living or X-ray-attenuated L3 larvae (Miller, 1971; Hotez, Trang and Cerami, 1987).
- Infective hookworm larvae fix complement via the alternative pathway *in vitro* (Klaaver-Wesseling, Vetter and Schoeman, 1982).
- Epidemiologic studies have identified populations of individuals who are predisposed to resistance against developing heavy hookworm infections despite multiple exposures (Schad and Anderson, 1985; Wakelin, 1985).
- Human volunteers exposed to hookworm larvae develop a cellular immune response to parasite antigen and develop eosinophil stimulation and eosinophilia, presumably in association with the biosynthesis and release of interleukin 5 (White, Maxwell and Gallin, 1986; Maxwell *et al.*, 1987).
- Worm-specific humoral antibodies can be measured in human volunteers experimentally infected with either *N. americanus* (Ball and Bartlett, 1969; Ogilve *et al.*, 1978; Maxwell *et al.*, 1987) or *A. ceylanicum* (Carroll and Grove, 1986).

An equal weight of evidence, however, argues that humans do not develop naturally acquired immunity to hookworm infection. For instance, although infected human volunteers develop hookworm-specific humoral antibodies they do not develop resistance with repeated exposure (Ottesen, 1990). An immunoepidemiologic analysis of *N. americanus* infections in a rural village in Papua New Guinea where prevalence is 80% (Pritchard *et al.*, 1990), supports this observation. Whereas significant correlations were found between the development of antibody to parasite excretory/secretory antigens and egg production as well as between antiworm collagen and the age of the host, these findings were thought to reflect the worm burden at the time of the study and the cumulative exposure to infection, respectively (Pritchard *et al.*, 1990). There is no evidence to suggest that either humoral antibody response can regulate populations of intestinal hookworms (Pritchard *et al.*, 1990).

The absence of protective antibodies in humans may reflect the hookworm's adroitness for immune evasion and escape. L3 larvae shed surface antigens (Klaver-Wesseling, Vetter and Visser, 1978), including the antigens shed on the L2 cuticular surface during exsheathment. Pritchard (1990) postulated that the sheath could function as an 'antigen smoke-screen' once shed in the dermis. The adult hookworm may use its proteases to degrade secretory IgA, and the presence of surface membrane-associated antigens on the L4 and adult stage of the parasite may suggest the presence of a protective surface coat (Pritchard, 1990). The surface coat may prevent gut mucosal mast cell recognition and deposition of mast cell proteases that would otherwise degrade deeper lying structural parasite collagens (Pritchard, McKean and Rogan, 1988; McKean and Pritchard, 1989). Recently, a peptide that blocks both neutrophil and eosinophil attachment has been isolated and cloned from the adult hookworm *Ancylostoma caninum* (Moyle *et al.*, 1994). Efforts are underway in several laboratories to identify antigens from larval and adult stages of hookworms which, when administered as a subunit vaccine, may overcome these immune evasion mechanisms.

Given the long history of the hookworm's association with man, which for *Ancylostoma* spp. began with domestication of the dog (Cameron, 1956), it is reasonable to speculate that as yet unidentified non-immune or innate resistance factors have importance. These conceivably could include the elaboration of cutaneous inflammatory mediators (e.g. eicosanoids, cytokines) that affect host entry and hemoglobin polymorphisms that prevent parasite-derived hemoglobinase degradation. For *A. duodenale*, arrested development is also a means by which parasite populations are regulated.

10.6 CLINICAL FEATURES

10.6.1 LARVAL INVASION AND MIGRATION

The papular vesicular dermatitis ('ground itch'), accompanied by intense burning and itching, usually develops at the cutaneous site where hookworm larvae enter. The lesions frequently develop on the hands and feet and subside within days to weeks in the absence of secondary pyogenic infection. A second urticarial rash will then often develop in association with larval somatic migration. Cough and dyspnea with asthma-like wheezing occur usually one to two weeks after skin invasion in association with larval migration through the lungs. Hookworm pneumonitis that results from worms rupturing through blood capillaries and into the air sacs is usually less severe than the pneumonitis associated with ascariasis and strongyloidiasis. This migratory phase is associated with the onset eosinophilia which reaches peak levels 35–65 days after the infection but precedes the arrival of larvae into the intestine (Ottesen, 1990).

An unusual outbreak of ground itch followed by pulmonary symptoms was described in which 27 young men from the same village began playing *Kabaddi*, a game associated with prolonged body contact on very slushy and muddy ground (Koshy *et al.*, 1978). The men immediately experienced intense itching on their feet that spread to the whole body, forcing them to shorten their game, run to their village wells to pour water over themselves, and travel several kilometers to receive corticosteroids and antihistaminic drugs from a local hospital. Generalized pruritis lasted with a mean duration of 6.5 days, and was followed by an onset of cough, dyspnea and wheezing in association with larval pulmonary migration (Koshy *et al.*, 1978). Pulmonary symptoms continued for an average of 3 months and were followed by the appearance of hookworm ova in the stool. A 24-h stool collection after anthelminthic treatment revealed hundreds of *A. duodenale* adult worms.

A similar immediate hypersensitivity-like syndrome, known as 'Wakana disease', occurs with the ingestion of large numbers of L3 *A. duodenale* larvae (Yoshida, Nakanishi and Mitani, 1958). This clinical condition consists of nausea and vomiting, cough, dyspnea and eosinophilia, one to several days following larval ingestion. The onset of symptoms coincides with the period of larval development in the intestinal mucosa (Faust, Russell and Jung, 1971).

Skin invasion by L3 zoonotic hookworm larvae, particularly those of *A. braziliense*, results in 'creeping eruption' also known as cutaneous larva migrans of hookworm origin. These larvae produce an erythematous papule at the site of entry but do not enter the dermis. Unable to penetrate the basement membrane of the epidermal–dermal junction of human skin, they migrate laterally in the deep epidermis several millimeters to centimeters per day to produce winding cutaneous tunnels within several days. Tunnel formation is accompanied by intense pruritis and often secondary bacterial invasion. Creeping eruption is common during the summer months in the southern United States, particularly among workers who repair plumbing under summer cottages (Faust, Russell and Jung, 1971).

10.6.2 INTESTINAL PARASITISM AND ANEMIA

The gastrointestinal symptoms that accompany the appearance of hookworms in the gut such as abdominal pain, nausea and anorexia are non-specific and, as Gilles (1990) points out, in the tropics these can be attributed to other concurrent infections. With moderate or severe infections, pica (clay or dirt eating) appears to relieve some of these symptoms, especially epigastric pain.

Approximately 10 to 20 weeks after exposure to infective larvae (except in cases where larvae undergo facultative growth arrest) the anemia of hookworm disease begins to appear. As indicated above, the degree and severity of anemia reflects a number of factors, including the host iron reserves and dietary intake, the overall nutritional status of the host, the number and sex of the adult hookworms present and the species of hookworm. The symptoms associated with anemia include dyspnea on exertion, palpitations, fatigue and impotence. Many patients report difficulties in concentration and that they are no longer able to work. Some patients develop aching in their thighs or calves while walking (Gilles, 1990). Severe anemia can lead to angina pectoris and even high output cardiac failure. The physical signs of hookworm anemia include new cardiac flow murmurs, pale sclerae, koilonychia or concavity of the fingernails and hypothermia. The skin can take on an unusual pale green-yellow pallor known as chlorosis which, in black patients, may manifest as depigmentation (Crosby, 1987b). The hemorrhagic properties of adult hookworms have been exploited to advantage by administering adult parasites (*A. duodenale*) via nasogastric tube to a child suffering from congenital polycythemia (Walterspiel *et al.*, 1985).

Superimposed on this clinical picture of anemia are the effects of protein-losing enteropathy which impart a kwashiorkor-like appearance – edema of the face, particularly periorbital edema, dermatitis, pot belly and sparse hair (Hotez, 1989; Smilllie and Augustine, 1926). These patients are often susceptible to bacterial and viral infections, including measles (Kofoid and Tucker, 1921).

Children who suffer from anemia secondary to hookworm disease exhibit delays in intellectual development. Based on measurements of intelligence quotient, the degree of mental retardation in children has been shown to be in proportion to the intensity of hookworm infection (Smillie and Spencer, 1926). They offered a compelling description of the child with severe hookworm disease:

> . . . both the mental and physical reactions are very slow. Little interest is taken in surroundings. The child does not run and play with other children. He is dull, apathetic, unable to concentrate upon his school problems, and apparently does not hear when spoken to, though slowly comprehending and gradually fulfilling appointed tasks. One has the impression that the child is living in another, entirely separate world, and is only remotely in contact with the everyday world about him. Every teacher of a southern rural school in the hookworm area has noted the immediate and almost startling improvement in mental alertness that occurs

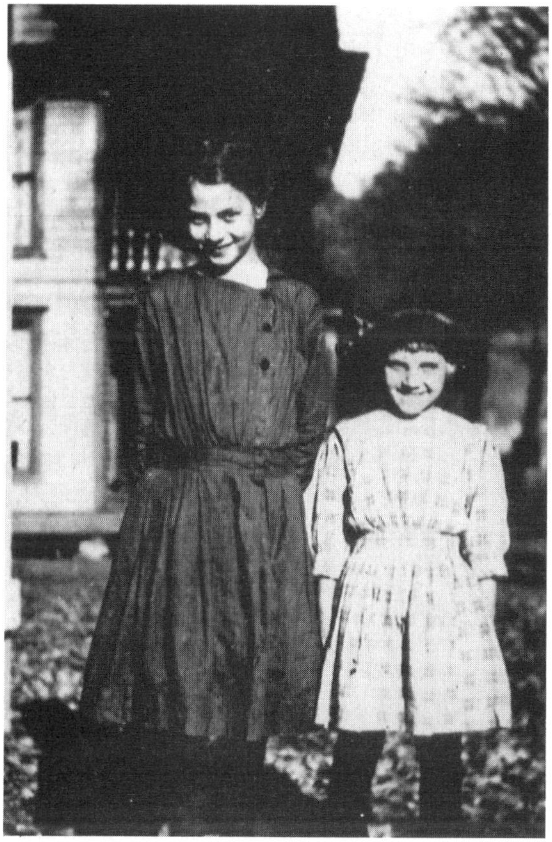

Figure 10.5 Two teenage girls of the same age in North Carolina in the early part of this century. The girl at the right was heavily infected with *N. americanus*. (Source: Shaplen, 1964.)

following treatment of these heavily infested children.

As shown in Figure 10.5, childhood hookworm infection also causes delays in physical growth that is particularly apparent at about the time of puberty when a striking divergence between infected and non-infected children emerges, as the former fall off the growth curve (Smillie and Augustine, 1926). Puberty is frequently delayed. Treatment with even a single dose of albendazole has been shown to reverse this trend and improve growth and physical fitness of children in Kenya with hookworm infection (Stephenson *et al.*, 1989; 1990).

10.6.3 NEONATAL AND INFANT HOOKWORM INFECTION

A syndrome of anemia with very pale complexion, melena, diarrhea, and anorexia, associated with a high mortality (3–6%) has been reported in infants infected with *A. duodenale*, particularly in parts of North China (Yu and Shen, 1990; Wang, 1988) and India (Nawalinski, Schad and Chowdhury, 1978). Of 158 cases of neonatal ancylostomiasis reported from China, 17% of the infants developed hookworm disease within three months and 44% within six months (Yu and Shen, 1990). Possible sources of infection that were cited included contaminated soil, contaminated sandbags or wheat-stem bundles and contaminated sand-filled adsorbent diapers (Yu and Shen, 1990; Wang, 1988).

Schad (1990) has reviewed the evidence that neonatal ancylostomiasis also occurs via transmammary or lactogenic transmission. Although vertical transmission of hookworm larvae in milk or colostrum is a well documented route of infection for dogs and other mammals, the evidence that it occurs in humans is still largely circumstantial (Hotez, 1989). The high prevalence of ancylostomiasis in nursing infants who do not have soil contact is often striking. In contrast, evidence for lactogenic infection with *N. americanus* has not been found (Schad, 1990), and in areas where both *A. duodenale* and *N. americanus* are endemic, only the former is associated with neonatal infection (Nawalinski, Schad and Chowdhury, 1978).

10.7 DIAGNOSIS

The diagnosis of syndromes caused by migrating larvae including ground itch, cutaneous larva migrans and pneumonitis are usually made on the basis of clinical criteria. The cutaneous manifestations require differentiation from cercarial dermatitis ('swimmer's itch') and other causes of creeping eruption, such as larva currens secondary to cutaneous migration of *Strongyloides stercoralis*. The pulmonary and early intestinal migrations caused by hookworm larvae cause manifestations that are often similar to other helminthic causes of pneumonitis and some immediate hypersensitivity syndromes.

Although heavy intestinal hookworm infection can be suspected by identifying melanotic stools, light-microscopic analysis of feces must be carried out to look for hookworm eggs. In general, the examination of three microscopic films of unconcentrated feces is adequate to diagnose clinically important hookworm infection (Faust, Russell and Jung, 1971). Fecal concentration techniques such as flotation with zinc sulfate or brine and sedimentation with formalin-ether will add sensitivity and facilitate detection of light hookworm infections. These concentration techniques are not acceptable for quantitative egg estimates, however (Beaver, 1975), and may lead the clinician to overestimate their clinical importance on the basis of egg yield (Faust, Russell and Jung, 1971).

There are several standard and reliable quantitative egg counting techniques which permit a direct estimate of hookworm egg output and an indirect measure of worm burden (Beaver, 1975). The correlation of egg output with worm burden is not direct and is influenced by fecundity that varies in response to intestinal worm crowding (Krupp, 1961), age of infection (Beaver, 1975) and host resistance (Miller, 1971). The three major quantitative techniques are the Stoll dilutional method (Stoll and Hausheer, 1926), the Beaver direct-smear method (Beaver, 1950) and the Kato cellophane-covered thick film method. The advantages and caveats of each method has been reviewed (Beaver, 1975).

Hookworm ova of *Ancylostoma* spp. and *N. americanus* are morphologically similar. Genus differentiation requires rearing and recovering L3 larvae by Harada–Mori filter paper and charcoal cultures (Harada and Mori, 1955; Beaver, Malek and Little, 1964; Hotez *et al.*, 1990a) and differentiation by light microscopy. Immunodiagnostic methods such as immediate hypersensitivity skin tests, hemagglutination inhibition, complement fixation, immunofluorescence and enzyme immunoassay have been developed (Ottesen, 1990), but require sources of parasite antigen that are not easily nor commercially available. These methods also do not always distinguish species or genuses during mixed infections. The identification of major cuticular and excretory/secretory antigens of *N. americanus* (Pritchard, 1990) and *Ancylostoma* spp. (Hotez, Trang and Cerami, 1987) will facilitate the development of specific immunodiagnostic reagents.

10.8 TREATMENT

A number of chemical anthelminthics are available for removing adult hookworms from the human small intestine. Many of these agents have appeared on the market only in the past few years. They are generally well tolerated, effective, and have a spectrum of activity that is broad enough to eradicate other common intestinal nematodes. These properties make some of these anthelminthics useful for mass application (Sturchler, 1982), by treating either all members of a community (mass chemotherapy) or a population which is at particularly high risk (targeted chemotherapy). The observation that certain individuals are predisposed to acquiring heavy hookworm burdens (Schad and Anderson, 1985), emphasizes the feasibility of targeted chemotherapy.

Aside from reinfection, there are several unique features about the biology of human hookworms that could potentially hinder attempts to apply the principles of mass or targeted chemotherapy:

- Canine and feline animal reservoirs harbor *A. caninum* and *A. ceylanicum*. Both parasites can develop to adulthood in humans.

- There is little or no evidence that the available anthelminthics will eradicate populations of arrested larvae. Viable arrested larvae have the capacity to repopulate the intestine months after conventional anthelminthic chemotherapy, or gain access to breast milk in preparation for vertical transfer.
- Benzimidazoles such as mebendazole and albendazole are embryotoxic and teratogenic in laboratory animals (Rossignol, 1990). Their safety has not been established in infants and neonates who are susceptible to infection with *A. duodenale*. These compounds are also relatively expensive.

The major anthelminthic agents used in the treatment of human hookworm infection are as follows:

- *Pyrantel pamoate* is a cyclic amidine that causes ganglionic blockade in the parasite (Rossignol, 1990). It is available in suspension and has been reported to be effective against neonatal ancylostomiasis (Wang, 1988). For *A. duodenale* infections a single dose may be adequate, whereas three consecutive doses may be required for *N. americanus* infections (Rossignol, 1990).
- *Mebendazole*, a benzimidazole microtubule inhibitor, is effective against both species of hookworms as well as other intestinal nematodes and some parasitic platyhelminths (Rossignol, 1990). Cure rates range up to 97% when administered as a 100 mg dose twice daily for three consecutive days; a single dose does not achieve an adequate cure rate (Rossignol, 1990).
- *Albendazole*, another benzimidazole, has been reported to be highly effective as a single 400 mg dose against both *A. duodenale* and *N. americanus* (Rossignol, 1990). Although albendazole is larvicidal for *N. americanus* (Cline *et al.*, 1984), it may not eradicate tissue-dwelling arrested larvae.
- *Levamisole hydrochloride* is effective against both species. Bone marrow suppression has been reported and it is not recommended in patients with underlying blood dyscrasias.
- *Bephenium hydroxynaphthoate, tetrachloroethylene,* and *metrifonate* are second-line agents in the treatment of hookworm infection and will not be discussed here.

10.9 PREVENTION AND CONTROL

A combination program of sanitation with appropriate disposal of human feces, health education and mass or targeted chemotherapy, has traditionally been implemented in order to eradicate hookworm infection. Although this kind of eradication program is often effective in reducing worm burdens, it is not routinely implemented in developing countries because of expense and the high incidence of reinfection. Moreover, it does not offer a means to eradicate populations of arrested larvae in human tissues. Wearing shoes or other footwear is not an effective control measure as all aspects of the skin are susceptible to larval penetration (Katz, 1975), compliance is poor and, for *A. duodenale*, oral ingestion is a common means of acquiring infection.

Better understanding of the biochemistry of helminth tissue invasion and the molecular biology of hookworm infection may ultimately provide the basis for rational vaccine development. These studies are hampered, however, by the absence of inexpensive animal models or *in vitro* culture methods, sufficient quantities of parasite material for biochemical analysis and a means to construct and analyse genetic mutants. The information explosion that has occurred in nematode cell biology, neurobiology and molecular genetics as a result of cell lineage, gene mapping and transgenic nematode construct studies on *C. elegans* has yet to benefit hookworm research.

ACKNOWLEDGEMENTS

I would like to thank Professors G. A. Schad and Frank Richards for their advice, encouragement and thoughtful discussions. This work was supported by a Culpeper Medical Scientist Scholarship, NIHR 29 AI32726, and a Clinical Research grant from the March of Dimes.

REFERENCES

Alho, A. M. and Underhill, C. B. (1989) The hyaluronate receptor is preferentially expressed on proliferating epithelial cells. *J. Cell Biol.*, **108**, 1557–65.

Ball, P. A. J. and Bartlett, A. (1969) Serological reactions to infection with *Necator americanus*. *Trans. Roy. Soc. Trop. Med. Hyg.*, **63**, 362–9.

Banwell, J. and Schad, G. A. (1984) Hookworm infection, in *Tropical and Geographical Medicine*, McGraw-Hill, New York.

Beaver, P. C. (1950) The standardization of fecal smears for estimating egg production and worm burden. *J. Parasit.*, **36**, 451–6.

Beaver, P. C. (1956) Larva migrans. *Exp. Parasit.*, **5**, 587–621.

Beaver, P. C. (1975) Biology of soil-transmitted helminths: the massive infection. *Hlth Lab. Sci.*, **12**, 116–25.

Beaver, P. C., Malek, E. A. and Little, M. D. (1964), Development of *Spirometra* and *Paragonimus* eggs in Harada–Mori cultures. *J. Parasit.*, **50**, 664–6.

Beaver, P. C., Yoshida, Y. and Ash, L. R. (1964), Mating of *Ancylostoma caninum* in relation to blood loss in the host. *J. Parasit.*, **50**, 286–93.

Blackman, V., Marsden, P. D., Banwell, J. and Hall Craggs, M. (1965) Albumin metabolism in hookworm anaemias. *Trans. Roy. Soc. Trop. Med. Hyg.*, **59**, 472–82.

Cameron, T. W. M. (1956) *Parasites and Parasitism*, Methuen & Co., London.

Cappello, M., Clyne, L., MacPhedran, P. and Hotez, P. J. (1993) *Ancylostoma* factor Xa inhibitor: partial isolation and identification as the predominant hookworm anticoagulant. *J. Infect. Dis.*, **167**, 1474–7.

Carroll, S. M. and Grove, D. I. (1986) Experimental infections of humans with *Ancylostoma ceylanicum*: clinical, parasitological, haematological and immunological findings. *Trop. Geog. Med.*, **38**, 38–45.

Carroll, S. M., Howse, D. J. and Grove, D. I. (1984) The anticoagulant effects of the hookworm, *Ancylostoma ceylanicum*: observations on human and dog blood in vitro and infected dogs in vivo. *Thromb. Haemost.*, **51**, 222–7.

Castro, G. A., Behnke, J. M. and Weisbrodt, N. W. (1990) Hookworm infection and malabsorption: a critical review, in *Hookworm Disease, Current Status and Future Directions*, Taylor and Francis, London, pp. 265–80.

Chernin, E. (1954) Problems in tropical public health among workers at a jute mill near Calcutta. II. A study of intestinal parasites in the labor force. *Am. J. Trop. Med. Hyg.*, **3**, 94–106.

Chowdhury, A. B. and Schad, G. A. (1972) *Ancylostoma ceylanicum*: a parasite of man in Calcutta and environs. *Am. J. Trop. Med. Hyg.*, **21**, 300–1.

Cline, B. L., Little, M. D., Bartholomew, R. K. and Halsey, N. A. (1984) Larvicidal activity of albendazole against *Necator americanus* in human volunteers. *Am. J. Trop. Med. Hyg.*, **33**, 387–94.

Cort, W. W. and Otto, G. F. (1940) Immunity in hookworm disease. *Rev. Gastroent.*, **7**, 2–14.

Cort, W. W., Ackert, J. E., Augustine, D. L. and Payne, F. K. (1922) Investigations on the control of hookworm disease. II. The description of an apparatus for isolating infective hookworm larvae from soil. *Am. J. Hyg.*, **2**, 1–16.

Croese, J., Prociv, P., Maguire, E. J. and Crawford, A. P. (1990) Eosinophilic enteritis presenting as surgical emergencies: a report of six cases. *Med. J. Austral.*, **153**, 415–17.

Croese, J., Loukas, A., Opdebeeck, J. *et al.* (1994). Human enteric infection with canine hookworms. *Ann. Intern. Med.*, **120**, 369–74.

Croll, N. A. and Smith, J. M. (1972) Mechanisms of thermopositive behaviour in larval hookworms. *J. Parasit.*, **58**, 891–6.

Croll, N. A. and Matthews, B. E. (1977) *Biology of Nematodes*. John Wiley and Sons, New York, pp. 59, 144, 145.

Crompton, D. W. T. and Stephenson, L. S. (1990) Hookworm infection, nutritional status and productivity, in *Hookworm Disease, Current Status and Future Directions*. Taylor and Francis, London, pp. 231–64.

Crosby, W. H. (1987a) The deadly hookworm, why did the Puerto Ricans die? *Arch. Intern. Med.*, **142**, 577–8.

Crosby, W. H. (1987b) What became of chlorosis? *J. Am. Med. Ass.*, **257**, 2799–800.

Eiff, J. A. (1966) Nature of an anticoagulant from the cephalic glands of *Ancylostoma caninum*. *J. Parasit.*, **52**, 833–43.

El Naggar, H. (1987) PhD Thesis, University of Pennsylvania.

Ettling, J. (1981) *The Germ of Laziness*, Harvard University Press, Cambridge, Mass.

Faust, E. C., Russell, P. F. and Jung, R. C. (1971) *Craig and Faust's Clinical Parasitology*, 8th edn, Lea and Febiger, Philadelphia.

Foster, A. O. (1935) The immunity of dogs to *Ancylostoma caninum*. *Am. J. Hyg.*, **22**, 65–105.

Foster, A. O. and Landsberg, J. W. (1934) The nature and cause of hookworm anemia. *Am. J. Hyg.*, **20**, 259–90.

Garside, P. and Behnke, J. M. (1989) *Ancylostoma ceylanicum* in the hamster: observations on the host–parasite relationship during primary infection. *Parasitology*, **98**, 283–9.

Georgi, L. L., Albert, P. S. and Riddle, D. L. (1990) *daf-1*, a *C. elegans* gene controlling dauer larva development encodes a novel receptor protein kinase. *Cell*, **61**, 635–45.

Gilles, H. M. (1985) Selective primary health care: strategies for control of disease in the developing world. XVII. Hookworm infection and anemia. *Rev. Infect. Dis.*, **7**, 111–18.

Gilles, H. M. (1990) Naturally acquired infections: what's needed? in *Hookworm Disease, Current Status and Future Directions*, Taylor and Francis, London, pp. 221–30.

Gilles, H. M., Watson-Williams, E. J. and Ball, P. A. J. (1964) Hookworm infection and anemia. An epidemiological, clinical and laboratory study. *Quart. J. Med.*, **33**, 1–24.

Gilman, R. H. (1982) Hookworm disease: host–pathogen biology. *Rev. Infect. Dis.*, **4**, 824–9.

Goodey, T. (1925) Observations on certain conditions requisite for skin penetration by infective larvae of strongyloides and ankylostomes. *J. Helminth.*, **3**, 51–62.

Harada, Y. and Mori, O. (1955) A new method for culturing hookworm. *Yanago Acta Medica*, **1**, 177–9.

Hawdon, J. M. and Schad, G. A. (1990) Serum-stimulated feeding in vitro by third-stage infective larvae of the canine hookworm *Ancylostoma caninum*. *J. Parasit.*, **76**, 394–8.

Hawdon, J. M. and Schad, G. A. (1991) Albumin and a dialyzable serum factor stimulate feeding in vitro by third-stage larvae of the canine hookworm *Ancylostoma caninum*. *J. Parasit.*, **77**, 587–91.

Hawdon, J. M., Volk, S. W., Pritchard, D. I. and Schad, G. A. (1992) Resumption of feeding in vitro by hookworm third-stage larvae: a comparative study. *J. Parasit.*, **77**, 587–91.

Hoagland, K. E. and Schad, G. A. (1978) *Necator americanus* and *Ancylostoma duodenale*: life history parameters and epidemiological implications of two sympatric hookworms on humans. *Exp. Parasit.*, **44**, 36–49.

Hotez, P. J. (1989) Hookworm disease in children. *Pediat. Infect. Dis. J.*, **8**, 516–20.

Hotez, P. J. and Cerami, A. (1983) Secretion of an proteolytic anticoagulant by *Ancylostoma* hookworms. *J. Exp. Med.*, **157**, 1594–603.

Hotez, P. J., Hawdon, J. and Schad, G. A. (1993) Hookworm larval infectivity, arrest, and amphiparatenesis: the *Caenorhabditis elegans* Daf-c paradigm. *Parasit. Today*, **9**, 23–6.

Hotez, P. J., Trang, N. L. and Cerami, A. (1987) Hookworm antigens: the potential for vaccination. *Parasit. Today*, **3**, 247–9.

Hotez, P. J., Trang, N. L. McKerrow, J. H. and Cerami, A. (1985) Isolation and characterization of a protease from the hookworm *Ancylostoma caninum*. *J. Biol. Chem.*, **260**, 7343–8.

Hotez, P. J., Hawdon, J., Cox, N. *et al.* (1990a) An apparatus for modified Harada–Mori cultures of third-stage hookworm larvae. *J. Helminth. Soc. Wash.*, **57**, 167–9.

Hotez, P. J., Haggerty, J., Hawdon, J. *et al.* (1990b) Infective *Ancylostoma* hookworm larval metalloproteases and their functions in tissue invasion and ecdysis. *Infect. Immun.*, **58**, 3883–92.

Hotez, P. J., Narasimhan, S., Haggerty, J. *et al.* (1992) Hyaluronidase from *Ancylostoma* hookworm larvae and its function as a virulence factor in cutaneous larva migrans. *Infect. Immun.*, **60**, 1018–23.

Hotez, P. J., Cappello, M., Hawdon, J. *et al.* (1994) Hyaluronidases of the gastrointestinal invasive nematodes *Ancylostoma caninum* and *Anisakis simplex*: their possible function in the pathogenesis of human zoonoses. *J. Infect. Dis.*, **170**, 918–26.

Joe, L. K. and Siang, T. K. (1959) Human intestinal helminths obtained from autopsies in Djakarta, Indonesia. *Am. J. Trop. Med. Hyg.*, **8**, 518–23.

Kalkofen, U. P. (1970) Attachment and feeding behavior of *Ancylostoma caninum*. *Z. Parasitenk.*, **33**, 339–54.

Kalkofen, U. P. (1974) Intestinal trauma resulting from feeding activities of *Ancylostoma caninum*. *Am. J. Trop. Med. Hyg.*, **23**, 1046–53.

Kalmon, E. H. (1954) Creeping eruption associated with transient pulmonary infiltrates. *Radiology*, **62**, 221–6.

Katz, M. (1975) Parasitic infections. *J. Pediat.*, **87**, 165–78.

Kerr, K. B. (1936) Studies on acquired immunity to the dog hookworm. *Ancylostoma caninum*. *Am. J. Hyg.*, **23**, 381–406.

Kirby-Smith, J. L., Dove, W. E. and White, G. F. (1926) Creeping eruption, *Arch. Dermatol. Syphil.*, **13**, 137–73.

Klaver-Wesseling, J. C. M., Vetter, J. C. M. Schoeman, E. N. (1982) The *in-vitro* interaction between several components of the canine immune system and infective larvae of *Ancylostoma caninum. Parasite Immun.*, **4**, 227–32.

Klaver-Wesseling, J. C. M., Vetter, J. C. M. and Visser, W. K. (1978) A comparative in vitro study of antibody to different stages of the hookworm *Ancylostoma caninum. Z. Parasitenk.*, **56**, 147–57.

Kofoid, C. A. and Tucker, J. B. (1921) On the relationship of infection by hookworms to the incidence of morbidity and mortality, in 22 842 men of the US Army at Camp Bowie, Texas. *Am. J. Hyg.*, **1**, 79–117.

Komiya, Y. and Yasuraoka, Y. (1966) The biology of hookworms. *Prog. Med. Parasit. Japan*, **3**, 4–114.

Koshy, A., Raina, V., Sharma, M. P. *et al.* (1978) An unusual outbreak of hookworm disease in north India. *Am. J. Trop. Med. Hyg.*, **27**, 42–5.

Krupp, I. M. (1961) Effects of crowding and of superinfection on habitat selection and egg production in *Ancylostoma caninum. J. Parasit.*, **47**, 957–61.

Kuriakose, E. T. (1963) Mooren's ulcer. *Am. J. Ophthal.*, **55**, 1064–9.

Lee, C. C. (1970) *Ancylostoma caninum*: intestinal pigment granules. *Exp. Parasit.*, **27**, 246–55.

Lee, K. T., Little, M. D. and Beaver, P. C. (1975) Intracellular (muscle-fiber) habitat of *Ancylostoma caninum* in some mammalian hosts. *J. Parasit.*, **65**, 460–1.

Little, M. D., Halsey, N. A., Cline, B. L. and Katz, S. P. (1983) *Ancylostoma* larva in a muscle fiber of a man following cutaneous larva migrans. *Am. J. Trop. Med. Hyg.*, **32**, 1285–8.

Loeb, L. and Smith, A. J. (1904) The presence of a substance inhibiting coagulation of blood in *Ancylostoma. Proc. Path. Soc. Phil.*, **7**, 173–8.

Looss, A. (1901) On the penetration of *Ancylostoma* larvae into the human skin. *Centralblatt Bakteriol. Parasitenk.*, **29**, 733–9.

Lozoff, B. and Brittenham, G. M. (1987) Behavioral alterations in iron-deficiency. *Hemat. Oncol. Clin. N. Amer.*, **1**, 419–64.

Mackler, B., Person, R., Miller, L. H. (1978) Iron deficiency in the rat: biochemical studies of brain metabolism. *Pediat. Res.*, **12**, 217–20.

Malinconico, S. M., Katz, J. B. and Budzynski, A. Z. (1984) Hementin: anti-coagulant protease from the salivary gland of the leech *Haementeria ghilianii. J. Lab. Clin. Med.*, **104**, 842–54.

Martin, L. K. (1972) Hookworm in Georgia. II. Survey of intestinal helminth infections in members of rural households of southeastern Georgia. *Am. J. Trop. Med. Hyg.*, **21**, 930–43.

Matthews, B. E. (1972) Invasion of skin by larvae of the cat hookworm *Ancylostoma tubaeforme. Parasitology*, **65**, 457–67.

Matthews, B. E. (1975) Mechanism of skin penetration by *Ancylostoma tubaeforme. Parasitology*, **70**, 25–38.

Matthews, B. E. (1982) Skin penetration by *Necator americanus* larvae. *Z. Parasitenk.*, **68**, 81–6.

Maxwell, C., Hussain, R., Nutman, T. B. *et al.* (1987) Clinical and immunologic responses of normal human volunteers to low dose hookworm (*Necator americanus*) infection. *Am. J. Trop. Med. Hyg.*, **37**, 126–34.

McCoy, O. R. (1931) Immunity reactions of the dog against hookworm (*Ancylostoma caninum*) under conditions of repeated infection. *Am. J. Hyg.*, **14**, 268–303.

McKean, P. G. and Pritchard, D. I. (1989) The action of a mast cell protease on the cuticular collagens of *Necator americanus. Parasite Immun.*, **11**, 293–7.

Miller, T. A. (1965) Influence of age and sex on susceptibility of dogs to primary infection with *Ancylostoma caninum. J. Parasit.*, **51**, 701–4.

Miller, T. A. (1971) Vaccination against the canine hookworm disease. *Adv. Parasit.*, **9**, 153–83.

Miller, T. A. (1978) Industrial development and field use of the canine hookworm vaccine. *Adv. Parasit.*, **16**, 333–42.

Miller, T. A. (1979) Hookworm infection in man. *Adv. Parasit.*, **17**, 315–84.

Miyake, K., Underhill, C. B., Lesley, J. and Kincade, P. W. (1990) Hyaluronate can function as a cell adhesion molecule and CD44 participates in hyaluronate recognition. *J. Exp. Med.*, **172**, 69–75.

Muhleisen, J. P. (1953) Demonstration of pulmonary migration of the causative organism of creeping eruption. *Ann. Intern. Med.*, **38**, 595–600.

Moyle, M., Foster, D. L., McGrath, D. E. *et al.* (1994) A hookworm glycoprotein that inhibits neutrophil function is a ligand of the integrin CD 11/CD 18. *J. Biol. Chem.* (in press).

Nawalinski, T. A. and Schad, G. A. (1974) Arrested development in *Ancylostoma duodenale*: course of self-induced infection in Man. *Am. J. Trop. Med. Hyg.*, **23**, 895–8.

Nawalinski, T., Schad, G. A. and Chowdhury, A. B. (1978) Population biology of hookworms in children in rural West Bengal. I. General parasitological observations. *Am. J. Trop. Med. Hyg.*, **27**, 1152–61.

Nutt, E., Gasic, T., Radkey, J. *et al.* (1988) The amino acid sequence of antistasin. *J. Biol. Chem.*, **263**, 10162–7.

Ogilve, B. M., Bartlett, A., Godfrey, R. C. *et al.* (1978) Antibody responses in self-infections with *Necator americanus*. *Trans. Roy. Soc. Trop. Med. Hyg.*, **72**, 66–71.

Oski, F. A. (1979) The nonhematologic manifestations of iron deficiency. *Am. J. Dis. Child.*, **133**, 315–22.

Ottesen, E. A. (1990) Immune responses in human hookworm infection, in *Hookworm Disease, Current Status and Future Directions*, Taylor and Francis, London, pp. 404–16.

Oya, Y. and Noguchi, I. (1977) Some properties of hemoglobin protease from *Ancylostoma caninum*. *Japan. J. Parasit.*, **26**, 307–13.

Peduzzi, R. and Piffaretti, J. C. (1983) *Ancylostoma duodenale* and the Saint Gothard anemia. *Lancet*, **287**, 1942–5.

Pollitt, E. and Leibel, R. L. (1976) Iron deficiency and behavior. *J. Pediat.*, **88**, 372–81.

Pritchard, D. I., McKean, P. G. and Rogan, M. T. (1988) Cuticle preparations from *Necator americanus* and their immunogenicity in the infected host. *Mol. Biochem. Parasit.*, **28**, 275–84.

Pritchard, D. I. (1990) *Necator americanus*: antigens and immunological targets, in *Hookworm Disease, Current Status and Future Directions*, Taylor and Francis, London, pp. 340–50.

Pritchard, D. I., Quinnell, R. J., Slater, F. G. *et al.* (1990) Epidemiology and immunology of *Necator americanus* infection in a community in Papua New Guinea: humoral responses to excretory-secretory and cuticular collagen antigens. *Parasitology*, **100**, 317–26.

Prociv, P. and Croese, J. (1990) Human eosinophilic enteritis caused by dog hookworm *Ancylostoma caninum*. *Lancet*, **335**, 1299–302.

Reeves, J. D., Vichinsky, E., Addiego, J. and Lubin, B. H. (1984) Iron deficiency in health and disease. *Adv. Pediat.*, **30**, 281–318.

Rep, B. H., Van Joost, K. S. and Vetter, J. C. M. (1971), Pathogenicity of *Ancylostoma ceylanicum*. *Trop. Geog. Med.*, **23**, 183–92.

Ribeiro, J. M. C. (1987) Role of saliva in blood-feeding by arthropods. *Ann. Rev. Entomol.*, **32**, 463–7.

Roche, M. and Layrisse, M. (1966) Nature and causes of hookworm anemia. *Am. J. Trop. Med. Hyg.*, **15**, 1029–102.

Rossignol, J. F. (1990) Chemotherapy: present status, in *Hookworm Disease, Current Status and Future Directions*, Taylor and Francis, London, pp. 281–90.

Salafsky, B., Fusco, A. C. and Siddiqui, A. (1990) *Necator americanus*: factors influencing skin penetration by larvae, in *Hookworm Disease, Current Status and Future Directions*, Taylor and Francis, London, pp. 329–39.

Schad, G. A. (1979) *Ancylostoma duodenale*: maintenance through six generations in helminth-naive pups. *Exp. Parasit.*, **47**, 246–53.

Schad, G. A. (1994) Hookworms: pets to humans. *Ann. Intern. Med.*, **120**, 434–5.

Schad, G. A. (1990) Hypobiosis and related phenomena in hookworm infection, in *Hookworm Disease, Current Status and Future Directions*, Taylor and Francis, London, pp. 71–88.

Schad, G. A. (1991) Historical introduction (submitted for publication).

Schad, G. A. and Anderson, R. M. (1985) Predisposition to hookworm infection. *Science*, **228**, 1537–40.

Schad, G. A. and Banwell, J. G. (1984) Hookworms, in *Tropical and Geographical Medicine* (eds K. S. Warren and A. A. F. Mahmoud), McGraw-Hill Book Co., New York, pp. 359–72.

Schad, G. A., Chowdhury, A. F., Dean, C. G. *et al.* (1973) Arrested development in human hookworm infections: an adaption to a seasonally unfavorable external environment. *Science*, **180**, 502–4.

Schad, G. A., Murrell, K. D. and Fayer, R. (1984) Paratenesis in *Ancylostoma duodenale* suggests possible meat-borne human infection. *Trans. R. Soc. Trop. Med. Hyg.*, **78**, 203–4.

Shaplen, R. (1964) *Toward The Well-Being of Mankind, Fifty Years of The Rockefeller Foundation*. Doubleday & Company, Inc., Garden City, NY, pp. 25, 27.

Shelmire, B. (1928) Experimental creeping eruption from a cat and dog hookworm (*A. braziliense*). *J. Am. Med. Assoc.*, **91**, 938–43.

Smillie, W. G. and Augustine, D. L. (1926) Hookworm infestation: the effect of varying intensities on the physical condition of school children. *Am. J. Dis. Child.*, **31**, 151–68.

Smillie, W. G. and Spencer, C. R. (1926) Mental retardation in school children infested with hookworms. *J. Educ. Psychol.*, **17**, 314–21.

Smith, G. and Schad, G. A. (1989) *Ancylostoma duodenale* and *Necator americanus*: effect of temperature on egg development and mortality. *Parasitology*, **99**, 127–32.

Spellman, G. G. and Nossel, H. L. (1971) Anticoagulant activity of dog hookworm. *Am. J. Physiol.*, **220**, 922–7.

Stephenson, L. S., Latham, M. C., Kinoti, S. N. *et al.* (1990) Improvements in physical fitness of

Kenyan schoolboys infected with hookworm, *Trichuris trichiura, Ascaris lumbricoides* following a single dose of albendazole. *Trans. R. Soc. Trop. Med. Hyg.*, **84**, 277–82.

Stephenson, L. S., Latham, M. C., Kurz, K. M. *et al.* (1989) Treatment with a single dose of albendazole improves growth of Kenyan schoolchildren with hookworm, *Trichuris trichiura*, and *Ascaris lumbricoides* infections. *Am. J. Trop. Med. Hyg.*, **41**, 78–87.

Stiles, C. W. (1902) A new species of hookworm (*Uncinaria americana*) parasitic in man. *Am. Med.*, **3**, 777–8.

Stoll, N. R. (1923) Investigations on the control of hookworm disease. XV. An effective method of counting hookworm eggs in feces. *Am. J. Hyg.*, **3**, 59–70.

Stoll, N. R. (1962) On endemic hookworm, where do we stand today? *Exp. Parasit.*, **12**, 241–52.

Stoll, N. R. and Hausheer, W. C. (1926) Concerning two options in dilution egg counting: small drop and displacement. *Am. J. Hyg.*, **6**, 134–45.

Stone, W. and Smith, F. W. (1973) Infection of mammalian hosts by milk-borne nematode larvae: a review. *Exp. Parasit.*, **34**, 306–12.

Sturchler, D. (1982) Chemotherapy of human intestinal helminthiases: a review, with particular reference to community treatment. *Adv. Pharm. Chemother.*, **19**, 129–54.

Sulica, V. I., Berberian, B. and Kao, G. F. (1988) Histopathologic findings of cutaneous larva migrans. *J. Cutan. Pathol.*, **15**, 346.

Thorson, R. E. (1956a) Proteolytic activity in extracts of the esophagus of adults of *Ancylostoma caninum* and the effect of immune serum on this activity. *J. Parasit.*, **42**, 21–5.

Thorson, R. E. (1956b) The effect of extracts of the amphidial glands, excretory glands, and esophagus of adults of *Ancylostoma caninum* on the coagulation of dog's blood. *J. Parasit.*, **42**, 26–30.

Udonsi, J. K. (1984) Changes in lipid contents of infective third-stage larvae of *Necator americanus* during desiccation and revival. *Z. Parasitenk.*, **70**, 81–5.

Van Der Gaag, R., Abdillahi, H., Stilma, J. S. and Vetter, J. C. M. (1983) Circulating antibodies against corneal epithelium and hookworm in patients with Mooren's ulcer from Sierra Leone. *Br. J. Ophthalmol.*, **67**, 623–8.

Velasquez, C. C. and Cabrera, B. C. (1968) *Ancylostoma ceylanicum* (Looss 1911) in a Filipino woman. *J. Parasit.*, **54**, 430–1.

Vetter, J. C. M., Leegwater, V. D. and Linden, M. E. (1977) Skin penetration of infective hookworm larvae. I. The path of migration of infective larvae of *Ancylostoma braziliense* in canine skin. *Z. Parasitenk.*, **53**, 255–62.

Vetter, J. C. M., Vingerhoed, J., Schoeman, E. and Wauters, H. W. (1985) Chemotactic attraction of infective hookworm larvae of *Ancylostoma caninum* by a serum dog factor. *Z. Parasitenk.*, **71**, 539–43.

Wakelin, D. (1985) Genetic control of immunity to helminth infections. *Parasit. Today*, **1**, 17–23.

Walterspiel, J. N., Buchanan, G. R., Schad, G. A. and Carpentieri, U. (1985) Erythropoietin-induced congenital erythrocytosis: treatment with myelosuppressive agents and hookworm infestations. *J. Pediat.*, **107**, 575–7.

Wang, C. I. (1988) Parasitic diarrhoeas in China. *Parasit. Today*, **4**, 284–7.

White, C. J., Maxwell, C. J. and Gallin, J. I. (1986) Changes in the structural and functional properties of human eosinophils during experimental hookworm infection. *J. Infect. Dis.*, **154**, 778–83.

Yorke, W. and Maplestone, P. A. (1926) *The Nematode Parasites of Vertebrates*. J. & A. Churchill, London.

Yoshida, Y., Nakanishi, Y. and Mitani, W. (1958) Experimental studies on the infection modes of *Ancylostoma duodenale* and *Necator americanus* to the definitive host. *Jap. J. Parasit.*, **7**, 102–12.

Yoshida, Y., Okamoto, K. and Chiu, J.-K. (1971) Experimental infection of man with *Ancylostoma ceylanicum*. *Chin. J. Microbiol.*, **4**, 157–67.

Yu, S.-H. and Shen, W.-X. (1990) Hookworm infection and disease in China, in *Hookworm Disease, Current Status and New Directions*. Taylor and Francis, London, pp. 44–54.

ELEVEN

Capillaria philippinensis and *Trichostrongylus orientalis*

J. H. Cross

Intestinal helminthic infections are the most common of the parasitic diseases in humans. More than one-half of the world's population have worms and in most cases man and his worms tolerate each other very well. It is only on rare occasions that this balance is disturbed and man suffers from the relationship. In this chapter, two nematode parasites are to be presented; both could be considered exotic since relatively few people are exposed to these infections. One (*Trichostrongylus orientalis*) can be considered an old timer since it has been known for many years and is not considered a very serious pathogen. The second species (*Capillaria philippinensis*), however, is relatively new to science and untreated infection may lead to death of the host.

11.1 *CAPILLARIA PHILIPPINENSIS*

Capillaria philippinensis is one of only three *Capillaria* species sporadically occurring in humans. *C. hepatica* is found in liver tissue of rodents and less than 50 human infections have been reported. *C. aerophilia* is found in the epithelial lining of the cat lungs and only 10 human infections have been reported. *C. philippinensis*, on the other hand, was first reported in humans and now believed to be a natural parasite of the intestinal tract of fish-eating birds. The parasite is new to man, has been involved in epidemics, is known to cause death if untreated and has been reported from several widespread areas of the world.

The first report of the disease was from a village in Ilocos Norte, Northern Luzon in the Philippines. A middle-aged male school teacher from the village died of intractable diarrhea, emaciation and cachexia (Chitwood, Valasquez and Salazar, 1964). Tiny nematodes with the appearance of a *Capillaria* species were recovered at autopsy. In 1965 a number of middle-aged males experienced a similar disease in another village called Pudoc West, Ilocos Sur. When an unusual number of people began to die, the Philippine Health Department was informed and the epidemic investigated. During the epidemic, 229 cases of intestinal capillariasis occurred in Pudoc West alone, and 60 people died (Detels *et al.*, 1969). The disease spread to other villages and in all known endemic areas in Northern Luzon over 1300 cases were documented and 90 people died between 1967 and 1968. The number of cases and deaths decreased after 1969, but the disease continues to be seen. In the Philippines a total of 1884 cases have been documented up to December 1990. In addition to

The opinions or assertions contained herein are the private ones of the author and are not to be construed as official or reflecting the views of the US Department of Defense or the Uniformed Services University of the Health Sciences.

Enteric Infection 2. Intestinal helminths. Edited by M.J.G. Farthing, G.T. Keusch and D. Wakelin. Published in 1995 by Chapman and Hall, London. ISBN 0 412 39140 6

Northern Luzon, another epidemic emerged in Southern Leyte in the Central Philippines in early 1980, but records of cases and deaths have not been kept in this area. A great many interesting superstitions and beliefs evolved during the epidemic in Northern Luzon and some of these have been reported elsewhere (Cross and Bhaibulaya, 1983).

The disease is also endemic in Thailand. The first case was reported in 1972 (Pradatsundarasar *et al.*, 1973) and a number of subsequent cases reported by Bhaibulaya (1975). An epidemic involving over 100 people occurred in 1981 resulting in nine deaths (Cross and Bhaibulaya, 1983). The parasitosis is now reported from other countries: Japan, four cases, Egypt two cases and Iran and Taiwan one case each.

11.1.1 TAXONOMY

Capillaria species are members of the Order Enoplida, superfamily Trichinelloidea and the family Trichuridae. They are closely related to *Trichinella* and *Trichuris* species. There are over 250 species of *Capillaria* on record characterized primarily by a long thin anterior and a slightly wider posterior end. The anterior end contains the esophagus which is surrounded by a large number of esophageal glands called stichocytes. The entire structure is called a stichosome. Males have a single sheathed copulatory spicule, terminal or subterminal anus and a small caudal alae or bursa-like structure at the tail. The female vulva is usually mid-body at the junction of the esophagus or stichosome. Female worms may produce bipolar peanut-shaped or barrel-shaped eggs or thin-shelled eggs. Some females are larviparous. Most *Capillaria* species have a direct life cycle but some have an indirect cycle utilizing an intermediate host.

Capillaria philippinensis was described as a species by Chitwood, Valasquez and salazar, 1968 from specimens collected from human autopsies. Male worms (Figure 11.1) measure 1.5–3.9 mm in length, and 3–5 μm, 23–28 μm and 18 μm respectively at the widest part of the anterior end, at the stichosome and at the cloaca. The male spicule ranges from 230–300 μm and the unspined spicular sheath over 400 μm. The anus is subterminal and there are ventrolateral expansions containing

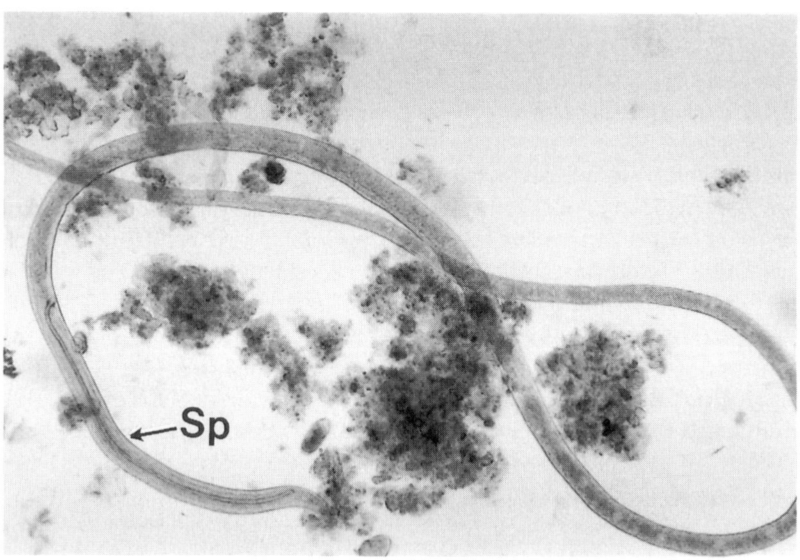

Figure 11.1 Male *Capillaria philippinensis*; Sp = spicule. Bar = 0.25 mm.

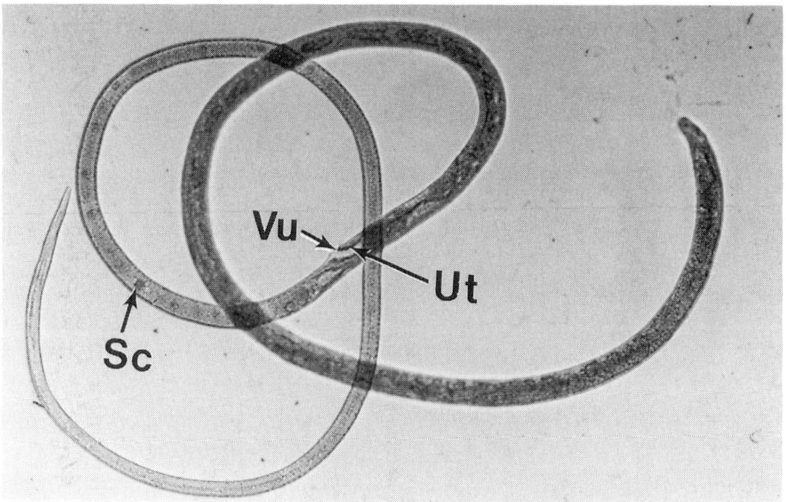

Figure 11.2 Young female *Capillaria philippinensis*; note salient vulva (Vu) and uterus (Ut). Sc = stichocytes. Bar = 0.25 mm.

two pairs of papillae. Females are longer and measure 2.33–5.3 mm. Width at the head is approximately 5–8 μm, 25 μm at the widest portion of the stichosome, 28–36 μm at the vulva and 29–47 μm post vulva. The vulva is salient and situated at the end of the esophagus (Figure 11.2). The anus is subterminal. The uterus of females may contain flattened bipolar, peanut-shaped, thick-shelled striated eggs, or thin-shelled eggs with or without embryos or larvae. Most females, however, produce single-cell peanut-shaped, thick-shelled eggs measuring 36–45 μm by 20 μm in size (Figure 11.3).

11.1.2 LIFE CYCLE

The life cycle of *C. philippinensis*, determined by laboratory experimentation, was found to be unique among nematode parasites. Eggs, readily found in the feces of patients, embryonated in water at ambient temperatures in 5–10 days. When fed to small freshwater/brackish water fish from endemic areas, the eggs hatched and the larvae doubled in size from 130–150 μm to 250–300 μm in about 3 weeks. Several species of fish were experimentally infected and one, *Hypseleotris bipartita*, which is often eaten raw by Filipinos, was the easiest to infect and maintain in the laboratory (Cross *et al.*, 1972). Several species of fish in Thailand have also been experimentally infected (Bhaibalaya, Indra-Ngarm and Anathapruit, 1979). *Macaca* species of monkeys were fed larvae from fish and they developed patent infections, but none manifested symptoms and none died. The parasite was able to multiply in the monkeys and autoinfection was confirmed. Mongolian gerbils (*Meriones unguiculatus*) were exposed to infection, developed patent infections and died in 6–7 weeks. Continued experimentation in the gerbils showed that larvae from fish develop into adults in 10–12 days and the adult females produce larvae. These larvae then develop into adults and the female worms of the second generation produce eggs which pass in the feces. The prepatent period is approximately 25 days. Infection of gerbils with two to three larvae produced patent infections and died with several thousand worms recovered at necropsy. Reproduction reaches peaks in 35–45 days at which time the gerbils usually die. Other studies

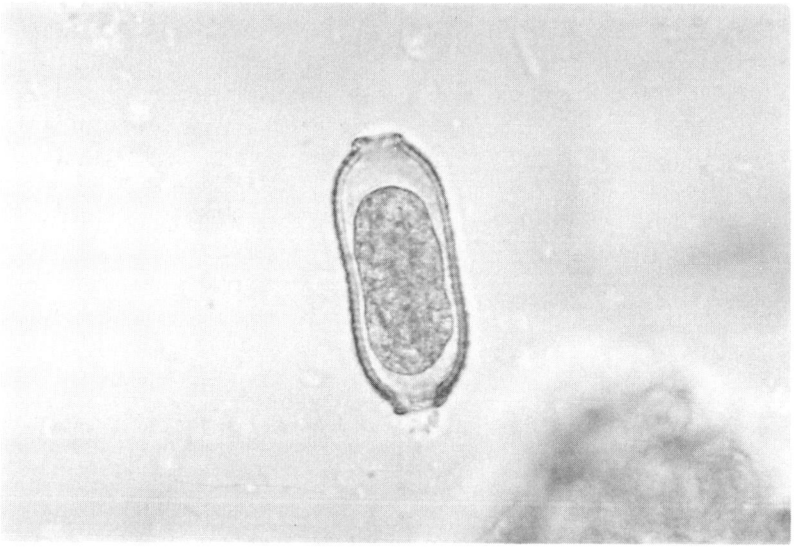

Figure 11.3 Unembryonated egg of *Capillaria philippinensis;* note striated cell and inconspicuous flattened bipolar plugs. Bar = 20 μm.

showed that transplanted egg-producing females from infected gerbils were able to switch to larvae producers in clean gerbils. In all infections, including human, there is always a small number of larviparous females present to build up and maintain the infection (Cross and Bhaibulaya, 1983). The transmission of the parasite by fish was confirmed in the Philippines by feeding naturally infected fish from lagoons to gerbils.

In studies in Thailand (Bhaibalaya and Indra-Ngarm, 1979), later confirmed in Taiwan (Cross and Basaca-Sevilla, 1983), showed that fish-eating birds could be infected with *C. philippinensis*. One bird in the Philippines has also been found naturally infected. It is now believed that *C. philippinensis* has a fish–bird life cycle and when humans eat infected freshwater fish uncooked they develop infections.

11.1.3 EPIDEMIOLOGY

When *C. philippinensis* emerged as a serious cause of public health problems in the Philippines, nothing was known about the parasite and how it was transmitted. Some *Capillaria* species have direct life cycles while others have indirect cycles utilizing an intermediate host. An intermediate host was suspected for *C. philippinensis* because of the unique eating habits of Filipinos living in the endemic area. The population's dietary habits are different from those of other Filipino groups in that the Ilocanos of Northern Luzon eat a great variety of raw foods. Animal life from the lagoons, such as shrimp, crabs, fish, clams and snails, is often eaten raw. Marine animal life, such as fish, squid, crabs and seaweed, is also eaten uncooked or cooked. Most of the animals eaten raw are usually small or more or less bite-sized. Large fish are usually cooked. The vital organs of goats, cows and water buffalo may be eaten raw, often by men while socially drinking local sugarcane wine or Philippine gin. Animal intestinal juice, cooked or uncooked, is used to season rice and other foods. Dog meat is also popular on special occasions; it is usually cooked.

Over 150 000 animal specimens from the endemic area were examined for *C. philippi-*

nensis and while *Capillaria* spp. and larvae were found in some mammals and fish none of the adult worms were *C. philippinensis*. Identification of the larvae to species could not be made, however.

Twice as many males (1334) acquired intestinal capillariasis as females (550). Although some children and elderly people were infected, most were aged between 20 and 40 years. Adult males eat more raw food, especially fish, from the lagoons than women and children. The men are farmers/fishermen and, after working the fields all day, stop at the lagoon on the way home to take a bath and check the fish traps. When hungry, a man will eat part of his catch uncooked and take the rest home for the family. At home the catch is usually cooked.

In Thailand the rural populations often eat raw fish from small streams and ponds. Most infections in Thailand are attributed to this practice. Some of the cases from Japan, Iran and Egypt have been associated with eating fish, but the source of infection in Taiwan is not known.

Since fish-eating birds have been incriminated as a possible natural host for *C. philippinensis*, it is now believed that birds, by their migratory habits, are responsible for disseminating the parasite. The birds spend the summer months in the far north where they mingle with birds from all parts of the world. If the infection is transmitted in this area, infected birds could carry the parasite back to the winter grounds in the south and transmit the infection to fish in that area. When humans eat these fish, of a size that birds can eat whole, infection, disease and death may develop within a month or two.

11.1.4 PATHOLOGY

Most of the pathology due to the parasite is found in the small intestine, primarily the jejunum. All stages of the nematode are found in the lumen (Figure 11.4) and in the glands, extending into the lamina propria (Figure 11.5). At one autopsy over 20 000 worms were estimated in one litre of bowel fluid (Cross and Bhaibulaya, 1983). Less than 15 autopsies were carried out on Filipinos (Canlas, Cabrera and Davis, 1967; Fresh *et al.*, 1972) and histologic examinations showed mucosal sloughing, denuded and flattened

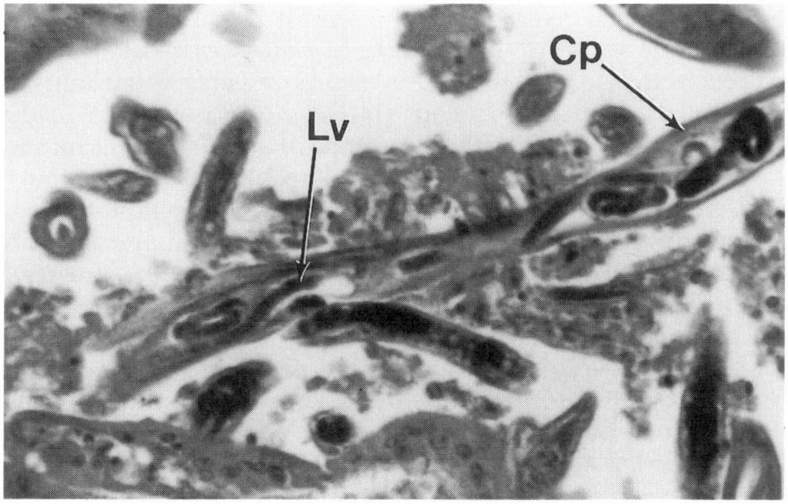

Figure 11.4 Sections of human small intestine at autopsy indicating sections of *Capillaria philippinensis* (Cp); note larvae (Lv) in the uterus of female worm. Bar = 0.4 mm.

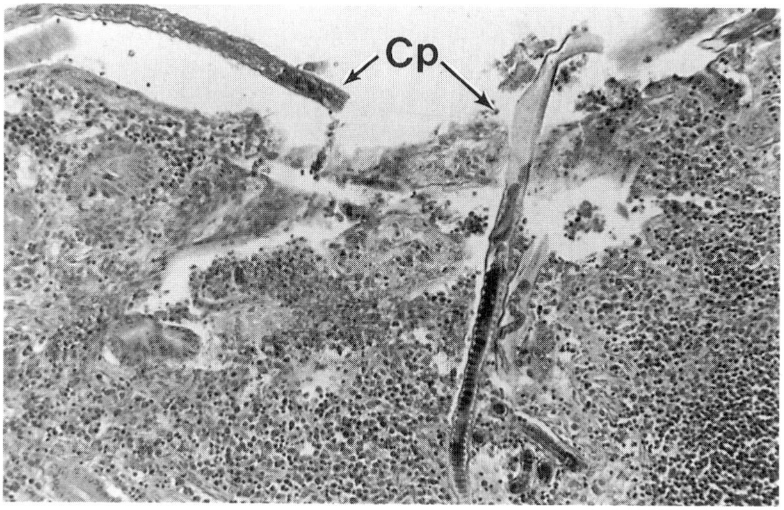

Figure 11.5 Section of human small intestine showing anterior end of *Capillaria philippinensis*; (Cp) note esophagus (E) or stichosome (Sc) consisting of columns of cells, stichocytes. Bar = 0.2 mm.

villi, atrophic crypts of Lieberkhun and depletion of the mucosal glands. Infiltration by plasma cells, lymphocytes, macrophages, neutrophils and eosinophils into the lamina propria was found. The parasite has not been found in any organ other than the intestine, except on one occasion when sections of a capillarid were found in the liver. There were some pathologic changes in other organs attributed to malnutrition and hypokalemia (Fresh *et al.*, 1972). Deaths were due to irreversible effects of electrolyte loss resulting in heart failure. Secondary bacterial infection and septicemia were responsible for deaths in some persons (Whalen *et al.*, 1969).

Jejunal biopsies from human and gerbil intestine taken at necropsy have been examined by electron microscopy. In human jejunun, the surface epithelium showed evidence of cell damage and abnormal extrusion and shedding of cells. The microvilli were scant and disorganized. The epithelium had complete loss of adhesion specialization and widespread separation of the epithelial cells. In gerbil tissue there were fine structural changes in the mucosa, direct mechanical compression and the appearance of a lytic substance at the anterior end of a worm in the tissue. Micro-ulcers were also seen adjacent to cuticular pores of the worm. These pathologic changes may be responsible in part for the malabsorption and loss of fluids, protein and electrolytes (Sun *et al.*, 1974).

11.1.5 CLINICAL FEATURES

It usually requires a few weeks after exposure to *C. philippinensis* before symptoms are manifested, probably coinciding with an increase in the worm population. It has been established that all those acquiring the infection eventually develop symptoms (Detels *et al.*, 1969). The first symptoms are diarrhea, irregular borborygmi and mild abdominal pain. As the disease progresses the diarrhea becomes more frequent with 8–10 voluminous stools per day, the abdominal pain intensifies and borborygmi increase. Vomiting, weight loss, body weakness, malaise, edema and anorexia develop. The patients are initially ambulatory but eventually become bed-ridden. After 2–3 months the patient becomes extremely weak, emaciated and exhibits pallor, dehydration and anasarca. Laboratory findings usually reveal the presence of eggs, larvae and adults of *C. philippinensis* in the stools. Plasma concentrations of total protein, potassium, carotene and calcium are low. There is malabsorption of fats and sugars and a protein-losing enteropathy (Dauz, Cabrera and Canlas, 1967; Whalen *et al.*, 1969). Patients at this time are critically ill and require immediate hospitalization and treatment. When the disease was first seen in the Philippines many patients died. Few patients die today because of early recognition of symptoms and immediate anthelmintic treatment.

11.1.6 DIAGNOSIS

In an endemic area such as Northern Luzon in the Philippines patients presenting with a gurgling stomach, diarrhea and abdominal pain are usually considered to be infected with *C. philippinensis*. The confirmed diagnosis, however, is detection of eggs (Figure 11.3), larvae (Figure 11.6) or adult parasites (Figures 11.1 and 11.2) in the stools. The parasite is generally found after a single direct stool examination; however, concentration techniques will increase diagnostic precision. Sometimes two or three stool examinations are required. The parasite may also be recovered by small intestine aspiration or biopsy. On occasions, when the parasite cannot be found, the patient may be given an anthelminthic following which the parasite may be recovered from feces. Serologic tests have been evaluated and found to be of little value (Banzon, Lewer and Yagore, 1975; Cross and Chi, 1978). Inexperienced technicians may confuse *C. philippinensis* eggs with those of *T. trichiura* (Figure 11.7).

11.1.7 TREATMENT

Fluid and electrolyte replacement, along with an antidiarrheal, an anthelminthic and a high protein diet, is necessary for those exhibiting signs and symptoms of a chronic infection. Thiabendazole, 25 mg/kg/day or 1 g/day for 30 days, was used during the epidemic and for the following few years. There were many side effects and relapses. At one time there

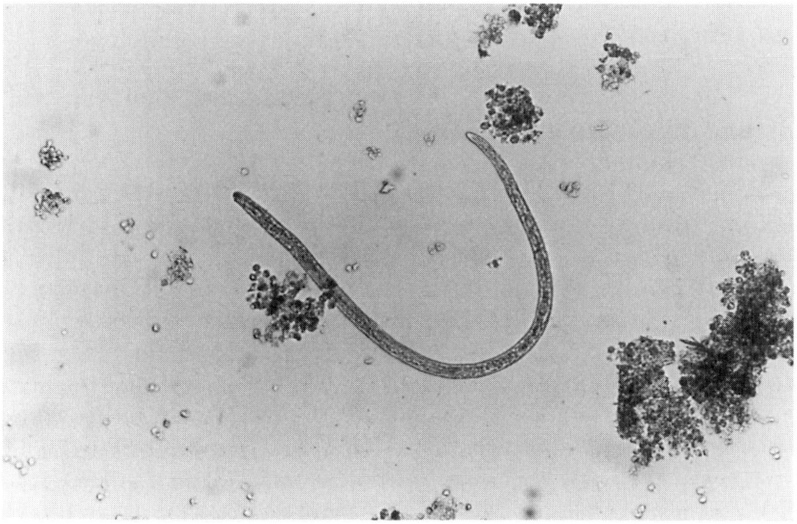

Figure 11.6 L2 larva of *Capillaria philippinensis* recovered from intestinal contents at autopsy. Bar = 0.25 mm.

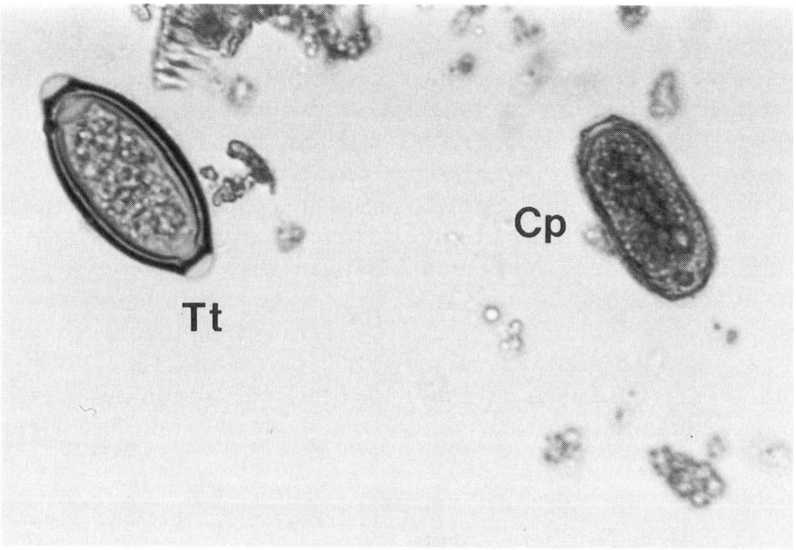

Figure 11.7 Eggs of *Trichuris trichiura* (Tt) and *Capillaria philippinensis* (Cp). The former is barrel-shaped, and larger with two prominent polar plugs. Bar = 25 μm.

were more relapses occurring than new cases (Singsong, 1974). One patient experienced 15 relapses over a 12-year period (Alcantara, Uylangco and Cross, 1985).

Mebendazole has replaced thiabendazole and, although relapses occur, they are infrequent. Mebendazole is given in dosages of 200 mg/day twice a day for 20 days for new cases and 30 days for those with a relapse history.

At the present time, albendazole is used in the Philippines and Thailand. The recommended dosage is 400 mg in divided doses for 10 days. Attempts to reduce treatment to 7 days has resulted in relapse in a few patients. Long-term treatment with thiabendazole and mebendazole is considered necessary since it is believed that these drugs have little effect on larval stages of the parasite. The drugs have more effect on the adult stages. Albendazole apparently affects the larval stages and can be given for shorter periods of time.

In the Philippines, patients are hospitalized during treatment. Many patients released early often return with a relapse. Once home they feel well and discontinue the medication. They often sell the remaining drug (most patients are very poor) or give it to a friend or relative with abdominal symptom. Thus therapy needs to be closely supervised.

11.1.8 PREVENTION AND CONTROL

It is extremely difficult to change eating habits that have been prevailing for generations. The control and prevention of capillariasis would be the avoidance of eating raw freshwater fish. The disease is considered a zoonosis which occurs in humans who eat small fish that are the diet of fish-eating birds. Educational programs informing populations of the potential dangers of eating the fish would be of value in known endemic areas. The treatment of all infected persons and the sanitary disposal of feces from these persons would prevent the spread. The washing in a lagoon of bed sheets contaminated with feces

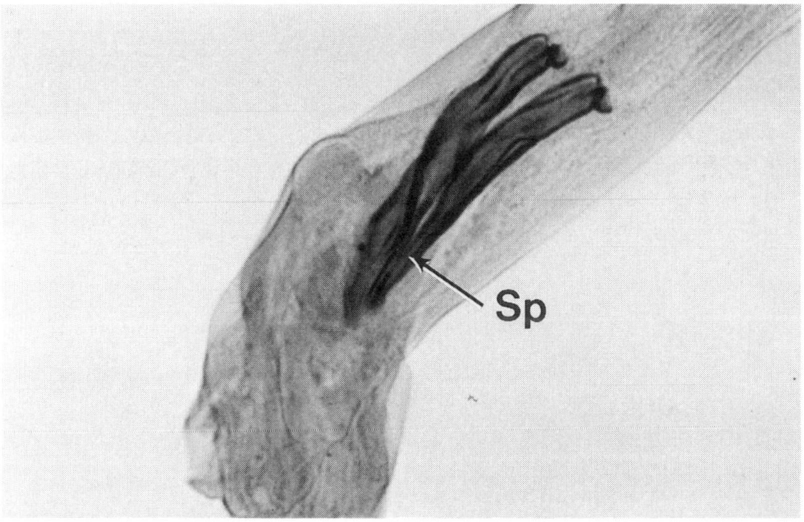

Figure 11.8 Posterior end of male *Trichostrongylus orientalis* showing characteristic pair of spicules (Sp). Bar = 40 μm.

from patients was probably responsible for infecting fish and the cause of the initial epidemic in Pudoc West. Recognition of symptoms and early treatment will prevent death.

11.2 *TRICHOSTRONGYLUS ORIENTALIS*

Trichostrongyliasis is caused by nematode species of *Trichostrongylus*. The nematodes are common intestinal parasites of herbivorous mammals, such as sheep, goats, bovines and other ruminants. Approximately 34 species are recognized and, of these, 10 have been reported in humans. *T. orientalis* is the most important in human medicine, but other species, such as *T. axei*, *T. colubriformis*, *T. skrjabini*, *T. vitrinus*, *T. probolurus*, *T. capricola*, *T. brevis*, *T. affinis* and *T. calcaratus*, are occasionally reported. Stoll (1947) estimated 5.5 million human *Trichostrongylus* infections worldwide, and Watson (1953), believing this an underestimation, increased the prevalence to 48 million.

11.2.1 TAXONOMY

Trichostrongylus is one of about 30 genera in the family Trichostrongylidae that parasitize animals including man. They belong to the superfamily Trichostrongyloidea, order Strongylorida, which characteristically have a caudal bursa and a pair of equal copulatory spicules in the males; the females have a complex ovejector with well developed sphincters. The trichostrongyles are small (2–30 mm, but usually 5–9 mm), slender worms with a small head without a buccal cavity or cervical papillae. The spicules are short and stout, brownish in color and ridged (Figure 11.8); the spicules are important in species identification. Eggs produced by females are thin-shelled, oval to elongated and hyaline, and resemble those produced by hookworms. They are longer and narrower than hookworms, and one or both ends may be pointed. They measure 81–104 by 40–48 μm (Figure 11.9).

11.2.2 LIFE CYCLE

Trichostrongylus orientalis reside in the small intestine where the female worms discharge

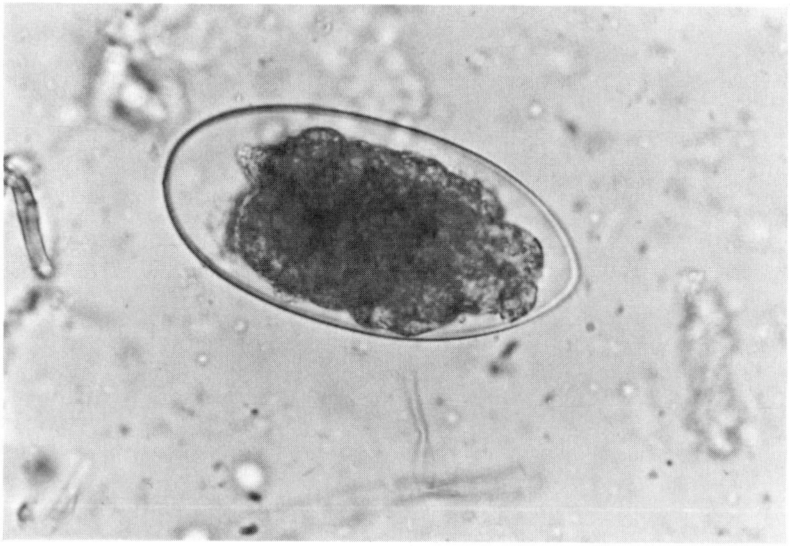

Figure 11.9 Egg of *Trichostrongylus orientalis* showing one end is pointed, the other rounded. Bar = 40 μm.

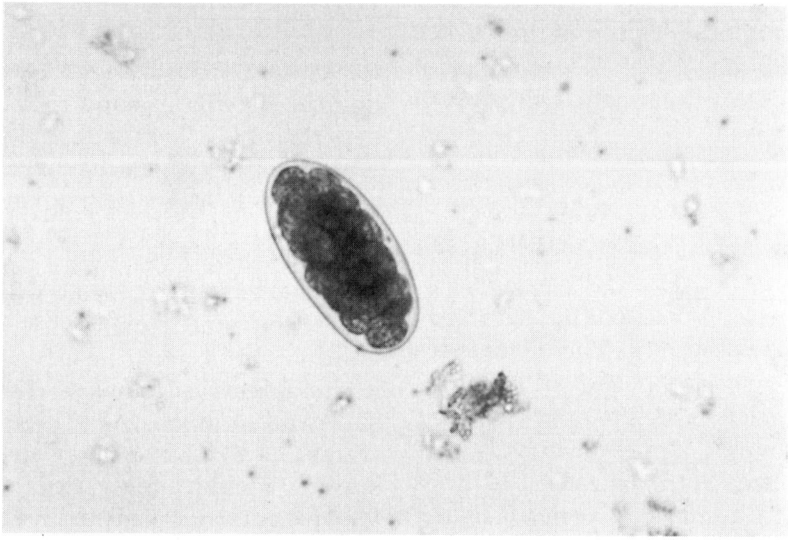

Figure 11.10 Egg of *Trichostrongylus orientalis* in morula stage with grape-like clusters of cells of equal size; ends of egg shell are rounded. Bar = 45μm.

100–200 eggs per day in the morula stage of development with individual divisions of equal size, circular and grape-like (Figure 11.10). The eggs are voided with the feces and under favorable conditions of temperature, oxygen and moisture, embryonate. In a day or more a first-stage rhabditoid larva hatches from the egg. In the fèces it molts into a second-stage rhabditiform larva, feeds on bacteria and molts again into an ensheathed third-stage filariform larva. This is the infective stage and migrates from the feces onto vegetation. This larva has a dorsal bend in the anal region and the postanal portion is attenuated and terminates in a minute knob.

Infection is usually acquired by larvae entering the host orally on contaminated blades of grass and vegetation. The larvae can live for long periods, even in stored materials, depending on environmental conditions. Upon reaching the small intestine, the larvae migrate into the mucosa and develop into adult males and females after two more molts in about 3–4 weeks.

11.2.3 EPIDEMIOLOGY

Trichostrongylus species are reported from a variety of animals throughout the world, but human infections are generally attributed to *T. orientalis*. Reports of human infections with this species are mainly from Iran, Japan and Korea, with a few sporadic reports from other areas of the world. Iran seems to be the most highly endemic area with overall infection rates of 67% in rural areas of Isfahan, Central Iran. Eight species of *Trichostrongylus* infect the population, with *T. colubriformis* and *T. orientalis* being the most common (Ghadirian and Arfaa, 1975). In the past, *T. orientalis* infections were not uncommon in Korea. In Pusan, 46% of outpatient stools were found positive for eggs (Soo, 1970) while 62% of stools from hospitalized patients in Taegu were positive (Choi *et al.*, 1971). In a survey among Korean military personnel, nearly 15% were found passing eggs of this parasite. *T. orientalis* was once common in Japan with infections being reported from widespread areas (Otsura and Ito, 1972). In Osaka, Nishimura *et al.* (1965) found 15% of schoolchildren infected. *T. axei* has also been reported in Japan, and Japan is the only area where *T. brevis* has been reported. At the present time, however, both are rare.

While other species of *Trichostrongylus* are considered parasites of herbivores, *T. orientalis* is considered a human parasite that occasionally infects other animals. Most *T. orientalis* infections occur where sanitary conditions are poor and where there is indiscriminate defecation. The prevalence rates are highest where human feces are used as fertilizer ('night soil'). This practice has been discouraged in Korea and, subsequently, infections in humans have decreased.

Humans acquire infections by eating contaminated vegetables. In Taegu, Korea, market and garden vegetables were examined for helminth ova and an average of 18% of the lettuce, young radishes and Chinese cabbage were contaminated with *Trichostrongylus* eggs (Choi and Lee, 1972). In Iran, Ghadirian and Arfaa (1975) attribute high prevalences of trichostrongyliasis to the people's habit of living close to their animals and the use of animal feces as fertilizer. Molding animal dung into cakes to use as fuel contaminates the hands of women who do not wash their hands before eating. In Isfahan where *T. orientalis* infection is common in humans, night soil is used to fertilize vegetables.

Penetration of the skin by infective-stage larvae is a possibility, but rare. It is not an important means of transmission of *Trichostrongylus* species. Larvae in drinking water is a source of infection, but not an important one.

11.2.4 PATHOLOGY

Trichostrongylus orientalis is known to invade the mucosa and when large numbers are present in the duodenum and upper jejunum, they may traumatize the mucosa causing desquamation and hemorrhage at the site of attachment. The worms are known to suck blood, but do not cause anemia. There may be a mild eosinophilia.

11.2.5 CLINICAL FEATURES

Most infections are asymptomatic, but when several hundred worms are present, there may be clinical manifestations. Most patients usually have multiple helminthic infections and symptoms cannot be attributed to *Trichostrongylus* alone (Ghadirian and Arfaa, 1975). Japanese workers have reported increased symptoms with an increase in number of eggs in the feces. Japanese patients experienced diarrhea, nausea, anorexia, weight loss, abdominal pain, headache and fatigue. There may also be eosinophilia and anemia (Otsura and Ito, 1972). Emaciation and dry skin also occur. Infections have been known to last for several years.

11.2.6 DIAGNOSIS

There are no specific clinical manifestations that will aid in the diagnosis; most infections are asymptomatic and symptoms that are present may be associated with other parasitoses. The parasitologic diagnosis is by finding *Trichostrongylus* eggs in the feces. Care must be taken to avoid confusion with other helminthic eggs, especially hookworm, which are usually smaller and more ovoid. Since the worms do not produce a large number of eggs, a stool concentration method should be used if the direct-smear stool examination is negative. Formalin-ethyl acetate concentration is of value as is the zinc sulfate flotation method. Eggs can also be seen in the Kato–Katz cellophane smear. Stool cultures are of value to recover filariform larvae which can be identified as *Trichostrongylus* spp. by the dorsal bend at the level of the anus and the minute knob at the end of the tail. Infective stage larvae may be introduced into animals and adult worms recovered at necropsy can be identified to species. The recovery of adult worms by duodenal aspiration is the quickest and simplest means of diagnosis. Adult worms may also be recovered from the feces following specific anthelminthic therapy.

11.2.7 TREATMENT

Most infected persons are usually not aware that they are infected and treatment may not be necessary. However, several anthelminthics are known to be effective: pyrantel pamoate, 11 mg/kg once daily; thiabendazole, 25 mg/kg twice a day for two days; mebendazole, 100 mg twice daily for 3 days (Seo *et al.*, 1977); albendazole may also be effective.

11.2.8 PREVENTION AND CONTROL

Infection with *T. orientalis* can be prevented by washing all vegetables and thorough cooking prior to eating. The ingestion of raw vegetables and the sucking of grass stalks in endemic areas should be avoided. Human feces, as well as animal feces, should not be used to fertilize vegetables raised for human or animal consumption. In areas where the use of night soil has been discouraged, such as in Japan and Korea, trichostrongyliasis has decreased. Good sanitary practices, washing of hands, eating cooked food and health education would aid in the control of this parasitosis.

REFERENCES

Alcantara, A. K., Uylangco, C. V. and Cross, J. H. (1985) An obstinate case of intestinal capillariasis. *Southeast Asian J. Trop. Med. Public Health*, **16**, 410–13.

Banzon, T. C., Lewerth, R. M. and Yagore, M. G. (1975) Serology of *Capillaria philippinensis* infection: reactivity of human sera to antigens prepared from *Capillaria obsignata* and other helminths. *Am. J. Trop. Med. Hyg.*, **24**, 256–63.

Bhaibulaya, M. and Indra–Ngarm, S. (1979). *Amaurornis phoenicurus* and *Ardeola bacchus* as experimental definitive hosts for *Capillaria philippinensis* in Thailand. *Int. J. Parasit.*, **9**, 321–2.

Bhaibulaya, M., Indra–Ngarm, S. and Anathapruit, M. (1979) Freshwater fishes of Thailand as experimental intermediate host for *Capillaria philippinensis*. *Int. J. Parasit.*, **9**, 105–8.

Bhaibulaya, M. (1975) Studies on capillariasis philippinensis in Thailand. I. Epidemiologic survey. *Rep. Thailand Nat. Res. Council*, p. 11.

Canlas, B. C., Cabrera, B. D. and Dauz, U. (1967) Human intestinal capillariasis. II. Pathological features. *ACTA Med. Philipp.* **4**, 84–91.

Chitwood, M. B., Valasquez, C. and Salazar, N. G. (1964) Physiological changes in a species of *Capillaria* (Trichuroidea) causing a fatal case of human intestinal capillariasis. *Proc. 1st. Int. Congr. Parasit.*, **2**, 797.

Chitwood, M. B., Valasquez, C. and Salazar, N. G. (1968) *Capillaria philippinensis sp. n.* (Nematoda: Trichinellida) from intestine of man in the Philippines. *J. Parasit.*, **54**, 368–71.

Choi, D. W. and Lee, S. (1972) Incidence of parasites found in vegetables collected from markets and vegetable gardens in Taegu area. *Korean J. Parasit.*, **10**, 44–51.

Choi, D. W., Park, S. D., Kim, J. W. *et al.* (1971) Intestinal parasite survey of Kyungpook National University Hospital patients. *Korean J. Parasit.*, **9**, 47–53.

Cross, J. H. and Bhaibulaya, M. (1983) Intestinal capillariasis in the Philippines and Thailand. In *Human Ecology and Infectious Diseases* (eds N. Croll and J. H. Cross), Academic Press, New York, pp. 103–36.

Cross, J. H. and Chi, J. C. H. (1978) The ELISA test in the detection of antibodies to some parasitic diseases in Asia. *Proc. 18th SEAMEO TROPMED Seminar: Current Concepts in the Diagnosis and Treatment of Parasitic and other Tropical Diseases in Southeast Asia*, Kuala Lumpur, 2–5 August 1977, pp. 178–82.

Cross, J. H., Banzon, T. C. M., Clarke, D. *et al.* (1972) Studies on the experimental transmission of *Capillaria philippinensis* in monkeys. *Trans. Roy. Soc. Trop. Med. Hyg.*, **66**, 819–27.

Cross, J. H. and Basaca–Sevilla, V. (1983) Experimental transmission of *Capillaria philippensis* to birds. *Trans. Roy. Soc. Trop. Med. Hyg.*, **77**, 511–24.

Dauz, U., Cabrera, B. D. and Canlas, G. (1967) Human intestinal capillariasis. I. Clinical features. *Acta Med. Philipp.*, **4**, 72–83.

Detels, R., Gutman, L., Jaramillo, J. *et al.* (1969) An epidemic of human intestinal capillariasis: a study in a barrio in North Luzon. *Am. J. Trop. Med. Hyg.*, **18**, 676–82.

Fresh, J. W., Cross, J. H., Reyes, V. *et al.* (1972) Necropsy findings in intestinal capillariasis. *Am. J. Trop. Med. Hyg.*, **21**, 169–73.

Ghadirian, E. and Arfaa, F. (1975) Present status of trichostrongyliasis in Iran. *Am. J. Trop. Med. Hyg.*, **24**, 935–41.

Nishimura, T., Okumura, T., Ishihara, Y. and Inamoto, T. (1965) Epidemiological studies on the *Trichostrongylus* infection in a rural area in Osaka Prefecture (I). *Jap. J. Parasit.*, **14**, 566–7.

Otsura, M. and Ito, J. (1972) Genus *Trichostrongylus* in Japan, in *Progress of Medical Zoology* (eds K. Morishita, K. Y. Kamiya and H. Matsuhayashi), Meguro Parasitological Museum, Tokyo, Vol. 4, pp. 425–62.

Pradatsundarasar, A., Pecharanond, K., Chintanawongs, C. and Ungthavorn, P. (1973) The first case of intestinal capillariasis in Thailand. *Southeast Asian J. Trop. Med. Public Hlth* **4**, 131–4.

Seo, B. S., Cho, S. Y., Kang, S. Y. and Chai, J. Y. (1977) Anthelminthic efficacy of methyl-5-benzoylbenzimidazole-2-carbamate (mebendazole) against multiple helminthic infections. *Korean J. Parasit.*, **15**, 11–16.

Singson, C. N. (1974) Recurrence in human intestinal capillariasis. *Philipp. J. Microbiol. Infect. Dis.*, **3**, 7–13.

Soo, B. S. (1970) Incidence of intestinal parasites with fecal examination on the out patients of Pusan University Hospital. *Korean J. Parasit.*, **8**, 71–5.

Stoll, N. R. (1947) This wormy world. *J. Parasit.*, **33**, 1–18.

Sun, S. C., Cross, J. H., Berg, H. S. *et al.* (1974) Ultrastructural studies of intestinal capillariasis *Capillaria philippinensis* in human and gerbil hosts. *Southeast Asian J. Trop. Med. Public Hlth*, **5**, 524–33.

Watson, J. M. (1953) Human trichostrongyliasis and its relationship to ankylostomiasis in Southern Iraq, with comments on world incidence. *Parasitology*, **43**, 102–9.

Whalen, G. E., Rosenberg, E. B., Strickland, G. T. *et al.* (1969) Intestinal capillariasis – a new disease in man. *Lancet*, **i**, 13–16.

TWELVE

Anisakis and *Oesophagostomum* spp. infection

G. C. Cook

12.1 ANISAKIASIS

Anisakiasis ('herring-worm', 'cod-worm', or 'seal-worm' disease) is a term used to describe several gastrointestinal infections caused by larval nematodes which belong to the subfamily Anisakidae. These are ingested in raw, lightly cooked, salted or pickled marine fish or squid. The principal affected geographical areas are Japan (Oshima, 1987), Holland (Thiel and Jansen, 1988) and California (Kliks, 1983). Whereas *Anisakis* is usually responsible in Japan and Holland, *Pseudoterranova* is more common in North America. In Japan and north America the third-stage (L3) larvae are consumed in *sushi* and *sashimi*, and in Holland, in 'green herrings'. In France, a retrospective study based on the experience of 32 laboratories with a special interest in parasitology, revealed 21 cases of anisakiasis between January 1985 and September 1987 (Hubert, Bacou and Belveze, 1989); in Belgium, six cases have recently been recorded after consumption of herrings marinated in vinegar (Verhamme and Ramboer, 1988). In the USA, 'cod-worm anisakiasis' (see below) is more common than 'anisakiasis' (Oshima, 1987).

The most common fish to be affected are herring, mackerel, salmon, cod and squid (*Anisakis*), and cod, halibut, flat fish, greenling and red snapper (*Pseudoterranova*) (Oshima, 1987). A simple method, which is useful in large-scale surveys, for recovering the larvae from the muscle of marine fish has been described (Brattey, 1988); following mechanical disintegration with a domestic food processor, the worms remain intact and then fluoresce brightly.

Adult anisakids occur in the intestinal tract of marine mammals (seals, porpoises, whales and dolphins, in the case of *Anisakis*; seals, fur-seals, walruses and sea lions in the case of *Pseudoterranova* (= *Phocanema* = *Terranova*)) (Oshima and Kliks, 1987) and less often in certain species of fish. *Anisakis simplex* was first recognized in 1908 (Ishikura and Namiki, 1989).

A great deal of confusion exists regarding appropriate nomenclature. Margolis (1977) has suggested that the term 'anisakiasis' should be restricted to infection with the larvae of *Anisakis*, and that 'non-specific anisakiasis' should be used for infection with anisakid larvae when the genus has not been identified; 'phocanemal (or terranoval) anisakiasis' is used for infections with larvae of the genus *Pseudoterranova* (Oshima, 1987). 'Pseudoterranoval anisakiasis' is an imprac-

Enteric Infection 2. Intestinal helminths. Edited by M.J.G. Farthing, G.T. Keusch and D. Wakelin. Published in 1995 by Chapman and Hall, London. ISBN 0 412 39140 6

tical name for clinicians, and thus 'cod-worm anisakiasis' is preferred.

12.1.1 AETIOLOGY

The usual cause of the disease is infection by L3 (or L4) larvae of *Anisakis simplex* (19–36 mm × 0.3–0.7 mm) or *Pseudoterranova decipiens* (25–50 mm × 0.3–1.2 mm); the former are white or milky in colour, possess an elongated pharynx, an intestine and a blunt tail with a longish mucron (>20 μm), whilst the latter are yellowish or brownish and (unlike *A. simplex*) have an anteriorly placed caecum. L2 *Anisakis* larvae (with a shorter pharynx and attenuated tail) rarely produce infection in humans. A technique utilizing multilocus electrophoresis has been used in a detailed evaluation of the relationship between adult *Anisakis* and their larvae obtained from the Mediterranean and north-east Atlantic Ocean (Orecchia *et al.*, 1986).

Figure 12.1 shows the life cycle of *A. simplex*. Eggs are passed in the faeces of the infected marine mammal and these hatch in cold water, liberating L2 larvae. These are, in turn, ingested by many forms of crustacea (krill) and it is in the haemocoel that L3 larvae develop. When the crustacea are swallowed by fish or squid the larvae are released(they do not undergo further development) and subsequently invade the body cavities and muscles, where they remain until their 'transport host' (there are 150 species) is devoured by a mammal. They develop into adult worms in the stomach of a marine mammal, but only very rarely in the human gastrointestinal tract (Kliks, 1983, 1986).

12.1.2 PATHOGENESIS AND PATHOLOGY

Larvae attach to the submucosa of the stomach or intestine causing ulceration and haemorrhage. Penetration of the intestinal wall can result in extra-intestinal infection (Thiel and Jansen, 1988). Figures 12.2 and 12.3 show an infected ileum. There is greater exudation from intestinal than gastric lesions. Mesentery, omentum and pancreas may be

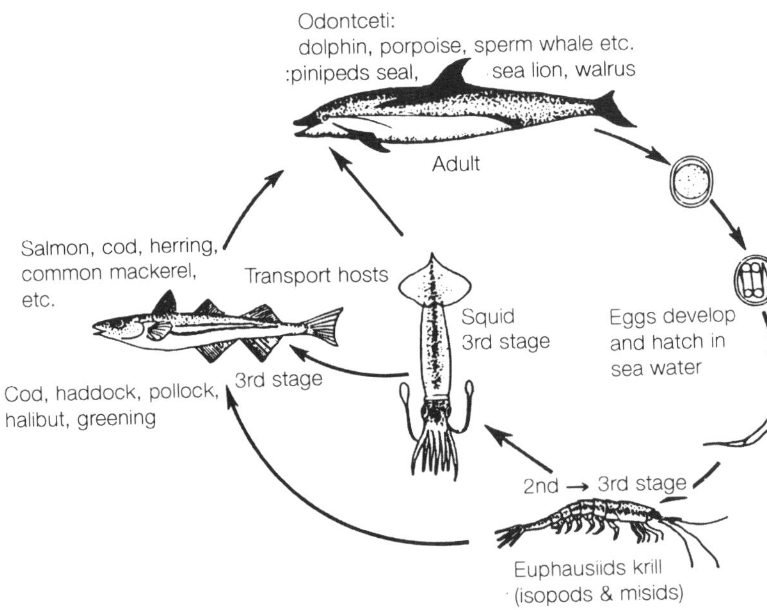

Figure 12.1 Life cycle of *Anisakis simplex*. (Source: Oshima, 1987.)

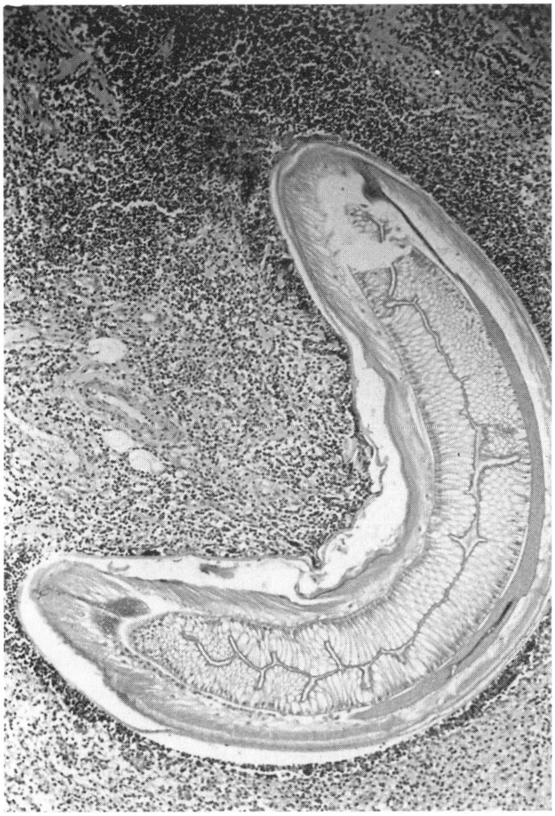

Figure 12.2 Section of an ileal specimen from an adult who presented with an acute appendicitis-like syndrome.

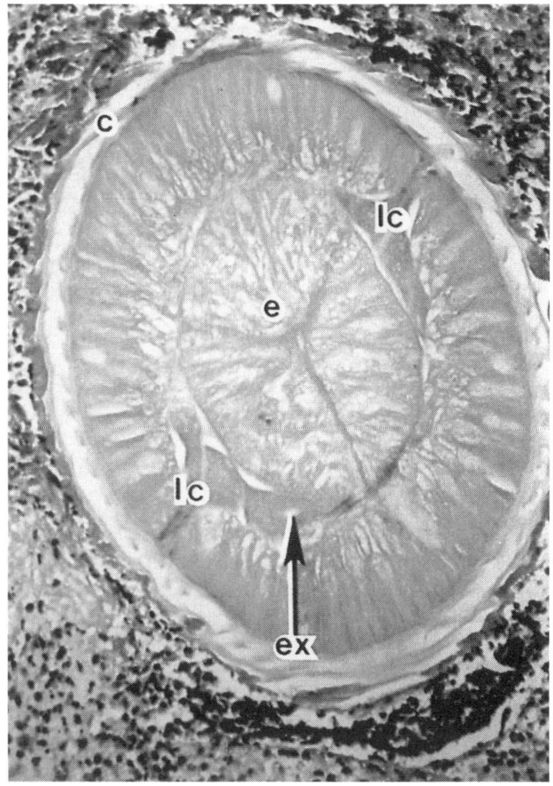

Figure 12.3 Larva of *Anisakis* sp. in a resected specimen of ileum. c = cuticle; lc = Y-shaped lateral chords; e = triradiated oesophagus; ex = excretory duct. (Source: Sakanari, Loinaz, Deardorff *et al.*, 1988.)

involved, and the lesions range from abscesses to eosinophilic granulomas (Hsiu *et al.*, 1986; Kliks, 1983, 1986). The larvae die within 10 days, after which the exudative inflammation slowly subsides, and an eosinophilic granuloma forms around the dead worm(s).

Gastric carcinoma is a common malignancy in Japan (in 1977, the overall rate was 52.3 per 100 000 men); gastric anisakiasis is also common (in 1988, 11 232 cases were recorded). As a result, an hypothesis has been assembled implicating *Anisakis* as a cocarcinogen in gastric carcinoma (Petithory *et al.*, 1990), but more work is required before this can possibly be accepted.

12.1.3 CLINICAL ASPECTS

A live worm may be coughed up within 48 h of a fish meal (McKerrow, Sakanari and Deardorff, 1988); occasionally, the worm may be felt in the oropharynx or proximal oesophagus where it produces a 'tingling sore-throat syndrome'. In the case of gastric anisakiasis (Ishikura and Namiki, 1989), an incubation period of 1–7 h (up to 20 h) after ingestion of infected fish or squid is followed by epigastric pain, nausea, vomiting and rarely haematemeses (Kliks, 1983; Hsiu *et al.*, 1986; Ikeda, Kumashiro and Kifune, 1989). An antral pseudotumour is a further manifestation. Ishikura *et al.* recorded 1523 and 223 cases of gastric and intestinal anisakiasis, respectively, in Japan in 1983 (Oshima, 1987).

Intestinal anisakiasis (Oshima, 1987) is usually caused by *Anisakis simplex*, and rarely *Pseudoterranova* larvae; 1–5 days after the infected meal, there is a sudden onset of abdominal pain with nausea and vomiting. Ileocaecal (Kliks, 1983) or appendiceal involvement may result from granuloma formation. There may be a mild fever and eosinophilia, but neither of these nor a leucocytosis are constant features. Intestinal obstruction is an occasional sequel (Verhamme and Ramboer, 1988). Presentation with a transient segmental colitis (barium enema may show an 'apple-core' lesion) has been recorded (Shirahama *et al.*, 1990). In some cases, the larvae escape from either the stomach or intestine and migrate into the peritoneal or pleural cavities. Peritonitis and death are rare sequelae. However, the majority of cases are self-limiting and the overall mortality rate low. Urticaria is a common symptom in individuals who eat marine fish; evidence has been presented from Japan indicating that this is a sensitivity reaction to antigens released by *Anisakis* larvae (Kasuya, Hamano and Izumi, 1990).

12.1.4 DIAGNOSIS

Clinical diagnosis is difficult (or impossible) unless a high 'index of suspicion' is maintained; a careful history with regard to raw or undercooked fish or squid ingestion is obviously essential. Misdiagnosis is common, and one report documented 153 such instances in one year at a hospital in Japan (Oshima, 1972). A peripheral blood eosinophilia is often present in the gastric (but not intestinal) form. Identification of larvae (and rarely adults) in vomit or biopsy material leads to a definitive diagnosis (Kliks, 1983; Verhamme and Ramboer, 1988); any surgical biopsy in which eosinophilic infiltration is a prominent feature should be regarded as suspicious. Gastric anisakiasis can usually be diagnosed using upper gastrointestinal endoscopy (Hsiu *et al.*, 1986; Kliks, 1986; Ikeda, Kumashiro and Kifune, 1989) as larvae are easily recognized and can be removed for parasitological identification. Biopsy of a 'pseudotumour' will reveal eosinophilic granuloma(s). Double-contrast radiology, or ultrasonography may also prove useful. Intestinal anisakiasis is difficult to diagnose, and may mimic appendicitis, ileus, or regional enteritis, often leading to laparotomy. Barium examination may reveal mucosal oedema and narrowing of the lumen of the terminal ileum with proximal dilatation. There may also be irregular thickening of the mucosa of the jejunum, ileum or colon. Small intestinal involvement may clinically resemble Crohn's disease (McKerrow, Sakanari and Deardorff, 1988; Sakanari *et al.*, 1988), whilst the gastric form can mimic peptic ulcer or cancer.

Serological diagnosis remains unreliable. Although *A. simplex*-specific IgE has been detected (Deardorff, Fukumura and Raybourne, 1986; Sakanari *et al.*, 1988; Yagihashi *et al.*, 1990), cross-reactions with antigens from other nematodes remains a serious problem. Nevertheless, serology can be of value in the assessment of therapy. *Anisakis simplex* antibodies have also been detected by radioallergosorbent analysis, ELISA and an immunofluorescent antibody assay (Sakanari *et al.*, 1988). Recently, monoclonal antibodies have been raised against antigen from *Anisakis* L1 larvae (Takahashi, Sato and Ishikura, 1986; Yagihashi *et al.*, 1990). There is therefore cause for optimism regarding more accurate pre-invasive diagnosis in the future (Ishikura and Namiki, 1989).

Other helminthic causes of eosinophilic granuloma of the small intestine include *Angiostrongylus costaricensis*, *Ascaris lumbricoides*, *Oesophagostomum* spp. pp. 169–71, and *Strongyloides stercoralis*.

12.1.5 MANAGEMENT

If the patient regurgitates and vomits the worm(s) the illness is self-limiting (Kliks, 1986). In the case of gastric anisakiasis, endoscopic removal of the larvae usually produces a satisfactory outcome (Deardorff, Fukumura and Raybourne, 1986; Ikeda, Kumashiro and Kifune (1989). In chronic infections, endoscopic removal of eosinophilic granuloma(s) is unnecessary. Intestinal anisakiasis does not usually require surgery, although this is not infrequently carried out (Verhamme and Ramboer, 1988) (see above). Management should be conservative, being dominated by fluid replacement and nutritional therapy, and complete cure is usual.

No anthelmintic agent has been shown to be of value in anisakiasis (Ishikura and Namiki, 1989). The benzimidazole compounds, especially albendazole, would seem most likely on *a priori* grounds to be effective chemotherapeutic agents, but proof is lacking.

12.1.6 PREVENTION

The disease may occur wherever raw or undercooked sea-fish is eaten. The obvious method for prevention is to avoid all raw or inadequately cooked, smoked, salted or marinated fish or squid. Adequate cooking (Kingston and Kilbourn, 1989) or pickling of fish prevents the disease, and the freezing of herrings at sea ($<-20°C$ for $\geqslant 60$ h) has, for example, eliminated the disease from Holland. The effect of commercial blast-freezing (to $-35°C$ for 15 h) on larval viability in salmon viscera has been assessed (Deardorff and Throm, 1988) and found to be entirely effective with no viable worms being detectable at or after 24 h.

The first recorded case in the USA was in 1958 (McKerrow, Sakanari and Deardorff, 1988). A clear cause–effect relationship between increased prevalence of the disease in the USA and the introduction of raw fish dishes has been suggested (Hsiu *et al.*, 1986; McKerrow, Sakanari and Deardorff, 1988). In practice, *sushi* served in professional *sushi* bars is rarely responsible for an *Anisakis* infection. It seems likely that the sharp increase in numbers of recognized cases of human anisakiasis is therefore related more to diagnostic advances (especially in endoscopy and radiology) than the commercialization of *sushi* (Oshima, 1987). However, a definite increase in the prevalence and intensity of *Pseudoterranova* in cod fillets caught off eastern Canada during the last 30 years has been recorded (Chandra and Khan, 1988). A further suggested factor to explain the increased prevalence is a popular movement for the protection of marine mammals (especially seals, sea lions and porpoises) in the coastal waters off Japan, and the western coast of the USA (McKerrow, Sakanari and Deardorff, 1988).

12.2 OESOPHAGOSTOMIASIS

This zoonotic nematode infection which is widely distributed throughout the tropics and subtropics also causes eosinophilic granulomas within the gastrointestinal tract, usually in the ileocaecal region. An animal reservoir is *not* required for completion of the life cycle. The first report of human disease was made in 1905 in southern Ethiopia (Polderman *et al.*, 1991). There seems no doubt that the infection is more common and widespread than is generally appreciated (Ross, Gibson and Harris, 1989a). In 1911, the eminent British helminthologist R. T. Leiper wrote:

> Andrew Foy, of West African medical staff, was good enough whilst on home leave to present to the London School of Tropical Medicine a tube containing a considerable number of species of *Necator americanus*, passed by a patient at Ibi, Northern Nigeria. In the course of routine examination of individual specimens, I have

been able to single count six examples of *Oesophagostomum apiostomum*.

12.2.1 AETIOLOGY AND LIFE CYCLE

At least three species of *Oesophagostomum* exist: *O. apiostomum* (*O. aculeatum*), *O. stephanostomum* and *O. bifurcum*; the former is a common parasite of subhuman primates in Africa (especially Uganda), the Philippines and China, and the latter two in Brazil, French Guiana and West Africa. Cattle, pigs, sheep and goats may also be infected by *Oesophagostomum* spp. Large series of human cases have been documented in northern Togo and northern Ghana (Polderman *et al.*, 1991); in rural areas around large towns in these regions, L3 larvae can be readily demonstrated in faecal samples (after incubation at room temperature) in up to 30% or more of the local inhabitants. Adult worms lie free within the lumen, or encysted within the mucosa in the caecum and colon; in addition to a mouth and oesophagus, they possess either a copulatory bursa (male: 0.8–1 cm × 0.35 mm) or vulva (female: 1 cm × 0.32 mm). Figure 12.4 shows the head of a female *O. bifurcum* by electron microscopy. Eggs (from which speciation is not possible) measure 60 × 40 μm in diameter and closely resemble those of hookworm (Chapter 10). After passage in faeces, the eggs hatch (in soil) to rhabditiform larvae; these develop to filariform larvae, and after being swallowed by a new host (via contaminated soil or water) pass to the caecum/colon, where, after mucosal invasion, they form submucosal cysts; they later re-enter the intestinal lumen and attach to the mucosa as adults.

12.2.2 PATHOGENESIS AND CLINICAL FACTORS

Eosinophilic granulomas are formed in the ileocaecal region. In the colon, the submucosal forms may cause polyposis with resultant dysentery and if they penetrate the bowel wall, peritonitis may ensue. There may also be tumour-like masses and abscesses. A recent report from Lome, Togo, has docu-

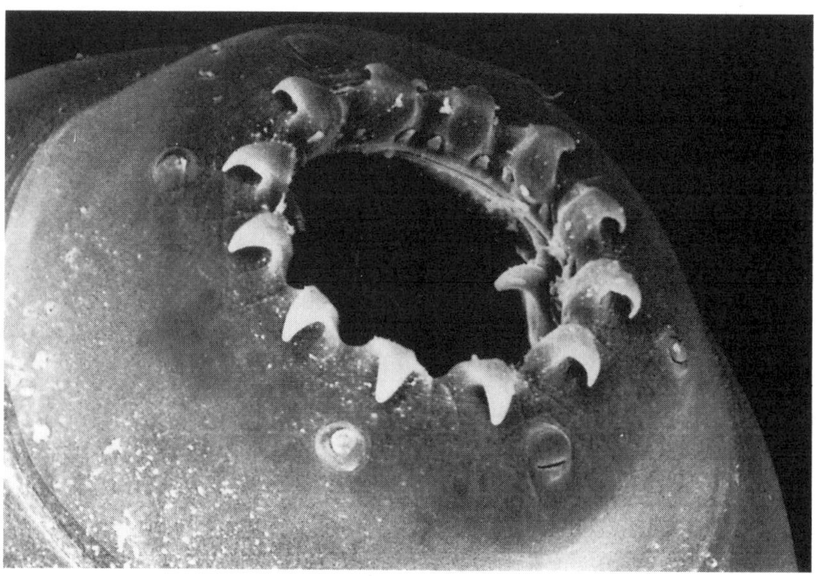

Figure 12.4 Scanning electron micrograph of the cephalic end of a female *Oesophagostomum bifurcum* recovered from human faeces in west Africa. (Source: Polderman, Krepal, Baeta *et al.*, 1991.)

mented 28 cases of 'pseudotumour' caused by *O. bifurcum* involving the upper intestine, ileum or appendix (Pages *et al.*, 1988). The stomach, ileum and abdominal wall may all be involved.

As with anisakiasis, right lower quadrant tenderness may mimic appendicitis; alternatively, it may be confused with carcinoma, or an inflammatory lesion, e.g. ileocaecal tuberculosis, amoeboma or pyomyositis. The adult worms do not cause symptoms; in northern Nigeria in 1913 they were demonstrated (as 'commensals') in 8 out of 200 jailed prisoners (Polderman *et al.*, 1991). Although rare, extra-intestinal involvement has been documented (Ross, Gibson and Harris, 1989a,b); these authors documented a solitary nodule caused by *O. bifurcum* on the back of a young woman who had lived for 3 months in Brunei. It is suggested that this resulted either from direct skin penetration, or possibly from haematogenous or lymphatic transmission from the gastrointestinal tract.

12.2.3 DIAGNOSIS

Laboratory diagnosis is by identification of the characteristic eggs, which must be carefully differentiated from those of *Necator americanus*; the presence of almost fully formed larvae (within the shell) should immediately lead to a suspicion that this is an *Oesophagostomum* spp., rather than hookworm infection.

12.2.4 MANAGEMENT

Drugs of choice are the benzimidazole compounds such as albendazole, mebendazole or thiabendazole. In one study, both albendazole (400 mg stat) and pyrantel pamoate (10 mg/kg stat) proved satisfactory in eliminating adult worms from the intestinal lumen (Polderman *et al.*, 1991).

Most helminthomas subside using conservative management, although complications (e.g. abscess(es), intestinal obstruction or peritonitis), or uncertainty of diagnosis may render laparotomy the correct course in management.

Although there is no work on a possible human vaccine, a recent report has documented partially successful vaccination in the eradication (measured by worm burden and faecal egg count) of a related species, *O. radiatum*, from cattle in Queensland, Australia (East and Bourne, 1988).

REFERENCES

Brattey, J. (1988) A simple technique for recovering larval ascaridoid nematodes from the flesh of marine fish. *J. Parasit.*, **74**, 735–7.

Chandra, C. V. and Khan, R. A. (1988) Nematode infestation of fillets from Atlantic cod, *Gadus morhua*, off eastern Canada. *J. Parasit.*, **74**, 1038–40.

Deardorff, T. L. and Throm, R. (1988) Commercial blast-freezing of third-stage *Anisakis simplex* larvae encapsulated in salmon and rockfish. *J. Parasit.*, **74**, 600–3.

Deardorff, T. L., Fukumura, T. and Raybourne, R. B. (1986) Invasive anisakiasis: a case report from Hawaii. *Gastroenterology* **90**, 1047–50.

East, I. J. and Bourne, A. S. (1988) A comparison of worm burden and faecal egg count for measuring the efficacy of vaccination against *Oesophagostomum radiatum*. *Int. J. Parasit.*, **18**, 863–4.

Hsiu, J.-G., Gamsey, A. J., Ives, C. E. *et al.* (1986) Gastric anisakiasis: report of a case with clinical, endoscopic, and histological findings. *Am. J. Gastroent.*, **81**, 1185–7.

Hubert, B., Bacou, J. and Belveze, H. (1989) Epidemiology of human anisakiasis: incidence and sources in France. *Am. J. Trop. Med. Hyg.*, **40**, 301–3.

Ikeda, K., Kumashiro, R. and Kifune, T. (1989) Nine cases of acute gastric anisakiasis. *Gastrointest. Endosc.*, **35**, 304–8.

Ishikura, H. and Namiki, M. (eds) (1989) *Gastric anisakiasis in Japan: epidemiology, diagnosis and treatment*, Springer-Verlag, Tokyo, Japan, pp. 144.

Kasuya, S., Hamano, H. and Izumi, S. (1990) Mackerel-induced urticaria and *Anisakis*. *Lancet*, **335**, 665.

Kingston, S. and Kilbourn, J. P. (1989) Diagnosis of a fourth reported case of intestinal anisakiasis in the United States? *Am. J. Clin. Pathol.*, **92**, 256.

Kliks, M. M. (1983) Anisakiasis in the western United States: Four new case reports from California. *Am. J. Trop. Med. Hyg.*, **32**, 526–32.

Kliks, M. M. (1986) Human anisakiasis: an update. *J. Am. Med. Assoc.*, **255**, 2605.

Margolis, L. (1977) Public health aspects of 'codworm' infection: a review. *J. Fish. Res. Board Can.*, **34**, 887–98.

McKerrow, J. H., Sakanari, J. and Deardorff, T. L. (1988) Anisakiasis: Revenge of the sushi parasite. *New Eng. J. Med.*, **319**, 1228–9.

Orecchia, P., Paggi, L., Mattiucci, S. *et al.* (1986) Electrophoretic identification of larvae and adults of *Anisakis* (Ascaridida: Anisakidae). *J. Helminth.*, **60**, 331–9.

Oshima, T. (1972) *Anisakis* and anisakiasis in Japan and adjacent area, in *Progress of Medical Parasitology in Japan*. Meguro Parasitological Museum, Tokyo, pp. 301–93.

Oshima, T. (1987) Anisakiasis – Is the sushi bar guilty? *Parasit. Today*, **3**, 44–8.

Oshima, T. and Kliks, M. (1987) Effects of marine mammal parasites on human health. *Int. J. Parasit.*, **17**, 415–21.

Pages, A., Kpodzro, K., Boeta, S. and Akpo-Allavo, K. (1988) La 'tumeur' de dapong: helminthiase à *Oesophagostome*. *Ann. Pathol.*, **8**, 332–5.

Petithory, J. C., Paugam, B., Buyet-Rousset, P. and Paugam, A. (1990) *Anisakis simplex*, a cofactor of gastric cancer? *Lancet*, **336**, 1002.

Polderman, A. M., Krepel, H. P., Baeta, S. *et al.* (1991) Oesophagostomiasis, a common infection of man in northern Togo and Ghana. *Am. J. Trop. Med. Hyg.*, **44**, 336–44.

Ross, R. A., Gibson, D. I. and Harris, E. A. (1989a) Cutaneous oesophagostomiasis in man. *J. Helminth.*, **63**, 261–2.

Ross, R. A., Gibson, D. I. and Harris, E. A. (1989b) Cutaneous oesophagostomiasis in man. *Trans. Roy. Soc. Trop. Med. Hyg.*, **83**, 394–5.

Sakanari, J. A., Loinaz, H. M., Deardorff, T. L. *et al.* (1988) Intestinal anisakiasis: a case diagnosed by morphologic and immunologic methods. *Am. J. Clin. Pathol.*, **90**, 107–13.

Shirahama, M., Koga, T., Uchida, S. *et al.* (1990) Colonic anisakiasis simulating carcinoma of the colon. *Am. J. Roentgen.*, **155**, 895.

Takahashi, S., Sato, N. and Ishikura, H. (1986) Establishment of monoclonal antibodies that discriminate the antigen distribution specifically found in *Anisakis* larvae (Type 1). *J. Parasit.*, **72**, 960–2.

Thiel, P. H. van and Jansen, J. (1988) Is the case of presumed gnathostomiasis in The Netherlands a peculiar autochthonous case of anisakiasis? *Acta Leidensia*, **57**, 75–7.

Verhamme, M. A. M. and Ramboer, C. H. R. (1988) Anisakiasis caused by herring in vinegar: a little known medical problem. *Gut*, **29**, 843–7.

Yagihashi, A., Sato, N., Takahashi, S. *et al.* (1990) A serodiagnostic assay by microenzyme-linked immunosorbent assay for human anisakiasis using a monoclonal antibody specific for *Anisakis* larvae antigen. *J. Infect. Dis.*, **161**, 995–8.

THIRTEEN

Taenia solium, *Taenia saginata* and *Hymenolepis nana*

A. Flisser

The adult tapeworms of *Taenia solium* and *Taenia saginata* are intestinal parasites exclusively of human beings, while *Hymenolepis nana* infects humans as well as mice. *T. solium* is called the pork tapeworm and *T. saginata* the beef tapeworm, because pigs and cattle are their main intermediate hosts, respectively. *H. nana* is the only cestode which does not have an obligatory requirement for an intermediate host. The definitive host is that which harbours the adult parasite and acquires infection after ingesting pork or beef infected with the larval stage or cysticercus, in the case of taeniasis, or by the ingestion of eggs, a flea or a beetle, which may act as intermediate hosts, in the case of hymenolepiasis. The intermediate host is the one which harbours the larval stage and infection is acquired after eating *Taenia* eggs.

In *H. nana* all the life cycle usually takes place in a single person since larval development occurs in the intestinal mucosa of the definitive host. Human beings may also harbor *T. solium* cysticerci in the brain, eyes, muscle and subcutaneous tissue, but are considered to be accidental intermediate hosts because infected human tissues are not eaten and so the infection is normally only perpetuated by infected pigs. These metazoan parasites are commonly named flatworms or tapeworms because of their ribbon-like appearance. They belong to the Phylum Platyhelminthes, Class Cestoda, Order Cyclophyllidea, Family Taeniidae or Hymenolepididae (Faust, Russell and Jung, 1970; Pawlowski, 1990; Pearse *et al.*, 1987; Schantz, 1989; Schmidt and Roberts, 1977; Vertser, 1967).

13.1 INTESTINAL CESTODE INFECTIONS IN PERSPECTIVE

Human taeniasis has been known since ancient Egyptian and Greek cultures. Many developments in the knowledge of these parasites arose during the eighteenth and nineteenth centuries (Grove, 1990; Wardle and McLeod, 1968). In recent times there have been relatively few publications regarding taeniasis and most deal with treatment and clinical aspects. Even the methodology routinely used for its diagnosis has not changed since the development of the formalin-ether sedimentation technique by Ritchie (Ritchie, 1948) in spite of its low sensitivity and specificity. Perhaps the decrease in research interest on taeniasis in this century has been because *T. solium*, the causative agent of human neurocysticercosis, was abolished from developed countries through improvements in sanitary infrastructure and health education (Gemmell *et al.*, 1983).

Enteric Infection 2. Intestinal helminths. Edited by M.J.G. Farthing, G.T. Keusch and D. Wakelin. Published in 1995 by Chapman and Hall, London. ISBN 0 412 39140 6

Also *T. saginata*, although a cosmopolitan parasite, does not cause severe disease but only an unpleasant sensation when evacuated. Furthermore, it was considered that intestinal adult cestodes did not induce a protective immune response in the definitive host which could expel the tapeworm (Chandler, 1939; Heyneman, 1963).

H. nana, on the contrary, has been exhaustively studied because it is a natural parasite of mice and therefore this system is used as an experimental model (Ito and Smyth, 1987).

In recent years, *T. solium* taeniasis regained importance because several studies indicate that tapeworm carriers are the main risk factor for acquiring cysticercosis (Cruz *et al.*, 1989, Diaz-Camacho *et al.*, 1990; Diaz-Camacho *et al.*, 1991; Lara–Aguilera *et al.*, 1992; Sarti *et al.*, 1988, 1992, 1994; Schantz *et al.*, 1992, 1994) and because neurocysticercosis is a major public health problem in many developing countries and is reappearing in developed countries (Earnest *et al.*, 1987; Flisser, 1988; Hitchcock, 1987; Richards *et al.*, 1985; Schantz *et al.*, 1992; Schenone, Villarroel and Rojas, 1982). Human neurocysticercosis may be a life-threatening disease. Patients present pleomorphic symptomatology and complex pathological manifestations which complicate its diagnosis and management. For further information dealing with neurocysticercosis excellent reviews have been published recently (Cook, 1988; del Brutto and Sotelo, 1988; Earnest *et al.*, 1987; Flisser, 1988, 1994; Flisser *et al.*, 1990; Leblanc *et al.*, 1986; Madrazo and Flisser, 1992).

13.2 HISTORICAL ASPECTS

Human taeniasis was recorded in early Egyptian culture where the infection was probably due to *T. saginata*, since Egyptians did not eat pork. Hippocrates, Aristotle and Threophrastus called them 'flatworms' meaning band or ribbon worm, while Romans, such as Celsus, Pliny the Elder and Galen, named them *lumbricus latus*, meaning broad or wide worm (Grove, 1990). *T. solium* was mistaken for *T. saginata* and *Diphyllobothrium latum* for two thousand years or more, until Tyson (1683) discovered and described the head of tapeworms and Redi (1684) published illustrations of the heads of dog and cat tapeworms.

13.3 BIOLOGY

An adult *Taenia* develops to maturity within three to four months after the ingestion of a cysticercus. *H. nana* matures between 20 to 30 days after the ingestion of eggs. Initially the scolex, which is approximately the size of a pin head, evaginates after being stimulated by bile and digestive enzymes. It attaches to the intestinal wall by its four suckers and rostellar hooks fasten into the intestinal mucosa (Cañedo, Laclette and Morales, 1982). *T. saginata* has an unarmed scolex because it lacks hooks. Proglottides or segments start to grow from the neck that follows the scolex and these form the strobila. *T. solium* measures 2–8 m long and *T. saginata* 4–12 m, while *H. nana*, the dwarf tapeworm, measures only 2–6 cm. *T. solium* contains approximately 1000 proglottides, *T. saginata* 2000 and *H. nana* 200. Proglottides close to the neck are immature because they have not yet developed sexual organs. Further back, the segments are sexually mature. Gravid proglottides are those farthest away from the scolex and resemble sacs full of eggs. Gravid *Taenia* proglottides contain around 60 000 eggs each and those of *Hymenolepis* 80–200 eggs. Gravid segments are released from the strobila and are evacuated with faeces in order to perpetuate the life cycle (Faust, Russell and Jung, 1970; Pawlowski, 1990; Pearse *et al.*, 1987; Schantz, 1989; Schmidt and Roberts, 1977; Vertser, 1967; Wardle and McLeod, 1968).

13.4 EPIDEMIOLOGY

Taeniasis due to *T. solium* has a highly variable prevalence in different regions of the world (Mahajan, 1982). Four million cases were reported in 1977 (Crompton and Joyner, 1980). In general, reports of *Taenia solium* taeniasis are scanty. Recently, the source of prevalence data for *T. solium* has shifted from coproscopical reports to community-based studies performed in endemic countries. A seroepidemiologic study performed in Ile de la Réunion showed correlation between human cysticercosis, taeniasis and epilepsy and between seropositive people, infected pigs and disposal of faeces (Michault *et al.*, 1990). A study performed in Taiwan showed that aboriginal but not non-aboriginal schoolchildren were infected with *Taenia* and suggested that it was due to ingestion of raw meat and viscera of wild animals among aborigines (Fan *et al.*, 1990). In Ecuador a large scale study demonstrated that population-based treatment of human taeniasis with a low dose of praziquantel is feasible and effective for short-term control of transmission of *Taenia solium* in hyperendemic areas (Cruz *et al.*, 1989).

In Mexico several epidemiological studies were performed which included demographic, environmental, medical history and diagnostic surveys for taeniasis and cysticercosis (Diaz-Camacho *et al.*, 1990; Diaz-Camacho *et al.*, 1991; Keilbach, de Aluja and Sarti, 1989; Sarti *et al.*, 1988, 1992). Risk factors associated with seropositivity included a history of passing tapeworm proglottides, frequent consumption of pork, poor personal and household hygiene and a history of seizures. Seropositive persons were significantly clustered within households, particularly in those that a member reported a history of having passed tapeworm proglottides or that had a positive coproscopic result for taeniid eggs. Swine cysticercosis was associated with leaving pigs freely roaming and deliberately using pig pens as a toilet area because the pigs would eat, and hence remove, the faeces.

The results of these surveys have identified community, behavioural and environmental practices that must be modified to prevent continued transmission of taeniasis and cysticercosis. They have shown that the immune response is a sensitive indicator of a tapeworm infection in a household or family and that it is easier to determine than the traditional search for taeniid eggs in stool. Most importantly, these studies have shown that the main risk factor for acquiring cysticercosis is the presence of a *Taenia* carrier in the close environment. Human neurocysticercosis has been the main indicator of the presence of *T. solium* because of its public health implications (Flisser, 1988; Gemmell *et al.*, 1983). Human cysticercosis has been reported with incidences that range from 1% to over 18% in many countries of Latin America, Asia and Africa where the disease is considered endemic (Flisser, 1988; Gajdusek, 1978; Gemmell *et al.*, 1983; Schenone, Villarroel and Rojas, 1982).

Recently, human cysticercosis has also been found in some developed countries (Earnest *et al.*, 1987; Hitchcock, 1987). A fourfold increase in annual numbers of neurocysticercosis cases occurred in Los Angeles county, USA, between 1973 and 1983 (Richards and Schantz, 1985; Schantz, 1991). Several cases were detected among three orthodox Jewish families in New York who do not eat pork (Schantz *et al.*, 1992). Recent studies in Mexico and South Africa have shown that neurocysticercosis is the most common cause of late onset epilepsy (Medina *et al.*, 1990; Van As and Joubert, 1991). In Indonesian West New Guinea, where the disease was introduced in 1971 (Gajdusek, 1978), neurocysticercosis ranked six years later as one of the major causes of mortality among adult Ekari people (Bending and Catford, 1983). Apparently it is reaching Papua New Guinea; 24% of burns cases admitted to the Hospital in Milne Bay Province were due to a fall into a fire during an epileptic fit (Barss and Wallace, 1983), which could have been caused by neurocysticercosis (Bending and Catford, 1983).

Taeniasis due to *T. saginata* is a cosmopolitan disease. Stoll reported 39 million cases (Stoll, 1947) and Crompton and Joyner (1980) found 61 million cases in 1977. *T. saginata* is widespread in most cattle-breeding countries of the world (Gemmell *et al.*, 1983; Pawlowski and Schultz, 1972). It is highly endemic, with a prevalence exceeding 10% of the human population in some countries of central and east Africa, the Near East and the Caucasian and south-central republics of the former USSR. Below 5% infection rates occur in many countries of Europe, south-east Asia and South America. In Canada, USA and Australia the prevalence is <0.1% (Pawlowski, 1990; Pawlowski and Schultz, 1972).

There are various sources of prevalence data. Most information is obtained from laboratory reports. For example, in the former USSR, based on 14 million samples, the mean prevalence of taeniasis was 0.6% in 1950 and 0.3% in 46 million stool samples in 1960 (Prokopenko, 1966). One and a half million coprologic studies performed between 1960 and 1989 in the Instituto Adolfo Lutz in São Paulo, Brazil yielded 0.5% of cases with taenia eggs (Dias *et al.*, 1991). Proglottides were obtained only in 355 cases; of those 311 could be specified, 88% were *T. saginata*. Another source of prevalence data is the consumption of taeniacides and taeniafuges. In France from April 1974 to March 1975, 407 000 doses of these drugs were sold and a prevalence of 0.75% was calculated (Doby, 1976). In the USA, physicians requested niclosamide from 1978 to 1981 for the treatment of 4414 cases of taeniasis and 6614 cases of hymenolepiasis (Schantz and McAuley, 1991). Prevalence may be also related to the frequency and financial consequences of beef cysticercosis. In highly endemic areas it is as high as 80%, while in Europe it ranges between 1 and 5%. In East Africa the development of a profitable beef industry has been inhibited by the high prevalence of cysticercosis (Pawlowski, 1990; Pawlowski and Schultz, 1972).

A new species of *Taenia* that infects humans is in the process of being defined. Adult worms of the Taiwan *Taenia* and the Indonesian *Taenia* are morphologically similar to *T. saginata*, but cysticerci have hooks like *T. solium* and are found in pigs but in the liver, not in muscles (Fan, 1988). These tapeworms are found in Asian Pacific regions, at least in Taiwan, Indonesia, Korea, Thailand and the Philippines (Fan, 1988; Fan *et al.*, 1989; Rhoads *et al.*, 1989). Studies on the zoonotic cycle of taeniasis in the Philippines indicated that people in this area had more opportunities of contact with *T. solium* than with *T. saginata* owing to the consumption of raw pork, but that tapeworms actually present in humans belonged exclusively to a species similar to the latter (Arambulo, Cabrera and Tongson, 1976; Ito, 1992). Furthermore, in these Asian countries, cysticercosis in humans is common; thus humans appear to be susceptible to both eggs and cysticerci of this Taiwan *Taenia* as they are to *T. solium* (Ito, 1992), although this has not been demonstrated.

H. nana infection is the most common of all cestodiases. Its global prevalence was reported as 20 million cases in 1947 (Stoll, 1947) and 29 million cases in 1977 (Crompton and Joyner, 1980), although up to 50 million infections have also been calculated (Pawlowski, 1990). Hymenolepiasis occurs most commonly where personal hygienic practices and the quality of sanitary facilities are poor (Willms, 1992). Infection rates are higher among children. Prevalence is especially high in warm and arid countries, as in the Mediterranean region, the Near East, the Indian subcontinent and South America. In these countries prevalence in children reaches 5 to 20% (Schantz, 1989). Hymenolepiasis may be one of the most common intestinal parasitic diseases where spread of soil-transmitted helminthiases is limited due to climatic conditions (Pawlowski, 1990). In developed countries with a temperate climate, individual cases of *H. nana* are reported occasionally (Willms, 1992). Several epidemic outbreaks have been described in orphanages and mental institutions of developed countries (Pawlowski, 1990; Schantz, 1989).

13.5 CLINICAL FEATURES

Most *Taenia* carriers are asymptomatic and only become aware of the infection as they notice proglottides passed with faeces or following spontaneous movement of *T. saginata* segments through the anus. The latter may result in the unpleasant sensation of creeping movements from a foreign body plus intense itching in the perineal area or even along the worm pathway on the skin of the thighs or legs (Schantz, 1989). Proglottides (up to 15) are released daily. Mild gastrointestinal symptoms may occur. Observations in 3110 patients revealed abdominal pain (35%), nausea (34%), weakness (25%), weight loss (21%), increased appetite (17%), headache (15%), constipation (9%), dizziness (8%), diarrhea (6%) and pruritus ani (4%) (Pawlowski and Schultz, 1972). Abdominal pain is usually vaguely located in the epigastrium or umbilical region and varies in intensity. Abdominal pain and nausea are probably due to distension or spasm of the intestinal wall as a reaction to tapeworm movements and are promptly relieved by eating. Hunger has been attributed to hypoglycaemia or as a result of irritation of the ileocaecal valve by tapeworm proglottides, while increased appetite is thought to have a psychological basis. No explanations regarding alterations of bowel movements have been proposed (Pawlowski and Schultz, 1972).

Other more infrequent clinical findings attributed to the worms include convulsions, syncope and allergic symptoms such as urticaria, pruritus and other skin disorders, but these are more likely to be due to concomitant infection with other intestinal parasites or to other causes. Blood eosinophilia has been reported in 5–46% of patients. Clinical manifestations are also related to age, sex and co-existing conditions (Pawlowski and Schultz, 1972; Schantz, 1989). Minor local inflammation results from attachment of the scolex to the mucosa in the upper part of the jejunum. As a result of worm migration to unusual sites or mechanical effects, particularly when multiple worms are present, various rare acute conditions or complications may occur, including appendicitis (Berry and Burrows, 1955; Panzeri, Castoldi and Undiano, 1965; Rousseau, Kerneis and Baron, 1969; Upton, 1980), invasion of the pancreatic and bile ducts (Plane, Ronceray and Dubin, 1980), intestinal obstruction or perforation (Lenoble and Dumontier, 1988), and vomiting of proglottides followed by aspiration (Schantz, 1989; Sterba and Dykova, 1979). Individual reactions to the infection differ widely and may be of a psychological nature as symptoms are often not reported until the patient becomes aware of being infected (Kociecka, 1987; Pawlowski and Schultz, 1972).

Although less information is available regarding *T. solium* taeniasis, reviews indicate that the symptomatology and pathology are less obvious, perhaps because tapeworms are smaller and less active and may remain unnoticed by carriers (Gemmell *et al.*, 1983; Pawlowski, 1990; Schantz, 1989; Yoshino, 1934a, b).

Most *H. nana* infections are asymptomatic and are probably caused by light or moderate worm numbers. Heavy infections frequently cause non-specific intestinal symptoms such as abdominal cramps, diarrhoea and anorexia. Dizziness, irritability and seizures have also been attributed to *H. nana* but may be related to other concomitant pathologic conditions (Dominguez-Sosa *et al.*, 1981; Pawlowski, 1990; Schantz, 1989). Developing cysticercoids destroy the villi that they occupy, heavy infections, therefore, may result in extensive enteritis (Schantz, 1989). Some symptoms are considered to be a result of toxic or allergic action of the parasite. For example 73% of Egyptian children that had an allergic eye disease (phlyctenular kerato-conjunctivitis) were infected with *H. nana*, while only 11% of children without eye disease had hymenolepiasis (Al-Hussaini *et al.*, 1979).

Symptomatology depends on the intensity and duration of the infection. It had been suggested that in the first year the disease is mainly subclinical, between one and five years some intestinal symptoms develop and after five years the general symptoms, such as loss of weight and weakness, are manifested. Infections with more than 3000 parasites or with 10 000 eggs/g faeces cause symptoms, whereas those with less than 1000 worms may only cause loose stools (Dominguez-Sosa *et al.*, 1981; Pawlowski, 1990). The extent of pathologic changes depends on the number of parasites present which is seemingly regulated by the immune status of the host, the presence of other diseases and nutritional status. Hymenolepiasis with high worm burdens is common in immunodeficient and undernourished children. In contrast, moderate infections are usually self-limiting and cleared by adolescence and are infrequent in healthy adults, including those living in endemic areas (Willms, 1992). This has been explained because *H. nana* infections induce humoral immunity and have an important cellular immune component (reviewed in Ito and Smyth, 1987).

13.6 DIAGNOSIS

Diagnosis of tapeworm infection is performed by coprological examination in order to identify eggs in stool samples (Faust, Russell and Jung, 1970; Gemmell *et al.*, 1983; Pawlowski, 1990; Penfold and Penfold, 1936; Schantz, 1989). This technique was first described by Ransom in 1856 (Ransom, 1856). Several variations of the techniques are available, the most commonly used are Faust's flotation and Ritchie's sedimentation techniques (Faust *et al.*, 1938; Faust, Russell and Jung, 1970; Ritchie, 1948). These assays have low sensitivity since they detect less than half of infected people by a single stool examination (Farahmadian *et al.*, 1973; Gemmell *et al.*, 1983; Hall *et al.*, 1981, Mazzotti, 1944a, b). Analyses in repeated stool samples increase the likelihood of detection of tapeworm carriers (Gemmell *et al.*, 1983; Sarti *et al.*, 1988). Perianal scraping has been reported to be relatively sensitive for diagnosing *Taenia* spp. infections (Mazzoti, 1944a, b; Rijpstra, Smith and Swellergrebel, 1981) although opposed results have also been reported (Beaver, Jung and Cupp, 1984; Sarti *et al.*, 1992). Decision on diagnosis of intestinal parasites may be facilitated with the use of algorithms (Vazquez-Tsuji *et al.*, 1987).

Eggs from both *Taenia* species are morphologically identical and their identification in faecal samples does not enable species specific diagnosis (Faust, Russell and Jung, 1970; Laclette *et al.*, 1982; Pawlowski, 1990). Observation of discharged proglottides with faeces is the initial diagnosis in many cases. *T. saginata* gravid proglottides may leave the host spontaneously, and thus infected people become aware of the presence of the parasite (Pawlowski, 1990; Schantz, 1989; Sterba and Dykova, 1979; Thornton, 1979; Willms, 1992). Apparently *T. solium* does not make its presence known in this way; however, *T. solium* proglottides may be motile in fresh faeces and capable of migrating outside the body (Beaver, Jung and Cupp, 1984; Yoshino, 1934a,b). Care should be taken when species-specific diagnosis is based solely on this parameter. An indication of the potential for *T. solium* to be discharged from the anus has been described by Beaver, Jung and Cupp, (1984) who quote that during 20 days a person in Colombia passed 102 *T. solium* proglottides in or on his faeces and on two occasions he collected motile proglottides from his thighs.

Species-specific diagnosis is routinely performed in clarified gravid proglottides when these are available and well preserved. *T. solium* has 7–16 lateral branches arising from the central uterus which redivide, while *T. saginata* has 14–32 primary branches (Beaver, Jung and Cupp, 1984; Elsdon-Dew and Proctor, 1965; Faust, Russell and Jung, 1970; Kuchenmeister, 1852; Pawlowski, 1990; Proctor, 1972; Schantz, 1989; Schmidt and Roberts, 1977; Verster, 1969). This diagnostic criterion can be misleading because there is an overlap in the number of primary branches, although it is possible to distinguish both species. Nevertheless, expertise is needed in order to define the number of primary uterine branches, which usually are not in overlapping numbers, in which case other parameters for species identification must be taken into account.

Other proglottid differences include the presence of an accessory ovary lobe in *T. solium* and of a vaginal sphincter in *T. saginata*, which are evident in mature or gravid proglottides (Beaver, Jung and Cupp, 1984; Verster, 1969). The presence or absence of hooks in the scolex is the most reliable difference between both species: *T. solium* has an armed scolex and *T. saginata* an unarmed one (Beaver, Jung and Cupp, 1984; Faust, Russell and Jung, 1970; Schmidt and Roberts, 1977). However, there are very low probabilities of obtaining the scolex after cestocidal treatment (Ahkami and Hadyan, 1969; Richards and Schantz, 1985; Rim *et al.*, 1979).

Diagnosis of *H. nana* infection is only possible by coprological examination since the tiny gravid proglottides are broken up in the intestine (Schantz, 1989). Flotation or concentration techniques should be performed in serial stool samples since egg output may be irregular and in low numbers and eggs are very fragile (Garcia-Rosales, Fragodos and Alvarez-Chacon, 1986; Pawlowski, 1990; Schantz, 1989).

Molecular methodologies have been recently applied to improve diagnosis. Detection of eggs in faeces has been standardized using DNA hybridization techniques (Flisser *et al.*, 1988). *T. saginata* eggs were detected with total genomic DNA as a radiolabelled probe in a hybridization dot blot assay. *T. saginata* DNA did not hybridize to *T. pisiformis* eggs, neither did *T. pisiformis* DNA hybridize to *T. saginata* eggs, and the DNA hybridization assay was also highly sensitive because as low as one *T. saginata* egg could be detected. Nevertheless some cross-hybridization between *T. saginata* DNA and *T. solium* DNA was found (Flisser *et al.*, 1988). Specific probes from genomic libraries have been reported for *T. solium* (McManus *et al.*, 1989; Rishi and McManus, 1987; Rishi and McManus, 1988) and *T. saginata* (Harrison, Delgado and Parkhouse, 1990) but have not been used yet to detect eggs. Different mobilities of glucose phosphate isomerase in extracts of *T. solium* and *T. saginata* submitted to electrophoresis have been described (Le Riche and Sewell, 1977).

Of great interest is the standardization of techniques to detect host-specific antibodies or parasite antigens in simple and more reliable assays than coprological examination and if possible even before the parasite is gravid and able to shed eggs or proglottides. Many studies have been performed with the aim of standardizing immunological methods for the diagnosis of *T. saginata* taeniasis; several techniques and antigens have been employed which resulted in diverse degrees of sensitivity and specificity (reviewed in Pawlowski and Schultz, 1972). In contrast, there is only one recent report that indicates that antibodies can be detected in individuals that harbour adult *T. solium* (Diaz *et al.*, 1992) in a Western blot assay that was originally standardized for antibody detection in patients with neurocysticercosis (Tsang, Brand and Boyer, 1989). Although these patients did not have neurological symptoms suggestive of neurocysticercosis, it is not possible to rule out the concomitant presence of cysticerci as a source of antigenic stimulus in people from endemic countries. Recombinant DNA technology has been used to obtain an antigen for *Taenia saginata* useful for immunodiagnosis of cattle cysticercosis that cross-reacts with infected swine; this antigen has been fully characterized (Zarlenga, Rhoads and Al-Yaman, 1994).

Anti-*H. nana* antibodies were detected by ELISA in 79 and 85% of young people and children of Peru and Mexico respectively, with intestinal hymenolepiasis (Castillo *et al.*, 1991; Gomez-Priego, Godinez-Hana and Gutierrez-Quiroz, 1991). False positive reactions were obtained in 30% and 72% serum samples respectively, from patients with hydatid disease, cysticercosis or taeniasis invalidating the assay for diagnostic purposes, mainly because hymenolepiasis is prevalent among populations living under conditions of poor hygiene where cysticercosis is also present. On the other hand cross-reactions are interesting to study in order to analyze antigenic similarities among these parasites or multiple parasitoses in the patients.

Parasite antibodies are usually searched for in serum. Recent studies indicate that saliva is also an appropriate source of antibodies in human neurocysticercosis and in experimental canine taeniasis (Feldman *et al.*, 1990; Kinder *et al.*, 1992). Analysis of human salivary antibody response should thus be considered for potential diagnostic use in taeniasis. An alternative for immunological diagnosis is the detection of parasite antigens in human faeces. Results in rats infected with *Hymenolepis diminuta* showed high specificity and sensitivity (Allan and Craig, 1989). When this assay was applied to human *T. solium* taeniasis, detection of coproantigens was 100% sensitive and no cross-reactivity with other helminths including *H. nana* was found, but it could not exclude *T. saginata* (Allan *et al.*, 1990). The assay was evaluated in field studies in China and Guatemala where it was specific and sensitive and was able to diagnose an individual who was negative by coproscopical studies and by cestocidal treatment but who passed several proglottides one day after treatment (Allan *et al.*, 1992). This ELISA in a dip stick presentation was also tested in field studies in Mexico and Guatemala. Results indicate that it is easy to perform and yields high degree of detection of taenia carriers confirmed by cestocidal treatment (Allan *et al.*, 1993). Coproantigen detection in patients with *T. saginata* yielded 85% sensitivity and 95% specificity by ELISA, although, as in the *T. solium* ELISA, no differentiation between both human parasites could be achieved (Desplazes *et al.*, 1991). ELISAs performed on faecal samples from dogs with *T. pisiformis* (Allan *et al.*, 1992) or *T. hydatigena* (Desplazes *et al.*, 1990) or rats with *H. diminuta* (Allan and Craig, 1989) experimental infections demonstrated coproantigens several weeks before patency. Results fluctuated in time and were independent from egg output after patency. Dog infections with 1000 to 4000 *Echinococcus granulosus* yielded higher optical density values than infections with 30 to 200 parasites (Allan *et al.*, 1992). ELISA became positive at 10 days after infection with over 10 000 worms and at 20 or 30 days when worm burden was lower (between 200 and 1000 or up to 10 000 parasites respectively) (Desplazes *et al.*, 1992). A similar correlation with parasite burden was found in Swiss foxes infected with *E. granulosus* (Desplazes *et al*, 1992). This information might be important for epidemiological surveys of human taeniasis in order to detect and treat prepatent infections and in hymenolepiasis where different intensities of infection are related to the clinical picture of the disease (Pawlowski, 1990). Furthermore, parasite antigens were not detected within 5 to 9 days after cestocidal treatment (Allan and Craig, 1989; Allan *et al.*, 1990; Desplazes *et al.*, 1990,

1991) and thus, can be a reliable monitor of drug efficacy.

Immunological methods have also been developed for the detection of eggs. A monoclonal antibody was raised against *E. granulosus* oncospheres and used in an immunofluorescence assay; 100% specificity and 73% sensitivity was obtained in infected dogs (Craig *et al.*, 1988). Interestingly, this assay detected *E. granulosus* eggs in soil samples inside Turkana huts and in water samples from open waterholes used by the people and their livestock (Craig *et al.*, 1988).

13.7 TREATMENT

At the beginning of the Christian era some Arab authors such as Serapion named tapeworms *cucurbitini* not only because of their resemblance to pumpkin seeds but because pumpkin seeds were one of the earliest remedies for tapeworm infections (Grove, 1990). During the 1950s mepacrine, tin compounds, paromomycin, acridine derivatives, dichlorophen, trichloropen, bithionol and extracts of *Aspidium* male fern were the drugs used for treatment of tapeworm infections (Gemmell *et al.*, 1983; Pawlowski and Schultz, 1979; Penfold, 1936). Progress in chemotherapy came with niclosamide, a chloronitrophenyl-chlorosalicylamide, which was introduced in 1960, and more recently with praziquantel, a synthetic acylated isoquinoline-pyrazine (Gonnert and Schraupstatter, 1960; Gonnert *et al.*, 1963; Groll, 1984; Thomas and Andrews, 1977; Pearson and Guerrant, 1983; deRezende, 1983). The effects of these drugs on parasites are diverse and precise knowledge of the mode of action is scanty. Praziquantel, paromomycin and tin compounds disrupt the worm's tegument (Pawlowski and Schultz, 1972; Thomas and Gonnert, 1977, Thomas, Andrews and Melhorn, 1982). Praziquantel also interferes with calcium channels (Coles, 1979) paralyzing the parasite (Garcia-Dominguez *et al.*, 1991), as does male fern extract (Sharma, Dubery and Iyer, 1980). Niclosamide uncouples oxidative phosphorylation and thus inhibits the uptake of oxygen and glucose (Sharma, Dubery and Iyer, 1980). The mode of action of pumpkin seeds, acridine derivatives and of paromomycin, an antibiotic found by serendipity to have anthelmintic activity (Salem and Al-Allaf, 1967), are not known (Pawlowski and Schultz, 1972).

Praziquantel and niclosamide are the drugs of choice for the treatment of taeniasis since they are now the best taeniacides (Pawlowski, 1990). Their efficacy has been extensively investigated (Gemmell *et al*, 1983; Gonnert and Schraufstatter, 1960; Groll, 1984, Pawlowski, 1990). Praziquantel and niclosamide are administered as a single oral dose in the morning before any meal and may be followed by a saline purge, although the need of the purge has been questioned (Richards and Schantz, 1985). Praziquantel is administered at 5 or 10 mg/kg and produces almost 100% cure rates, with few side effects such as mild and transient abdominal pain and in rare cases dizziness and skin rashes (Pawlowski, 1990; Schantz, 1989; Willms, 1992). Even a lower dose of 2.5 mg/kg showed full efficacy against *T. saginata* taeniasis (Pawlowski, 1991). Preliminary results in a community-based study indicate that 5 mg/kg had a lower efficacy than expected (Sarti, Flisser, Bronfman and Schantz, unpublished). Praziquantel is contraindicated for pregnant women, children younger than 2 years old and patients with cirrhosis (Willms, 1992).

Niclosamide is administered at 2 g total dose for adults in four 500 mg tablets that have to be well chewed and swallowed with a small amount of water. Dosages for children are proportionately lower, usually two or three tablets. The drug is well tolerated and toxic effects at therapeutic dosage have not been reported. A single treatment is effective in over 80–90% of cases. Niclosamide has no contraindications and can be used in pregnancy (Gonnert *et al.* 1963; Keeling, 1968;

Pawlowski, 1990; Perera, Western and Schultz; 1970; Schantz, 1989).

Paromomycin may also be used, in cases where the other two drugs are not available, at a single dose of 75 mg/kg with a maximum of 4 g after a meal. Mild side effects appear in 30–60% of cases, mainly diarrhoea and vomiting. This may, theoretically, be dangerous in cases of *T. solium* where it could lead to internal autoinfection and cysticercosis (Schantz, 1989).

Acridine derivatives, such as quinacrine, are still in use, at least in Asian countries (Chung Fan and Chiu, *et al*, 1985; Fan *et al.*, 1989; Rhoads *et al.*, 1989), despite the risk of intolerance and overdosage (Pawlowski and Schultz, 1972). These drugs should be reserved for refractory cases of *T. saginata* infection (Keeling, 1968).

A mixture of boiled areca nuts (75–150 g) and pumpkin seeds (50–100 g) used in Taiwan to treat 33 individuals with taeniasis was considered safe and effective (Chung and Ko, 1976). Areca nuts are presently used in China with high efficacy (Craig and Allan, personal communication). Albendazole, a benzimidazole derivative, is a potent and broad spectrum anthelmintic drug used in cases of multiple parasitic disease because of its effectiveness against intestinal cestodes and nematodes (Pene *et al.*, 1982). The recommended dose for treatment of tapeworms is 6.6 mg/kg (Willms, 1992). A single 400 mg dose yielded 65% cure rate in taeniasis, while 3-day dosages increased cure rate to 86% in 480 adult patients with single or mixed intestinal helminth infections (Jagota, 1986). Albendazole should not be used in children younger than 2 years old or during pregnancy, owing to the embryotoxic and teratogenic effects that have been observed in experimental animals (Marriner *et al.*, 1986; Willms, 1992).

Gastrografin (sodium and meglumine diatrizoates) a water-soluble contrast medium was found to cause the expulsion of *T. saginata*. Waki *et al.* (1986) discovered this by serendipity when they used the contrast medium to visualize tapeworms in the intestinal lumen radiologically and achieved 100% efficacy in the treatment of six *T. saginata* cases. Tapeworms were clearly seen by fluoroscopy as string-like radiolucent areas within the jejunum and showed active movements, appearing to move against the flow of gastrografin. Tapeworms were expelled alive, unfragmented and apparently not injured 20–50 m after treatment. The mode of action of gastrografin was examined but could not be defined (Waki *et al.*, 1986). In spite of this successful result, a recent report indicates that the use of gastrografin is expensive and since the insertion of the duodenal tube may cause discomfort, it is not recommended in cases of *T. saginata* infections, but might be taken into consideration in *T. solium* carriers in order to reduce risk of autoinfection (Ohnishi and Murata, 1990).

Chemotherapy can be considered successful if no proglottides reappear within four months after treatment. If necessary, drug administration can be repeated after a few weeks or if proglottides are released again after three to four months (Pawlowski, 1990; Schantz, 1989). Caution is required in patients with *T. solium* taeniasis because it is possible that even the low single dose of praziquantel used for treatment of taeniasis may exacerbate symptoms if that person also has cysticerci in the brain or the eyes (Gemmell *et al.*, 1983; Flisser *et al.*, 1993).

Detailed histological study of proglottides released by *T. solium* carriers before and after treatment with niclosamide showed that the drug did not damage the parasite's tegument, minimizing the possibilities of autoinfection due to release of eggs (Martinez-Baez, Martinez-Marañon and Molina-Pasquel, 1971) as suggested elsewhere (Ditzel and Schwartz, 1967; Perera, Western and Schultz, 1970). Praziquantel causes severe damage to proglottides (Thomas, Andrews and Melhorn, 1982) and thus in theory it can favour autoinfection. Nevertheless confirmation of internal autoinfection has never been obtained in *T. solium*. An abnormal degree of reverse peristalsis would be required to carry gravid proglottides from the distal small intestine to the stomach (Richards and Schantz, 1985). However, reflux of proglottides could occur during protracted emesis and they have been found in vomitus (Webbe, 1967). For this reason drugs which provoke nausea and vomiting should not be used in intestinal taeniasis (Pawlowski, 1990; Richards and Schantz, 1985; Schantz, 1989). Neither praziquantel nor niclosamide induce nausea or vomiting.

Treatment of hymenolepiasis was difficult until therapy with niclosamide was introduced in 1962. A dose of 60 to 80 mg/kg, with a maximum of 2 g daily, given for 5–7 consecutive days, is well tolerated and cures 90% of all infections (Pawlowski, 1990). Treatment with praziquantel is even more effective and much simpler as it needs only a single dose of 25 mg/kg by which it produces parasitological cure in 95% of infected children (Schantz, 1989). Whether treatment is performed with praziquantel or niclosamide, heavy infections may require a repeat course after 10 days. Follow-up faecal examinations are suggested every second week for at least three months after treatment, as *H. nana* infections may recur. Concomitant treatment of all infected family members and institution inmates greatly diminishes the risk or reinfection from external sources (Pawlowski, 1990).

Only recently has the effect of niclosamide and praziquantel been analysed in relation to their effects on destrobilation using *H. diminuta* infections in rats as the experimental model (Dixon and Arai, 1991). Interestingly, effective dosages determined 24 h after treatment agreed very closely with those in the literature. Nevertheless, when destrobilation was considered by analysing the number of regenerating worms in rats examined 8 days after treatment with either drug, it appeared that neither drug was as effective as previously reported. Fully effective dosage of niclosamide was 1500 mg/kg and of praziquantel, 30 mg/kg, i.e. 15 or 6–12 times higher, respectively, than the dosages recommended for both drugs (Dixon and Arai, 1991). This result, although obtained in a rat model, may explain failures reported in treatment of human tapeworm carriers.

13.8 IMMUNITY AGAINST INTESTINAL TAPEWORMS

There is substantial evidence to indicate that host-protective immunity can occur against *Hymenolepis* species in rodent models (reviewed by Ito and Smyth, 1987). Nevertheless, there have been few significant advances in the knowledge of the immunology of adult taeniid infections in humans (Gemmell *et al.*, 1983; Ito and Smyth, 1987; Lightowlers, Mitchell and Rickard, 1992). Furthermore, the evidence in favour of development of any acquired resistance to superinfection is poor and, where there is some evidence, immunity is inconsistent and incomplete (Lightowlers, Mitchell and Rickard, 1992; Miller, 1932; Rickard, Coman and Cannon, 1977) or even absent (Heath, Parmeter and Osborn, 1980). In contrast, immunity against the larval stage has been extensively studied (reviewed by Flisser, Perez-Montfort and Larralde, 1979 and by Lightowlers, Mitchell and Rickard, 1992). As recently stated by Lightowlers and co-workers (1992) 'in no other helminth infection are the beneficial effects of host anti-parasite immune responses so obvious as in larval cestode infections'. Also, there are no data regarding detection of oncospheral antibodies in human cases of *T. solium* taeniasis or cysticercosis or *T. saginata* taeniasis, whereas in dogs infected with *E. granulosus*, *T. hydatigena* or *T. pisiformis* oncospheral serum antibodies have been detected (Gasser *et al.*, 1988; Jenkins and Rickard, 1985). This finding suggests that some taeniid eggs may hatch in the gut of humans infected with the adult tapeworm and penetrate the host's tissues sufficiently to induce the anti-oncosphere immune response (Lightowlers, Mitchell and Rickard, 1992). As recently suggested by Lightowlers (personal communication), the presence of the intestinal stage of *T. solium* may protect the host from infection, or even autoinfection, against the larval stage.

13.9 PREVENTION AND CONTROL

The first article of volume 1, number 1 of the *Journal of Parasitology* dealt with the killing of *T. saginata* cysticerci in beef (Ransom, 1914). Many lines of basic and applied research have been undertaken. Results regarding the control of tapeworms in human beings by improving diagnosis and management as well as by defining prevalence rates and risk factors have been reviewed in this chapter. Not long ago all species of intestinal helminths, including taeniasis, were recognized as an important problem that could be solved with the use of broad-spectrum anthelmintics specially in school-age children (Halloran, Burdy and Pollitt, 1989). The main reason for the recognition is that intestinal helminth infections cause poor school participation and performance (Leslie and Jamison, 1990). Cost-benefit analyses of school-based interventions suggest that appropriate health and nutrition interventions in schools are likely to give very high-yield investments (Jamison and Leslie, 1990). As Warren (1991) stated recently:

> 19 of the 23 major human helmint infections can be treated with only 3 drugs: albendazole, praziquantel, and ivermectin. These drugs are so innocuous to the human host that mass chemotherapy can be employed without individual diagnosis, and since they do not require cold storage conditions or administration with needles and syringes, cost estimates for control programs of mass chemotherapy given in and by the school system would be in the range of one dollar per treated child per year. Protection provided over a 10 year period of schooling would cost only $10 per child.

Parallel to the application of the recently gained knowledge regarding the potential benefits of chemotherapy, research should be reinforced towards the understanding of the immune response of infected people against tapeworms. These investigations could improve immunodiagnostic methods and would focus especially on the development of an effective vaccine. Recently, a recombinant vaccine that showed 94% protection in an experimental trial was developed against the larval stage of *Taenia ovis* in sheep (Johnston *et al.*, 1989).

ACKNOWLEDGEMENTS

I should like to thank Lic. Erasto Brito and its library staff for providing many articles, and Dr M. Lightowlers for correcting the manuscript, providing helpful discussions, several articles and the proper environment to complete this chapter.

REFERENCES

Ahkami, S. and Hadyan, A. (1969) The appearance of the scolex of *Taenia saginata* in the stool after eradication of the parasite by niclosamide. *Z. Tropenmed. Parasiten.*, **20**, 341–5.

Al-Hussaini, M. K., Khalifa, Al-Ansary, A. T. A. *et al.* (1979) Phlyctenular eye disease in association with *Hymenolepis nana* in Egypt. *Br. J. Ophthal*, **63**, 627–31.

Allan, J. C. and Craig, P. S. (1989) Coproantigens in gut tapeworm infections: *Hymenolepis diminuta* in rats. *Parasit. Res.* **76**, 68–73.

Allan, J. C., Avila, G., García-Noval, J. *et al.* (1990) Immunodiagnosis of taeniasis by coproantigen detection. *Parasitology*, **101**, 473–7.

Allan, J. C., Craig, P. S., García, J. *et al.* (1992) Coproantigen detection for immunodiagnosis of echinococcosis and taeniasis in dogs and humans. *Parasitology*, **104**, 1–9.

Allan, J. C., Mercos, F., García-Noval, J. *et al.* (1993) Dipstick dot ELISA for the detection of *Taenia* coproantigens in humans. *Parasitology*, **107**, 79–85.

Arambulo, P. V., Cabrera, B. D. and Tongson, M. S. (1976) Studies on the zoonotic cycle of *Taenia saginata* taeniasis and cysticercosis in the Philippines. *Int. J. Zoon.*, **3**, 77–104.

Barss, P. and Wallace, K. (1983) Grass-skirt burns in Papua New Guinea. *Lancet*, (**April 2**), 733–4.

Beaver, P. C., Jung, R. C. and Cupp, E. W. (1984) *Clinical Parasitology*, Lea and Febiger, Philadelphia.

Bending, J. J. and Catford, J. C. (1983) Epidemic of burns in New Guinea due to cerebral cysticercosis. *Lancet*, (**April 23**), 922.

Berry, L. R. and Burrows, R. B. (1955) Appendicitis with cestodes. *Archs Pathol.*, **59**, 587–93.

Cañedo, L., Laclette, J. P. and Morales, E. (1982). Evagination of the metacestode of *Taenia solium*, in *Cysticercosis: Present State of Knowledge and Perspectives*, (eds A. Flisser, K. Willms, J. P. Laclette *et al.*), Academic Press, New York, pp. 363–73.

Castillo, R. M., Grados, P., Carcamo, C. *et al.* (1991) Effect of treatment on serum antibody to *Hymenolepis nana* detected by enzyme-linked immunosorbent assay. *J. Clin. Microbiol.*, **29**, 413–14.

Chandler, A. C. (1939) The effects of number and age of worms and development of primary and secondary infections with *Hymenolepis diminuta* in rats, and investigation into the true nature of 'premunition' in tapeworm infections. *Am. J. Hyg.*, **29**, 105.

Chung, W. C., Fan, P. C. and Chiu, H. M. (1985) [Survey of helminthic infections and treatment of *Taenia* species infection among aborigines in Chien-Shih District, Hsin-Chu County, northern Taiwan]. *Chung-Hua-Min-Kuo-Wei-Sheng-Wu-Chi-Mien-I-Hsueh-Tsa-Chih*, **18**, 96–103.

Chung, W. C. and Ko, B. C. (1976) Treatment of *Taenia saginata* infection with mixture of areca nuts and pumpkin seeds. *Chung-Hua-Min-Kuo-Wei-Sheng-Wu-Hsueh-Tsa-Chih*, **9**, 31–5.

Coles, G. C. (1979) The effect of praziquantel on *Schistosoma mansoni*. *J. Helminth.*, **53**, 31–3.

Cook, G. C. (1988) Neurocysticercosis: parasitology, clinical presentation, diagnosis and recent advances in management. *Q. J. Med. New Series*, **68**, 575–83.

Craig, P. S., Macpherson, C. N. L., Watson-Jones, D. L. *et al.* (1988) Immunodetection of *Echinococcus* eggs from naturally infected dogs and from environmental contamination sites in settlements in Turkana, Kenya. *Trans. Roy. Soc. Trop. Med. Hyg.*, **82**, 268–74.

Crompton, D. W. T. and Joyner, S. M. (1980) Worms and man, in *Parasitic Worms*, Wykeham Publ. Ltd (Taylor and Francis Group), London, pp. 177–90.

Cruz, M., Davis, A., Dixon, H. *et al.* (1989) Operational studies on the control of *Taenia solium* taeniasis/cysticercosis in Ecuador. *Bull. Wld. Hlth. Org.*, **67**, 401–7.

del Brutto, O. H. and Sotelo, J. (1988) Neurocysticercosis: an update. *Rev. Infect. Dis.*, **6**, 1075–87.

deRezende, G. L. (1983) Praziquantel: experiencia clinica mundial. *Bol. Chil. Parasit.*, **38**, 52–63.

Desplazes, P., Gottstein, B., Stingelin, Y. *et al.* (1990) Detection of *Taenia hydatigena* copro-antigens by ELISA in dogs. *Vet. Parasit.*, **36**, 91–103.

Desplazes, P., Eckert, J., Pawlowski, Z. S. *et al.* (1991) An enzyme-linked immunosorbent assay for diagnostic detection of *Taenia saginata* copro-antigens in humans. *Trans. Roy. Soc. Trop. Med. Hyg.*, **85**, 391–6.

Desplazes, P., Gottstein, B., Eckert, J. *et al.* (1992) Detection of *Echinococcus* coproantigens by enzyme-linked immunosorbent assay in dogs, dingoes and foxes. *Parasit. Res.*, **78**, 303–8.

Dias, R. M. D. S., Silva, M. I. P. G., Mangini, A. C. S. *et al.* (1991) Ocorrencia de *Taenia sp.* na populacao atendida no laboratorio central do Instituto Adolfo Lutz, São Paulo, SP, Brasil (1960/1989). *Rev. Inst. Med. Trop. São Paulo*, **33**, 147–51.

Diaz, J. F., Verastegui, M., Gilman, R. H. *et al.* (1992) Immunodiagnosis of human cysticercosis (*Taenia solium*): a field comparison of an antibody-enzyme-linked immunosorbent assay (ELISA), an antigen-ELISA, and an enzyme-linked immunoelectrotransfer blot (EITB) assay in Peru. *Am. J. Trop. Med. Hyg.*, **46**, 610–13.

Diaz-Camacho, S., Candil, A., Uribe, M. *et al.* (1990) Serology as an indicator of *Taenia solium* tapeworm infections in a rural community in Mexico. *Trans. Roy. Soc. Trop. Med. Hyg.*, **84**, 563–6.

Diaz-Camacho, S., Candil, A., Suate, V. *et al.* (1991) Epidemiological study and control of *Taenia solium* infections with praziquantel in a rural village of Mexico. *Am. J. Trop. Med. Hyg.*, **45**, 522–31.

Ditzel, J. and Schwartz, M. (1967) Worm cure without tears. The effect of niclosamide on taeniasis saginate in man. *Acta Med. Scand.*, **182**, 663–4.

Dixon, B. R. and Arai, H. P. (1991). Anthelmintic-induced destrobilation and its influence on calculated drug efficacy in *Hymenolepis diminuta* infections in rats. *J. Parasit.*, **77**, 769–74.

Doby, J. M. (1976) Fréquence de la teniase humaine par *Taenia saginata* en France. *Med. Malad. Infect.*, **6**, 477–83.

Dominguez-Sosa, D., Alvarez-Chacon, R., Wong-Chio, M. *et al.* (1981) Himenolepiasis pura. *Acta Ped. Mexico*, **2**, 86–8.

Earnest, M. P., Reller, L. B., Filley, C. M. *et al.* (1987) Neurocysticercosis in the United States:

35 cases and a review. *Rev. Infect. Dis.*, **9**, 961–79.

Elsdon-Dew, R. and Proctor, E. M. (1965) Distinction between *Taeniarhynchus saginata* and *Taenia solium*. *S. Afr. Sci.*, **61**, 215–17.

Fan, P. C. (1988) Taiwan *Taenia* and taeniasis. *Parasit. Today*, **4**, 86–8.

Fan, P. C., Lin, C. Y., Kosman, M. L. *et al.* (1989) Experimental infection of Indonesia *Taenia* (Samosir strain) in domestic animals. *Int. J. Parasit.*, **19**, 809–12.

Fan, P. C., Chung, W. C., Lin, C. Y. *et al.* (1990) Prevalence of taeniasis and enterobiasis among aboriginal children in mountainous areas of Taiwan. *Kao-Hsiung-I-Hsueh-Ko-Hsueh-Tsa-Chih*, **6**, 475–82.

Farahmandian, I., Sahba, G. H., Afraa, F. *et al.* (1973) A comparison of stool examination and mass treatment for indications of the prevalence of *Taenia saginata*. *Trop. Geog. Med.*, **25**, 171–3.

Faust, E. C., D'Antoni, J. S., Odom, V. *et al.* (1938) A critical study of clinical laboratory techniques for the diagnosis of protozoan cysts and helminth eggs in feces. *Am. J. Trop. Med.*, **18**, 169–83.

Faust, E. C., Russell, P. F. and Jung, R. C. 1970 *Craig and Faust's Clinical Parasitology*, Lea and Febiger, Philadelphia, pp. 502–7, 785–90.

Feldman, M., Plancarte, A., Sandoval, M. *et al.* (1990) Comparison of two assays (EIA and EITB) and two samples (saliva and serum) for the diagnosis of neurocysticercosis. *Trans. Roy. Soc. Trop. Med. Hyg.*, **84**, 559–62.

Flisser, A. (1988) Neurocysticercosis in Mexico. *Parasit. Today*, **4**, 131–7.

Fisser A. (1994) Taeniasis and cysticercosis due to *Taenia solium*, in *Progress in Clinical Parasitology* (ed. T. Sun), vol. 4, CRC Press Inc., Boca Raton, Florida, pp. 77–116.

Flisser, A., Perez-Montfort, R. and Larralde, C. (1979) The immunology of human and animal cysticercosis. A review. *Bull. Wld Hlth Org.*, **57**, 839–56.

Flisser, A., Reid, A., García-Zepeda, E. *et al.* (1988) Specific detection of *Taenia saginata* eggs by DNA hybridisation. *Lancet*, (**December 17**), 1429–30.

Flisser, A., Plancarte, A., Correa, D. *et al.* (1990) New approaches in the diagnosis of *Taenia solium* cysticercosis and taeniasis. *Ann. Parasit. Hum. Comp.*, **65**, 95–8.

Flisser, A., Madrazo, I., Plancarte, A. *et al.* (1993) Neurological symptoms in occult neurocysticercosis after a single taeniacidal dose of praziquantel. *Lancet*, **342**, 748.

Gajdusek, D. C. (1978) Introduction of *Taenia solium* into west New Guinea with a note on an epidemic of burns from cysticercus epilepsy in the Ekari people on the Wissel lakes area. *Papua New Guinea Med. J.*, **21**, 329–42.

Garcia-Dominguez, C., Correa, D., Rabiela, M. T. and Flisser, A. (1991) Praziquantel treatment of muscle *Taenia solium* cysticercosis. 4. Reversible *in vitro* effect. *Parasit. Res.*, **77**, 691–6.

Garcia-Rosales, J. J., Fragodos, M. A. and Alvarez-Chacon, R. (1986) Demostracion de la efectividad del metodo de Kato-Katz en la deteccion y cuantificacion de huevos de helmintos. *Rev. Mex. Patol. Clin.*, **33**, 143–51.

Gasser, R. B., Lightowlers, M. W., Obendorf, D. L. *et al* (1988) Evaluation of a serological test system for the diagnosis of natural *Echinococcus granulosus* infection in dogs using *E. granulosus* protoscolex and oncosphere antigens. *Aust. Vet. J.*, **65**, 369–73.

Gemmell, M., Matyas, Z., Pawlowski, Z. *et al.* (1983) *Guidelines for Surveillance, Prevention and Control of Taeniasis/Cysticercosis*. VPH/83.49. World Health Organization, Geneva, pp. 1–207.

Gomez-Priego, A., Godinez-Hana, A. L. and Gutierrez-Quiroz, M. (1991) Detection of serum antibodies in human *Hymenolepis* infection by enzyme immunoassay. *Trans. Roy. Soc. Trop. Med. Hyg.*, **85**, 645–7.

Gonnert, R., Johannis, J., Schraupstatter, E. *et al.* (1963) Konstitution und cestocide wirkung in der Yomesan-Reihe. *Med. Chem.*, **7**, 540–67.

Gonnert, R. and Schraupstatter, E. (1960) Experimentelle untersuchungen mit *N*-(2′-chlor-4′-nitrophenyl)-5-chlorsalicylamid, einem neuen bandwurmittel. *Arzneimittel-Forsch.*, **10**, 881–4.

Groll, E. (1984) Praziquantel. *Adv. Pharmac. Chemother.*, **20**, 219–38.

Grove, D. I. (1990) *A History of Human Helminthology*. CAB Intl., Oxon, UK, pp. 355–83.

Hall, A., Latham, M. C., Crompton, D. W. T. *et al.* (1981) *Taenia saginata* (cestoda) in western Kenya: the reliability of faecal examination in diagnosis. *Parasitology*, **83**, 91–101.

Halloran, M. E., Bundy, D. A. P. and Pollitt, E. (1989) Infectious disease and the UNESCO Basic Education Initiative. *Parasit. Today*, **5**, 359–62.

Harrison, L. J. S., Delgado, J. and Parkhouse, R. M. E. (1990) Differential diagnosis of *Taenia saginata* and *Taenia solium* with DNA probes. *Parasitology*, **100**, 459–61.

Heath, D. D., Parmeter, S. N. and Osborn, P. J. (1980) An attempt to immunise dogs against *Taenia hydatigena*. *Res. Vet. Sci.*, **29**, 388–9.

Heyneman, D. (1963) Host–parasite resistance patterns, some implications from experimental studies with helminths. *Ann. N. Y. Acad. Sci.*, **113**, 114.

Hitchcock, R. (1987) Cysticercosis in the UK. *J. Neurol. Neurosurg. Psychiat.*, **50**, 1080.

Ito, A. (1992) Cysticercosis in Asian-Pacific Regions. *Parasit. Today*, **8**, 182–3.

Ito, A. and Smyth, J. D. (1987) Adult cestodes-immunology of the lumen-dwelling cestode infections, in *Immune Responses in Parasitic Infections: Immunology, Immunopathology and Immunoprophylaxis: Trematodes and Cestodes*, vol 2 (ed. E. J. L. Soulsby), CRC Press Inc, Boca Raton, Florida, pp. 115–63.

Jagota, S. C. (1986) Albendazole, a broad-spectrum anthelmintic, in the treatment of intestinal nematode and cestode infection: a multicenter study in 480 patients. *Clin. Ther.*, **8**, 226–31.

Jamison, D. T. and Leslie, J. (1990) Health and nutrition considerations in education planning 2. The cost and effectiveness of school-based interventions. *Food Nutr. Bull.*, **12**, 204–14.

Jenkins, D. J. and Rickard, M. D. (1985) Specific antibody responses to *Taenia hydatigena*, *T. pisiformis* and *Echinococcus granulosus* infection in dogs. *Aust. Vet. J.*, **62**, 72–8.

Johnson, K. S., Harrison, G. B. L., Lightowlers, M. W. *et al.* (1989) Vaccination against ovine cysticercosis using a defined recombinant antigen. *Nature*, **338**, 585–7.

Keeling, J. E. (1968) The chemotherapy of cestode infections, in *Advances in Chemotherapy*, Vol 3 (eds A. Goldin, F. Hawking and R. Schnitler), Academic Press, New York, pp. 109–52.

Keilbach, N. M., de Aluja, A. S. and Sarti, E. (1989) A program to control taeniasis-cysticercosis (*T. solium*): experiences in a Mexican village. *Acta Leidensia*, **57**, 181–9.

Kinder, A., Carter, S. D., Allan, J. *et al.* (1992) Salivary and serum antibodies in experimental canine taeniasis. *Vet. Parasit.*, **41**, 321–7.

Kociecka, W. (1987) Intestinal cestodiases in *Intestinal Helminthic Infections* (ed. Z. S. Pawlowski) Baillière Tindall, London, Vol. 2, No. 3, pp. 677–94.

Kuchenmeister, F. (1852) Uber eine neuve *Taenia* des Menschen, *Taenia mediocanellata* hominis seu Zittavensis (mihi). *Dt. Klin.*, **4**, 101–3.

Laclette, J. P., Ornelas, Y., Merchant, M. T. *et al.* (1982) Ultrastructure of the surrounding envelopes of *Taenia solium* eggs, in *Cysticercosis: Present State of Knowledge and Perspectives* (eds A. Flisser, K. Willms, J. P. Laclette *et al.*), Academic Press, New York, pp. 375–87.

Lara-Aguilera, R., Mendoza, J. F., Martinez, J. L. *et al.* (1992) *Taenia solium* taeniasis and neurocysticercosis in a Mexican rural family. *Am. J. Trop. Med. Hyg.*, **46**, 85–9.

Le Riche, P. D. and Sewell, M. M. H. (1977) Differentiation of *Taenia saginata* and *Taenia solium* by enzyme electrophoresis. *Trans. Roy. Soc. Trop. Med. Hyg.*, **71**, 327–8.

Leblanc, R., Knowles, K. F., Melanson, D. *et al.* (1986) Neurocysticercosis: surgical and medical management with praziquantel. *Neurosurgery*, **18**, 419–27.

Lenoble, E. and Dumontier, C. (1988) [Perforations of the small intestine and intestinal parasitic diseases. Apropos of a case of peritonitis caused by the perforation of the small intestine combined with *Taenia saginata* infection]. *J. Chir. Paris*, **125**, 350–2.

Leslie, J. and Jamison, D. T. (1990) Health and nutrition considerations in education planning. 1. Educational consequences of health problems among school-age children. *Food Nutr. Bull.*, **12**, 191–203.

Lightowlers, M. W., Mitchell, G. F. and Rickard, M. D. (1992) Cestodes, in *Immunology and Molecular Biology of Parasitic Infections*, 3 edn. (eds K. S. Warren and N. Agabian), Blackwell Scientific, Oxford, pp. 436–70.

Madrazo, I. and Flisser, A. (1992) Parasitic infestation of the cerebrum: cysticercosis, in *Brain Surgery, Complication Avoidance and Management* (ed. J. M. L. Appuzo), Churchill Livingstone, New York, pp. 1419–30.

Mahajan, R. C. (1982) Geographical distribution of human cysticercosis, in *Cysticercosis: Present State of Knowledge and Perspectives* (eds A. Flisser, K. Willms, J. P. Laclette *et al.*), Academic Press, New York, pp. 39–46.

Marriner, S. E., Morris, D. L., Dickson, B. and Bogan, J. A. (1986) Pharmacokinetics of albendazole in man. *Eur. J. Clin. Pharmacol.*, **30**, 705–8.

Martinez-Baez, M., Martinez-Marañon, R. and Molina-Pasquel, C. (1971) Estudio histologico de proglotides de *Taenia solium* expulsados despues de la administracion de Yomesan. *Rev. Invest. Salud Publ.*, **31**, 152–62.

Mazzotti, L. (1944a) Observaciones en 10 individuos parasitados con *Taenia saginata*: Presencia de huevecillos en la region perianal y en otras regiones cutaneas. *Rev. Inst. Salub. Enferm. Trop. Mexico*, **5**, 207–13.

Mazzotti, L. (1944b) Presencia de huevecillos de *Taenia* en la region perianal. *Rev. Inst. Salub. Enferm. Trop. Mexico*, **5**, 153–5.

McManus, D. P., Garcia-Zepeda, E., Reid, A. *et al.* (1989) Human cysticercosis and taeniasis: molecular approaches for specific diagnosis and parasite identification. *Acta Leidensia*, **57**, 81–91.

Medina, M. T., Rosas, E., Rubio-Donnadieu, F. *et al.* (1990) Neurocysticercosis as the main cause of late-onset epilepsy in Mexico. *Archs. Int. Med.*, **150**, 325–7.

Michault, A., Duval, G., Bertil, G. *et al.* (1990) Etude seroepidemiologique de la cysticercose a l'Ile de la Réunion. *Bull. Soc. Pathol. Exp.*, **83**, 82–92.

Miller, H. M. (1932) Superinfection of cats with *Taenia taeniaeformis*. *J. Prev. Med.*, **6**, 17–29.

Ohnishi, K. and Murata, M. (1990) Intraduodenal 'Gastrografin' injection against *Taenia saginata* infection. *Lancet*, **336**, 880.

Panzeri, A., Castoldi, F. and Undiano, C. (1965) [Acute appendicitis due to taeniasis (*Taenia solium*)]. *Medicina, Panama*, **23**, 112–13.

Pawlowski, Z. S. (1990) Cestodiases: taeniasis, cysticercosis, dyphyllobothriasis, hymenolepiasis and others, in *Tropical and Geographical Medicine* (eds K. S. Warren and A. F. Mahmoud), 2nd edn, McGraw-Hill, New York, pp. 490–504.

Pawlowski, Z. S. (1991) Efficacy of low doses of praziquantel in taeniasis. *Acta Trop.*, **48**, 83–8.

Pawlowski, Z. S. and Schultz, M. G. (1972) Taeniasis and cysticercosis. *Adv. Parasit.*, **10**, 269–343.

Pearse, V., Pearse, J., Buchbaum, M. *et al.* (1987) *Living Invertebrates*, Blackwell Scientific Publ. California, pp. 242–6.

Pearson, R. D. and Guerrant, R. L. (1983) Praziquantel: a major advance in anthelmintic therapy. *Ann. Int. Med.*, **99**, 195–8.

Pene, P., Mojon, M., Garin, J. P. *et al.* (1982) Albendazole: a new broad spectrum anthelmintic. Double-blind multicenter clinical trial. *Am. J. Trop. Med. Hyg.*, **31**, 263–6.

Penfold, H. B. (1936) The treatment of patients infested with *Taenia saginata* with special reference to certain unusual results. *Med. J. Aust.*, **23**, 385–98.

Penfold, W. J. and Penfold, H. B. (1936) The diagnosis of *Taenia saginata* infestation. *Med. J. Aust.*, **23**, 318–21.

Perera, D., Western, K. A. and Schultz, M. G. (1970) Niclosamide treatment of cestodiasis. *Am. J. Trop. Med. Hyg.*, **19**, 610–12.

Plane, P., Ronceray, J. and Dubin, P. (1980) [Acute pancreatitis from obstruction of Wirsung's canal by *Taenia saginata*]. *J. Chir. Paris*, **117**, 193–4.

Proctor, E. M. (1972) Identification of tapeworms. *S. Afr. Med. J.*, **46**, 234.

Prokopenko, L. I. (1966) [Taeniasis and its control in USSR]. *Medskaja Parazitar Bol.*, **35**, 652–61.

Ransom, B. H. (1914) The destruction of the vitality of cysticercus bovis by freezing. *J. Parasit.*, **1**, 5–9.

Ransom, W. H. (1856) On the diagnosis and treatment for roundworm and on the occurrence of a new species of *Taenia* in the human body. *Med. Times Gaz., New Series*, **12**, 598–601.

Redi F. (1684) *Osservazioni intorno agli animal viventi che si trouvano negli animali viventi*, Piero Matini, Firenze, p. 244.

Rhoads, M. L., Murrell, K. D., Cross, J. H. and Fan, P. C. (1989) The serological response of pigs experimentally infected with a species of *Taenia* from Taiwan. *Vet. Parasit.* **30**, 279–85.

Richards, F. and Schantz, P. M. (1985) Treatment of *Taenia solium* infections. *Lancet*, **(June 1)**, 1264–5.

Richards, F., Schantz, P.M., Ruiz-Tiben, E. *et al* (1985) Cysticercosis en Los Angeles County. *J. Am. Med. Ass.*, **254**, 3444–8.

Rickard, M. D., Coman, B. J. and Cannon, R. M. (1977) Age resistance and acquired immunity to *Taenia pisiformis* infection in dogs. *Vet. Parasit.*, **3**, 1–9.

Rijpstra, A. C., Smith, A. M. and Swellengrebel, N. H. (1981) How and where to search for the ova of *Taenia saginata*. *Trop. Geog. Med.*, **13**, 160–6.

Rim, H. J., Park, S. B., Lee, J. S. *et al.* (1979) Therapeutic effects of praziquantel (Embay 8440) against *Taenia solium* infection. *Kor. J. Parasit.*, **17**, 67–72.

Rishi, A. K. and McManus, D. P. (1987) DNA probes which unambiguously distinguish *Taenia solium* from *T. saginata*. *Lancet*, **28**, 1275–6.

Rishi, A. K. and McManus, D. P. (1988) Molecular cloning of *Taenia solium* genomic DNA and characterization of taeniid cestodes by DNA analysis. *Parasitology*, **97**, 161–76.

Ritchie L. S. (1948) An ether sedimentation technique for routine stool examinations. *Bull. U.S. Army Med. Dept.*, **8**, 326.

Rousseau, C., Kerneis, J. P., Baron, A. *et al.* (1969) [Uveitis of undetermined etiology and parasitic appendicitis caused by *Taenia saginata*.] *Annls. Ocul. Paris*, **2**, 741–9.

Salem, H. H. and Al-Allaf, G. (1967) Paromomycin and *Taenia saginata*. *Lancet*, **ii**, 1360.

Sarti, E. J., Schantz, P. M., Lara, R. *et al* (1988) *Taenia solium* taeniasis and cysticercosis in a Mexican village. *Trop. Med. Parasit.*, **39**, 194–8.

Sarti, E., Schantz, P. M., Plancarte, A. *et al* (1992) Prevalence and risk factors for *Taenia solium* taeniasis and cysticercosis in humans and pigs in a village in Morelos, Mexico. *Am. J. Trop. Med. Hyg.*, **46**, 677–85.

Sarti, E., Schantz, P., Plancarte, A. *et al.* (1994) Epidemiologic investigation of *Taenia solium* taeniasis and cysticercosis in a rural village of Michoacan state, Mexico. *Trans. Roy. Soc. Trop. Med. Hyg.*, **88**, 49–52.

Schantz, P. M. (1989) Cestode diseases, in *Tropical Medicine and Parasitology* (eds R. Goldsmith and D. Heyneman), Appleton & Lange, Norwalk, Connecticut, pp. 485–518.

Schantz, P. M. (1991) Parasitic zoonoses in perspective. *Int. J. Parasit.*, **21**, 161–70.

Schantz, P. M. and McAuley, J. (1991) Current status of food-borne parasitic zoonoses in the United States. *Southeast Asian J. Trop. Med. Publ. Hlth (suppl.)*, **22**, 65–71.

Schantz, P. M., Moore, A. C., Muñoz, J. *et al.* (1992) Neurocysticercosis in an orthodox Jewish community in New York city. *New Engl. J. Med.*, **327**, 692–5.

Schantz, P. M., Sarti, E., Plancarte, A. *et al.* (1994) Community-based epidemiological investigation of cysticercosis due to *Taenia solium*: comparison of serological screening tests and clinical findings in two populations in Mexico. *Clin. Infect. Dis.*, **18**, 879–85.

Schenone, H., Villarroel, F. and Rojas, A. (1982) Epidemiology of human cysticercosis in Latin America, in *Cysticercosis: Present State of Knowledge and Perspectives* (eds A. Flisser, K. Willms, J. P. Laclette *et al.*), Academic Press, New York, pp. 25–38.

Schmidt, G. D. and Roberts, L. S. (1977) *Foundation of Parasitology*, C. V. Mosby Co., St Louis, pp. 354–79.

Sharma, S., Dubery, S. K. and Iyer, R. N. (1980) Chemotherapy of cestode infections. *Prog. Drug Res.*, **24**, 219–66.

Sterba, J. and Dykova, I. (1979) Symptomatology of taeniasis caused by *Taenia saginata*. *Folia Parasit. (Praha)*, **26**, 281–4.

Stoll, N. S. (1947). This wormy world. *J. Parasit.*, **32**, 1.

Thomas, H. and Andrews, P. (1977) Praziquantel – a new cestocide. *Pesticide Sci.*, **8**, 556–60.

Thomas, H. and Gonnert, R. (1977) The efficacy of praziquantel against cestodes in animals. *Z. Parazitenk.*, **52**, 117–28.

Thomas, H., Andrews, P. and Melhorn, H. (1982) New results on the effect of praziquantel in experimental cysticercosis. *Am. J. Trop. Med. Hyg.*, **31**, 803–10.

Thornton, H. (1979) Give yourself a tapeworm. *Vet. Rec.*, **104**, 287.

Tsang, V. C. W., Brand, A. J. and Boyer, A. E. (1989) An enzyme-linked immunoelectrotransfer blot assay by glycoprotein antigens for diagnosing human cysticercosis (*Taenia solium*). *J. Infect. Dis.*, **159**, 50–9.

Tyson, E. (1683) Lumbricus latus, or a discourse read before the Royal Society, of the jointed worm, wherein a great many mistakes of former writers concerning it, are remarked; its natural history from more exact observations is attempted; and the whole urged, as a difficulty against the doctrine of univocal generation. *Phil. Trans. Roy. Soc.*, **13**, 113–44.

Upton, A. C. (1950) Taenia proglottides in the appendix. Possible association with appendicitis. Report of cases. *Am. J. Clin. Pathol.*, **20**, 1117–20.

Van As, A. D. and Joubert, J. (1991) Neurocysticercosis in 578 black epileptic patients. *S. Afr. Med. J.*, **80**, 327–8.

Vazquez–Tsuji, O., Villafuerte, J. J., Velasco, O. *et al.* (1987) Algoritmos para el diagnostico de las parasitosis intestinales. *Infectologia*, **7**, 609–27.

Verster, A. (1967) Redescription of *Taenia solium* Linnaeus, 1758 and *Taenia saginata* Goeze, 1782. *Z. Parasitenk.*, **29**, 313–28.

Verster, A. (1969) A taxonomic revision of the genus *Taenia* Linnaeus, 1758 S. Str. *Onderstepoort J. Vet. Res.*, **36**, 3–58.

Waki, K., Oi, H., Takakashi, S. *et al.* (1986) Successful treatment of *Diphyllobothrium latum* and *Taenia saginata* infection by intraduodenal 'Gastrografin' injection. *Lancet*, (November 15), 1124–6.

Wardle, R. A. and McLeod, J. A. (1968) *The Zoology of Tapeworms*, Hafner Publ. Co., New York pp. 155–72, 388–427, 449–74.

Warren, K. (1991) Helminths and health of school-age children. *Lancet*, **338**, 686–7.

Webbe, G. (1967) The hatching and activation of taeniid ova in relation to the development of cysticercosis. *Z. Trop. Parasit.*, **18**, 354–69.

Willms, K. (1992) Cestodes (tapeworms), in *Infectious Diseases* (eds S. Gorbach, J. G. Bartlett and N. R. Blacklow), W. B. Saunders, Philadelphia, pp. 2021–37.

Yoshino, K. (1934a) On the evacuation of eggs from detached gravid proglottides of *Taenia solium* and on the structure of its eggs. *Taiwan Igakkai Zasshi*, **33**, 47–58.

Yoshino, K. (1934b) On the subjective symptoms caused by the parasitism of *Taenia solium* and its development in man. *Taiwan Igakkai Zasshi*, **33**, 183–94.

Zarlenga, D. S., Rhoads, M. L. and Al-Yaman, F. M. (1994) A *Taenia crassiceps* cDNA sequence encoding a putative immunodiagnostic antigen for bovine cysticercosis. *Mol. Bioch. Parisitol.* In press.

FOURTEEN

Small intestinal trematodes

P. Katelaris
and
M. J. G. Farthing

Many species of intestinal flukes have been found to infect humans but the pathogenicity of most of these remains unknown. Information regarding the epidemiology and pathogenicity of intestinal trematode infections is scant and it is difficult to estimate the importance of these infections to human populations. The World Health Organization (1981) estimated that approximately 50 million people were infected with one or more species of intestinal fluke. Most intestinal trematode infections have been reported from Asia, parts of Africa and the Middle East while occasional reports have come from elsewhere. The most commonly identified flukes belong to the families Fasciolidae (*Fasciolopsis buski*) and Heterophyidae (*Heterophyes heterophyes, Metagonimus yokogawai*).

14.1 *FASCIOLOPSIS BUSKI*

14.1.1 HISTORICAL ASPECTS

Infection with *F. buski* results in fasciolopsiasis. This fluke was first described by Busk in 1843 in the duodenum of a lascar sailor who died in London. The life cycle of the parasite was described in a Taiwanese pig by Nakagawa in 1921 and in humans by Barlow in 1925. *F. buski* has been known by a variety of names including *Distomum crassum* (Busk, 1859), *D. rathouisi* (Poirier, 1887), *Fasciolopsis rathouisi* (Poirier, 1886; Ward, 1903), *F. fulleborni* (Rodenwaldt, 1909) and *F. goddardi* (Ward, 1910).

14.1.2 MORPHOLOGY

F. buski, also known as the giant intestinal fluke, is the largest of the intestinal flukes and varies in size between 20 and 75 mm in length, 8 and 20 mm in breadth and 0.5 and 3 mm in thickness. It is a fleshy worm, usually elongate to ovoid in shape and a beefy red colour. The integument is spinose and there is no cephalic cone. The oral sucker (os) is about 0.5 mm in diameter nearby to the ventral sucker which is four times as large. The intestine includes prepharynx, pharynx, oesophagus and unbranched caeca. The highly dendritic testes lie one behind the other in the posterior half of the worm. The branched ovary is situated in the middle of the body. Finely granular 'vitelline' follicles extend from the level of the ventral sucker along the lateral field to the posterior end of the body. The large ovoid egg is yellowish-brown and has a clear thin shell with a small operculum at one end. Eggs measure about 80 by 135 μm and are unembryonated when

Enteric Infection 2. Intestinal helminths. Edited by M.J.G. Farthing, G.T. Keusch and D. Wakelin. Published in 1995 by Chapman and Hall, London. ISBN 0 412 39140 6

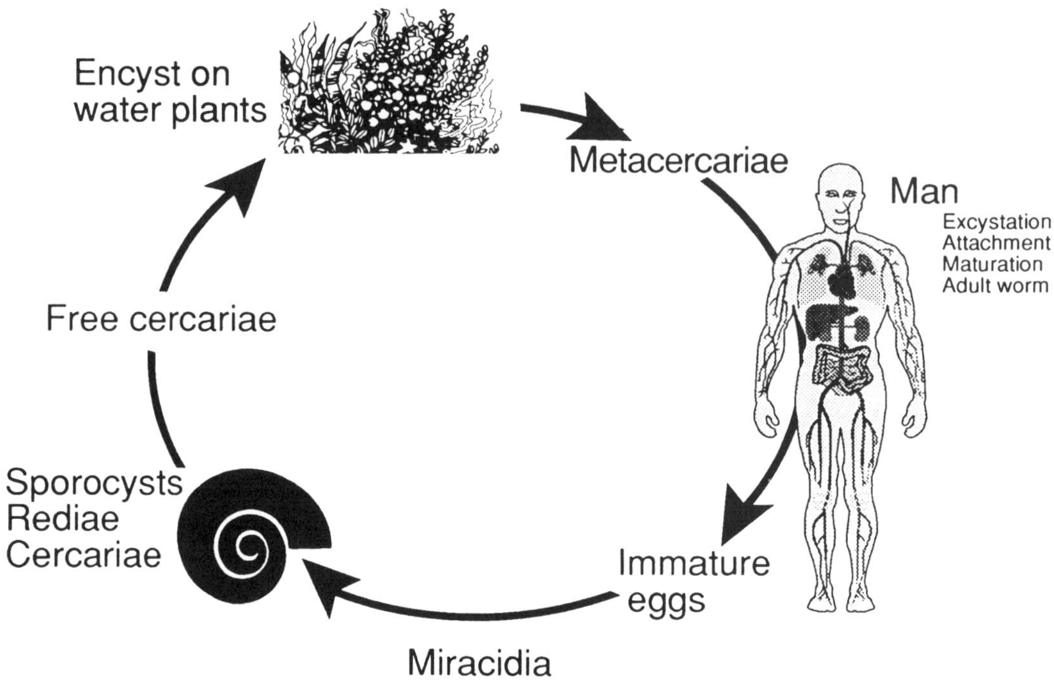

Figure 14.1 *Fasciolopsis buski* life cycle.

laid. These are very similar to eggs of *F. hepatica*.

14.1.3 LIFE CYCLE

The adult flukes are found in the small intestine of man, pigs and occasionally dogs (Strickland, 1984). Immature eggs are shed in faeces and on reaching fresh water, develop miracidia inside the shell within 3–8 weeks at a temperature of 25–30 °C. Upon hatching, the miracidia swim about in the water. On contact with the first intermediate host, an appropriate snail, miracidia penetrate soft tissues and within a period of a few weeks sporocysts, then first and second generation rediae and finally cercariae develop. The molluscan hosts in China, North Vietnam and Taiwan include *Segmentina hemisphaerula*, *Hippeutis cantori* and *Gyraulus* species. In India (Assam) and Thailand, *Segmentina trochoideus* is found as a host. The development time in the snail lasts approximately four weeks. The cercariae then swim out of the snail, encyst on water plants and develop into metacercariae. Edible water plants on which encystation occurs include water caltrop, water chestnut, water bamboo and watercress. Humans or pigs may become infected by eating raw stems, leaves or pods of these edible plants (Strickland, 1984). Humans may also become infected by biting off the hull or skin of these infected plants, where the metacercariae are encysted, before swallowing the raw plant. Excystation occurs in the duodenum and metacercariae attach to the intestinal wall and develop into adult worms in about three months. Each worm may discharge up to 25 000 eggs per day into the intestinal lumen. The life span of the fluke is about one year. The life cycle of *F. buski* is illustrated in Figure 14.1.

14.1.4 EPIDEMIOLOGY

F. buski is endemic in Taiwan, Thailand, Laos, Indonesia, Bangladesh, India (Assam and Bengal), parts of central and south China with reports of sporadic cases from other regions. Detailed epidemiological data of the distribution and prevalence of this parasite are lacking. Fasciolopsiasis is mostly confined to areas where people raise and eat edible freshwater plants and also farm pigs in regions where the molluscan intermediate hosts are plentiful. Raising swine near freshwater sources in which edible plants are grown facilitates the transferance of eggs in pig excreta to the water where the life cycle is continued (Cross, 1969). Use of human night soil for fertilizer also enhances transmission.

14.1.5 PATHOLOGY

The flukes attach to the duodenal and jejunal mucosa and may cause a mucus discharge. At the site of attachment the worms cause inflammation followed by local erosion. Haemorrhage may occur at the site of deep ulceration. Abscesses have also been observed in the bowel wall. A heavy worm load may induce an acute ileus or result in intestinal obstruction. In heavy infections attachment may not be confined to the duodenum and jejunum and worms may be found attached in the pyloric region of the stomach and also in the colon. Systemic features have been attributed to the absorption of toxic worm metabolites but are probably due to protein-losing enteropathy secondary to mucosal damage (Markell, Voge and John, 1986). This may result in oedema of the face and trunk.

14.1.6 CLINICAL FEATURES

Most infections are light and asymptomatic. Initial symptoms of infection may include diarrhoea and hunger pains. These symptoms occur towards the end of the incubation period and in light infections may be the only symptoms. In heavy infection the upper abdominal pain may mimic peptic ulcer and the patient may complain of weakness and lethargy. Diarrhoea may alternate with constipation initially but diarrhoea usually becomes persistent. The stools are typically a greenish-yellow colour, foul smelling and contain undigested food. In some patients, appetite is increased while in others there is anorexia, nausea and vomiting. Flukes are occasionally seen in the vomitus. Oedema of the face, abdominal wall and lower limbs is common and ascites often develops. The abdominal pain may become more generalized. In heavy infections the presentation may be with acute ileus or bowel obstruction. In severe cases extreme prostration may develop followed by death if the infection remains untreated (Rahman, Idris and Azad Khan, 1981).

14.1.7 DIAGNOSIS

The diagnosis is made by identifying the characteristic eggs in stool samples. The eggs must be differentiated from those of *Echinostoma* spp. and also *Fasciola* spp. Diagnosis may also occasionally be made by finding the adult flukes in faeces or vomitus. Nonspecific laboratory findings may include a leucocytosis with eosinophilia. Other laboratory abnormalities depend on the duration and severity of the diarrhoea.

14.1.8 TREATMENT

Praziquantel is the drug of choice for fasciolopsiasis. The drug causes contraction and vacuolization of the tegument of the fluke. A single dose of 15 mg/kg in the evening is usually sufficient but higher doses have been used (Harinasuta, Bunnag and Radomyos, 1984). The flukes are expelled the following day. This treatment is very effective with almost complete cure rates. Side-effects may include headaches, dizziness, drowsiness, nausea, abdominal pain, pruritus and myalgia but are usually short-lived (<48 h) and mild (Bunnag, Harinasuta and Radomyos, 1983). In untreated light infection there may be spontaneous resolution within one year if reinfection has not occurred. Untreated heavy infection may cause severe morbidity and result in death.

14.1.9 PREVENTION

Metacercariae are killed by immersion of the infected water plants in boiling water for a few seconds. In endemic areas where water plants are eaten raw, washing the whole plant in clean water followed by peeling of the outer layer and rewashing the plant in clean water provides some safeguard against individual infection. At the community level, health education combined with altered agricultural practices may result in a reduction of the prevalence of infection in endemic areas. Cessation of the use of human night soil as fertilizer combined with the introduction of modern methods of pig husbandry (which prevent pig excrement contaminating pond water and includes the use of commercial feed rather than the use of water plants) may result in a reduction in the prevalence of infection. These measures combined with mass treatment of infected populations and demographic changes due to urbanization appear to have eradicated the infection in some areas of Thailand and Taiwan. Eradication of water caltrop in an area of Thailand resulted in elimination of the infection (Ratnaubol and Hasbamrur, 1963).

14.2 *HETEROPHYES HETEROPHYES*

Several species of heterophyid flukes have been identified from humans. Of these, *H. heterophyes* and *Metagonimus yokogawai* are the most common.

14.2.1 HISTORICAL ASPECTS

H. heterophyes is a minute fluke first described by Bilharz at an autopsy in Cairo in 1851. Onji and Nishio reported the infection in Japanese in 1915 and named the fluke *Heterophyes nocens*. *H. heterophyes* has also been known as *Distoma heterophyes* (Siebold, 1852) and *Heterophyes aegyptiaca* (Cobbold, 1866).

14.2.2 MORPHOLOGY

This tiny fluke measures 1–1.7 mm in length and 0.3–0.7 mm in breadth. It is pyriform with a broadly rounded posterior end. The integumentary scales are narrow and close to one another and more numerous anteriorly. The oral sucker is minute (90 μm diameter). The larger ventral sucker (230 μm) is thick walled and muscular and lies in the anterior part of the middle third of the body. The two oval testes lie at the posterior end in a slightly oblique plane. The small ovary is globose and lies in the anterior portion of the posterior third of the body. The eggs are light brown in colour, operculate and ovoidal measuring 28–30 by 15–17 μm. These eggs resemble those of *M. yokogawai* but have a thicker shell.

14.2.3 LIFE CYCLE

The adult flukes attach to the small intestinal mucosa in the jejunum and upper ileum. Fully mature eggs containing ciliated miracidia are excreted in the faeces. These hatch only after ingestion by the appropriate brackish water or freshwater snail (*Pironella conica* in Egypt, *Cerithidia cingulata* in Japan). In this first intermediate host one or two generations of sporocysts develop and cercariae eventually emerge. These then encyst in the second intermediate host, brackish or freshwater fish, to become infective metacercariae. These second intermediate hosts are mullet (*Mugil cephalus, M. capito*), *Tilapia nilotica* and *Aphanius fasciatus* in Egypt and mullet, minnow (*Gambusia affinis*) and *Asanthogobius* spp. in

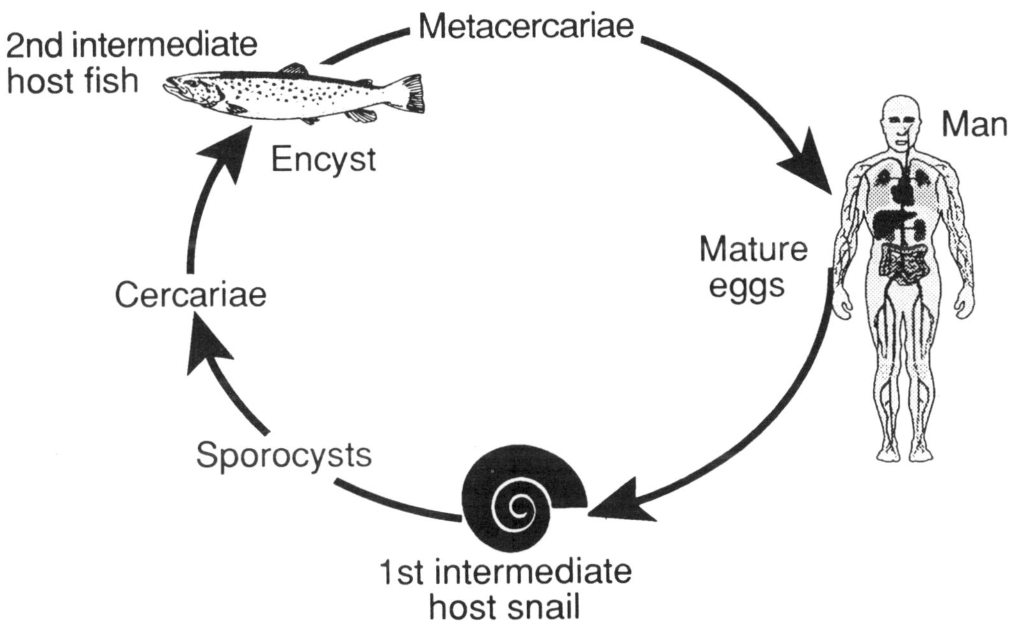

Figure 14.2 *Heterophyes heterophyes* life cycle.

Japan. Man, the definitive host, becomes infected by eating these parasitized fish raw, inadequately cooked or inadequately preserved. Metacerceriae are able to live up to 7 days in salted fish. *H. heterophyes* has also been found to infect cats, dogs, foxes and other fish-eating mammals from endemic areas. In some areas, human faecal contamination of water, in particular by fishermen, is a human source for the continuation of the life cycle. The life cycle of *H. heterophyes* is illustrated in Figure 14.2.

14.2.4 EPIDEMIOLOGY

The fluke is probably most common along the Nile Delta of Egypt. There is some evidence suggesting that the prevalence of *H. heterophyes* may be declining in this region (Taraschewski, 1985). It is also found in Turkey, Tunisia and Iran (Massoud, Jalali and Reza, 1981) and has been described in Europe, (Taraschewski and Nicolaidou, 1987). In Asia, foci of infection have been identified in south and central China, Indonesia, the Philippines, Japan and Korea (Chyu, 1969). Infection had been found in dogs in India. The distribution of infection may be more extensive than is recognized. Prevalence data is sparse and confused by the difficulty in differentiating this species in the egg stage from many other heterophyid flukes also acquired from the ingestion of raw fish.

14.2.5 PATHOLOGY

Attachment of flukes to the small intestinal mucosa results in inflammation and superficial necrosis at the sites of attachment. Eggs and occasionally mature flukes may enter the systemic circulation via the mesenteric lymphatics and blood vessels to cause serious systemic sequelae, particularly in the heart and central nervous system. This is thought to be due to embolic occlusion of blood vessels by the eggs and an associated inflammatory tissue response. High IgE in serum but not intestinal fluid has been reported in subjects with heterophyiasis (el-Ganayni *et al.*, 1989).

14.2.6 CLINICAL FEATURES

Light infection may be asymptomatic. In symptomatic cases symptoms begin after ingestion and a pre-patent period which averages nine days. Mild intermittent diarrhoea with mucus, sometimes associated with colicky abdominal pain, and dyspepsia are often present. Systemic spread of the parasite may cause myocarditis which may result in cardiac failure. In the Philippines in particular, deaths due to heterophyid myocarditis have been reported not infrequently (Kean and Breslau, 1964). Localization to the cerebral vasculature may cause a syndrome resembling cerebral haemorrhage (Sheir El-Shabrawy and Aboul-Enein, 1970; Tantachumrun and Kliks, 1978).

14.2.7 DIAGNOSIS

Diagnosis is based on the identification of the characteristic eggs in stools. However, as these may be difficult to distinguish from other heterophyid eggs and also resemble somewhat the eggs of *Clonorchis* and *Opisthorchis* eggs, the definitive diagnosis may only be made by identification of adult flukes recovered after antihelminthic therapy (Radomyos, Bunnag and Harinasuta, 1984). As *H. heterophyes* and *M. yokagawai* have relatively short lives, the diagnosis can be excluded in a subject who has not eaten potentially infectious fish within the last year.

14.2.8 TREATMENT

Praziquantel is the drug of choice. A single dose of 15–25 mg/kg is usually adequate. Contraction, vacuolization and bleb formation has been observed in the tegument of worms incubated with praziquantel (Taraschewski *et al.*, 1986).

14.2.9 PREVENTION

Avoidance of the consumption of raw fish or of inadequately cooked, salted or pickled fish is adequate to prevent infection in individuals. Health education is required to help alter existing practices. Efforts to reduce infection in mammalian reservoir hosts, such as dogs and cats, would also be beneficial.

14.3 *METAGONIMUS YOKOGAWAI*

M. yokogawai is another of the species of heterophyids and is closely related to *H. heterophyes*.

14.3.1 HISTORICAL ASPECTS

In 1911 Yokogawa obtained larvae from experimentally infected dogs and adult worms from a case of human infection in Taiwan. These specimens he sent to Katsurada who named the fluke *Heterophyes yokogawai* but later changed it to *Metagonimus yokogawai*.

14.3.2 MORPHOLOGY

The fluke measures 1–2.5 mm in length by 0.4–0.7 mm in breadth. It closely resembles *H. heterophyes* in size, shape and habitat. The ventral sucker is situated to the right of the mid-line with its long axis in a diagonal plane and this is a distinctive feature. The eggs measure 26–28 μm by 15–17 μm and are extremely difficult to differentiate from those of *H. heterophyes*. These eggs are fully mature when laid.

14.3.3 LIFE CYCLE

The life cycle of *M. yokogawai* resembles that of *H. heterophyes*. The first intermediate host is the snail (*Semisulcospira libertina* and related molluscan species) which ingest the fully mature eggs. In this host they undergo development with one or two generations of sporocysts before the emergence from the snail of characteristic cercariae. After swimming freely the cercariae become encysted under the scales, in the skin or in the flesh of freshwater fish. These second intermediate hosts include several species of freshwater fish particularly trout, known as sweetfish (*Plectoglossus altivelis* and *Odontobutis obscurus*), salmon (*Salmo perryi* and *Tribolodon hakonensis*), carp and loach (Chai and Lee, 1990). Encysted cercariae develop into metacercariae in these fish. Ingestion of these fish raw or undercooked is the mode of transmission of human infection. Faecal contamination of water in which these fish live maintains the life cycle of this parasite. Other fish-eating mammals such as dogs and cats act as reservoirs. Pelicans may also be an important reservoir host.

14.3.4 EPIDEMIOLOGY

The similarity of the eggs of *M. yokogawai* to other heterophyids and to *Clonorchis* make accurate assessment of the distribution of this fluke difficult, but it is probably the most common intestinal fluke in Asia (Chai and Lee, 1990). In Japan, Taiwan and Korea infection has been ascribed to the ingestion of raw or undercooked sweet oriental trout and other freshwater fish. In areas of endemic foci of infection a considerable proportion of the population may be infected: up to 50% in some areas in Japan and 20% in Korea (Cho, Kang and Lee 1984). Infection has also been described in China, some areas of Russia, including Siberia, as well in the Balkan states, Israel and Spain. Infection causing chronic, intermittent diarrhoea has been reported in travellers to endemic areas (Goldsmith, 1978).

14.3.5 PATHOLOGY

Attachment of the larval flukes to the small intestinal epithelium results in local inflammation and a granulomatous reaction which may become encapsulated. There may be an eosinophilic and neutrophilic infiltrate around eggs deposited in the gut mucosa. As in heterophyiasis, eggs may permeate the mesenteric lymphatics and be carried via the blood stream to the myocardium or brain where granulomatous changes may cause local effects.

A mouse model of infection has been used to study structural and functional intestinal mucosal abnormalities induced by *M. yokogawai*. Inflammation and villous atrophy were seen in the proximal jejunum 2–4 weeks after infection. This was associated with decreased activity of brush border disaccharidases (sucrase, lactase, maltase and trehalase) and aminopeptidase at this site. Enzyme activities recovered three weeks after infection. Mice treated after one week had earlier recovery of enzyme activities (Hong *et al.*, 1991). In experimental infection of cats and dogs, juvenile worms were found initially in the intestinal crypts. Adult flukes were found in the intervillous spaces. Mucosal damage, including villus shortening, goblet cell depletion, inflammation and brush border shortening was noted. These pathological findings regressed after four weeks despite persistance of adult flukes (Cho, Kang and Lee, 1984).

Immunogold labelling of adult worms, using IgG raised from experimentally infected cats, has shown concentration of gold labelling on the tegumental syncytium as well as the cytoplasm of tegumental cells and the epithelial lamella of the caecum (Ahn, Rim and Kim, 1991).

14.3.6 CLINICAL FEATURES

The clinical features of infection with *M. yokogawai* are similar to those of *H. heterophyes*.

phyes. The infection may be asymptomatic particularly in chronically infected subjects. Mild diarrhoea with the passage of excess mucus is common but severe abdominal pain, watery diarrhoea and prostration may follow ingestion of a single parasitized raw fish in a previously uninfected individual (Cho, Kang and Lee, 1984). Embolization of eggs to the heart or brain may cause serious sequelae in these organs.

14.3.7 DIAGNOSIS

The definitive diagnosis of *M. yokogawai* can only be made by identification of adult flukes expelled following antihelmintic therapy as the eggs are virtually indistinguishable from those of *H. heterophyes*. Scanning electron microscopy has been used to distinguish heterophyid eggs from those of opisthorchiid flukes in epidemiological research in order to determine species prevalence in particular regions (Ditrich, Giboda and Sterba, 1990).

14.3.8 TREATMENT

Praziquantel in a single dose of 15–25 mg/kg is effective treatment. Contraction and vacuolization of the tegument is observed in ultrastructural studies following incubation of the fluke in media containing praziquantel (Melhorn, Kajima and Rim, 1983).

14.3.9 PREVENTION

Avoidance of the consumption of raw or inadequately cooked freshwater fish will prevent infection. Prevention of faecal contamination of fresh water in which intermediate hosts live will interrupt the life cycle of this parasite.

14.4 OTHER HETEROPHYID INFECTIONS IN HUMANS

A variety of other heterophyid species, found almost exclusively in Asia and the Pacific region, have been shown to infect humans (Seo, Hong and Chai, 1981, Pearson and Ow-Yang, 1982; Radomyos, Bunnag and Harinasuta, 1983; Chai and Lee, 1990). There may be a high prevalence of intestinal fluke infection in regions of endemic foci; in Laos, 44% of villagers from one area had eggs of small flukes in stool specimens (Ditrich, Scholz and Giboda, 1990). Infection is associated with the ingestion of raw or partially cooked freshwater fish. Other mammals and fish-eating birds are reservoirs of infection. The best predictor of the existence of foci of intestinal fluke infection and their species composition appears to be the presence of the second intermediate host fish (Ditrich, Scholz and Giboda, 1990). Most of these flukes appear to produce similar intestinal lesions to those caused by *H. heterophyes* and *M. yokogawai*. Treatment with praziquantel appears similarly effective.

ACKNOWLEDGEMENTS

The authors gratefully acknowledge the support of the Wellcome Trust.

REFERENCES

Ahn, H., Rim, H. J. and Kim, S. J. (1991) Antigenic localities in the tissues of *Metagonimus yokogawai* observed by immunogoldlabelling method. *Kisaengchunghak-Chapchi*, **29**, 245–57.

Bunnag, D., Harinasuta, T. and Radomyos, P. (1983) Clinical trial of praziquantel on *Fasiolopsiasis buski*. *Southeast Asian J. Trop. Med. Public Hlth*, **14**, 216–19.

Chai, J. Y. and Lee, S. H. (1990) Intestinal trematodes of humans in Korea: Metagonimus, heterophyids and echinostomes. *Kisaengchunghak-Chapchi*, **28**, 103–22.

Cho, S. Y., Kang, S. Y. and Lee, J. B. (1984) Metagonimiasis in Korea. *Arzneimittel-Forsch.*, **34**, 1211–13.

Chyu, I. (1969) Heterophyidae infection in Korea, in *Proceedings of the 4th Southeast Asian Seminar on Parasitology and Tropical Medicine: Schistosomiasis and other Snail-transmitted Helminthiasis* (ed. C. Harinasuta), Manila, Philippines, pp. 201–8.

Cross, J. H. (1969) Fasiolopsiasis in southeast Asia and the Far East, in *Proceedings of the 4th Southeast Asian Seminar on Parasitology and Tropical Medicine: Schistosomiasis and other Snail-transmitted Helminthiasis* (ed. C. Harinasuta), Manila, Philippines, pp. 177–99.

Ditrich, O., Giboda, M. and Sterba, J. (1990) Species determination of eggs of opisthorchiid and heterophyid flukes using scanning electron microscopy. *Angew. Parasit.*, **31**, 3–9.

Ditrich, O., Scholz, T. and Giboda, M. (1990) Occurrence of some medically important flukes (Trematoda: Opisthorchiidae and Heterophyidae) in Nam Ngum water reservoir, Laos. *Southeast Asian J. Trop. Med. Public Hlth*, **21**, 482–8.

el-Ganayni, G. A., Youssef, M. F., Handousa, A. E. *et al.* (1989) Serum and intestinal immunoglobulins in heterophyiasis. *J. Egypt. Soc. Parasit.*, **19**, 219–23.

Goldsmith, R. S. (1978) Chronic diarrhoea in returning travelers: intestinal parasitic infection with the fluke *Metagonimus yokogawai*. *South. Med. J.*, **71**, 1513–15.

Harinasuta, T., Bunnag, D. and Radomyos, P. (1984) Efficacy of praziquantel on fasciolopsiasis. *Arzneimittel-Forsch.*, **34**, 1214–15.

Hong, S. T., Yu, J. R., Myong, N. H. *et al.* (1991) Activities of brush border membrane bound enzymes of the small intestine in *Megagonimus yokogawai* infection in mice. *Kisaengchunghak-Chapchi*, **29**, 9–20.

Kean, B. H. and Breslau, R. C. (1964) Parasites of the human heart, in *Cardiac Heterophyidiasis* (eds B. H. Kean and R. C. Breslau), Grune & Stratton, New York, pp. 95–103.

Markell, E. K., Voge, M. and John, D. T. (1986) *Medical Parasitology*. 6th edn, W. B. Saunders Co., Philadelphia.

Massoud, J., Jalali, H. and Reza, M. (1981) Studies on trematodes of the family Heterophyidae (Odhner 1914) in Iran. Preliminary epidemiological surveys in man and carnivores in Khuzestan. *J. Helminth.*, **55**, 255–60.

Mehlhorn, H., Kojima, S., Rim, H. J. *et al.* (1983) Ultrastructural investigations on the effects of praziquantel on human trematodes from Asia: *Clonorchis sinensis, Metagonimus yokogawai, Opisthorchis viverrini, Paragonimus westermani* and *Schistosoma japonicum*. *Arzneimittel-forsch.*, **33**, 91–8.

Pearson, J. C. and Ow-Yang, C. K. (1982) New species of *Haplorchis* from southeast Asia, together with keys to the Haplorchis-Group of heterophyid trematodes of the region. *Southeast Asian J. Trop. Med. Public Hlth*, **13**, 35–60.

Radomyos, P., Bunnag, D. and Harinasuta, T. (1983) *Haplorchis pumilio* (Looss) infection in man in northeastern Thailand. *Southeast Asian J. Trop. Med. Public Hlth*, **14**, 223–7.

Radomyos, P., Bunnag, D. and Harinasuta, T. (1984) Worms recovered in stools following praziquantel treatment. *Arzneimittel-forsch.*, **34**, 1186–8.

Rahman, K. M., Idris, M. D. and Azad Khan, A. K. (1981) A study of fasciolopsiasis in Bangladesh. *Am. J. Trop. Med. Hyg.*, **84**, 81.

Ratnaubol, K. and Hasbamrur, C. (1963) A survey for the presence of *Fasciolopsis buski* at Bang Kun Sri after eradication of the water-caltrop. *Med. J. Chulalongkorn Hosp. Med. Sch.*, **10**, 4–8.

Seo, B. S., Hong, S. Y. and Chai, J. Y. (1981) Studies on intestinal trematodes in Korea. III. Natural human infections of *Pygidiopsis summa* and *Heterophyes heterophyes nocens*. *Seoul J. Med.*, **22**, 228–35.

Sheir, Z. M. and El-Shabrawy Aboul-Enein, M. (1970) Demographic clinical and therapeutic appraisal of heterophyiasis. *J. Trop. Med. Hyg.*, **73**, 148.

Strickland, G. T. (1984) *Hunter's Tropical Medicine*, 6th edn, WB Saunders Co, Philadelphia.

Tantachumrun, T. and Kliks, M. (1978) Heterophyid infection in human ileum: report of three cases. *Southeast Asian J. Trop. Med. Public Hlth*, **9**, 228–31.

Taraschewski, H. (1985) Investigations on the prevalence of Heterophyes species in twelve populations of the first intermediate host in Egypt and Sudan. *J. Trop. Med. Hyg.*, **88**, 265–71.

Taraschewski, H., and Nicolaidou, A. (1987) Heterophyes species in Greece: record of *H. heterophyes, H. aequalis* and *H. dispar* from the first intermediate host, *Pironella conica*. *J. Helminth.*, **61**, 28–32.

Taraschewski, H., Mehlhorn, H., Bunnag, D. *et al.* (1986) Effects of praziquantel on human intestinal flukes (*Fasciolopsis buski* and *Heterophyes heterophyes*). *Zentbl. Bakt. Mikrob. Hyg.*, **262**, 542–50.

World Health Organization (1981) Intestinal protozoan and helminthic infections. *Technical Report Series*, WHO, Geneva, p. 666.

FIFTEEN

Trichuris trichiura

E. S. Cooper

The whipworm, *Trichuris trichiura*, is one of the most common human parasites. Because there is little doubt that it is practically harmless to the individual host when infection is light, there has been much reluctance to accept that heavy infections give rise to a specific disease, although this has now been well established for over forty years (Jung and Beaver, 1951). Because this nematode combines an extremely high prevalence rate in some communities (sometimes over 90%) with a highly aggregated frequency distribution within the same host population, it provides a good example of a most successful parasite life strategy. To physicians, trichuriasis exemplifies the difference between the ease of the temporary eradication of an individual infection and the difficulty of the control of transmission in a real, overcrowded human community.

15.1 HISTORICAL ASPECTS

Trichuris species occur as parasites of many mammalian hosts (Beer, 1971), including primates, rodents, domestic animals and camels, but excluding the equines. The eggs of a *Trichuris* parasite have recently been described in the 30 000-year-old coprolites (fossilized faeces) of a rodent in South America (Ferreira *et al.*, 1991). Also in that continent, *Trichuris trichiura* was found to be an inhabitant of the gut of an Inca boy, whose body was preserved through freezing on a mountain in Chile for 500 years (Pizzi and Schenone, 1954). Since the body was pre-Colombian, this is suggestive evidence that the human parasite may have accompanied the migration of man from Asia to the Americas some 15 000 years ago. *T. trichiura* has also been noted in the intestine of a preserved Han dynasty (260 BC – AD 220) cadaver in China. The parasitosis is known from specimens dating from around 500 BC to the present day to have been endemic throughout Europe (Bundy and Cooper, 1989).

Although a number of authors expressed the suspicion that the parasite might have more importance in human pathology than was generally assigned to it (Musgrave, Clegg and Polk, 1908), the first compelling and rigorous description of a specific disease was that of Jung and Beaver in 1951. These authors described 352 children in Louisiana with colonic inflammation and diarrhoea, and they proved that the dysentery was not due to amoebiasis but was related to the concentration of *Trichuris* eggs in the stool. The paper of Gilman *et al.* (1983) is a further landmark in clinical description, with its emphasis on the predictable nutritional cost of such intensity of infection as to show worms in the rectal mucosa. Studies by Bundy (Bundy, 1986) concentrated for the first time on the epidemiology and population biology of the parasitosis, with their

Enteric Infection 2. Intestinal helminths. Edited by M.J.G. Farthing, G.T. Keusch and D. Wakelin. Published in 1995 by Chapman and Hall, London. ISBN 0 412 39140 6

implications for control of transmission in whole communities.

15.2 BIOLOGY

Trichuris trichiura is a member of the nematode superfamily Trichuroidea, and is therefore quite closely related to the pathogen *Trichinella spiralis*. The genus is also often called *Trichocephalus*, especially in French and Spanish medical literature. The adult (Figure 15.1) is shaped like a whip, with the handle representing the wider posterior section containing the reproductive organs and the intestine, while the long, fine anterior part, called the stichosome, contains the long pharynx, lined with secretory cells called stichocytes. The whole worm is about 4 cm long. The male has a curled posterior end. The eggs are thick-walled and barrel-shaped, with a plug at each pole.

The eggs, passed in the faeces, contain a zygote and are not infectious until embryonation, which takes place in the soil over 2–4 weeks. The egg now contains the L1 larva. Following human ingestion, the larva is released from the egg in the small intestine, and passes into the large intestine. It penetrates the epithelium in the mucosal crypts, most probably of the caecum, although penetration in the small intestine is also a possibility (Miller, 1947). The caecum is the usual site of full development of the worm, and the terminal ileum, more distal colon and rectum are only involved in the most intense infections.

The larva develops by moulting, and the adult develops from the L4 stage, by now having migrated with the epithelial cells up the sides of the crypts. The anterior part of the adult lies in a tunnel within the epithelium between the mouths of the crypts, while the posterior part is free in the lumen. At the extreme anterior end is a stylet. The sex ratio of the adults is close to unity. Copulation occurs during momentary contact and each female produces up to 20 000 eggs per day. The life expectancy of an adult worm is

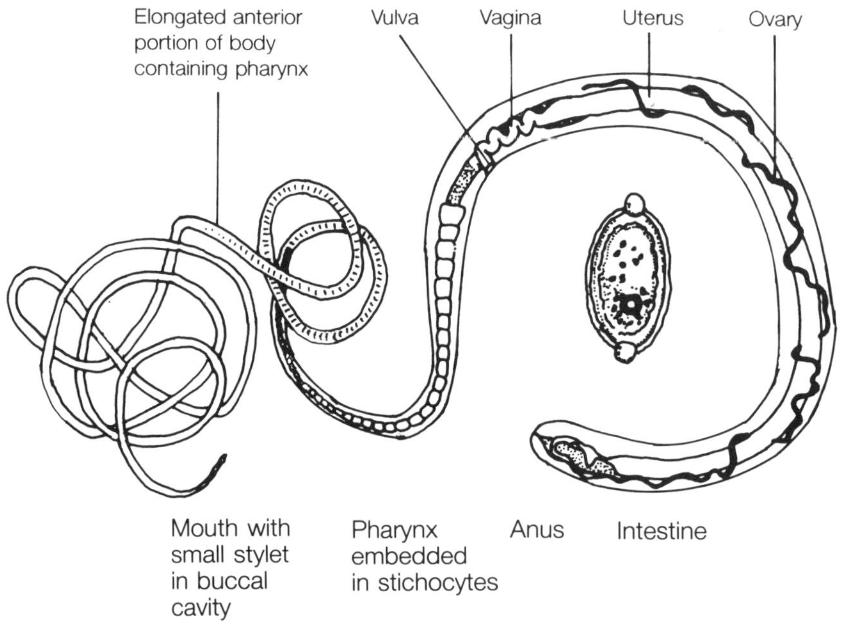

Figure 15.1 An adult female worm and egg of *Trichuris trichiura*. (Source: Whitfield, 1982.)

unknown but has been estimated at 1–3 years (Bundy and Cooper, 1989).

15.2.1 POPULATION BIOLOGY

As with the other geohelminthiases, the most heavily parasitized hosts contribute most to the contamination of the soil with eggs, and therefore to the onward transmission of the infection. Anderson and May (1982) described simple, deterministic mathematical models of the dynamics of transmission of geohelminths, which were applied by Bundy to *Trichuris trichiura* (Bundy *et al.*, 1985a). Because of the effectiveness and safety of the carbamated benzimidazole drugs, worm burdens (in expulsion stool collections) and reinfection could be studied in the field, allowing the estimation of the parameters for these models. The important characteristics of the population dynamics of trichuriasis have been reviewed by Bundy and Cooper (1989) but are briefly summarized here.

Where prevalence is high it remains so throughout life. Mean intensity, however, has a convex profile when plotted against host age, peaking between two and ten years. The relationship between the prevalence and the mean intensity of a geohelminth infection is non-linear, with the number of worms per person increasing steeply after an infection rate of about 80% of the population has been achieved. Since the mean worm burden is usually higher in trichuriasis than ascariasis, in a widely infected community reduction in mean intensity is associated with even less reduction in prevalence than in ascariasis. The practical consequence of this is relative difficulty in control by community chemotherapy. Furthermore, the overdispersion of the frequency distribution within any age-class is higher in trichuriasis than ascariasis (measured by the negative binomial distribution having a smaller exponent k) (see section 15.2.3). This again makes control more difficult. Finally, the predisposition of individuals in villages to re-acquire infection at a similar intensity to that which they had before, whether high or low, has been shown in longitudinal studies (Bundy and Cooper, 1988).

15.2.2 IMMUNOLOGY

Descriptive data on the immunological response of the host to the parasite have been published only within the last few years; moreover, functional explanations of the immune response are still awaited. Roach and her colleagues (1988) showed the recognition of mouse *Trichuris* (*T. muris*) excretory–secretory antigen by antibodies in the sera of humans infected by *T. trichiura*. The humoral immune profile of humans infected with *T. trichiura* has now been described by Lillywhite *et al.* (1991). Specific IgA, IgE, IgG_1, IgG_2 and IgG_4 antibodies were detected in sera. Blocking with *Ascaris* antigens was used to show the specificity of the responses. Despite this immunogenicity, the nematode conspicuously fails to produce a cell-mediated inflammatory response in the intestinal mucosa (MacDonald *et al.*, 1991), at least in intense, symptomatic infections. It is possible that it is the very absence of the mucosal cell-mediated response that predisposes to the intense infection; examination of the cellular response in lightly infected or apparently resistant subjects would be needed to resolve this. Cooper *et al.* (1991) showed a mucosal immune response in heavily infected children that may be pathogenic but is not protective: this is an IgE-mediated local anaphylaxis. In conclusion, there appears to be a relatively stable immunological equilibrium between parasite and host which needs, and is currently receiving, more investigation.

15.3 EPIDEMIOLOGY

Bundy and Cooper (1989) have estimated world prevalence of the nematode infection at 800 million by combining sample prevalences from published surveys with country and continental population data from the World Bank (1987). Without China, for which data were lacking, the estimate was 550 million. The crude estimate of 800 million was reached by assuming that China's prevalence was similar to that of the rest of Asia.

Neither infection itself, nor the clinical disease associated with intense infection, are exclusively tropical. Repeated clinical reports have come from Malaysia, South Africa and the Caribbean, but many physicians continue to believe that clinical trichuriasis is rare in tropical Africa, despite such reports as that of Jung and Jelliffe (1952) and Harland (1986). Ratard *et al.* (1991) reported on a national survey in Cameroon involving 49 distinct communities in ten provinces. In nine provinces the prevalence of *Trichuris* exceeded that of *Ascaris*. By province, the lowest prevalence for trichuriasis was 3.1% and the highest 97.3%. The difference was better explained by climate, favouring the extreme humidity of the equatorial zone, than by any other variable. However, such factors as overcrowding and poverty become important when the geographical scale is enlarged to distinguish microhabitats (Kan, 1985; Bundy and Cooper, 1988).

For an estimate of the epidemiology of morbidity, rather than simply of infection, a study of one village in the Caribbean suggested that the attributable risk of intense trichuriasis as a factor in chronic diarrhoea was of the order of 23% (Cooper and Bundy, 1986). Walsh and Warren (1979) had provided a world estimate for detectable morbidity ascribable to trichuriasis as 1 per 5000 total population. In this village, admittedly a single community with hyperendemic geohelminth transmission, this estimate of world population morbidity was exceeded 50-fold.

15.4 PATHOGENESIS

The whipworm is invasive, but only as far as the single layer of columnar epithelial cells lining the intestinal mucosa. There are, however, systemic effects of infection. The finger clubbing that is a feature of the most intense infections (see section 15.5.4) is the most unequivocal demonstration that a systemically mediated signal has passed from the infected bowel mucosa to a remote part of the host's body.

15.4.1 COLONIC MUCOSA

Flexible colonoscopy and ileoscopy, in which the tip of the colonoscope is passed through the ileocaecal valve, allow direct access to the area colonized by adult *T. trichiura*. The macroscopically visible colitis is not severe; there is oedema but little friability and no ulceration. Mucosal biopsies are easily obtained and the histology and immunohistochemistry of the colonic and rectal mucosa have now been described in some detail (MacDonald *et al.*, 1991). Routine histological sections are indistinguishable from those obtained from 'disease controls', i.e. worm-free children from the same community with mucoid diarrhoea or colonic or rectal polyps who also underwent colonoscopy and mucosal biopsy. From the mildness of the inflammatory change it can be inferred that T cells *in situ* are not activated to produce interleukin-2 (IL2) and interferon-gamma (IFNγ) in the presence of the worms, since none of the expected tissue responses to these lymphokines is in progress. There is, in fact, no increase in the number of intraepithelial lymphocytes although the proportion bearing gamma-delta receptors is reduced. The percentage of CD4+ lamina propria cells in *Trichuris* dysentery syndrome (TDS) is also reduced. Cells bearing the receptor for IL2, (CD25+ cells) are not increased. The epithelium also fails to show the consequences expected of a local T-cell activation.

Despite the apparent lack of T-cell activation, there are two indications of an inflammatory response to trichuriasis within the lamina propria: increased numbers of macrophages, with evidence of their production of cytokines, and an IgE-mediated mucosal mast cell response. Both of these have consequences which are costly to the host.

Two separate studies (Cooper *et al.*, 1990b, and unpublished data) of TDS colonic biopsies and biopsies from disease controls (necessarily more heterogeneous) have shown consistent results, with complete separation of the populations in proportion of calprotectin-staining lamina propria cells, detected using the monoclonal antibody MAC387. This is a marker for cells of the monocyte/macrophage series (Flavell, Jones and Wright, 1987), which are evidently twice as numerous in the lamina propria in TDS. Immunostaining using anti-tumour necrosis factor α (TNFα) has also shown a highly significant difference in positive cells. We may conclude at this point, therefore, that, despite the absence of T cell-mediated immunopathology, there is an inflammatory response in the mucosa, with an increase in TNF-producing cells and an increase in macrophages, which may or may not be the same cells.

Immunohistochemical examination of formalin-fixed caecal mucosal biopsies showed a 10-fold increase in the proportion of lamina propria cells with surface IgE in those children with intense trichuriasis, compared with uninfected children with non-specific mucoid diarrhoea (Cooper *et al.*, 1991). About 10% of the lamina propria cells were positive to the peroxidase-conjugated anti-human IgE monoclonal antibody; the expectation is that many of these cells will be mucosal mast cells. Direct staining for mast cells with Alcian blue on tissue fixed in Carnoy's medium has confirmed an increase in their numbers in trichuriasis. The cells in trichuriasis stained more lightly than in controls, however, and granules were also seen in the intercellular spaces. The implication is that these more abundant mast cells were also degranulating. The degranulation was corroborated by electron microscopy on rectal biopsies in trichuriasis.

15.4.2 INTESTINAL FUNCTION

Recently the leakage of protein across the mucosal surface of the gut in severe trichuriasis has been investigated. This was assessed as the clearance of plasma into stool of alpha$_1$-antitrypsin (Cooper *et al.*, 1992). In control children the mean clearance was 17 ml of plasma per day, but in 29 children with intense trichuriasis an average of 113 ml (SD 45) was cleared by the gut (Whyte, Cooper and Robinson, 1991). This represents about 7 g of protein. A typical daily dietary intake for a 10 kg, stunted Jamaican child from Kingston is 25–30 g protein (Walker, Powell and Grantham–McGregor, 1990), so the average enteric loss can be estimated at around one quarter of the intake.

The leakage of protein across the intestinal mucosa is not the only manifestation of the loss of mucosal integrity. There is also an abnormally high permeability to molecules of the size of a disaccharide, shown by the lactulose–rhamnose differential sugar absorption test (Sanderson *et al.*, 1987). The lactulose–rhamnose ratios of all of 20 children with *Trichuris* dysentery syndrome were found to be abnormally high (Finzi–Smith, Cooper and Bennett, 1991); 18 of these children were retested after treatment, when estimations of height velocity indicated that they were in a recovery growth-spurt. In children with trichuriasis, it appeared to be the increased lactulose absorption that diminished on treatment, rather than the monosaccharide absorption that increased. This result is consistent with the findings of protein leakage from plasma, and suggests that the tight junctions between enterocytes in the small intestine are involved. The protein-losing enteropathy described above could be of small or large bowel origin; but if the disaccharide permeability effect originates in the large intestine, then it is in contrast to other forms of intestinal inflammation, such as Crohn's disease (Lobley *et al.*, 1990). Both protein loss and intestinal permeability are significantly correlated with worm burden.

15.4.3 SYSTEMIC EFFECTS

Gilman *et al.* (1983) reported that children with severe trichuriasis had low serum albumin concentrations, which returned to normal, similar to local control children, after their recovery. Although protein-losing enteropathy may have made some contribution to this depression of circulating albumin, it is likely to represent an acute phase inflammatory response (Grimble, 1989). Cooper *et al.* (1990b) showed an elevation in plasma TNF in *Trichuris* dysentery syndrome (TDS), which would be consistent with such a response. Gilman and his colleagues also showed an increased urinary excretion of hydroxyproline accompanying recovery, which would suggest an increased synthesis of collagen, and which was accompanied by a catch-up phase in nutritional status.

15.5 CLINICAL FEATURES

The great majority of people, adults or children, who harbour a few adult whipworms in their caecum appear to be completely asymptomatic. It is difficult to believe that their health is in any way compromised. Furthermore, there is no threat of the few caecal parasites becoming more abundant and hence pathogenic in the future, as is the case with *Strongyloides stercoralis*, because *Trichuris* cannot reproduce itself in its host. Only continued exposure to infected soil produces further risk.

By contrast, when worm loads exceed about 50–150 worms, which usually implies that the infection is no longer confined to the proximal colon, there are associated gastrointestinal symptoms. With several hundred or thousand worms there is a clinical pancolitis and a clear chronic illness. This has been called 'massive infantile trichuriasis' (Kourí and Valdes Díaz, 1952), '*Trichuris* colitis' (Cooper and Bundy, 1989) or, perhaps best, '*Trichuris* dysentery syndrome' (TDS) (Ramsey, 1962).

The three principal features of TDS are chronic diarrhoea, anaemia and growth retardation.

Gastrointestinal symptoms include:

- Anorexia
- Pica
- Lower abdominal pain
- Mucoid diarrhoea
- Dysentery
- Rectal prolapse.

Systemic secondary effects include:

- Iron deficiency
- Anaemia
- Linear growth retardation
- Clubbing of fingers and toes
- Body wasting if dysentery is *severe*.

15.5.1 DIARRHOEA

The stool in TDS is invariably full of mucus. In most cases there is also obvious blood. Sometimes the stools, although very frequent (4–12 per day), are of small volume and may consist of nothing but mucus, blood and earth or small stones that a child may have ingested. However, the stools are often watery too, suggesting a secretory diarrhoea. It was this which led Mathan and Baker (1970) to perform jejunal biopsies in Indian children with this syndrome (with negative results). When the stools are copious and watery, they also tend to have a curious acrid smell which some say is virtually diagnostic of trichuriasis.

Rectal prolapse is a well-known symptom of intense trichuriasis. Its occurrence was reported in 11 of 13 studies of the clinical features of trichuriasis (reviewed in Bundy and Cooper, 1989), with an average case frequency of 34%.

15.5.2 ANAEMIA

Anaemia in the *Trichuris* dysentery syndrome can be very severe. However, anaemia is a clear example of the non-linearity of the relationship of morbidity to the prevalence of infection. Two community-wide studies (Otto, 1935; Greenberg and Cline, 1979) showed a complete lack of association between trichuriasis and anaemia, but then low-intensity infections greatly predominated in their surveys.

The mechanism of blood loss in severe trichuriasis is likely to be both by gross loss from the inflamed rectum and by passage of red cells across the entire lower intestinal epithelium, rendered permeable by the anaphylactic inflammation. Leakage of red cells across the colonic epithelium was likewise considered by Beer, Sansom and Taylor (1974) to be the probable mechanism of blood loss in trichuriasis in the pig.

15.5.3 GROWTH RETARDATION

Among the 13 studies of clinical trichuriasis reviewed by Bundy and Cooper (1989), only four recorded children's height-for-age. These four were from the Caribbean, South America, South Africa and Malaysia and recorded a mean of 71% as the incidence of height-for-age shorter than two standard deviation scores below the median. Cooper and Bundy (1986) have pointed out that growth retardation can occur when symptoms of colitis are mild, with an infection intensity of around 100 worms. (See Figure 15.2.)

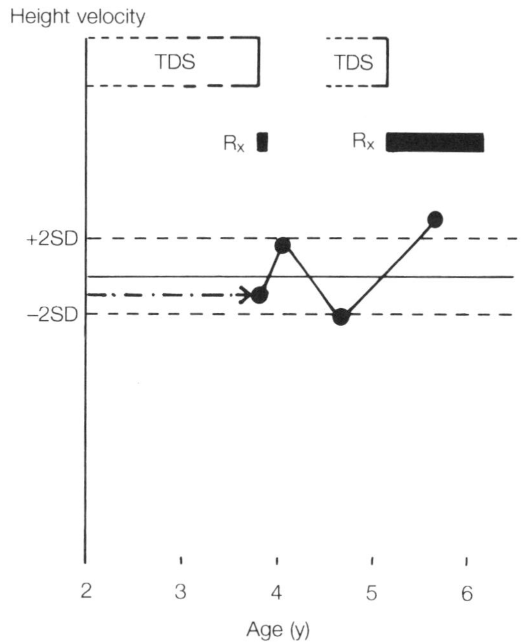

Figure 15.2 Height velocity in a child with *Trichuris* dysentery syndrome relapsing after initial therapy.

Figure 15.2 shows the height velocity in a child with TDS. This stunted child had a history of chronic dysentery for at least two years. On admission, his height was −3.2 SD by reference to a British standard (Tanner and Whitehouse, 1976). In the figure, however, height *velocity*, not attained height, is shown. The mean, +2 SD and −2 SD Tanner–Whitehouse height velocities for age provide the *y*-axis scale and are shown as horizontal lines. Initial treatment was with a 3-day course of mebendazole. Symptoms resolved and height velocity increased. However, after being lost to follow-up, the child presented again more than one year later with a history of recurrence of the syndrome. His height velocity had fallen, but returned to an above-normal value ('catch-up' growth) following retreatment, which was sustained

Table 15.1 Frequencies of finger clubbing and rectal prolapse at different cut-offs of infection intensity in a set of 45 cases of *Trichuris* dysentery syndrome

Intensity (Adult T. trichiura*)*	*Clubbing (%)*	*Prolapse (%)*
>1	15/45(33)	15/45(33)
>200	15/37(41)	14/37(38)
>400	14/32(44)	12/32(38)
>600	14/31(45)	12/31(39)
>800	14/27(52)	11/27(41)
>1000	11/19(58)	9/19(47)
>2000	4/6 (67)	2/6 (33)

by repetition of the anthelmintic course in 3-month cycles.

Most of our evidence for the specific retardation of growth in the TDS is indirect, and depends on the reversal of growth retardation upon treatment of the helminthiasis (Cooper *et al.*, 1990a). Exceptionally high growth velocities are achieved in a recovery or 'catch-up' phase, even though the child's environment and available diet remain unchanged.

15.5.4 FINGER CLUBBING

This is not a disability, but it is important because it is systemically mediated. Bowie, Morison and Ireland (1978) described clubbing as a specific manifestation of intense trichuriasis, and it was mentioned in four other of the 13 clinical studies reviewed by Bundy and Cooper (1989), having a mean incidence of 40%. The changes are reversible with treatment. As shown in Table 15.1, finger clubbing is strongly correlated with the intensity of infection. Even the occurrence of rectal prolapse is not so well predicted by infection intensity.

15.6 DIAGNOSIS

The clinical suspicion of trichuriasis rests on a history of mucoid diarrhoea for many months in a child who is living in, or who has come from, an endemic area. Clinical features which strongly suggest the diagnosis are growth retardation, finger clubbing, rectal prolapse, a history of awaking from sleep with the need to defaecate, a history of eating earth, or visible dirt in the stool. The specificity of frank dysentery will depend on the prevalence of amoebiasis in the region, since this may cause the passage of similar stools.

Confirmation of TDS may be obained by proctoscopy (Gilman *et al.*, 1983), inspecting for adult worms in the mucosa. They will not be present in the lower rectum in any but the most intense infections. This is a quicker, more direct and more specific way than microscopy of a stool sample for the clinician to decide whether TDS is the principal diagnosis. Stool microscopy should be quantitative (eggs per gram) or semiquantitative. The modified Kato thick smear method (Martin and Beaver, 1968) is recommended.

15.7 TREATMENT

Many anthelmintics (such as piperazine and levamisole), which are effective against ascariasis, fail in trichuriasis. In the past, hexylresorcinol by enema, dithiazinine and thiabendazole (a non-carbamate benzimidazole) were recommended as they are partially effective, but they may now be considered as quite obsolete. Chanco and Vidad (1978) have summarized the history of chemotherapy against *Trichuris* before the advent of the benzimidazole carbamates (albendazole, mebendazole, flubendazole, etc.). These drugs are highly effective and, at least with multiple dosage regimens, will virtually ensure complete expulsion of the worm from the host (Van den Bossche, Lette and Horig, 1982; Royal Society of Medicine, 1984; Rossignol and Maisonneuve, 1984). Bundy *et al.* (1985b) showed that the temporal pattern of the expulsion of *T. trichiura* was similar following either albendazole or mebendazole.

The benzimidazole carbamates are broad-spectrum anthelminics and effective against the other common geohelminth infections. Oxantel is another effective drug, specific for trichuriasis, with a quite different mode of action, paralysing the worms through nicotine-like membrane depolarization. During such expulsion the worms are not only paralysed but also metabolically inactivated, since they are unable to incorporate [^{35}S]-labelled methionine (unpublished observation). Oxantel is given in combination with pyrantel, a broad-spectrum anthelmintic. The disadvantage of this combination, especially in mass applications, is that the dose must be calculated against body weight, whereas with the benzimidazole carbamates a fixed dose is given. The only clear advantage is that in mixed infections treatment does not lead to the ectopic migration of *Ascaris*, which is one of the few undesirable effects of the benzimidazoles (Kan and Sinniah, 1983).

With the benzimidazole carbamates, single-dose therapy is convenient for control programmes and for treating asymptomatic infection; for symptomatic cases, however, three-day courses will increase the probability of complete expulsion from the colon and so are to be preferred. Benzimidazole drugs appear to be safe but their use in pregnancy is contraindicated because of uncertainty over possible teratogenicity. There is also caution over their use in the first year of life, although clinical judgement should be used in the relatively unlikely event of a symptomatic infection at this age.

15.7.1 DOSAGE

Albendazole is formulated as 200 mg tablets or 100 mg/5 ml suspension. It has most often been used as a single dose of 400 mg. The usual multiple dosage is 400 mg daily for three consecutive days. Mebendazole is formulated as a 500 mg tablet which may be given for single dose treatment, or as 100 mg tablets or 100 mg/5 ml suspension. The usual dose is 100 mg twice daily for three days. Oxantel–pyrantel is formulated as a suspension of 50 mg/ml of each ingredient, with a recommended single dose of each ingredient of 10 mg/kg body weight. The dose may need to be repeated several times for complete expulsion of worms in a heavy infection.

15.8 PREVENTION AND CONTROL

The principles of control in trichuriasis, ascariasis and hookworm infection are similar. Public health campaigns should take advantage of knowledge of local prevalences and estimated morbidity rates of each parasite in choosing the chemotherapeutic agent when mass chemotherapy is part of the chosen strategy. A broad-spectrum drug may be more expensive than some ascaricides, but will control three helminthiases simultaneously.

15.8.1 SANITATION

The separation of faeces from soil by disposal in pit latrines, septic tanks or sewers will interrupt the life cycles. In communities with high levels of such sanitation the parasitic geohelminths cease to be a problem. However, the size of the world's population living in slums and shanty towns is increasing, which implies that the appropriate habitat for intestinal parasites is also expanding. In urban slum areas there are problems of space, organization and land tenure. In low-lying land or on seashores, which naturally tend to attract aggregations of dwellings, the digging of conventional pit latrines may be impossible because of the water table. Sewerage is an expensive capital project requiring industrialization to support it. Even the low-cost alternatives may not be practical. These problems do not make a case for abandoning attempts at improving sanitation, but they suggest that progress will be difficult and slow.

15.8.2 VACCINATION

Naturally acquired immunity in trichuriasis is clearly incomplete (Cooper *et al.*, 1991). If stimulation of this immunity will involve increased mucosal T-cell activation (Shiddo *et al.*, 1990), there may be inflammatory consequences which may themselves cause undesirable side-effects (Cooper *et al.*, 1992). Clearly, the biological problem is itself a difficult one. Apart from this, it seems unlikely that the appropriate investment to solve it will be made in a disease which is not fatal or epidemic, and which involves members of the global population who have the least power, influence or franchise.

15.8.3 CHEMOTHERAPY AT THE COMMUNITY LEVEL

Appropriate anthelmintics are already available, immediately effective and apparently safe. However, random, mass chemotherapy may produce disappointing results if parasite population dynamics are not taken into account (Anderson and May, 1982). A rational and cost-effective strategy is the targeting of 2–10-year-old children, since this age class contains about 90% of all heavily infected individuals in a community (Bundy *et al.*, 1987). These, therefore, contribute the greatest number of infective stages to the soil for onward transmission. Fortunately, this is the segment of the population most heavily infected with *Ascaris* too. A cycle of retreatment needs to be established, since the models of Anderson and May predict a rapid rebound to the pretreatment equilibria of the system once chemotherapy stops. Control by targeted chemotherapy alone may well be cost-beneficial in terms of the improvement in community health, but it can only have a lasting effect if it is combined with improvements in sanitation.

ACKNOWLEDGEMENTS

I thank the Wellcome Trust both for personal support and for its sustained support of research into trichuriasis.

REFERENCES

Anderson, R. M. and May, R. M. (1982) Population dynamics of human helminth infections: control by chemotherapy. *Nature*, **297**, 557–63.

Beer, R. J. S. (1971) Whipworms of domestic animals. *Vet. Bull., London*, **41**, 343–9.

Beer, R. J. S., Sansom, S. F. and Taylor, P. J. (1974) Erythrocyte losses from pigs with experimental *Trichuris suis* infections measured with a whole body counter. *J. Comp. Pathol.*, **84**, 331–46.

Bowie, M. D., Morison, A. and Ireland, J. D. (1978) Clubbing and whipworm infestation. *Archs Dis. Child.*, **53**, 411–13.

Bundy, D. A. P. (1986) Epidemiological aspects of *Trichuris* and trichuriasis in Caribbean communities. *Trans. Roy. Soc. Trop. Med. Hyg.*, **80**, 702–18.

Bundy, D. A. P. and Cooper, E. S. (1988) The evidence for predisposition in trichuriasis in humans: comparison of institutional and community studies. *Ann. Trop. Med. Parasit.*, **82**, 251–6.

Bundy, D. A. P. and Cooper, E. S. (1989) *Trichuris* and trichuriasis in humans. *Adv. Parasit.*, **28**, 107–73.

Bundy, D. A. P., Thompson, D. E., Cooper, E. S. *et al.* (1985a) Population dynamics and chemotherapeutic control of *Trichuris trichiura* infection of children in Jamaica and St Lucia. *Trans. Roy. Soc. Trop. Med. Hyg.*, **79**, 759–64.

Bundy, D. A. P., Thompson, D. E., Cooper, E. S. and Blanchard, J. (1985b) Rate of expulsion of *Trichuris trichiura* with multiple and single dose regimens of albendazole. *Trans. Roy. Soc. Trop. Med. Hyg.* **79**, 641–4.

Bundy, D. A. P., Cooper, E. S., Thompson, D. E. *et al.* (1987) Age-related prevalence and intensity of *Trichuris trichiura* infection in a St Lucian community. *Trans. Roy. Soc. Trop. Med. Hyg.*, **81**, 85–94.

Chanco, P. P. and Vidad, J. Y. (1978) A review of trichuriasis, its incidence, pathogenicity and treatment. *Drugs*, **15** (Suppl.), 87–93.

Cooper, E. S. and Bundy, D. A. P. (1986) Trichuriasis in St Lucia, in *Diarrhoea and Malnutrition in Childhood* (eds J. A. Walker-Smith and A. S. McNeish), Butterworths, London, pp. 91–6.

Cooper, E. S. and Bundy, D. A. P. (1987) Trichuriasis. *Clin. Trop. Med. Comm. Dis.*, **2**, 629–43.

Cooper, E. S., Bundy, D. A. P., MacDonald, T. T. and Golden, M. H. N. (1990a) Growth suppression in the *Trichuris* dysentery syndrome. *Eur. J. Clin. Nutr.*, **44**, 138–47.

Cooper, E., Spencer, J., Murch, S. *et al.* (1990b) *Bull. Soc. Fr. Parasit.*, (*Suppl.*, 2), 347.

Cooper, E. S., Spencer, J. M., Whyte-Alleng, C. A. M. *et al.* (1991) Immediate hypersensitivity in the colon of children with *Trichuris* dysentery. *Lancet*, **338**, 1104–7.

Cooper, E. S., Whyte-Alleng, C. A. M., Finzi-Smith, J. S. and MacDonald, T. T. (1992) Intestinal nematode infections in children: the pathophysiological price paid. *Parasitology* (suppl.), **104**, S91–S103.

Ferreira, L. F., Aranjo, A., Confalonieri, U. *et al.* (1991) Trichuris eggs in animal coprolites dated from 30 000 years ago, *J. Parasit.*, **77**, 491–3.

Finzi-Smith, J., Cooper E. and Bennett, F. (1991) Intestinal permeability, diet and growth. *Lancet*, **338**, 1404.

Flavell, D. J., Jones, D. B. and Wright, D. H. (1987) Identification of tissue histiocytes on paraffin sections by a new monoclonal antibody. *J. Histochem. Cytochem.*, **35**, 1217–26.

Gilman, R. H., Chong, Y. H., Davis, C. *et al.* (1983) The adverse consequences of heavy *Trichuris* infection. *Trans. Roy. Soc. Trop. Med. Hyg.*, **77**, 432–8.

Greenberg, E. R. and Cline, B. L. (1979) Is trichuriasis associated with iron deficiency anaemia? *Am. J. Trop. Med. Hyg.*, **28**, 770–2.

Grimble, R. F. (1989), Cytokines: their relevance to nutrition. *Eur. J. Clin. Nutr.*, **43**, 217–30.

Harland, P. S. E. G. (1986) Trichuriasis in Africa and the Caribbean, in *Diarrhoea and Malnutrition in Childhood* (eds J. A. Walker-Smith and A. S. McNeish), Butterworths, London, pp. 85–90.

Jung, R. C. and Beaver, P. C. (1951) Clinical observations on *Trichocephalus trichiuris* (whipworm) infestation in children. *Pediatrics*, **8**, 548–57.

Jung, R. C. and Jelliffe, D. B. (1952) The clinical picture and treatment of whipworm infection. *W. Afr. Med. J.*, **1**, 11–15.

Kan, S. P. (1985) Soil-transmitted helminthiasis in Selangor, Malaysia. *Med. J. Malaysia*, **37**, 180–90.

Kan, S. P. and Sinniah, B. (1983) Comparison of the efficacy of single doses of oxantel pamoate alone and in combination with mebendazole in the treatment of mixed *Trichuris trichiura* infections, in *Collected Papers on the Control of Soil-transmitted Helminthiases*, Vol. II, The Asian Parasite Control Organisation, Tokyo, pp. 126–9.

Kourí, P. and Valdes Díaz, R. (1952) Concepto actual sobre el papel patógeno del *Tricocéfalo dispar (Trichuris trichiura)*. *Revta Kuba Med. Trop.*, **8**, 37–41.

Lillywhite, J. E., Bundy, D. A. P., Didier, J. M. *et al.* (1991) Humoral immune responses in human infection with the whipworm, *Trichuris trichiura*. *Parasite Immun.*, **13**, 491–6.

Lobley, R. W., Burrows, P. C., Warwick, R., Dawson, D. J. and Holmes, R. (1990) Simultaneous assessment of intestinal permeability and lactose tolerance with orally administered raffinose, lactose and 1-arabinose. *Clin. Sci.*, **79**, 173–83.

MacDonald, T. T., Choy, M. Y., Spencer, J. *et al.* (1991) The histopathology and immunohistochemistry of the caecum in children with the Trichuris dysentery syndrome. *J. Clin. Path.*, **44**, 194–9.

Martin, L. K. and Beaver, P. C. (1968) Evaluation of Kato thick smear technique for quantitative diagnosis of helminth infections. *Am. J. Trop. Med. Hyg.*, **17**, 381–91.

Mathan, V. I. and Baker, S. J. (1970) Whipworm disease: intestinal structure and function of patients with severe *Trichuris trichiura* infection. *Am. J. Dig. Dis.*, **15**, 913–18.

Miller, M. J. (1947) Studies on the life cycle of *Trichocephalus vulpis*, the whipworm of dogs. *Can. J. Res. D.*, **25**, 1–11.

Musgrave, W. E., Clegg, M. T. and Polk, M. (1908) Trichocephaliasis (with a report of four cases, including one fatal case). *Philip. J. Sci.*, **3**, 545–66.

Otto, G. F. (1935) Blood studies on *Trichuris*-infested and worm-free children in Louisiana. *Am. J. Trop. Med.*, **15**, 693–704.

Pizzi, T. and Shenone, H. (1954). Hallazo de huevos de *Trichuris trichiura* en contenido intestinal de un cuerpo arqueológico Incaiaco. *Boln Chil. Parasit.*, **9**, 73–5 [Abs in *Trop. Dis. Bull.*, (1961), **58**, 492–3].

Ramsey, F. C. (1962) Trichuris dysentery syndrome. *W. Ind. Med. J.*, **11**, 235–9.

Ratard, R. C., Kouemeni, L. E., Ekani Bessala, M. M. *et al.* (1991) Ascariasis and trichuriasis in Cameroon. *Trans. Roy. Soc. Trop. Med. Hyg.*, **85**, 84–8.

Roach, T. I. A., Wakelin, D., Else, K. J. and Bundy, D. A. P. (1988) Antigenic cross-reactivity between the human whipworm, *Trichuris trichiura*, and the mouse trichuroids *Trichuris muris* and *Trichinella spiralis*. *Parasite Immun.*, **10**, 279–91.

Rossignol, J. F. and Maisonneuve, H. (1984) Benzimidazoles in the treatment of trichuriasis: a review. *Ann. Trop. Med. Parasit.*, **78**, 135–44.

Royal Society of Medicine (1984) *Albendazole and Helminthiasis*, International Congress and Symposium Series No. 61. RSM, London.

Sanderson, I. R., Boulton, P., Menzies, I. S. and Walker-Smith, J. A. (1987) Improvement of abnormal lactulose/rhamnose permeability in active Crohn's disease of the small bowel by an elemental diet. *Gut*, **28**, 1073–6.

Shiddo, S., Ilardi, I., Mussa, C. *et al.* (1990) Reinfection of Somali children with *Trichuris trichiura* after chemotherapy: relevance of immunostimulation. *Trans. Roy. Soc. Trop. Med. Hyg.*, **84**, 832–9.

Tanner, J. M. and Whitehouse, R. H. (1976) Clinical longitudinal standards for height, weight, height velocity, weight velocity, and stages of puberty. *Archs Dis. Child.*, **51**, 170–9.

Van den Bossche, H. R., Lette, F. and Horig, C. (1982) Mebendazole and related anthelmintics. *Adv. Pharmac. Chemother.*, **19**, 67–128.

Walker, S. P., Powell, C. A. and Grantham-McGregor, S. M. (1990) Dietary intakes and activity levels in stunted and non-stunted children in Kingston, Jamaica. *Eur. J. Clin. Nutr.*, **44**, 527–34.

Walsh, J. A. and Warren, K. S. (1979) Selective primary health care. *N. Engl. J. Med.*, **301**, 967–74.

Whitfield, P. J. (1982) Parasitic helminths, in *Modern Parasitology* (ed. F. E. G. Cox), Basil Blackwell, Oxford, pp. 34–83.

Whyte, C. A. M., Cooper, E. S. and Robinson, R. D. (1991) Protein-losing enteropathy and trichuriasis. *W. Ind. Med. J.*, **40** (suppl. 1), 59–60.

World Bank (1987) *World Bank Atlas*, 1986. World Bank, Washington.

SIXTEEN

Enterobius vermicularis infection

G. C. Cook

Enterobiasis (threadworm, or pinworm disease) is caused by the small nematode *Enterobius vermicularis* (Cook, 1980, 1990a). It occurs world-wide and is certainly not limited to the tropics; children are more often affected than adults. It is arguably the most common helminthic infection of humans, this is certainly the case in north–west Europe and the USA, where prevalence rates of up to 100% have been recorded (Cook, 1980; 1990a). It is especially common in family groups, institutions, asylums, schools and army camps, particularly when there is overcrowding. *E. vermicularis* infection is an ancient human affliction: eggs have been visualized in a coprolite from western Utah, carbon-dated to 7837 BC.

E. vermicularis infection is usually considered to be a nuisance, rather than a serious disease; however, health disturbances (especially in children) are significant (section 16.3). In an uncomplicated case, management is usually simple though elimination of the parasite from a family group or institution often poses substantial problems.

Infection usually occurs by ingestion of eggs via contaminated hands, food and, less commonly, water. Local mechanical stimulation by migrating worms and local irritation caused by them (or their deposited eggs) produces the classical symptom pruritus ani. Local scratching results in finger contamination, autoinfection, and further spread to the environment.

16.1 EPIDEMIOLOGY

One estimate puts the total number of individuals infected at one billion (Nagar, 1987). It is the most common helminthic infection in north-west Europe and the USA. It is unusual in children <2 years of age. Prevalence is highest amongst young schoolchildren (5–10 years) living in overcrowded conditions where rates of infection as high as 80–90% have been documented at summer camps or crowded institutions. Sex incidence is similar and no social class is exempt, although personal hygiene and exposure to infected individuals is obviously important. Transmission is common in families of infected children. Handling of infected children's clothing or bedding can convey infection.

In England, a report from Liverpool has documented infection in 11 out of 20 children in an orthopaedic ward (Ashford, Hart and Williams, 1988), all of whom were asymptomatic. In south California prevalence rates of 11.6–43% have been recorded (Wagner and Eby, 1983). A large study carried out at nine kindergartens or pre-schools in the

Enteric Infection 2. Intestinal helminths. Edited by M.J.G. Farthing, G.T. Keusch and D. Wakelin. Published in 1995 by Chapman and Hall, London. ISBN 0 412 39140 6

western suburbs of Brisbane, Western Australia in 1986, showed an overall prevalence rate of 32% (Novak *et al.*, 1987). The maximum rate (43%) occurred in the 6–12-year-old group. Another estimate put the number of infected primary schoolchildren in the USA at 20–30%, but this percentage might be decreasing (Vermund and MacLeod, 1988); in this study which was carried out in New York City, data recorded between 1971 and 1986 showed a sharp decline in newly diagnosed cases from 248 to 38 – a rate of 8% per year.

Infection rates have been recorded in some developing countries. For example, 624 children were examined at Basrah, Iraq (Mahdi and Al-Khfaji, 1990); 56 infections were recorded (9%), and infection was most common in those <5 years old. In another study, 1167 faecal samples from 0.6–6-year-old children at a hospital at Riyadh, Saudi Arabia, yielded *E. vermicularis* in 85 (4.2%) (Bolbol *et al.*, 1989). However, examination of faecal samples always gives a low yield for this infection (section 16.4).

In south-west Puerto Rico, a prevalence survey of intestinal helminthic infections in 852 children produced only two positive results (Rivera-Marrero, 1986), although only faecal samples were examined and the true rate was therefore underestimated. In Macao City, Taiwan (again using faecal samples), only 39 (0.3%) out of 1309 children had a positive result (Chac-Tai, 1989).

A recent survey looked at infection in a southern Indian fishing community (Haswell-Elkins *et al.*, 1987), where the overall infection rate was 74.3%. Certain individuals tended to reacquire a significantly higher level of infection, relative to other members of the community, following mass anthelmintic chemotherapy (Haswell-Elkins, Elkins and Anderson, 1987).

Clearly, British and other travellers to unsophisticated environments in developing countries are often exposed to an unusually high prevalence rate of this helminthic infection.

A high prevalence has also been reported in homosexual men (Weller, 1985; Cook, 1990a). However, there are no data to suggest that this constitutes an 'opportunist' infection in the context of HIV infection.

16.2 PATHOGENESIS AND PATHOLOGY

E. vermicularis was probably first seen by Carl Linneaus in 1758, and originally named *Oxyuris vermicularis*; the disease was then termed oxyuriasis. Although related species can infect some animals, *E. vermicularis* is normally confined to humans, although infection has occasionally been reported in chimpanzees, gibbons and marmosets. Recent evidence suggests that *E. vermicularis* lives sympatrically with a newly identified species, *E. gregorii*, in the UK and France (Chittenden and Ashford, 1987). The fact that the latter organism could be readily detected in a group of Liverpool University students suggested to these authors that both species are probably widespread in the UK.

The adult female measures 9–12 × 0.5 mm (Figure 16.1). There are three labia, and a lateral pair of cephalic wing-like alae. The muscular oesophagus terminates in a bulb; the posterior tip is attenuated, and constitutes the posterior one-third of the organism. The reproductive system is T-shaped, the slit-like vulva opening at the base of the T, near the junction of the anterior and middle thirds of the body; in cross-section, characteristic eggs can be demonstrated within the uteri. The adult males are much smaller (length 2.5 mm) and possess a ventrally curved tail, with caudal alae, and a single large copulatory spicule.

The life cycle of *E. vermicularis* takes place entirely within the lumen of the gastrointestinal tract, there being no visceral component as occurs in hookworm and *Ascaris lumbricoides* infection. After ingestion, the eggs hatch in the upper small intestine with the liberation of larvae (140–150 μm in length).

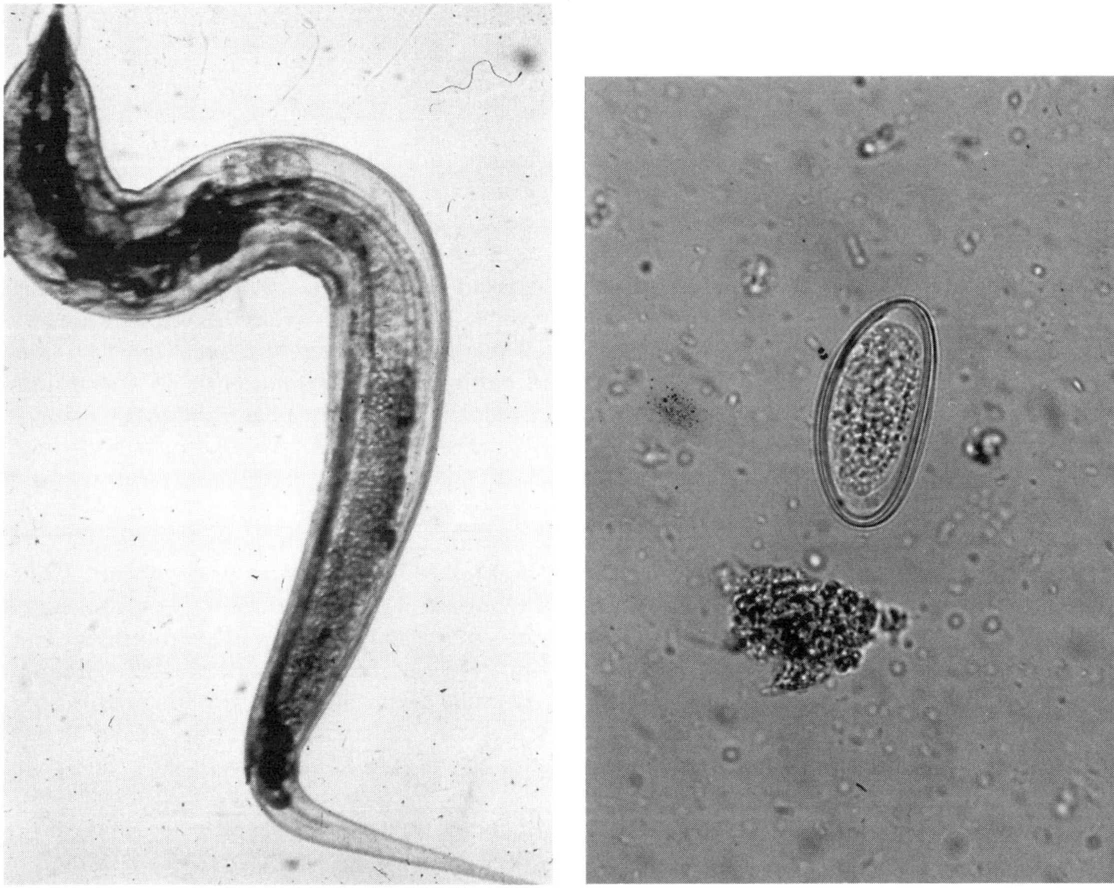

Figure 16.1 An adult female *E. vermicularis* (left) and a single egg in a faecal sample (right).

These migrate to the ileum, caecum and appendix, moult *en route* and develop into adults. Adult female worms settle in the lower ileum (where copulation occurs), caecum, appendix or ascending colon; minute ulcerations may develop at the site(s) of attachment. Haemorrhage and secondary infection can cause small ulcers and submucosal abscesses. Most infected patients harbour a few to several hundred adult worms. Female worms move at the rate of 6–7 cm in in 30 min. The adult females live for 37–93 days and the males for around 7 weeks; oviposition begins at 5 weeks. When the ovary is full of eggs, the gravid female worms migrate from the colon, and through the anus. Eggs are laid whilst they traverse the perianal or perineal skin. They are expelled by uterine contraction, death and disintegration of the worm, or disruption during scratching. About 11 000 eggs, which are ovoid (50–54 μm × 20–27 μm), asymmetrically flattened on one side, and almost colourless (Figure 16.1), are produced by a single gravid female worm. The shell contains a thick, outer, albuminous layer (this brings about adherence to environmental objects), a thin hyaline layer and an embryonic membrane. At the time of oviposition, the larvae are still immature and therefore not infective. Atmospheric oxygen hastens development, and they become infective at body temperature within 6 h. Egg survival is greatest at low temperature and high humidity. In warm, dry conditions, they begin to lose infectivity after 1–2 days. The whole cycle takes between two and four weeks.

There are four possible methods of transmission:

- direct infection from the anal and perianal regions by finger-nail contamination (autoinfection), and from soiled night clothes;
- exposure to viable eggs on soiled bed linen and other contaminated objects in the environment;
- via contaminated dust from bed clothes, pyjamas, toys, furniture, and cat and dog fur (there is no good evidence for a canine or feline reservoir (Cook, 1989)) containing embryonated eggs to the nose or mouth;
- retroinfection; after hatching on the anal mucosa, the larvae migrate into the sigmoid colon and from thence to the caecum.

In one study (Editorial, 1974), 119, 305, and 5000 eggs ft^2 were detected on the walls of a school hall, classroom and lavatory, respectively.

16.2.1 COMPLICATED INFECTIONS

Rarely, adult worms traverse the female genital tract and reach the peritoneum. Alternatively they may enter the peritoneal cavity via a perforation in the bowel wall, e.g. in appendicitis, diverticulitis or intestinal malignancy. The role of haematogenous spread is unclear. Dead worms and eggs (which remain identifiable long after death of the adults) surrounded by a granulomatous reaction (lymphocytes and a few eosinophils predominate) (Figure 16.2), have been demonstrated in the vaginal wall, cervix, endometrium, fallopian tubes (Saffos and Rhatigan, 1977; Nagar, 1987), ovary and peritoneum. Direct infection following abdominal operations has also been recorded. Migration to ectopic sites can give rise to diagnostic difficulty (Chandrasoma and Mendis, 1977). Eosinophilic granuloma of the colon (Bijlmer, 1946; Shiraki *et al.*, 1974) and omentum has been de-

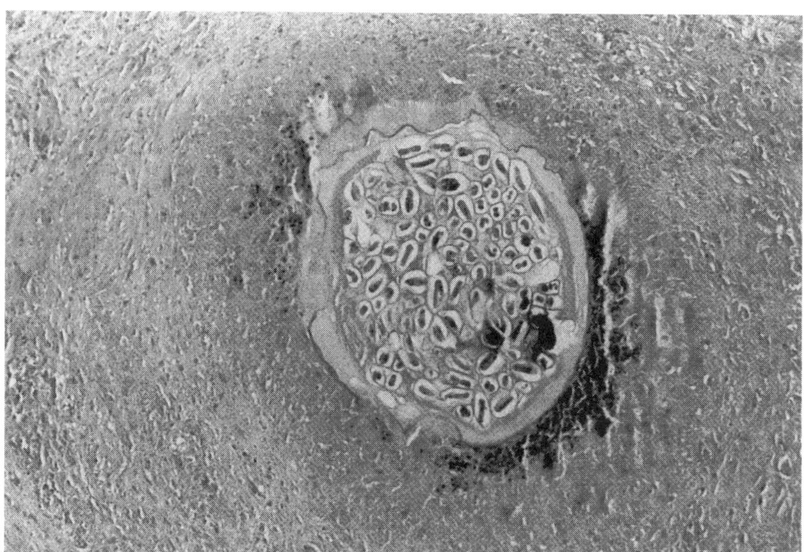

Figure 16.2 A necrotizing granuloma containing an adult *E. vermicularis* at the centre. (Source: Mondou and Gnepp, 1989.)

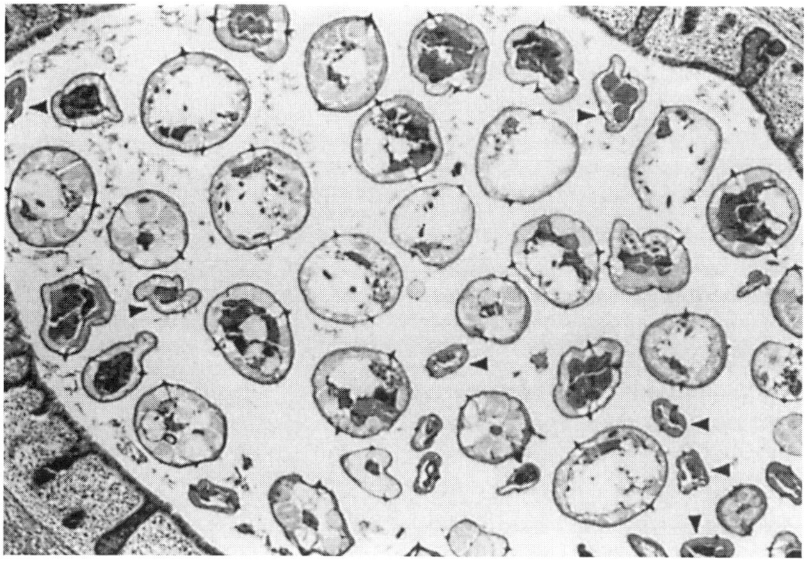

Figure 16.3 Male (arrowed) and female adults of *E. vermicularis* within the lumen of a resected appendix. (Source: Williams and Dixon, 1988.)

scribed. Other sites of ectopic infection include the liver (Mondou and Gnepp, 1989), spleen, kidney and lung (Mayers and Purvis, 1970; Beaver, Kriz and Lan, 1973). Chronic pelvic peritonitis has also been described. A report from Seville, Spain, has documented the presence of two *E. vermicularis* worms within a macerated embryo removed at endometrial curettage of a missed abortion (Mendoza *et al.*, 1987); eggs were recovered from the vagina and endometrium of the infected woman. The authors concluded that this 'provides further evidence for the invading capacity of *E. vermicularis*'. Other rare sites at which *E. vermicularis* has been documented include the external auditory meatus and conjunctival sac, the route of infection presumably being via contaminated fingers.

Granulomas have frequently been mistaken for those produced by *Schistosoma* spp. (the causative organisms in schistosomiasis or bilharzia). Peritoneal involvement may be confused both at laparotomy and macroscopically, with tuberculosis or metastatic neoplasia due to the presence of white or yellowish nodules.

Whether *E. vermicularis* is causatively related to *acute* appendicitis remains the subject of a great deal of controversy (Mayers and Purvis, 1970; Budd and Armstrong, 1987, 1988; Nagar, 1987; Williams and Dixon, 1988; Gupta *et al.*, 1989). The occasional presence of *E. vermicularis* in the appendix has been recognized since 1724 (Nagar, 1987) and it has been implicated in the pathogenesis of acute appendicitis since 1907. Figure 16.3 shows male and female *E. vermicularis* in the human appendix. At Bristol, England, during a five-year period, 1419 appendices were resected from individuals with clinical evidence of acute appendicitis, and a further 110 during the course of another surgical procedure (Budd and Armstrong, 1987). *E. vermicularis* was present in 38 (2.7%) of those with clinical appendicitis (but none of the other conditions); it was most common in appendices exhibiting chronic inflammation, and those which were histologically normal; only rarely was this nematode present when there was histological evidence of acute appendicitis. These authors concluded that 'although *E. vermicularis* may have a causal role in appendicular pain and chronic inflammation, it is rarely related to acute appendicitis'.

In a study from Leeds, England, examination of 199 appendices containing *E. vermicularis* revealed male worms in 116 and females in 20 (Williams and Dixon, 1988); the remainder contained mixed infections. Whilst there was no association between the sex of the worm and appendiceal inflammation, the latter was frequently seen in association with luminal ova which were present in 25. The conclusion from this survey was that eggs released from female *E. vermicularis* might give rise to luminal appendiceal obstruction.

At Allahabad, India, 2921 appendicectomies were carried out during a 25-year period and all specimens were subjected to histological examination (Gupta *et al.*, 1989). In 153 (5%) cases a significant pathological abnormality was documented, and in 75 (2.5%) this involved a parasite: *E. vermicularis* (41), *Entamoeba histolytica* (17), *Ascaris lumbricoides* (13), *A. lumbricoides* and *Trichuris trichiura* (2), and *Taenia* spp. (2). By use of a toluidine blue staining technique, mast cell numbers have been counted in 22 histologically normal appendices, and 22 containing *E. vermicularis* (Crow and Howe, 1988); the correlation between presence of mast cells and infection was not significant.

A report from China has described a fatal case of *E. vermicularis* infection in a chimpanzee (*Pan troglodytes*) (Zhang, Ji and McManus, 1990). The nematode was present in mesenteric lymph glands, mesenteric lymphatics, and hepatic and pulmonary vasculature. The authors concluded (from the histological appearances) that *E. vermicularis* probably gained access to these organs via the 'lymphatic or haematogenous pathway'.

16.3 CLINICAL ASPECTS

The majority of infections are asymptomatic. When symptoms result from an infection,

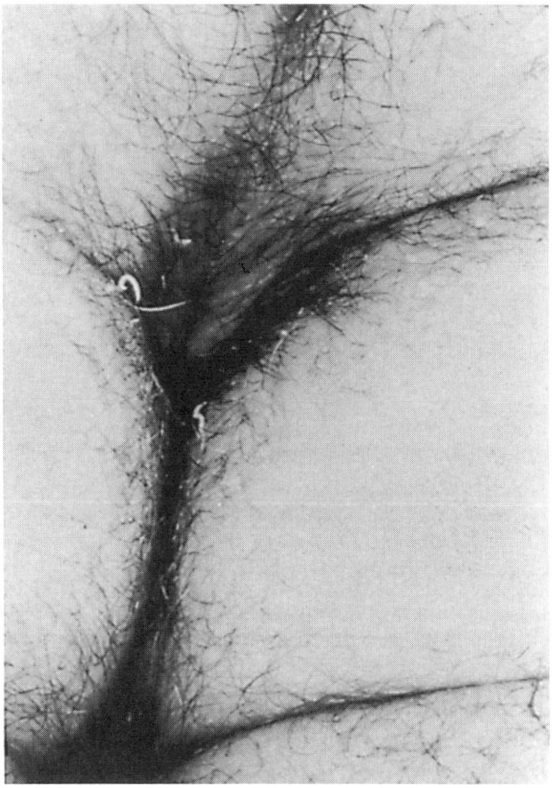

Figure 16.4 *E. vermicularis* on the perianal region of a homosexual man; folliculitis of the buttocks is also present. (Source: Fiumaru and Tang, 1986.)

pruritus ani and perineal pruritus are the most common. Other symptoms include a local tickling sensation and acute pain. These symptoms tend to be worse at night and may produce insomnia, restlessness and tiredness. Infected children may develop anorexia, weight loss, poor concentration, irritability, emotional instability and enuresis. Secondary (eczematous) bacterial dermatitis and folliculitis (Fiumara and Tang, 1986) may complicate these local lesions (Figure 16.4). There may be skin trauma, excoriation and secondary infection (Chaudhry and Longworth, 1989). Observers in Israel have concluded that *E. vermicularis*-induced pruritus is more common in patients with underlying dermatological disease (Ganor, 1987);

18 out of 25 children with either pruritus ani or pruritus vulvae had one of the following: psoriasis, atopic dermatitis, contact dermatitis, neurodermatitis or seborrhoeic dermatitis, and in most cases there was no evidence of local disease in the perianal or perivulval regions. Suggestions have been made that abdominal pain (including colic) can result from an *E. vermicularis* infection (Brewster, 1989). Nail biting and thumb sucking have also been associated.

In prepubertal girls, vulvovaginitis is a recognized sequel when adult worms have migrated to the vagina (Arsenault and Gerbie, 1986). Acute urinary infection, enuresis and incontinence have also been attributed to infection (Mayers and Purvis, 1970). Vaginal discharge (with or without endometritis) has also been recorded (McKay, 1989). Although some have postulated that *E. vermicularis* transports *Escherichia coli* and other coliform bacteria into the female bladder and urinary tract (perineal scratching might also induce introital colonization), the frequency and importance of this remains unclear (Simon, 1974). *Chronic* genitourinary infection with *E. vermicularis* has been recorded in India (Singh and Samantaray, 1989). A 20-year-old married Moslem woman experienced 'burning on micturition and crawling sensations in her vagina and urethra'. She was subsequently shown to have profuse pyuria, and eggs and larvae of *E. vermicularis* were repeatedly documented in her urine and vaginal discharge. Various systemic and oral regimens of antimicrobials and anthelmintics had failed to improve her symptoms, but local applications of a piperazine solution (section 16.5) for 8 days produced a cure. These authors concluded that the focus of infection was probably in the vagina and not the intestinal tract.

Acute appendicitis resulting from an *E. vermicularis* infection is probably rare (see section 16.2.1). Other symptoms which have been attributed to *E. vermicularis* infection include nymphomania, keratoconjunctivitis, abdominal pain, nose picking, tooth grinding and nightmares (Editorial, 1974). However, not all investigators have been able to document such exotic and/or bizarre symptoms (Mayers and Purvis, 1970).

Parents can become distraught at the thought that their child is suffering from 'worms'.

16.4 DIAGNOSIS

This depends on accurate identification of adult worms and/or eggs. They may be visualized in the perianal region or vagina, usually at night (Hood, 1989). Diagnosis can be made by application of a strip of Sellotape to the anus and then sticking this on to a microscope slide when visualization of worms and eggs is straightforward (debris can be cleared with a drop of toluene). This procedure is best applied before the individual under investigation either defaecates or bathes on waking in the morning. The buttocks are spread and the tape pressed several times against the anal or perianal skin. There is no doubt that repeat investigation on separate days gives a higher yield of positive results: 90% of infections can be detected with three swabs; six consecutive negative swabs on separate days virtually excludes the diagnosis.

Other diagnostic systems (using glass or wool applicators or Cellophane), some supplied in proprietary form (which may be sent to the laboratory by post), are available. One such technique ('Sterile pinworm collector', Starplex Scientific, Mississauga, Ontario) utilizes a transparent adhesive strip, which is placed across the anus and is then examined microscopically. Eggs may also be detected in perianal scrapings or swabs, or from beneath the fingernails. A group of workers at Cairo, Egypt, found that a 'modified perianal oil swab' technique was superior to other methods (Khalil *et al.*, 1987). After perianal swab-

Table 16.1 Some chemotherapeutic agents used against *E. vermicularis* infection

Drug	*Dose**	*Toxicity*
Mebendazole	100 mg	Rarely, abdominal pain/diarrhoea; contraindicated in pregnancy
Albendazole†	400 mg (or 10–14 mg/kg)	Rarely, abdominal pain/diarrhoea; contraindicated in pregnancy
Piperazine‡ [Expressed as hydrate]	Adults and children over 12 years 2 g; children under 2 years 50–75 mg/kg; 2–4 years 750 mg, 5–12 years 1.5 g Dose given once daily for 7 days. Piperazine preparations are available for 'over the counter' treatment	Neurotoxicity, cerebellar ataxia, vomiting, diarrhoea, urticaria, tremor, dizziness, visceral disturbances, weakness; contraindicated in renal and liver disease and epilepsy
Pyrantel embonate	10 mg/kg (maximum 1 g) Repeat 6-weekly	Nausea, vomiting, diarrhoea, cramps, headaches, dizziness, drowsiness, transient elevation of transaminase concentrations
Viprynium (pyvinium) embonate	5 mg base/kg (maximum 350 mg)	Nausea, vomiting, cramps; stains garments and skin

* A second dose after 1–2 weeks is often required. In recurrent or 'resistant' infections, repeat chemotherapy every 2 months might occasionally be needed, and in those subjected to constant exposure, e.g. school children and teachers, a repeat dose every 2–4 months has been advocated.
† This agent is only available on a named patient basis.
‡ Should not be used concurrently with a phenothiazine.

bing, adhesive Sellotape was applied and the latter was fixed on a clean glass slide, a drop of cedar oil added, and examination carried out under low-power magnification.

Faecal material obtained by digital rectal examination occasionally yields a positive result (section 16.1). Faeces should be mixed with normal saline and examined under a coverslip. In a heavy infection, female worms may be adherent to a faecal bolus. However, routine examination of a faecal sample gives a positive diagnosis in only 5–15% of infected individuals. Occasionally adult worms are visualized, usually accidentally, during colonoscopy (Goldenberg and Marignani, 1990). Rarely *E. vermicularis* eggs are incidentally found in a Papanicolaou-stained vaginal smear, and in urine (Adungo, Odingo and Pamba, 1986; Singh and Samantaray, 1989). In the former report from Kenya, *E. vermicularis* was demonstrated in urine specimens from three girls aged 5, 7 and 10 years (Adungo, Odingo and Pamba, 1986).

Infection is *not* accompanied by a peripheral blood eosinophilia or iron deficiency anaemia.

16.5 MANAGEMENT

Table 16.1 summarizes some of the chemotherapeutic agents which have been used to eradicate an *E. vermicularis* infection (Cook, 1990b). Chemotherapy for the entire family is often recommended, because asymptomatic infection in other members can act as a reservoir of infection; this is especially necessary when there are several small children in the family. In geographical areas with a high prevalence of *E. vermicularis*, chemotherapy should be given at frequent intervals to achieve a long-term reduction in overall infection within the community (Haswell-

Elkins, Elkins and Anderson, 1987). Antipruritic ointments can produce symptomatic relief.

The benzimidazole compounds are the most effective chemotherapeutic agents available. These inhibit microtubule function in the adult worms and cause glycogen depletion. Single-dose mebendazole is usually effective, although some physicians recommend repeating this one week later. This agent is poorly absorbed and therefore luminal concentration is high. It is free of serious side-effects, although abdominal pain and diarrhoea have occasionally been reported. Results suggest that albendazole is probably more effective (see below). The benzimidazole compounds are not recommended during pregnancy, because teratogenicity has been reported in experimental studies.

Alternative chemotherapeutic agents (Table 16.1) are piperazine, pyrantel embonate and viprynium (pyrvinium) embonate. In Peru, ivermectin has produced an 85% cure rate (Naquira *et al.*, 1989). A herbal remedy (*Artemisia herba-alba* extract) proved valuable in Iraq (Al-Waili, 1988).

Many comparative trials of chemotherapeutic agents have been carried out (Cook, 1980, 1990b). In Egypt, 13 (81.5%) out of 16 cases were cured with single-dose mebendazole, but only 10 (62.5%) out of 16 with piperazine (Khalil *et al.*, 1987). In India, however, 58 (60%) out of 97 patients responded to single-dose mebendazole whereas 95 (96%) out of 99 were cured with pyrantel (Sarmah, 1988). Albendazole produced a 100% cure rate in a trial concurrently carried out in several countries, and involving 141 patients (Coulaud and Rossignol, 1984); a similar result was documented in 29 children treated in Brazil (Neto *et al.*, 1985). Others have also reported a 100% cure rate using this agent (Goldsmith, 1988). Although albendazole is therefore probably the most effective chemotherapeutic agent, it is not readily available in several countries (UK included).

The correct choice of chemotherapeutic agent for use in an *E. vermicularis* infection in pregnancy has recently received attention (Leach, 1990). When immediate eradication is considered important and/or natural eradication (by scrupulous attention to personal hygiene, etc.) is in doubt, piperazine seems to be a reasonable choice. Whenever possible, however, this should be delayed until after the first trimester.

Parents should be reassured that *E. vermicularis* infection is not a serious disease.

16.6 PREVENTION AND CONTROL

Prophylaxis is largely dependent on personal hygiene and the cleanliness of living quarters. As with head lice, the stigma attached to an *E. vermicularis* infection is unjustified and unfair. Infection occurs in the highest strata of society, where standards of hygiene, nutritional status, etc. are excellent. An increase in public health education will eventually break down this barrier.

During treatment, reinfection must obviously be prevented. Careful hand washing and finger scrubbing (fingernails must be kept as short as possible) after defaecation and before meals is essential in prevention of infection, and in prophylaxis. Children should wear gloves whilst sleeping. In practice eradication from a family circle may prove very difficult and repeated courses of chemotherapy (for a year or more) are occasionally required. Ideally, bed covers, sleeping garments and hand towels should be changed daily and the bedroom floor kept clean. These procedures must be adopted by all in the family or institution.

Household detergents have little effect on the viability of *E. vermicularis* eggs. Use of a damp cloth moistened with an antibacterial agent or bleach to clean a bathroom merely serves to spread any (viable) eggs which are present (Ibarra, 1989). Simple laundering of clothes and linen is adequate to disinfect them; such items should not be shaken, because this disseminates infective eggs. Food should be covered in order to limit contamination with dust-borne eggs.

Meticulous attention to hygienic measures, especially in childhood, will reduce the prevalence not only of *E. vermicularis*, but also the potentially more serious *Toxocara canis* infection, for which dogs form an important reservoir (Cook, 1989).

In an era when child sexual abuse is major headline news, an increase in awareness of the importance of *E. vermicularis* infection in the production of anal and vulval symptoms is clearly of paramount importance (Ibarra, 1989).

REFERENCES

Adungo, N. I., Ondijo, S. O. and Pamba, H. O. (1986) Observation of *Enterobius vermicularis* ova in urine: 3 case reports. *East Afr. Med. J.*, **63**, 676–8.

Al-Waili, N. S. (1988) *Artemisia herba-alba* extract for treating *Enterobius vermicularis* infection. *Trans. Roy. Soc. Trop. Med. Hyg.*, **82**, 626.

Arsenault, P. S. and Gerbie, A. B. (1986) Vulvovaginitis in the pre-adolescent girl. *Pediat. Ann.*, **15**, 577–9; 583–5.

Ashford, R. W., Hart, C. A. and Williams, R. G. (1988) *Enterobius vermicularis* infection in a children's ward. *J. Hosp. Infect.*, **12**, 221–4.

Beaver, P. C., Kriz, J. J. and Lau, T. J. (1973) Pulmonary nodule caused by *Enterobius vermicularis*. *Am. J. Trop. Med. Hyg.*, **22**, 711–13.

Bijlmer, J. (1946) An exceptional case of oxyuriasis of the intestinal wall. *J. Parasit.*, **32**, 359–66.

Bolbol, A. S., Mostafa, S. D., Al–Sekait, M. and Al–Nasser, A. A. (1989) Pattern of intestinal parasitic infection in preschool children in Riyadh, Saudi Arabia. *J. Hyg. Epidem. Microbiol. Immun.*, **33**, 253–9.

Brewster, D. H. (1989) *Enterobius vermicularis*: a possible cause of intestinal colic? *J. Roy. Coll. Gen. Pract.*, **39**, 387–8.

Budd, J. S. and Armstrong, C. (1987) Role of *Enterobius vermicularis* in the aetiology of appendicitis. *Br. J. Surg.*, **74**, 748–9.

Budd, J. S. and Armstrong, C. P. (1988) The correlation between gross appearance of the appendix at appendicectomy and histological examination. *Ann. Roy. Coll. Surg. Enol.*, **70**, 395–6.

Chac–Tai, C. (1989) Prevalence of intestinal helminth infections among Chinese schoolchildren in Macao City. *Trans. Roy. Soc. Trop. Med. Hyg.*, **83**, 238.

Chandrasoma, P. T. and Mendis, K. N. (1977) *Enterobius vermicularis* in ectopic sites. *Am. J. Trop. Med. Hyg.*, **26**, 644–9.

Chaudhry, A. Z. and Longworth, D. L. (1989) Cutaneous manifestations of intestinal helminthic infections. *System Mycoses Parasit. Dis.*, **7**, 275–90.

Chittenden, A. M. and Ashford, R. W. (1987) *Enterobius gregorii* Hugot 1983; first report in the U.K. *Ann. Trop. Med. Parasit.*, **81**, 195–8.

Cook, G. C. (1980) *Tropical Gastroenterology*, Oxford University Press, Oxford, pp. 443–4.

Cook, G. C. (1989) Canine-associated zoonoses: an unacceptable hazard to human health. *Quart J. Med.*, **70**, 5–26.

Cook, G. C. (1990a) *Parasitic Disease in Clinical Practice*, Springer-Verlag, London, Berlin, pp. 114–16.

Cook, G. C. (1990b) Threadworm infection and its treatment. *Pharm. J.*, **244**, 765–7.

Coulaud, J. P. and Rossignol, J. F. (1984) Albendazole: a new single dose anthelmintic. *Acta Tropica*, **41**, 87–90.

Crow, J. and Howe, S. (1988) Mast cell numbers in appendices with threadworm infestation. *J. Pathol.*, **154**, 347–51.

Editorial (1974) Children's worms. *Br. Med. J.*, **4**, 3.

Fiumara, N. J. and Tang, S. (1986) Folliculitis of the buttocks and pinworms: a case report. *Sexually Transmitted Dis.*, **13**, 45–6.

Ganor, S. (1987) In whom does pinworm infection itch? *Int. J. Dermat.*, **26**, 667.

Goldenberg, S. P. and Marignani, P. (1990) The endoscopic diagnosis of colonic enterobiasis. *Gastrointest. Endosc.*, **36**, 309–10.

Goldsmith, R. S. (1988) Recent advances in the treatment of helminthic infections: ivermectin, albendazole, and praziquantel, in *Parasitic Infections* (eds J. H. Leech, M. A. Sande and R. K. Root), Churchill Livingstone, New York, Edinburgh, pp. 327–47.

Gupta, S. C., Gupta, A. K., Keswani, N. K. *et al.* (1989) Pathology of tropical appendicitis. *J. Clin. Pathol.*, **42**, 1169–72.

Haswell-Elkins, M. R., Elkins, D. B. and Anderson, R. M. (1987) Evidence for predisposition in humans to infection with *Ascaris*, hookwoom, *Enterobius* and *Trichuris* in a South Indian fishing community. *Parasitology*, **95**, 323–37.

Haswell-Elkins, M. R., Elkins, D. B., Manjula, K. *et al.* (1987) The distribution and abundance of *Enterobius vermicularis* in a South Indian fishing community. *Parasitology*, **95**, 339–54.

Hood, C. (1989) *Enterobius vermicularis*. *Practitioner*, **233**, 503.

Ibarra, J. (1989) Towards a viable approach to the threadworm problem. *Health at School*, **5**, 54–7.

Khalil, H. M., Okbi, L. A. el., Sarwat. M. A. *et al.* (1987) Modifications in diagnosis and treatment of *Enterobius vermicularis*. *J. Egypt Soc. Parasit.*, **17**, 643–50.

Leach, F. N. (1990) Management of threadworm infestation during pregnancy. *Arch. Dis. Child.*, **65**, 399–400.

Mahdi, N. K. and Al-Khfaji, A. A. (1990) Prevalence and seasonal variation of enterobiasis in children of Iraq. *Southeast Asian J. Trop. Med. Public Hlth*, **21**, 135–8.

Mayers, C. D. and Purvis, R. J. (1970) Manifestations of pinworms. *Can. Med. Ass. J.*, **12**, 489–93.

McKay, T. (1989) *Enterobius vermicularis* infection causing endometritis and persistent vaginal discharge in three siblings. *N. Z. Med. J.*, **102**, 56.

Mendoza, E., Jorda, M., Rafel, E. *et al.* (1987) Invasion of human embryo by *Enterobius vermicularis*. *Arch. Pathol. Lab. Med.*, **111**, 761–2.

Mondou, E. N. and Gnepp, D. R. (1989) Hepatic granuloma resulting from *Enterobius vermicularis*. *Am. J. Clin. Pathol.*, **91**, 97–100.

Nagar, H. (1987) Surgical aspects of parasitic disease in childhood. *J. Pediat. Surg.*, **22**, 325–31.

Naquira, C., Jimenez, G., Guerra, J. G. *et al.* (1989) Ivermectin for human strongyloidiasis and other intestinal helminths. *Am. J. Trop. Med. Hyg.*, **40**, 304–9.

Neto, V. A., Castilho, V. L. P., Moreira, A. A. B. *et al.* (1985) Effácia do albendazol no tratamento da enterobíase. *Rev. Inst. Med. Trop, São Paulo*, **27**, 143–4.

Novak, C., Walker, T., Wood, D. and Prociv, P. (1987) Enterobiasis in the suburbs. *Med. J. Aust.*, **147**, 414.

Rivera-Marrero, C. A. (1986) Prevalence and intensity of helminth infections in southwest Puerto Rico. *J. Parasit.*, **72**, 787–8.

Saffos, R. O. and Rhatigan, R. M. (1977) Unilateral salpingitis due to *Enterobius vermicularis*. *Am. J. Clin. Pathol.*, **67**, 296–9.

Sarmah, H. C. (1988) A randomized controlled trial of pyrantel and mebendazole in children with enterobiasis and concomitant ascariasis. *Indian Pediat.*, **25**, 544–7.

Shiraki, T., Otsuru, M., Kenmotsu, M. *et al.* (1974) Invasion of *Enterobius vermicularis* into the human tissues – a report of 4 cases of eosinophilic granulomas caused by adult *Enterobius* in the intestines and their adjacent tissues. *Jap. J. Parasit.*, **23**, 125–37.

Simon, R. D. (1974) Pinworm infestation and urinary tract infection in young girls. *Am. J. Dis. Child.*, **128**, 21–2.

Singh, S. and Samantaray, J. C. (1989) Topical anthelmintic treatment of recurrent genitourinary enterobiasis. *Genitourin. Med.*, **65**, 284–6.

Vermund, S. H. and MacLeod, S. (1988) Is pinworm a vanishing infection? Laboratory surveillance in a New York City Medical Center from 1971 to 1986. *Am. J. Dis. Child.*, **142**, 566–8.

Wagner, E. D. and Eby, W. C. (1983) Pinworm prevalence in California elementary school children, and diagnostic methods. *Am. J. Trop. Med. Hyg.*, **32**, 998–1001.

Weller, I. V. D. (1985) The gay bowel. *Gut*, **26**, 869–75.

Williams, D. J. and Dixon, M. F. (1988) Sex, *Enterobius vermicularis* and the appendix. *Br. J. Surg.*, **75**, 1225–6.

Zhang, G.-W., Ji, X.-R. and McManus, D. P. (1990) The presence of pinworms (*Enterobius* sp.) in the mesenteric lymph nodes, liver and lungs of a chimpanzee, *Pan troglodytes*. *J. Helminth.*, **64**, 29–34.

SEVENTEEN

Abdominal angiostrongylosis

P. Morera

Abdominal angiostrongylosis, caused by *Angiostrongylus costaricensis* (Morera and Céspedes, 1971) or *Morerastrongylus costaricensis* (Chabaud, 1972), is a parasitic disease characterized by a granulomatous inflammatory reaction with heavy eosinophilic infiltration of the intestinal wall, especially in the ileocecal region. Ectopic localizations of the nematode cause liver and testicular lesions.

Although the parasite was described in 1971 (Morera and Céspedes, 1971), the disease has been observed in Costa Rican children since 1952. Subsequently, the definitive and intermediate hosts were identified and the life cycle was elucidated (Morera, 1973). Since then, human cases of the disease have been reported from Mexico to Argentina, including some Caribbean Islands. More recently an autochthonous case of the disease has been reported from Africa. In addition, naturally infected cotton rats (*Sigmodon hispidus*) have been found in the USA.

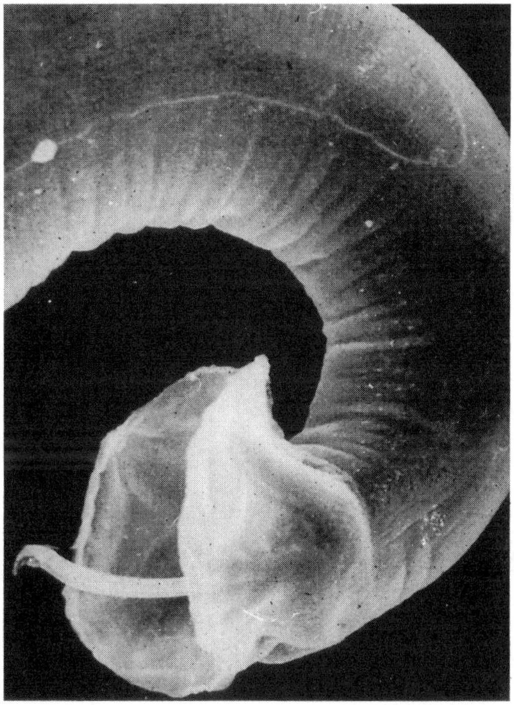

Figure 17.1 Caudal end of a male *Angiostrongylus costaricensis* showing the copulatory bursa and the spicules arising from the bottom of it.

17.1 ETIOLOGY

17.1.1 MORPHOLOGY

A. costaricensis is a filiform nematode that normally lives within the mesenteric arteries of the definitive host. The male is 20 mm long with a copulatory bursa and two spicules approximately 300 mm in length (Figure 17.1). The female is 33 mm long, and the anus and the vulva are located near the caudal end (Figure 17.2).

Enteric Infection 2. Intestinal helminths. Edited by M.J.G. Farthing, G.T. Keusch and D. Wakelin. Published in 1995 by Chapman and Hall, London. ISBN 0 412 39140 6

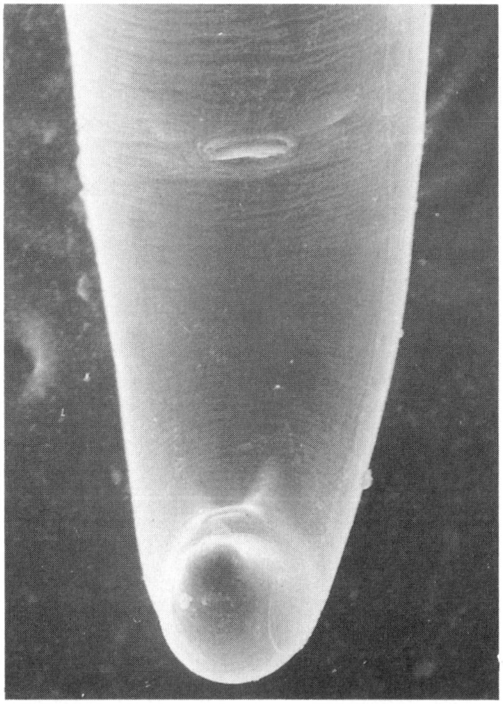

Figure 17.2 Caudal end of a female showing the vulva or gonopore (g) and the anus (a) near the tip of the tail.

17.1.2 DEVELOPMENT

In the natural definitive host (often rodents) the adult worms live within the ileocecal branches of the anterior mesenteric artery. Here, the female oviposit and the eggs are carried out by the blood stream into the intestinal wall, where they embryonate (Figure 17.3). The first stage larvae hatch, migrate to the lumen through the intestinal wall, and reach the soil within the rat feces. The molluscan intermediate host, usually veronicellid slugs, become infected by eating the rat feces. Two molts take place in the molluscan fibromuscular tissues, and after 18 days the infective third stage larva matures; these larvae could remain within the mollusc for several months or could be shed with its mucus secretion. The definitive mammalian host becomes infected by eating

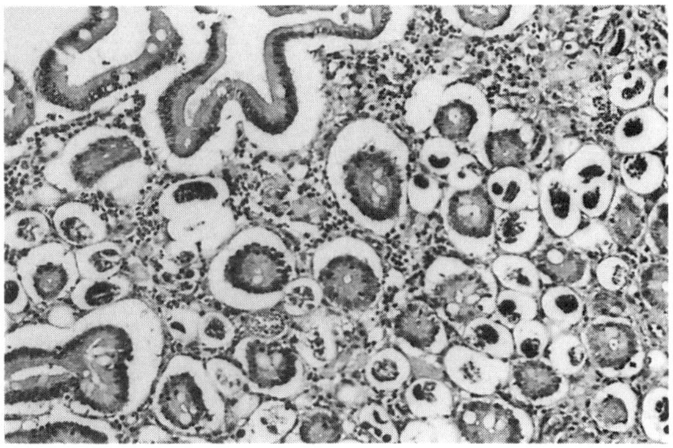

Figure 17.3 Section of the intestinal wall (cecum) of cotton rat showing eggs and embryos scattered in the small vessels of connective tissue.

the infected mollusc. The prepatent period is 24 days.

17.2 EPIDEMIOLOGY

17.2.1 DISTRIBUTION AND PREVALENCE

The disease has been reported from Mexico to Argentina, including some Caribbean Islands. However, it has often been found as a result of routine examination of surgical specimens in pathology departments. In addition, naturally infected cotton rats have been found in the USA (Uberlaker and Hall, 1979). Although human cases have been observed in the Continental USA we do not know whether the cases are autochthonous or not. Recently, the first human African case has been reported (Baird *et al.*, 1987).

In areas where clinical knowledge and the methodology for laboratory diagnosis have been improved, it is becoming clear that this is quite a prevalent parasitic disease. In 1993, more than 650 cases were diagnosed in Costa Rica (population 3 million), to give a probably underestimated, rate of 21.6 cases per 100 000 persons per year. In that country, its distribution is universal, from sea level to an altitude of 2000 m. We think that in areas where physicians are unaware of the problem, most clinical and subclinical cases probably go unrecognized or misdiagnosed.

Although the cotton rat (*Sigmodon hispidus*) is considered the most important definitive host, other reports of 11 additional rodent species, one case of coati (*Nasua narica*) in Costa Rica (Monge, Arroyo and Solano, 1978), and of marmosets (*Saguinus mystax*) from Iquitos, Peru (Sly *et al.*, 1982) have found these species to be naturally infected. Studies carried out in Costa Rica showed that the highest infection rate found for *S. hispidus* was 43.2%, similar to that found in Panama (35.0%) for the same species (Tesh *et al.*, 1973).

At least two species of veronicellid slugs in Costa Rica, one in Ecuador and one in Brazil are naturally infected with *A. costaricensis*: 50% of 6025 slugs from 20 Costa Rican localities, from sea level to an altitude of 2000 m, were found to be infected (Morera, 1985). More than 16 000 infective larvae were counted in a single specimen.

Thus, the opportunities for humans to become infected are high.

17.2.2 TRANSMISSION

Although several molluscs are naturally infected, veronicellid slugs are considered the main intermediate hosts. There is no evidence that persons intentionally eat slugs; however, small ones deeply hidden in salad greens could be finely chopped and inadvertently eaten raw. In addition, several cases are known of ingestion of these molluscs by infants. Nevertheless, most human infections are probably caused by ingestion of the infective larvae shed in the secretion of the molluscs. Slugs have been found in ripe fruits that have fallen to the ground. The characteristic mucus trails left by the molluscs can be observed throughout the endemic areas. The propensity for small children to put things in their mouths could explain why they show the highest infection rates.

17.3 PATHOLOGY AND CLINICAL FEATURES

In most cases, the lesions are located in the ileocecal region. They have also been observed in the hepatic flexure, descending colon, regional lymph nodes, liver and testicles.

Two major pathogenetic mechanisms are clearly distinguishable in the infections caused by *A. costaricensis*. The adult worms living within the mesenteric arteries (Figure 17.4) damage the endothelium inducing thrombosis and, consequently, necrosis of the tissues formerly supplied by the vessel. Secondly, eggs, embryos and larvae, as well as excretion/secretion products, produce an inflammatory reaction. Combinations of these phenomena, as well as the patient's susceptibility, and the number and localization of parasites, determine the clinicopathologic differences, ranging from cases in which only the appendix is damaged to those in which major surgery is required.

The gross examination of surgical specimens reveals a rigid and thickened intestinal wall with yellowish foci on the serosal surface and in the mesentery. The intestinal lumen is

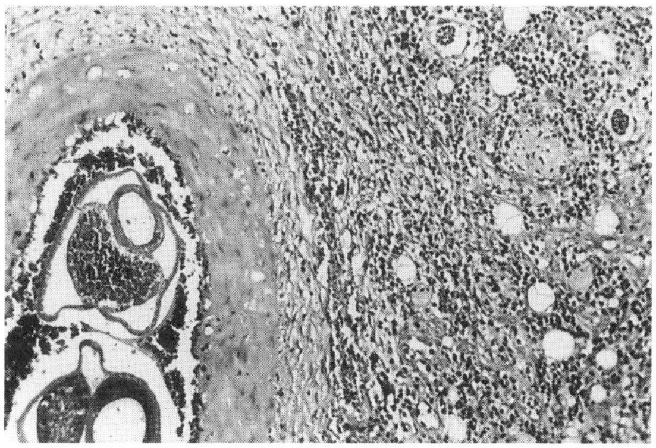

Figure 17.4 Section of human tissue (cecum) showing cross-sections of adult parasites (A) within an artery. Two embryos are also observed (B). The tissue is heavily infiltrated by inflammatory reaction: most cells are eosinophils.

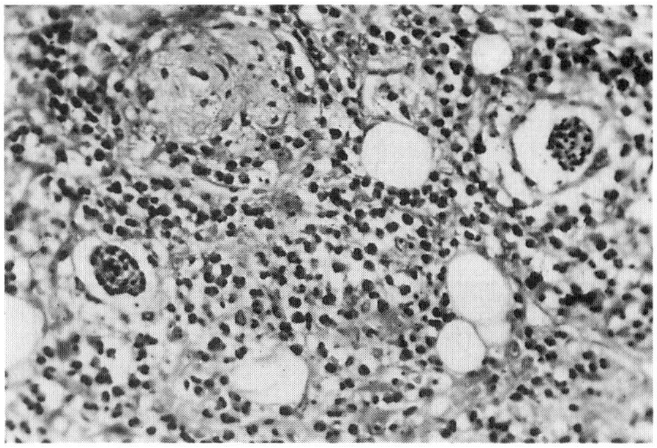

Figure 17.5 The section shows two embryos (arrows) within small vessels of the intestinal wall and heavy eosinophilic infiltration.

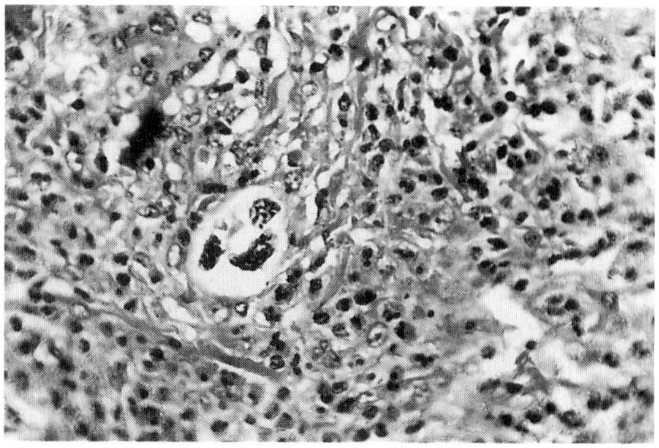

Figure 17.6 Young L1 larva coiled in a small portal vessel; the normal architecture of the liver is masked by the inflammatory reaction.

reduced, sometimes causing partial or complete obstruction. Necrotic areas can perforate. In many cases, even though only an appendicectomy is performed, the surgeon observes lesions of the cecum.

Histopathology demonstrates granulomatous inflammatory reaction with heavy eosinophilic infiltration, especially in the mucosa and submucosa; the serosa and muscular layers are often involved to a lesser degree. Eggs, embryos and larvae appear in small cavities lined by endothelium (Figure 17.5). Unfertilized eggs usually degenerate and are difficult to recognize. These structures as well as the excretion/secretion antigens are easily identified by immunochemical techniques. Large areas of necrosis are caused by arterial thrombosis. Eggs and embryos are present in the mesenteric lymph nodes, which also show reticuloendothelial hyperplasia and eosinophilic infiltration.

Hepatic lesions caused by *A. costaricensis* are similar to those caused by *Toxocara canis* (Morera *et al.*, 1982). However, the finding of eggs, embryos (Figure 17.6) and even adult worms in the hepatic parenchyma establishes the diagnosis.

In excised necrotic testicles histologically showing extensive parenchymal hemorrhagic necrosis, worms could be observed obstructing the arteries of the spermatic cord (Ruiz and Morera, 1983).

Abdominal angiostrongylosis predominantly affects children. From 116 patients studied in a pediatric hospital, 53% were of school age, 37% were of preschool age and 10% were infants. Of these patients, 64% were male and 34% female (Loría-Cortes and Lobo-Sanahuja, 1980).

When the worms are located in the ileocecal region, most patients complain of pain in the right iliac fossa and the right flank. Palpation in this area often causes pain. Rectal examination is also painful in about one half of the cases, and most patients present with fever ranging from 38 to 38.5°C (100.4°F to 101.3°F), but rarely accompanied by chills. In chronic cases, a mild fever may persist for several weeks. Anorexia, vomiting and constipation are also present in about 50% of patients. A very important finding is a tumor-like mass that, if present, can be palpated in the lower right quadrant and may be confused with a malignancy.

Although a few patients have no hematologic abnormalities, leukocytosis and eosinophilia are usually present. White blood cell counts usually range between 15 000 and

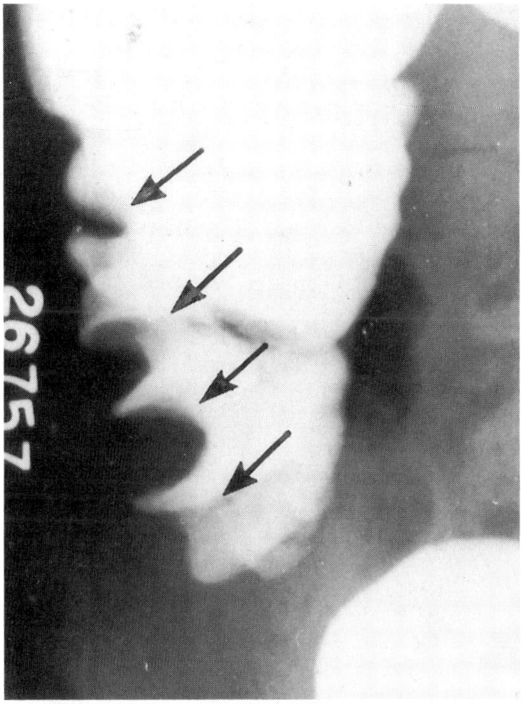

Figure 17.7 X-ray of the cecal region showing filling defects (arrows) of the intestinal lumen.

50 000/mm^3 and eosinophilia from 20% to 50%. The leukocytosis has been as high as 169 000/mm^3 with a 91% eosinophilia.

A barium follow-through or barium enema examination is often helpful in making the diagnosis. Radiological changes are localized in the terminal ileum, cecum appendix and ascending colon. The contrast medium shows incomplete filling (Figure 17.7) and irritability of the involved areas. The lumen is reduced by the thickening of the intestinal wall.

Sometimes the patient complains of pain in the upper right quadrant; in these cases, the liver is almost always enlarged and tender to palpation. At laparoscopy, small yellowish spots are seen on the surface of the liver. Most patients have hepatic involvement along with intestinal angiostrongylosis.

When the testicle is involved, the most remarkable findings are acute pain, accompanied by redness that later changes to purple. Eosinophilia and leukocytosis are also conspicuous. All patients with testicular necrosis have been misdiagnosed as having testicular torsion and the correct diagnosis was only made following surgery.

17.4 DIAGNOSIS

In infected rats, the L1 larvae can be easily identified in the stools; however, this is not true in humans. In man an immunological test should therefore be used to confirm suspected cases. Immunoelectrophoresis and Ouchterlony immunodiffusion tests give good results (Sauerbrey, 1977); however, an inexpensive and rapid latex bead agglutination test also gives high sensitivity and specificity rates.

17.5 TREATMENT

Surgery, when necessary, is the treatment of choice for abdominal angiostrongylosis. However, as knowledge of this often self-limiting disease increases, more non-surgical cases are being followed. Three drugs, diethylcarbamazine, thiabendazole and albendazole, have been used with 'remission' of symptoms reported. However, there was no objective evidence to prove that cure was attributable to the drugs. In fact, *in vitro* and *in vivo* trials in experimentally infected rats demonstrate that the parasites are excited by the drugs instead of killed, causing erratic migrations and worsening of the lesions (Morera and Bontempo, 1985). Thus, chemotherapy is not recommended until experimental studies demonstrate a more efficacious drug. Non-surgical patients should therefore be observed carefully: while some may have remission of symptoms, others could eventually develop an acute syndrome that requires surgery.

REFERENCES

Baird, J. K., Neafie, R. C., Lanoie, L. and Connor, D. H. (1987) Abdominal angiostrongyliasis in an African man. *Am. J. Trop. Med. Hyg.*, **37**, 353–6.

Chabaud, A. (1972) *Stefankostrongylus dubosti* n. sp. parasite du potamogales et essai de classification des nématodes Angiostrongylinae. *Ann. Parasit.*, **47**, 735–44.

Loría-Cortes, R. and Lobo-Sanahuja, J. F. (1980) Clinical abdominal angiostrongylosis. A study of 116 children with intestinal eosinophilic granuloma caused by *Angiostrongylus costaricensis*. *Am. J. Trop. Med. Hyg.*, **29**, 538–44.

Monge, E., Arroyo, R., and Solano, E. (1978) A new definitive host of *Angiostrongylus costaricensis* Morera and Cespedes, 1971. *J. Parasit.*, **64**, 34.

Morera, P. (1985) Angiostrongiliasis abdominal: transmisión y observaciones sobre su posible control, in *Control and Eradication of Infections Diseases*. Int. Symp. PAHO/WHO copublication series no. 1, pp. 230–5.

Morera, P. and Céspedes, R. (1971) *Angiostrongylus costaricensis* n. sp. (Nematoda: Metastrongylidae) a new lungworm occurring in man in Costa Rica. *Rev. Biol. Trop.*, **18**, 173–85.

Morera, P. (1973) Life history and redescription of *Angiostrongylus costaricensis* Morera and Céspedes 1971. *Am. J. Trop. Med. Hyg*, **22**, 613–21.

Morera, P. and Bontempo, I. (1985) Acción de algunos antihelmínticos sobre *Angiostrongylus costaricensis*. *Rev. Med. Hosp. Nal. Niños Costa Rica*, **20**, 165–74.

Morera. P., Pérez, F., Mora, F. and Castro, L. (1982) Visceral larva migrans-like syndrome caused by *Angiostrongylus costaricensis*. *Am. J. Trop. Med. Hyg.*, **31**, 67–70.

Ruiz, P. J. and Morera, P. (1983) Spermatic artery obstruction caused by *Angiostrongylus costaricensis* Morera and Céspedes 1971. *Am. J. Trop. Med. Hyg.*, **32**, 1458–9.

Sauerbrey, M. (1977) A precipitin test for the diagnosis of human abdominal angiostrongyliasis. *Am. J. Trop. Med. Hyg.*, **26**, 1156–8.

Sly, D. L., Toft, J. D., Gardiner, G. H. and London, W. T. (1982) Spontaneous occurrence of *Angiostrongylus costaricensis* in marmosets (*Saguinus mystax*). *Lab. Anim. Sci.*, **32**, 286–8.

Tesh, R., Ackerman, L., Dietz, W. and Williams, J. (1973) *Angiostrongylus costaricensis* in Panama. Prevalence and pathological findings in wild rodents infected with the parasite. *Am. J. Trop. Med. Hyg.*, **22**, 348–56.

Uberlaker, J. E. and Hall, N. M. (1979) First report of *Angiostrongylus costaricensis* Morera and Céspedes 1971 in the United States. *J. Parasitol.*, **65**, 307.

EIGHTEEN

Schistosomiasis

G. R. Olds
and
P. M. Wiest

18.1 SCHISTOSOME SPECIES

Schistosomes are metazoan parasites which infect 200–300 million humans worldwide (Mahmoud and Wahab, 1990). These digenetic trematodes live as separate male and female worms within the vascular system of the mammalian host and use freshwater snails as intermediate hosts. Five major schistosome species infect humans. *Schistosoma mansoni* and *S. japonicum* account for the majority of intestinal and hepatic pathology induced by schistosomes and together are a leading cause of hepatic fibrosis worldwide (Dunn and Kamel, 1981). *Schistosoma mansoni* is found in Africa and South America while the Far Eastern species, *S. japonicum*, is found in China, the Philippines, Indonesia and formerly in Japan and Formosa. *Schistosoma haematobium* primarily affects the human urinary tract and thus it will not be discussed in detail in this book on enteric infections. *Schistosoma intercalcatum* and *S. mekongi* are less prevalent in the world and are restricted to West Africa and the Mekong river basin of South-East Asia, respectively. They will be discussed briefly at the end of the chapter.

18.2 HISTORICAL ASPECTS

We know from mummified remains in Egypt and China that schistosomes have infected man for thousands of years (Mahmoud and Wahab, 1990). Early Egyptians described the symptoms caused by *S. haematobium* in hieroglyphics, including haematuria (Katz, Despommier and Gwadz, 1982). They even recognized that the disease was associated with the Nile River. The causative agent for schistosomiasis, however, was not discovered until 1852 when a German physician, Theodor Bilharz, discovered the adult worms of *S. haematobium* in an autopsy performed in Egypt (Bilharz, 1853). As a result, schistosomiasis is known throughout much of Europe and Africa as bilharziasis. The British physician Manson described a case of *S. mansoni* in a traveler to the West Indies (Manson, 1902)) and definitively differentiated this species from that described by Bilharz (*S. haematobium*). The hepatic/intestinal African species was named in his honor. In 1903 the classical hepatic lesion associated with schistosomiasis was described by Symmers (Symmers, 1903) and termed 'clay pipe stem' cirrhosis for its unusual appearance on gross examination of the organ. This was later changed to clay pipe stem 'fibrosis', since microscopic sections of the liver did not show micronodular cirrhosis or bridging necrosis characteristic of other forms of cirrhotic liver disease (due to alcohol, hepatitis B, carbon tetrachloride, etc.).

Enteric Infection 2. Intestinal helminths. Edited by M.J.G. Farthing, G.T. Keusch and D. Wakelin. Published in 1995 by Chapman and Hall, London. ISBN 0 412 39140 6

The eggs of the Far Eastern species, *S. japonicum*, were first noted by Majima at an autopsy finding, but the adult worms were not found (Majima, 1888)). He did, however, correctly connect these eggs with the patient's unique type of liver fibrosis. The first description of the adult worms of this species was made by Katsurada who also described the clinical manifestations of acute infection including Katayama fever (Katsurada, 1904)). The first complete life cycle of any species of schistosome was published a decade earlier by Miyairi and Suzuki who also correctly identified the *Oncomelania* species of snails as the intermediate host for *S. japonicum* (Miyairi and Suzuki, 1914). A similar observation was made for *Biomphalaria glabrata* snails by Leiper for *S. mansoni* (Leiper, 1918).

The first successful treatment of schistosomiasis was tartar emetic which was used in patients in the Sudan in 1916. Because only a small subset of the infected population ever develop clinical illness and because of the toxicity of tartar emetic, some medical historians speculate that more people died as a result of therapy than would have died from untreated schistosomiasis (Warren, 1992). This unsatisfactory situation remained until the mid 1960s when less toxic agents were developed. It was not however until the 1970s that effective oral non-toxic therapy became available, culminating with praziquantel (Andrews, 1985). This drug currently forms the basis for most national control programs for schistosomiasis.

18.3 EPIDEMIOLOGY

Schistosomiasis is a disease transmitted by specific species of freshwater snails to man. As a result, the distribution within an endemic country is largely determined by the microecology of these molluscs. Transmission can occur throughout the year or be seasonal. In temperate regions such as China, seasonal temperature (summer and winter) dramatically affects transmission. Similarly, in areas with distinct wet and dry seasons, seasonal rainfall may have a significant effect.

Schistosomiasis is primarily a disease of school-age children and young adults (Mahmoud and Wahab, 1990; Butterworth *et al.*, 1989). Both the prevalence and intensity of infection peak at 10–20 years of age in individuals chronically exposed to the parasite, followed by a decrease in older individuals. This decline is due in some cases to decreased water contact but in general is largely a result of the development of resistance to reinfection (Anderson, 1987; Butterworth, 1990) following chronic (5–10 years) exposure. In areas where rice farming or fishing are major occupational exposures to schistosomiasis, a second smaller peak in prevalence of infection is observed in 30–40 year old persons. Peak morbidity as manifested by hepatosplenomegaly also peaks in adolescence and is generally maximal a few years after peak prevalence and intensity of infection. The prevalence of hepatic fibrosis as determined by ultrasonography generally peaks during the fourth and fifth decades of life.

While *S. mansoni* is almost exclusively a human pathogen, *S. japonicum* infects a variety of mammalian hosts. As a result, effective control programs concentrating on treating human cases has changed the current prevalence and intensity of infection with *S. mansoni* and schistosome induced morbidity (Grysells and Polderman, 1991). In *S. japonicum*, transmission and prevalence of human infections have been reduced; however, non-human reservoirs continue to excrete eggs into the environment thus maintaining infection in the snail population. Thus, serious consideration must be given to control of infection of non-human reservoirs or snail control if a significant impact on transmission of *S. japonicum* is to occur.

18.4 LIFE CYCLE

The life cycle of schistosomes is shown in Figure 18.1. The infective stage for humans is called the cercaria (Wilson, 1987). The organisms swim in fresh water and have a long slender body attached to a bifurcated tail. The cercaria are shed from a snail into water where the parasite actively seeks a mammalian host. The time of cercarial shedding is species-dependent, being maximal at mid-day for *S. mansoni* and at night for *S. japonicum*. With all schistosome species, humans become infected through contact with water. A more detailed diagram of this process is shown in Figure 18.2. During infection, the cercarial body rapidly penetrates the skin leaving the tail behind. Proteolytic enzymes are released from penetration glands which facilitate cercarial invasion. Over the next hours, the cercariae transform into parasitic larvae called schistosomula (Stirewalt, 1974). At this stage, schistosomula are still vulnerable to host immune attack but by the time they evolve to fully grown adult worms they are totally resistant to host immune responses. The complete mechanism of immune evasion is unknown. Numerous means to evade host defenses have been proposed and include acquisition of host antigens, suppression of the host's immune response, membrane turnover, antigenic variation and intrinsic changes in the parasite's surface (Damian, 1987; Pearce and Sher, 1987). Parasites migrate to the lungs and then ultimately to the portal sinusoids of the liver. During this period the parasites undergo rapid growth into adolescent worms. In the liver, the male and female worms become sexually mature, pair and migrate to the mesenteric veins. Egg-laying commences with each female producing from 200 to 3000 eggs per day, depending on the species. The eggs are laid within the vasculature and eventually pass through the intestinal wall into the stool where they are carried in the faeces into the environment. The average life span of an individual worm has been estimated to be from 3 to 10 years but individuals have been found with active infection 30 years or more after leaving an endemic area (Warren, Mahmoud and Cummings, 1974). Approximately two-thirds of the eggs exit the body in the stool; the remaining eggs become deposited in host tissue. Unfortunately, eggs within tissue elicit an immune response which is responsible for most of the pathology observed in schistosomiasis. As a result, schistosomiasis is often considered primarily an immunologic disease (Olds, 1988).

Following defecation, eggs hatch upon contact with fresh water, releasing ciliated motile miracidia. These free-living organisms then locate and penetrate a specific snail intermediate host (Jourdane and Theron, 1987). Within the snail, asexual reproduction takes place and, in a few weeks, thousands of infective cercariae emerge.

A highly successful parasite such as the schistosome often evolves mechanisms which optimize the parasitic condition of the host (Butterworth *et al.*, 1989). It is highly advantageous on a population basis for parasites to distribute themselves throughout the entire human population and not to infect any single host with an overwhelming parasite burden. The adult schistosome appears to do this by evoking in the host a modest level of resistance to new cercarial challenge. The adult remains impervious to these immunologic mechanisms. Since these worms are incapable of multiplying within man, this results in the majority of infected individuals being only lightly infected. This conforms to the observation that both the prevalence and intensity of infection decreases in older individuals chronically exposed to the parasite. An understanding of this process forms the basis for most of the current research on a vaccine against this parasite (Olds, 1988; Butterworth, 1992).

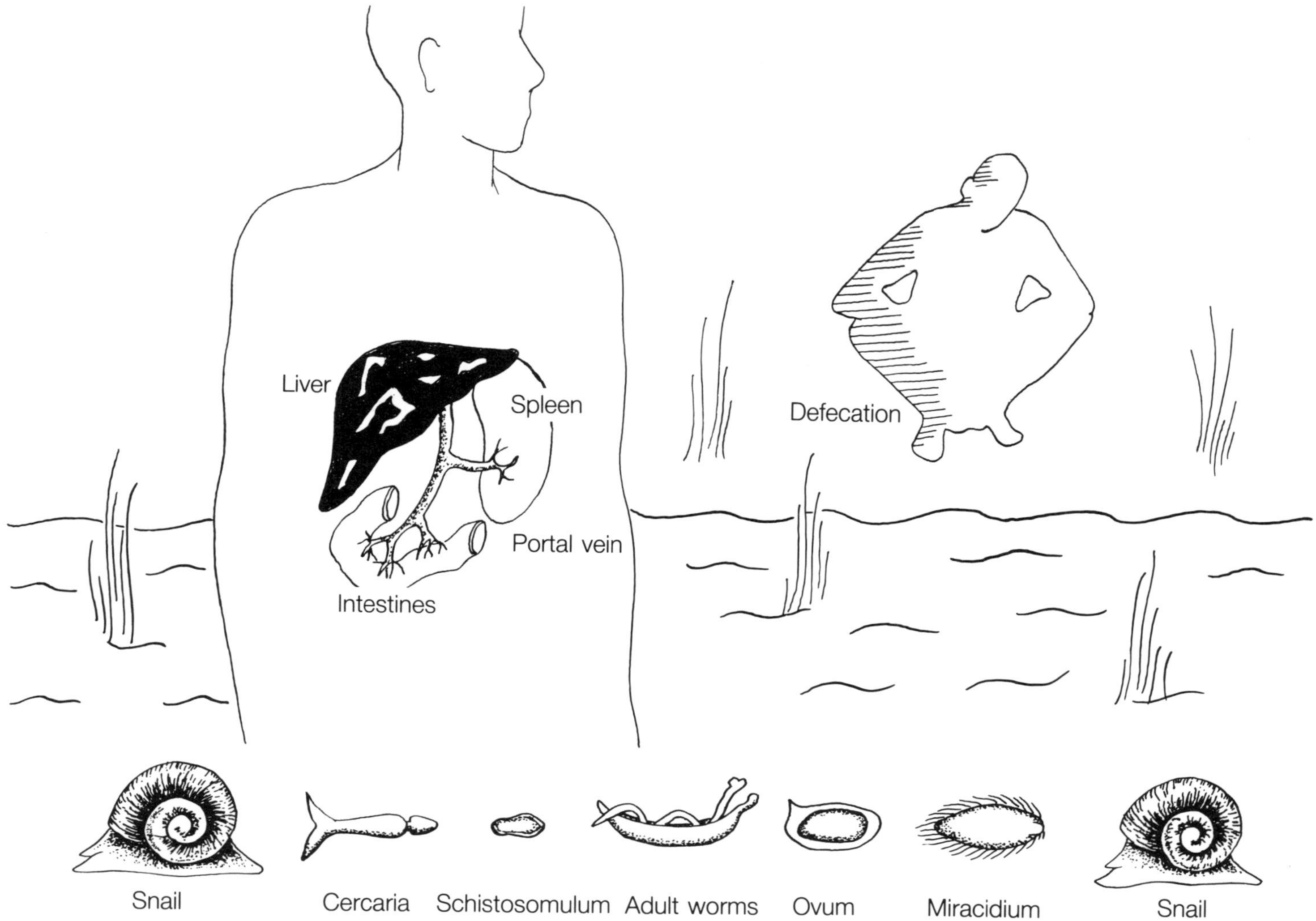

Figure 18.1 Life cycle of *Schistosoma mansoni*. (Drawn by M.E. Gorden.)

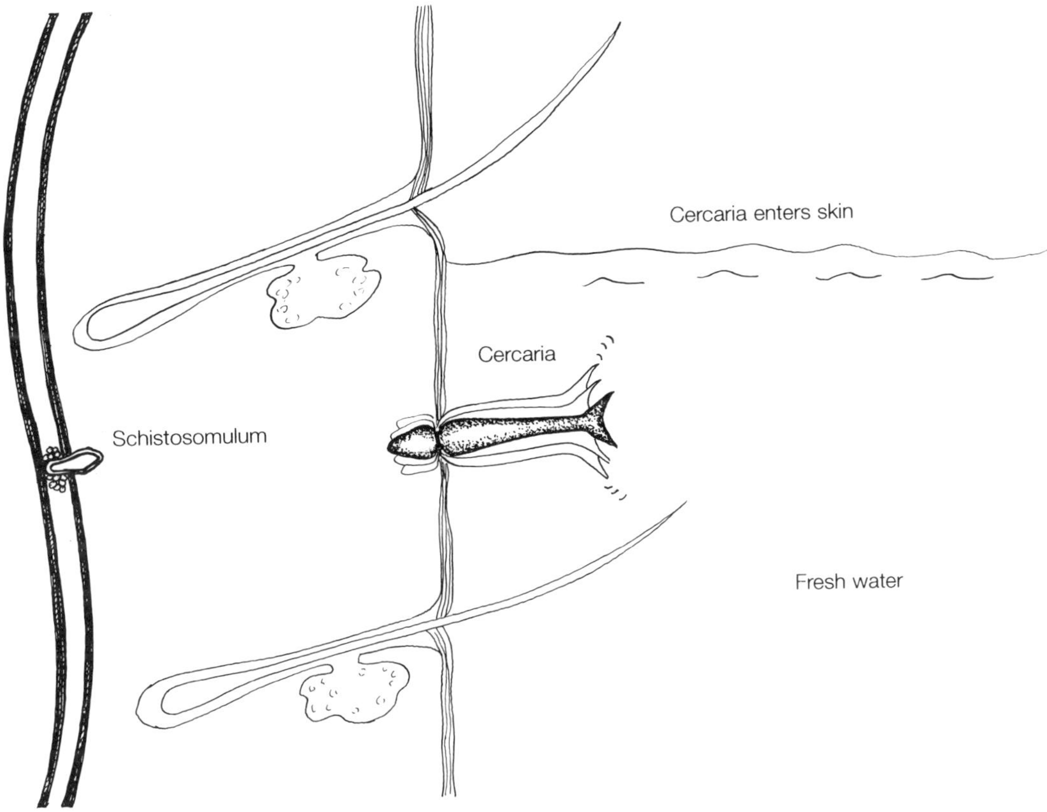

Figure 18.2 Human infection by schistosome cercaria. (Drawn by M. E. Gorden.)

18.5 IMMUNOPATHOLOGY

The major pathological sequelae in patients infected with schistosomes are due to the inflammatory reaction elicited by eggs trapped within host tissues (Boros, 1989). This response attempts to destroy these highly immunogenic foci but at a cost to adjacent tissues as shown in Figure 18.3. Both *S. mansoni* and *S. japonicum* adult worms produce eggs, some of which are carried downstream in the portal circulation to the liver where they become trapped in the presinusoidal spaces. Single eggs of *S. mansoni* are trapped in the liver while aggregates of 6–8 eggs of *S. japonicum* are often found (Warren, 1987). Enzymes and antigens are released by the miracidia within the eggs. These molecules, termed soluble egg antigens (SEA), evoke a vigorous delayed hypersensitivity response by the host and are the basis for the immunopathology observed in schistosomiasis (Boros and Warren, 1970).

The host response to SEA leads to formation of a granuloma that surrounds the egg (Warren, 1982). The egg granuloma in both *S. japonicum* and *S. mansoni* is composed of macrophages, T lymphocytes and eosinophils, a few plasma cells and later fibroblasts. These cells ultimately destroy the egg. After years of chronic hepatic inflammation, patients may present with the characteristic Symmer's clay pipe stem fibrosis. The linear thick deposits of collagen and glycosaminoglycans resemble clay pipes macroscopically (Dunn and Kamel, 1981; von Lichtenberg, 1987). Fibrosis follows the granulomatous host response and occurs mostly at the site of

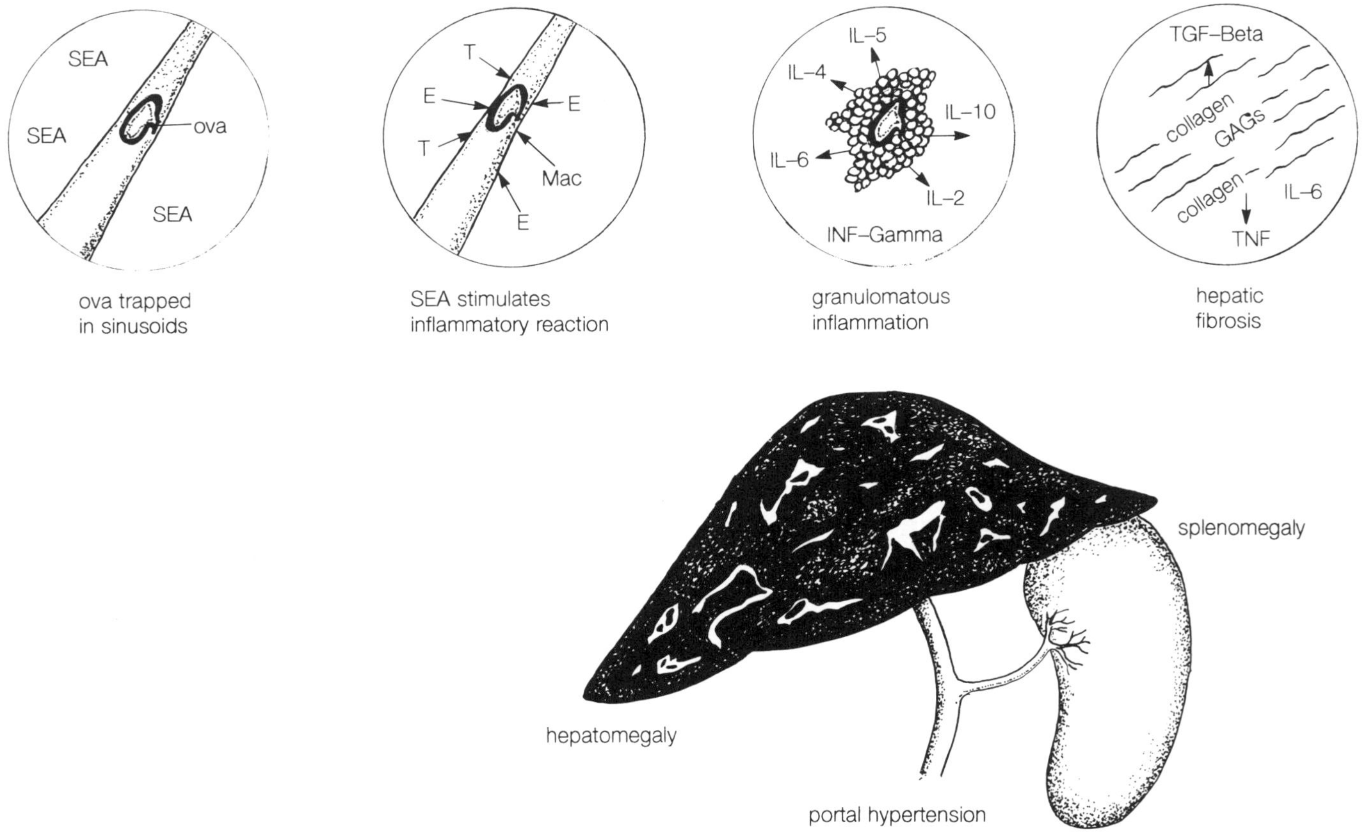

Figure 18.3 Immunopathogenesis in schistosomiasis. SEA = soluble egg antigens; T = T-lymphocyte; E = Eosinophil; Mac = Macrophage; Il = interleukin; INF = interferon; TGF = transforming growth factor; TNF = tumour necrosis factor; GAG = glycosaminoglycans. (Produced by M. E. Gordon.)

resolving granulomas. Fibrotic bands can also occur around portal veins distant from granulomas. In contrast to most other causes of liver disease, the hepatic parenchyma and function is largely spared until very late in infection. The location of these deposits, however, leads to mechanical obstruction of portal blood flow. This results in elevated portal pressures, increased collateral blood flow and ultimately to bleeding esophageal varices, a major cause of morbidity and mortality.

Splenomegaly also occurs in most individuals and can be massive on occasion. Splenic enlargement results from both portal hypertension and chronic lymphocytic infiltration (von Lichtenberg, 1987). Granulomas also form around eggs transversing the intestinal wall. This inflammatory reaction can lead to chronic colitis and gastrointestinal blood loss (Cheever *et al.*, 1978). In *S. mansoni* infection, colonic inflammation can become excessive, particularly in children, and lead to an unusual form of polyposis (Lehman *et al.*, 1970). Finally when portal hypertension and collateral blood flow become severe, eggs bypass the liver through these channels and become deposited in the lungs as small pulmonary emboli (Shaw and Ghareeb, 1968). This leads to a fibro-obstructive process similar to that observed in the liver. Thus, in countries where hepatic forms of schistosomiasis are common, pulmonary fibrosis, pulmonary hypertension and cor pulmonale constitute the second leading morbid sequelae of infection.

The immunology of the egg granuloma has been studied extensively in experimental animals both *in vivo* and *in vitro* (Colley, 1987). *In vitro* models of human granulomas have also been developed (Goes *et al.*, 1991). Soluble egg antigens (SEA) secreted by the ova are processed by tissue macrophages and stimulate helper T cells (probably both Th 1 early and Th 2 CD4+ cells later) (Mathew and Boros, 1986; Yamashita and Boros, 1990; Grzych *et al.*, 1991; Henderson *et al.*, 1991; Scott *et al.*, 1989). This process is mediated by a variety of cytokines including IL-2, gamma interferon, IL-10 and, to a greater extent, IL-4, IL-5 and IL-6. IL-5 is believed to be primarily responsible for the eosinophilia observed with this parasite (Sector, Steward and Colley, 1990). The connection between granulomatous inflammation and hepatic fibrosis is less clear. In experimental animals no direct correlation has been observed between the size of granulomas and the resultant deposits of collagen and glycosaminoglycans for *S. japonicum* but, in infection with *S. mansoni*, those strains with the largest granulomas also develop the most hepatic fibrosis (Cheever *et al.*, 1984, 1987). Recent studies have demonstrated that isolated intact cultured egg granulomas produce fibrogenic growth factors that stimulate fibroblasts to proliferate and synthesize collagen and fibronectin and regulate fibrosis (Prakash and Wyler, 1991). This has led to the concept that hepatic fibrosis is mediated by a different set of cytokines than those which regulate granulomatous inflammation. These include TGF-β, TNFα and IL-6 (Andus, Bauer and Gerok, 1991; Kresina, Quincy and Zern, 1992).

Despite these immunopathogenic events, the majority of individuals infected with *S. mansoni* or *S. japonicum* do not develop severe hepatosplenic disease even after years of infection. A partial explanation for this observation is that most humans and experimental animals are capable of down-regulating these immunopathogenic responses to trapped ova during chronic parasitism. This process has been termed immune modulation and has been the focus of intense investigation for several years (Boros, 1989; Olds, 1988; Warren, 1977).

A variety of immunoregulatory mechanisms has been demonstrated to mediate this response both *in vitro* and *in vivo*. In *S. mansoni* infection, cellular immune mechanisms appear to dominate while in *S. japonicum* infection regulatory idiotypic and anti-idiotypic interactions have been described (Olds *et al.*, 1986; Colley, 1981; Stavitsky, 1987). Much of the work has been based on animal models. In humans, children modulate the size of granulomatous inflammation over time as determined on rectal biopsy (Rocklin *et al.*, 1980). This correlates with decreased *in vitro* response to SEA. Indirect evidence for immune modulation in humans includes the observation that in endemic areas for schistosomiasis, hepatic enlargement (largely the result of granulomatous inflammation), is more common in chronically infected children than in adults. Furthermore, lymphoid cells from acutely infected individuals respond more vigorously to stimulation with SEA than cells obtained from chronically infected hosts (Warren, 1977; Olds, 1986). Immune responses to SEA are always more vigorous in individuals following successful chemotherapy than while they are actively infected. In addition, *in vitro* granulomas are smaller in size if cells are obtained from chronically infected patients than when the cells come from acutely infected individuals or those obtained after successful parasitologic cure (Boros, 1989; Doughty *et al.*, 1984). The exact mechanism for immune modulation in humans is unknown but recent evidence suggests this process is part of a regulatory immune network (idiotypes and anti-idiotypes) (Colley, 1990). These observations have led to the concept that the subset of individuals who go on to develop severe and often fatal hepatic pathology are those who fail to modulate granulomatous inflammation and subsequent fibrosis following chronic parasitism. This hypothesis is supported by the fact that those who develop severe pathology in both *S. mansoni* and *S. japonicum* infection appear to have specific HLA-D locus haplotypes and that patients with hepatosplenic disease have different (and often more vigorous) immune responses to egg antigens than matched individuals without overt pathology (Sasazuki *et al.*, 1980).

The present immunopathology of schistosomiasis may, however, be affected by current control efforts. Whereas in the past schistosomiasis was characterized by chronic infection, the widespread use of community-based chemotherapy will soon change this pattern to that of repeated acute infections followed by parasitological cure. What effect this will have on these beneficial immunologic adjustments is unclear. The effect of curative chemotherapy on pathology has only recently been studied. In general, hepatic enlargement appears reversible following treatment, particularly in children (Sleigh *et al.*, 1986). Hepatic enlargement may, however, take several years to resolve. The same is generally true of splenic enlargement. The effect of curative chemotherapy on hepatic fibrosis is still unclear. Some studies have reported reversibility of hepatic fibrosis as determined by ultrasonography (Homeida *et al.*, 1991; Mohamed-Ali *et al.*, 1991). Others suggest that fibrogenesis is arrested by treatment but resolves only slowly if at all over time. Finally, it has been suggested that fibrosis can progress despite successful treatment (Cheever and Deb, 1989). If this were true, then current national control strategies would be expected to have little or no effect on hepatic fibrosis. These issues along with the effect of repeated reinfection have yet to be definitely resolved.

18.6 OTHER SCHISTOSOME-INDUCED MORBIDITY

The major clinical manifestations of schistosomiasis are due to the host's response to eggs lodged in the liver. Schistosomes can, however, induce other syndromes. Schistosome dermatitis occurs during skin invasion by cercariae during which the parasite dies within the dermis. This results in a typical skin rash called 'swimmer's itch'. This syndrome is a sensitization phenomenon since it occurs in previously exposed individuals.

Several weeks after infection, individuals can develop a serum sickness-like syndrome termed Katayama fever (von Lichtenberg, 1987). This is most commonly observed in individuals infected with *S. japonicum* and occurs soon after the onset of egg deposition. Occasionally this condition is seen earlier with massive exposure. It is thought to be an antigen–antibody complex-mediated process due to massive challenge of newly produced egg antigens. Individuals occasionally die during this complication of infection. Fortunately, most individuals in endemic areas do not develop this clinical syndrome.

Several other sequelae may occur in schistosomiasis. In cerebral schistosomiasis, patients develop seizures or other changes in consciousness. This often occurs in *S. japonicum* infection and is due to deposition of eggs within the brain. It is suggested that adult worms migrate aberrantly to the brain but worms have never been identified in this location. Transverse myelitis has also been reported usually due to *S. mansoni* (Lechtenberg and Vaida, 1977). Nephrotic syndrome is another complication of schistosomiasis in which kidney biopsies demonstrate antigen–antibody complexes (Andrade and Rocha, 1979). This condition generally responds to successful chemotherapy. Eggs may also be deposited in the lungs with development of pulmonary hypertension.

Although more difficult to quantitate because of coexistence of polyparasites and malnutrition, schistosomiasis appears to have a profound effect on childhood growth and development (Stephenson, 1987). This is particularly true if schistosome infection occurs during the adolescent growth spurt. *S. japonicum* infection in adolescence, for example, has been associated with a 6–8 cm stunting in height and a 2–3 kg difference in weight as compared with uninfected controls (McGarvey *et al.*, 1993). Some of these effects are reversible with successful chemotherapy particularly in young children but concern exists that potential catch-up growth will be impossible after adolescence.

18.7 CLINICAL FEATURES

Schistosome dermatitis occurs within hours of penetration of the skin by cercariae and consists of a maculopapular pruritic rash. In human schistosomes, the reaction is usually mild and escapes unnoticed. In contrast, infection with cercariae that normally infect birds may lead to an intense dermatitis and is common in the Great Lakes of north central USA.

In Katayama fever or acute schistosomiasis, especially in infection with *S. japonicum*, the patient develops characteristic clinical features weeks after primary infection. Patients may have an acute onset of fever, chills, headache, sweating, hepatosplenomegaly, lymphadenopathy and peripheral eosinophilia. Most symptoms and signs disappear after a few weeks, but death may occur.

Most individuals with chronic schistosomiasis are lightly infected and thus asymptomatic. Several community-based studies suggest that infected patients may complain of fatigue, crampy abdominal pain or diarrhea. The most common clinical manifestation of schistosomiasis is hepatosplenomegaly (Dunn and Kamel, 1981; von Lichtenberg, 1987). Typically no other signs of liver disease are found. In severe cases of chronic schistosomiasis, patients present with signs of porto-systemic shunting, ascites and/or hematemesis. These individuals have generally been infected for many years or may represent end-stage disease without active infection. The end stage of hepatosplenic schistosomiasis occurs with new onset jaundice and ascites followed by liver failure. It is unclear whether this represents the natural progression of schistosomiasis or reflects in some individuals other insults such as underlying infection with hepatitis B virus (HBV).

Schistosomiasis should be suspected in cases of hepatomegaly since other forms of chronic liver disease are often associated with a small shrunken liver at the time of portosystemic shunting. Splenic enlargement alone is not a helpful differentiating feature since it can occur in all forms of chronic liver disease. The presence of a massively enlarged, firm spleen in the presence of an enlarged liver is highly suggestive of schistosomiasis. Since HBV is endemic in all areas with schistosomiasis, liver disease due to both of these pathogens is common. In general, liver biochemical tests are normal in schistosomiasis until late in the disease. In addition, hepatic encephalopathy is also uncommon in schistosomiasis until late. All of these features help distinguish schistosomal liver disease from other hepatic insults. The management of hematemesis is usually conservative, particularly when the degree of reversibility is not known. Sclerotherapy is effective and is preferred to surgical shunting procedures. Splenectomy is rarely indicated in schistosomiasis because of the potential reversibility following curative therapy.

Pulmonary hypertension with or without cor pulmonale is a very late complication of collateral blood flow and has been particularly well described in *S. mansoni* and *S. haematobium* infections (Shaw and Ghareeb, 1968). It occurs in *S. mansoni* infection, the setting of long-standing hepatic disease.

A special note should be made of the association between schistosomiasis and salmonella, particularly *Salmonella typhi* or *Salmonella paratyphi A* or *B*. Patients with schistosomiasis have an increased frequency of salmonella infection and often fail standard antibacterial treatment regimens. It is thought that salmonella are sequestered in the gut or tegument of the schistosome where they are protected from antibiotics (Young *et al.*, 1973). In addition, schistosomes may alter the immunological response of the host to these bacterial pathogens allowing development of chronic salmonellosis (Muniz-Junqueira, Prata and Tosta, 1992). Successful treatment of schistosomiasis is required for bacteriologic cure of patients infected with salmonella.

In general, patients come to the attention of a physician with hepatic or splenic enlargement, unexplained eosinophilia, increased plasma IgE concentrations, bloody diarrhea or anemia, all of which are commonly present during chronic infection with schistosomes. Occasional patients will present with recent onset seizures or transverse myelitis or have a clinical picture consistent with Katayama fever such as fever, headache, adenopathy and eosinophilia.

18.8 DIAGNOSIS

Schistosomiasis can generally be diagnosed by finding eggs during routine stool examination (Peters and Kazura, 1987). The shape and size of the eggs are characteristic for each species of schistosome which allows easy identification. More than one stool examination may be required to diagnose schistosomiasis, particularly in light infections. If several stools are negative and the diagnosis is still suspected, rectal snips can be obtained on sigmoidoscopy to increase sensitivity. Tissue from these superficial biopsies can be crushed between slides and examined for the presence of eggs. Care must be taken to distinguish live from old calcific ova. The latter can persist, particularly those of *S. japonicum*, for many years and does not represent current infection. Serology is helpful in diagnosing acute schistosomiasis (Katayama fever) or cerebral schistosomiasis when stool examinations are negative. It is also helpful in diagnosing schistosomiasis in travellers or temporary residents of an endemic area (Peace Corps workers or soldiers, for example). Serology is not helpful in individuals who live in endemic areas since most serologic tests remain positive for many years after parasitologic cure.

The diagnosis of schistosome-induced liver disease requires special consideration. Unfortunately, several hepatic pathogens may coexist within the same patient. The long-term prognosis as well as the expected response to antischistosome therapy depends on these contributory factors. Liver disease due to schistosomiasis can be suspected non-invasively by observing characteristic patterns with abdominal ultrasonography or computerized tomography (Mohamed-Ali *et al.*, 1991). Thickened portal veins are seen on ultrasonography and represent periportal fibrosis. These findings have been validated by liver biopsy. These non-invasive tests cannot, however, determine the contribution of other hepatic pathogens. Up to one-third of patients suspected of having pure schistosomal-induced liver disease are found, on open wedge biopsy, to have additionally micronodular cirrhosis, generally caused by HBV. These individuals would be expected to have a worse long-term prognosis than those with only schistosomiasis and may fail to improve following treatment with praziquantel. Although double infections may be suspected from elevated transaminases and bilirubin as well as hepatitis B and C serology, patients usually require a confirmatory liver biopsy. Unfortunately thin needle biopsies may not demonstrate clay pipe stem fibrosis since this process is unevenly distributed throughout the liver and easily missed with small tissue samples. An open liver biopsy may be required to evaluate thoroughly a patient with suspected schistosome-induced liver disease.

18.9 TREATMENT

All schistosome species can be successfully treated with praziquantel (King and Mahmoud, 1989). *S. mansoni* can also be treated with oxamniquine but drug tolerance and resistance has increasingly been reported (Foster, 1987). The dose of praziquantel for *S. mansoni* and *S. japonicum* infections are different. *S. mansoni* is generally treated in the USA with a 25 mg/kg dose given twice separated by 4–6 h. Most national control programs use a single 40 mg/kg dose because compliance is higher. This higher dose, however, is associated with a slightly higher frequency of nausea and vomiting. The recommended treatment dose against *S. japonicum* is 3×20 mg/kg doses separated by 4–6 h. Again, in the field, 2×25 mg/kg doses are generally used for operational reasons. Pregnant and lactating women are not treated but definitive studies on the detrimental effects of praziquantel in these situations have not been performed.

The mechanism of action of praziquantel against adult worms is not known. Early effects on schistosomes include tetany, membrane depolarization, Ca^{2+} influx and damage of the surface tegument (Andrews, 1985). Recent studies indicate that an intact immune response is necessary for parasite killing by praziquantel (Brindley and Sher, 1990). Praziquantel was significantly less active against schistosomes in immunocompromised hosts than in normal animals. In animals depleted of B cells, parasite killing due to praziquantel was dramatically reduced. This defect could be restored upon adoptive transfer of immune serum. These data suggest that praziquantel exposes parasite antigens which allows killing of adult schistosomes by the host's immune response.

Because of this interaction between schistosome drugs and the host immune system, it is difficult to interpret treatment failure in the individual patient. Occasional individuals fail to be cured by standard doses of praziquantel even on repeated administration and adequate blood concentrations. When schistosome eggs are collected from these individuals and passed through snails into laboratory animals, no change in praziquantel sensitivity was observed. As a result, treatment failures may well represent immunologic host defects rather than the development of drug resistance by the worm. Recent studies have demonstrated, however, that relative resistance to praziquantel can be induced in *Schistosoma mansoni* in the murine model (Fallon and Doenhoff, 1994). It is thus essential that all patients treated with praziquantel have close follow-up in order to assure parasitic cure.

18.10 PREVENTION AND CONTROL

Travelers to schistosome endemic countries should be cautioned against swimming or walking in fresh water. Waterproof footwear is effective protection. The military is currently working on a topical barrier to prevent cercarial penetration but it is not yet commercially available. Many national control programs have focused on the use of praziquantel although Brazil uses oxamniquine (Brindley and Sher, 1990). The strategy of most successful programs is based on annual community surveillance and treatment of positive cases. Snail control is expensive and only marginally effective when used alone (Utroska *et al.*, 1989). As a result, molluscicides are currently used only as an adjunct to community-based chemotherapy in problem areas. When funds are limited, programs generally focus on treatment of school-aged children where the bulk of the morbidity and infection are found. These individuals also represent the major source of environmental contamination in exclusively human schistosome species (*S. mansoni* and *S. haematobium*). Unfortunately, current screening techniques (single stool sample examined by a local medical technician) still miss a significant percentage of the lightly infected population. In addition, even when the prevalence decreases, the cost of screening remains high unless only target populations are used (school-aged children). If the cost of praziquantel could be reduced significantly in the future, mass chemotherapy will probably be the control measure of choice. This will be true particularly if it can be combined with treatment for other intestinal parasites (Anderson and Medley, 1985).

18.11 OTHER SCHISTOSOME SPECIES

18.11.1 *S. MEKONGI*

S. mekongi is a newly described schistosome species found along the Mekong River watershed. It is currently endemic in Cambodia, Viet Nam and Laos. This schistosome species may be found in the USA in patients who have emigrated from south-east Asia (Klumpp and Chu, 1987). It is generally considered to be less pathogenic than *S. japonicum* but severe fibrotic liver disease has been described. The eggs are similar to those of *S. japonicum*. Praziquantel is the drug of choice for treatment.

18.11.2 *S. INTERCALCATUM*

S. intercalcatum is a relatively new species of schistosome found in parts of west and central Africa (Hofstetter *et al.*, 1981). The ova of *S. intercalcatum* are similar to those of *S. haematobium*. Infection with *S. intercalcatum* should be suspected in a patient who has a stool specimen positive for *S. haematobium*. *S. haematobium* eggs can rarely appear in the stool and the ova of the two species can be differentiated morphologically by an expert. Fortunately the urine is generally free of ova in *S. intercalcatum* which can aid in making the diagnosis. The clinical features and pathology of this infection are still unclear but infection can be successfully treated with praziquantel.

REFERENCES

Anderson, R. M. (1987) Determinants of infection in human schistosomiasis, in *Baillière's Clinical Tropical Medicine and Communicable Diseases: Schistosomiasis*, Vol. 2 (ed. A. A. F. Mahmoud), Baillière Tindall, London, pp. 279–300.

Anderson, R. M. and Medley, G. F. (1985) Community control of helminth infections of man by mass and selective chemotherapy. *Parasitology*, **90**, 629–60.

Andrade, Z. A. and Rocha, H. (1979) Schistosomal glomerulopathy. *Kidney Int.*, **16**, 23–9.

Andrews, P. (1985) Praziquantel: mechanisms of antischistosomal activity. *Pharmac. Ther.*, **29**, 129–56.

Andus, T., Bauer, J. and Gerok, W. (1991) Effects of cytokines on the liver. *Hepatology*, **13**, 364–75.

Bilharz, T. (1853) A study on human helminthography, derived from information by letter from Dr. Bilharz in Cairo, along with remarks by Prof. Th. V. Siebold in Breslau. *Zoology*, **4**, 53–71.

Boros, D. L. (1989) Immunopathology of *Schistosoma mansoni* infection. *Clin. Microbiol. Rev.*, **2**, 250–69.

Boros, D. L. and Warren, K. S. (1970) Delayed hypersensitivity granuloma formation and dermal reaction induced and elicited by a soluble factor isolated from *Schistosoma mansoni* eggs. *J. Exp. Med.*, **132**, 488–507.

Brindley, P. J. and Sher, A. (1990) Immunological involvement in the efficacy of Praziquantel. *Exp. Parasit.*, **71**, 245–8.

Butterworth, A. E. (1990) Studies on human schistosomiasis: chemotherapy, immunity and morbidity. *Ann. Parasit. Hum. Comp.*, **65** (suppl. 1), 53–7.

Butterworth, A. E. (1992) Vaccines against schistosomiasis: Where do we stand? *Trans. Roy. Soc. Trop. Med. Hyg.*, **86**, 1–2.

Butterworth, A. E., Corbett, E. L., Dunne, D. W. *et al.* (1989) Immunity and morbidity in human schistosomiasis, in *New Strategies in Parasitology* (ed. K. P. W. J. McAdam), Churchill Livingstone, Edinburgh, pp. 193–216.

Cheever, A. W. and Deb, S. (1989) Persistence of hepatic fibrosis and tissue eggs following treatment of *Schistosomiasis japonicum* infected mice. *Am. J. Trop. Med. Hyg.* **40**, 620–8.

Cheever, A. W., Duvall, R. H., Hallach, T. A., Jr. (1984) Differences in hepatic fibrosis and granuloma size in several strains of mice infected with *Schistosoma japonicum*. *Am. J. Trop. Med. Hyg.* **33**, 602–7.

Cheever, A. W., Kamel, I. A., Elui, A. M. *et al.* (1978) *Schistosoma mansoni* and *S. haematobium* infection in Egypt III: Extrahepatic pathology. *Am. J. Trop. Med. Hyg.*, **27**, 55–75.

Cheever, A. W., Duvall, R. H., Hallak, T. A., Jr *et al.* (1987) Variation of hepatic fibrosis and granuloma size among mouse strains infected with *Schistosoma mansoni*. *Am. J. Trop. Med. Hyg.*, **37**, 85–97.

Colley, D. L. (1981) Immune responses and immunoregulation in experimental and clinical schistosomiasis, in *Parasitic Diseases*, Vol 1 (ed. J.M. Mansfield), Marcel-Dekker, New York, pp. 1–83.

Colley, D. C. (1987) Dynamics of the human immune response to schistosomiasis, in *Clinical Tropical Medicine and Communicable Disease*, Vol 2(2) (ed. A. A. F. Mahmoud), Baillière Tindall, London, 315–32.

Colley, D. L. (1990) Occurrence, roles and uses of idiotypes and anti-idiotypes in parasitic diseases, in *Idiotypic Network and Diseases* (eds J. Cernyad and J. Mierncap), American Society for Microbiology, Washington, DC. pp. 71–95.

Damian, R. T. (1987) Molecular mimicry revisited. *Parasit. Today*, **3**, 263–6.

Doughty, B. L., Ottesen, E. A., Nash, T. E. and Phillips, S. M. (1984) Delayed hypersensitivity granuloma formation around *Schistosoma mansoni* eggs *in vitro*. III. Granuloma formation and modulation in human schistosomiasis mansoni. *J. Immunol.*, **133**, 993–7.

Dunn, M. A. and Kamel, R. (1981) Hepatic schistosomiasis. *Hepatology*, **1**, 653–61.

Fallon., P. G. and Doenhoff, M. J. (1994) Drug-resistant schistosomiasis: resistance to praziquantel and oxaminiquine induced in *Schistosoma mansoni* in mice is drug specific. *Am. J. Trop. Med. Hyg.* **51**(1), 83–8.

Foster, R. (1987) A review of clinical experience with oxamniquine. *Trans. Roy. Soc. Trop. Med.*, **81**, 55–9.

Goes, A. M., Gazzinelli, G., Rocha, R. *et al.* (1991) Granulomatous hypersensitivity to *Schistosoma mansoni* egg antigens in human schistosomiasis III. In vitro granuloma modulation induced by immune complexes. *Am. J. Trop. Med. Hyg.*, **44**, 434–43.

Grysells, B. and Polderman, A. M. (1991) Morbidity due to schistosomiasis mansoni, and its control in Subsaharan Africa. *Parasit. Today*, **7**, 244–9.

Grzych, J. M., Pearce, E., Cheever, A. *et al.* (1991) Egg deposition is the major stimulus for the production of TH2 cytokines in murine schistosomiasis mansoni. *J. Immunol.*, **146**, 1322–7.

Henderson, G. S., Conary, J. T., Summar, M. *et al.* (1991) In vivo molecular analysis of lymph-

okines involved in the murine immune response during Schistosoma mansoni infection. I. IL-4 mRNA, not IL-2 mRNA is abundant in the granulomatous livers and mesenteric lymph nodes of infected mice *J. Immunol.*, **147**, 992–7.

Hofstetter, M., Nash, T. E., Cheever, A. W. *et al.* (1981) Infection with *Schistosoma mekongi* in Southeast Asian Refugees. *J. Inf. Dis.*, **144**, 420–6.

Homeida, M. A., Tom, I. E., Nash, T. and Bennett, J. L. (1991) Association of the therapeutic activity of praziquantel with the reversal of Symmer's fibrosis induced by *Schistosoma mansoni. Am. J. Trop. Med. Hyg.*, **45**, 360–5.

Jourdane, J. and Theron, A. (1987) Larval development: eggs to cercariae, in *The Biology of Schistosomes from Genes to Latrines* (eds D. Rollinson and A. J. B. Simpson), Academic Press, London, pp. 83–106.

Katsurada, F. (1904) The etiology of parasitic disease. *Iji Shinbun*, **669**, 1325–32.

Katz, M., Despommier, D. D. and Gwadz, R. (1982) Schistosomiasis, in *Parasitic Diseases*, Springer–Verlag, New York, NY, pp. 94–105.

King, C. H. and Mahmoud, A. A. F. (1989) Drugs five years later: Praziquantel. *Ann. Int. Med.*, **110**, 290–6.

Klumpp, R. K. and Chu, K. Y. (1987) Focal mollusciciding: an effective way to augment chemotherapy of schistosomiasis. *Parasit. Today* **3**, 74–6.

Kresina, T. F., Quincy, H. D. and Zern, M. A. (1992) Cytokines, hepatic fibrosis and schistosomiasis. *RI Med. J.* **75**, 191–5.

Lechtenberg, R. and Vaida, G. A. (1977) Schistosomiasis of the spinal cord. *Neurology* **27**, 55–9.

Lehman, J. S., Farid, Z., Bassily, S. *et al.* (1970) Intestinal protein loss in schistosomal polyposis of the colon. *Gastroenterology*, **59**, 433–56.

Leiper, R. T. (1918) *Researches on Egyptian Bilharziosis*. John Bale Son and Danielsson, London.

Mahmoud, A. A. F. and Wahab, M. F. A. (1990) Schistosomiasis, in *Tropical and Geographical Medicine* (eds K. S. Warren and A. A. F. Mahmoud), 2nd edn, McGraw-Hill, New York, NY, pp. 458–72.

Majima, T. (1888) A strange case of liver cirrhosis caused by parasite ova. *Tokyo Ig Za*, **2**, 898–901.

Manson, P. (1902) Report of the case of bilharzia from the West Indies. *Br. Med. J.*, **2**, 1894–5.

Mathew, R. C. and Boros, D. L. (1986) Anti L3T4 antibody treatment suppresses hepatic granuloma formation and abrogates antigen-induced interleukin-2 production in *Schistosoma mansoni. Inf. Immun.*, **54**, 820–6.

McGarvey, S. T., Wu, G., Zhang, S., Wang, Y. *et al.* (1993) Child growth nutritional status and schistosomiasis japonica in Jiangxi, China. *Am. J. Trop. Med. Hyg.*, **48**, 547–53.

Miyairi, K. and Suzuki, M. (1914) Der Zwischenwirt der *Schistosomiasis japonicum* Katsurada. *M. Heilunger der Medizinischen FakulM. Heilunger der Medizinischen Fakultat Kalrserchen Universitat Kyusohu*, **1**, 187–97.

Mohamed-Ali, Q., Doehring-Schwerdtferger, E., Abdel-Rahim, I. M. *et al.* (1991) Ultrasonographic investigation of periportal fibrosis in children with *Schistosoma mansoni* infection: reversibility of morbidity seven months after treatment with Praziquantel. *Am. J. Trop. Med. Hyg.*, **44**, 444–51.

Muniz-Junqueira, M. I., Prata, A. and Tosta, C. E. (1992) Phagocyte and bactericidal function of mouse macrophages to *Salmonella typhimurium* in schistosomiasis mansoni. *Am. J. Trop. Med. Hyg.*, **46**, 132–6.

Olds, G. R. (1988) Immunopathology and resistance in helminthic infections, in *Parasitic Infections. Contemporary Issues in Infectious Diseases* (eds J. H. Leech, M. A. Sande, R. K. Root), Churchill Livingstone, New York, pp. 61–80.

Olds, G. R. and Kresina, T. F. (1985) Network interactions in *Schistosoma japonicum* infection. Identification and characterization of a serologically distinct immunoregulatory auto-anti-idiotypic antibody population. *J. Clin. Invest.*, **76**, 2338–47.

Olds, G. R. and Stavitsky, A. B. (1986) Mechanisms of in vivo modulation of granulomatous inflammation in murine schistosomiasis japonicum. *Infect. Immun.*, **52**, 513–18.

Pearce, E. J. and Sher, A. (1987) Mechanisms of immune evasion in schistosomiasis. *Microbiol. Immun.*, **8**, 219–32.

Peters, P. A. S. and Kazura, J. W. (1987) Update on diagnostic methods for schistosomiasis, in *Baillière's Clinical Tropical Medicine and Communicable Disease*, vol. 2(2) (ed. A. A. F. Mahmoud), Baillière Tindall, London, pp. 419–33.

Prakash, S. and Wyler, D. J. (1991) Fibroblast stimulation in schistosomiasis. XI. Purification to apparent homogeneity of fibroblast-stimulating factor-1, an acidic heparin-binding growth factor produced by schistosomal egg granulomas. *J. Immun.*, **146**, 1679–84.

Rocklin, R. E., Brown A. P., Warren K. S. *et al.* (1980) Factors that modify the cellular-immune response in patients infected by *Schistosoma mansoni. J. Immunol.*, **125**, 1916–23.

Sasazuki, T., Ohta, N., Kaneska, R. and Kohina, S. (1980) Association between HLA haplotype and low responsiveness to schistosomal worm antigen in man. *J. Exp. Med.*, **152**, 2148.

Scott, P., Reave, E., Cheever, A. W. *et al.* (1989) Role of cytokines and CD4+ T-cell subsets in the regulation of parasite immunity and disease. *Immun. Rev.*, **112**, 161–82.

Secor, W. E., Steward, S. J. and Colley, D. G. (1990) Eosinophils and immune mechanisms. VI. The synergistic combination of GM-CSF and IL-5 accounts for eosinophil stimulation promoter. *J. Immun.*, **144**, 1484–9.

Shaw, A. F. B. and Ghareeb, A. A. (1968) The pathogenesis of pulmonary schistosomiasis in Egypt with special reference to Ayerza's disease. *J. Path. Bact.*, **46**, 401.

Sher, A., Coffman, R. L., Hienz, S. *et al.* (1990) Interleukin-5 is required for the blood and tissue eosinophilia but not granuloma formation induced by infection with *Schistosoma mansoni*. *Proc. Natl. Acad. Sci. USA*, **87**, 61–5.

Sleigh, A. C., Hoff, R., Mott, K. E. *et al.* (1986) Manson's schistosomiasis in Brazil: 11 year evaluation of successful disease control with oxamniquine. *Lancet*, **i**, 635–7.

Stavitsky, A. B. (1987) Immune regulation in schistosomiasis japonica. *Immun. Today*, **8**, 228–33.

Stephenson, L. S. (1987) *The Impact of Helminth Infections on Human Nutrition*. Taylor and Francis, London.

Stirewalt, M. A. (1974) *Schistosoma mansoni*: cercariae to schistosomula. *Adv. Parasit.*, **12**, 115–82.

Symmers, W. St C. (1903) Note on a new form of liver cirrhosis due to the presence of the ova of bilharzia haematobia. *J. Path. Bact.*, **9**, 237–9.

Utroska, J. A., Chen, M. G., Dixon, H. *et al.* (1989) An estimate of global needs for Praziquantel within schistosomiasis control programs. *WHO/Schisto* 89.102 Riv. **1**, 15.

von Lichtenberg, F. (1987) Consequences of infections with schistosomes, in *The Biology of Schistosomes from Genes to Latrines* (eds D. Rollinson and A. J. B. Simpson), Academic Press, London, pp. 185–232.

Warren, K. S. (1977) Modulation of immunopathology and disease in schistosomiasis. *Am. J. Trop. Med. Hyg.*, **S26**, 113–19.

Warren, K. S. (1982) The secret to the pathogenesis of schistosomiasis: in vivo models. *Immun. Rev.*, **61**, 189–213.

Warren, K. S. (1987) Schistosomiasis japonica. *Clinics Gastroent.*, **7**, 77–85.

Warren, K. S. (1992) A brief history of schistosomiasis. *RI Med. J.*, **75** (176–7).

Warren, K. S., Mahmoud, A. A. F., Cummings, P. *et al.* (1974) Schistosomiasis mansoni in Yemeni in California: Duration of infection, presence of disease, therapeutic management. *Am. J. Trop. Med. Hyg.*, **23**, 902–29.

Wilson, R. A. (1987) Cercariae to liver worms: development and migration in the mammalian host, in *The Biology of Schistosomes from Genes to Latrines* (eds D. Rollinson and A. J. B. Simpson), Academic Press, London, pp. 83–106.

Yamashita, T. and Boros, D. L. (1990) Changing patterns of lymphocyte proliferation, IL-2 production and utilization, and IL-2 receptor expression in mice infected with *Schistosoma mansoni*. *J. Immun.*, **145**, 724–31.

Young, S. W., Higashi, G., Kamal, R. *et al.* (1973) Interaction of salmonellae and schistosomes in host–parasite relations. *Trans. Roy. Soc. Trop. Med. Hyg.*, **67**, 797–802.

NINETEEN

Intestinal helminths – new approaches to diagnosis

D. I. Pritchard, P. J. Tighe
and
E. E. Billett

The diagnosis of human intestinal helminthiases is largely dependent on the accurate identification of ova, larvae or (in the case of some cestodes) proglottids in the evacuated faeces of the infected host (Tables 19.1–3). However, there are problems associated with diagnosis based on the gross morphology of these life-cycle stages, but there have been recent developments which could revolutionize the field of diagnostic metazoan parasitology. Using modern technology, it is already possible to detect some infections in prepatency, and it may soon be possible to identify infections accurately using either immunological or nucleic acid probes, and to determine parasite loads in the infected host. Having said this, experienced field parasitologists will no doubt be tempted to query the necessity for such accuracy in diagnosis, as broad spectrum chemotherapy is equally capable of removing a number of parasite species simultaneously. This is a perfectly valid point, but the following section justifying the requirement for new approaches will be succinct, as we consider it the responsibility of the clinician or researcher to decide on the degree of accuracy of their diagnosis. Instead, this chapter will concentrate on a description of the 'art of the possible', and not necessarily the 'probable'.

19.1 REQUIREMENT FOR NEW TECHNIQUES

New techniques are considered to be desirable for many reasons. The processing of faecal matter for the diagnosis and quantitation of infection is both a laborious and unpleasant task, usually carried out in what would be described by some as relatively primitive conditions (Figure 19.1).

For the *detection* of infection, a known quantity (approximately 1 g) of faeces is normally processed in such a way (e.g. formalin-ether) as to allow the concentration of ova and the detection of light infections. However, multiple inspection is often required and egg excretory patterns can be erratic.

For the accurate *quantitation* of infection, full post-chemotherapy faecal samples are required, to allow worms to be removed by sieving and counted. As with any human population, problems of compliance inevitably arise, especially as chemotherapy is

Enteric Infection 2. Intestinal helminths. Edited by M.J.G. Farthing, G.T. Keusch and D. Wakelin. Published in 1995 by Chapman and Hall, London. ISBN 0 412 39140 6

Table 19.1 Established methods of diagnosis of common intestinal nematodes of man

	A. lumbricoides	*E. vermicularis*	*T. trichiura*	Hookworms (*N. americanus*, *A. duodenale*)	*Stronglyoides stercoralis*
Usual method of diagnosis	Bile-stained, thick-shelled ova (1 cell stage in faeces)	Smooth, thick-shelled egg on perianal skin	Characteristic egg (with mucoid plugs at poles) in faeces	Thin-shelled egg at 4–8 cell stage in faeces	Characteristic L1 larva (short buccal chamber, prominent genital primordium)
Problems with diagnosis	Eggs decorticate; * infertile eggs are inconspicuous and do not float in zinc sulphate	Eggs not seen in faeces	Rarely presents a problem	Eggs of 2 species indistinguishable; may hatch in faeces, larva similar to *S. stercoralis*	Larvae passed sporadically in small numbers
Prospective diagnostic antigens	L2, L3 and adult ES products† Adult cuticular collagen‡			Adult ES products§	Larval ES products‖
Morphology of faecal stage	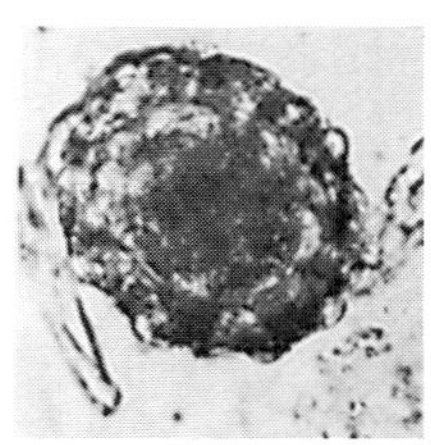	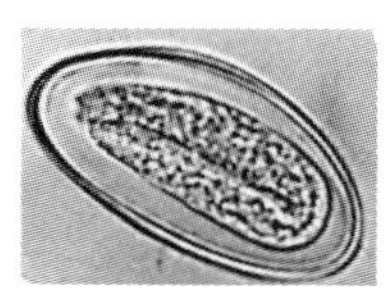	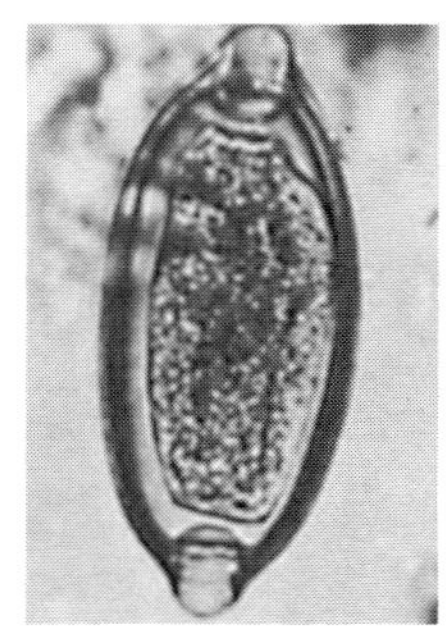	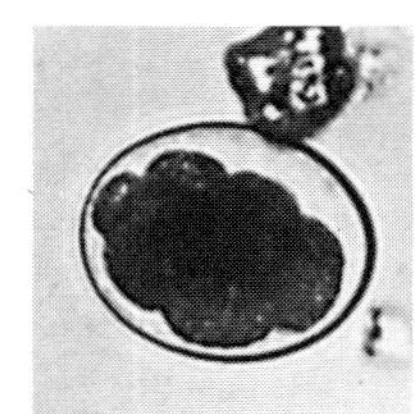	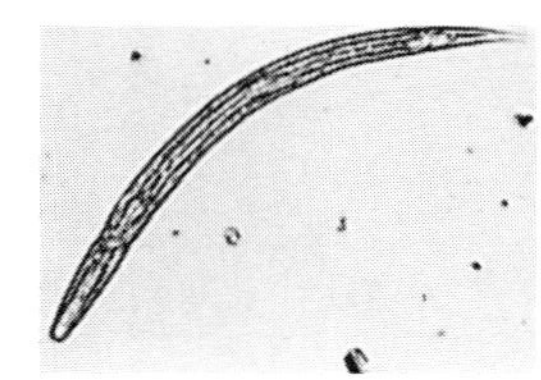

Sources: * Kennedy *et al.* (1987); † Kennedy and Qureshi (1986); ‡ Martin and Pasternak (1986); § Pritchard *et al.* (1990); ‖Carr and Pritchard (1987).

Table 19.2 Established methods of diagnosis of the common intestinal cestodes of man

	Diphylobothrium latum	*Taenia saginata*	*Taenia solium*	*Hymenolepis nana*	*Hymenolepis diminuta*	*Dipylidium caninum*
Usual method of diagnosis	Ovoid, operculate yellow/brown ova in faeces (knob at abopercular end); proglottids passed occasionally	Gravid proglottids in faeces; yellow/brown thick shelled ova with oncosphere may be found in faeces	As for *T. saginata*	Spheroidal, pale thin-shelled eggs in faeces; oncosphere has 2 polar thickenings, with 4–8 filaments	Large, ovoid yellowish, moderately thick-shelled egg in faeces, with oncosphere	Gravid proglottids containing egg clusters
Problems with diagnosis	Ova similar to those of *Paragonimus*	Ova identical to *T. solium*	Ova identical to *T. saginata;* ova less likely to be found in faeces	Ova sometimes confused with *H. diminuta*	Not to be confused with *H. nana;* no polar filaments	Proglottids resemble food particles
Prospective diagnostic antigens		*Taenia*-specific coproantigens; detectable prior to patency*	As for *T. saginata*		*H. diminuta* specific coproantigens†	
Morphology of faecal stage	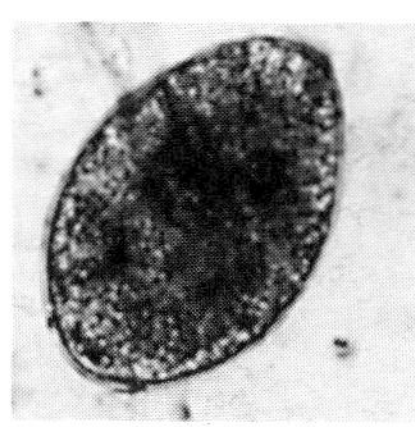	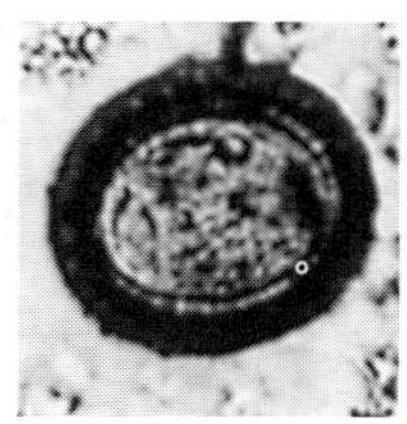	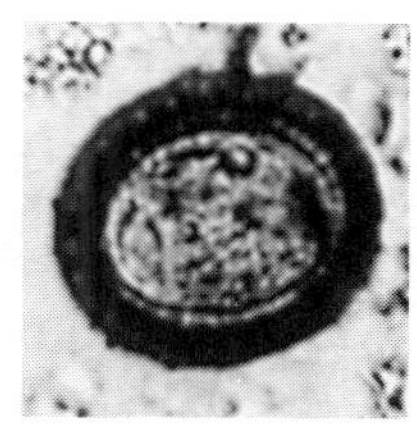	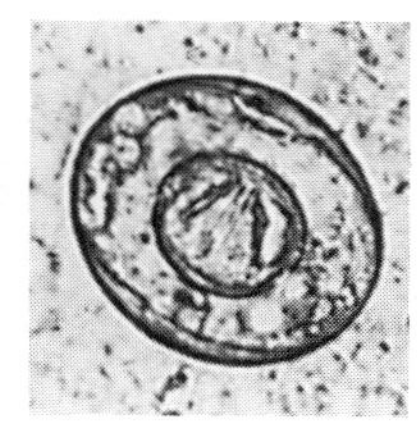	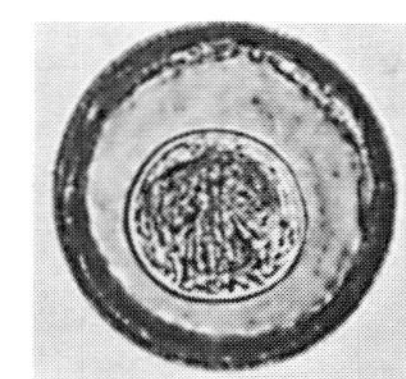	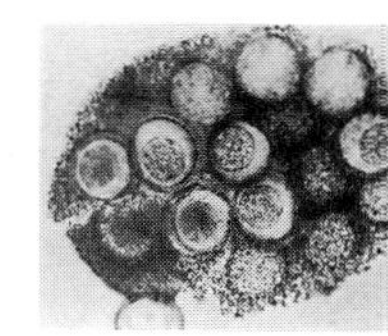

Sources: * Allan *et al.* (1990); † Allan and Craig (1989).

Table 19.3 Established methods of diagnosis of the common intestinal trematodes of man

	Fasciolopsis buski	*Echinostoma ilocanum*	*Heterophyes heterophyes*	*Metagonimus yokogawai*
Usual method of diagnosis	Unembryonated operculated ova	Unembryonated operculated ova	Embryonated operculated ova	Embryonated operculated ova
Problems with diagnosis	The ova of *F. buski*, *E. ilocanum* and *F. hepatica* are similar in size and shape and cannot be easily distinguished. These ova contain an undifferentiated embryo when shed. Ova of *H. heterophyes*, *M. yokogawai* and *O. sinensis* are similarly difficult to differentiate, and contain a fully formed miracidium when shed.			
Morpholoy of a typical trematode ovum (*F. buski*)	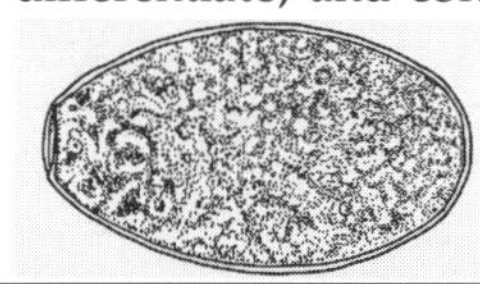			

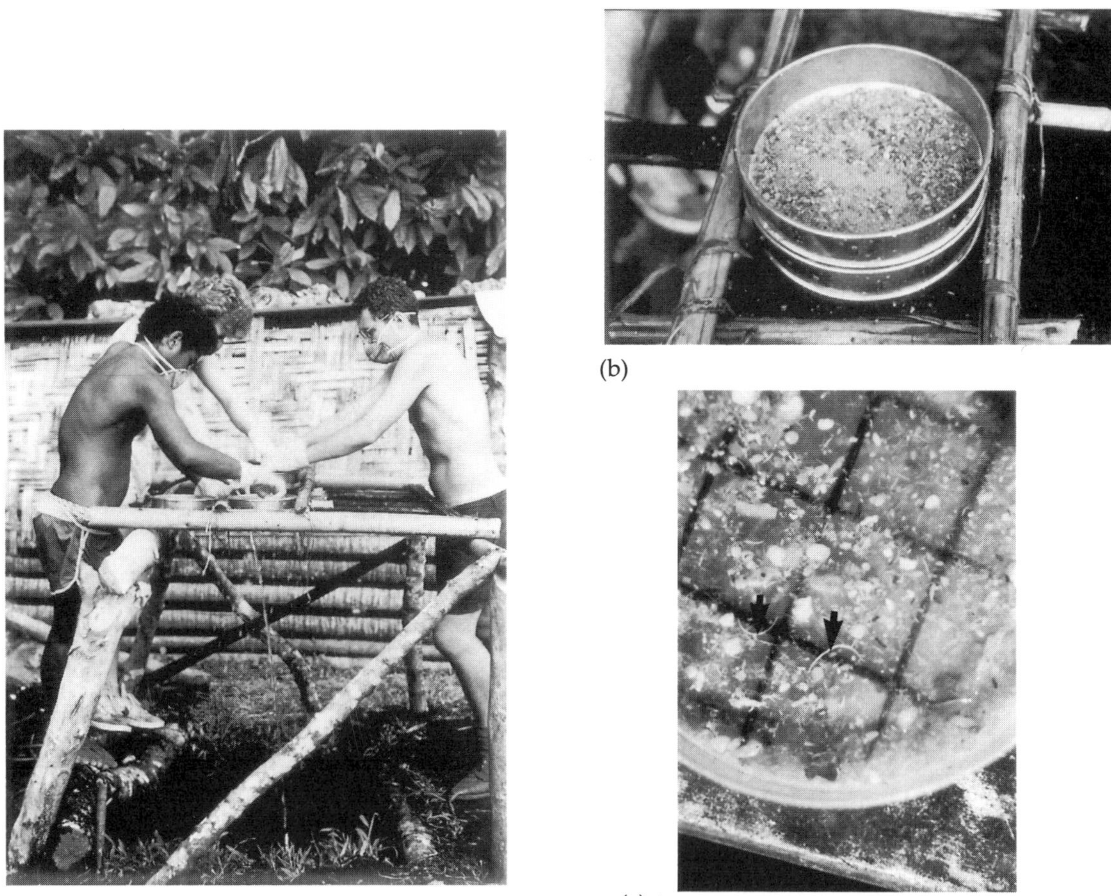

Figure 19.1 The processing of human faecal matter for the diagnosis and quantification of infection. (a) Sieving human faecal (following chemotherapy) matter through a series of graded sieves. (b) Retention of undigested food matter on the upper (coarse) sieve. (c) Recovery of *Necator americanus* from sieved faecal matter. The hookworms are arrowed. (Source: Pritchard *et al.*, 1990.)

usually effective over a protracted time period.

Therefore, new techniques (such as the faecal or coproantigen technique described in section 19.2.1) designed to simplify this procedure would be considered advantageous to the clinical/epidemiologist, particularly if such techniques were able to assess worm burdens, based on a small single sample. This development would also allow the rapid processing of samples. In our experience, with full compliance, the collection and processing of 200 samples for the assessment of eggs per gram (epg) occupies 7 days, while the assessment of the same number of samples for worm burdens occupies 20 days. This is before the samples are even counted (Pritchard *et al.*, 1990).

The *accuracy of detection* could be considered important in situations where the ova of two species are indistinguishable, yet their epidemiology and susceptibility to chemotherapy are distinct. Examples here include taeniasis and hookworm infection.

Many diagnostic techniques currently in use either depend on parasite patency (the detection of ova or larvae), or the presence of circulating antibody. However, each of these parameters has the drawback of an intrinsic lag-phase, and the presence of circulating antibodies would not necessarily be indicative of current infection (due to their protracted half-lives in the blood). Therefore, it would be advantageous in many situations to detect and remove infections before they establish and induce pathology (e.g. in occult toxocariasis and in immunocompromised individuals); it is likely that such methods would be based on the detection of antigen and would have to be very sensitive.

Using currently available techniques, the detection of *light infections* is dependent on the concentration of faeces. As this requires specialized chemicals and equipment, clinicians in underdeveloped countries often resort to the more simple Kato smear. Therefore, a need exists for a relatively simple 'user friendly' technique for the detection of light infections.

Smith (1983) stated that one of the greatest problems in identifying intestinal parasitic infections accurately was the lack of experienced technicians. The development of relatively simple and objective assays would therefore be of great advantage.

New approaches under development fall into two main categories; the detection of *antigens* and the detection of *nucleic acids*. The former category is immunologically based and can be further subdivided into the detection of antigen in faeces (coproantigen), and the detection of circulating antigen in the blood of the infected host. The choice of technique will depend on its sensitivity and specificity for the endemic pathogen population, and on the ease of sampling. For example, the willingness of communities to give blood or faecal samples varies according to local customs and beliefs. (One obvious advantage of techniques based on blood sampling is that you are absolutely sure of the derivation of your sample.)

19.2 IMMUNOLOGICAL TECHNIQUES

19.2.1 THE DETECTION OF FAECAL OR COPROANTIGENS

Powerful immunological techniques to detect small quantities of faecal antigens derived from pathogens were first developed by microbiologists, and used for the diagnosis of, for example, rotavirus in cattle (Ellens and de Leeuw, 1977), the reovirus-like agent of human infantile gastroenteritis (Yolken *et al.*, 1977) and *Clostridium perfringens* Type A (Jackson, Yip Chuck and Brodsky, 1985). This type of approach was soon adopted by parasitologists and used to detect, for example, coproantigens released during infections with the protozoans *Giardia lamblia* (Green, Miles and Warhurst, 1985) and *Entamoeba histolytica* (Baumann and Gottstein, 1987).

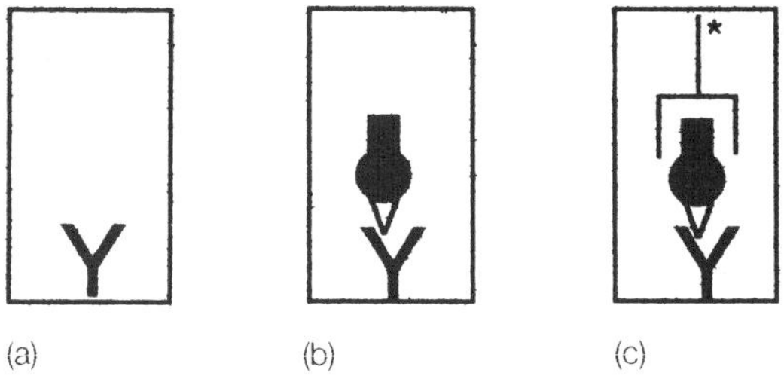

Figure 19.2 Basic format of an antigen-capture ELISA. (a) = Wells of polystyrene ELISA plates are coated with affinity-pure antibody (Y) Free, unbound antibody is washed away. (b) = Uncoated sites are blocked with 50% fetal calf serum (FCS), then the faecal sample added in 50% FCS. Antigen (▽) is captured by the bound antibody. Free, unbound antigen is washed away. (c) = A second epitope on the captured antigen (■) is detected using a labelled (isotope, enzyme, dye) second antibody (⊐—*).

More recently, diagnostic coproantigen detection has been successfully applied to *Taenia hydatigena* infection in dogs. (Deplazes *et al.*, 1990), *Hymenolepis diminuta* infection in rats (Machnicka and Krawczuk, 1988; Allan and Craig, 1989) and *Taenia saginata* and *Taenia solium* infections in humans (Allan *et al.*, 1990).

(a) Methodology

Antigen capture ELISA

The most popular method used to date for the detection of coproantigen has been the antigen capture ELISA technique (Figure 19.2). This technique usually involves the coating of individual wells of a polystyrene ELISA plate with either a monoclonal or affinity-purified polyclonal antibody against the antigen of interest. The plate is then blocked (usually with fetal calf serum), to prevent non-specific interactions, followed by the application of aqueous (phosphate-buffered saline) or detergent (0.3% Tween) extracts of the faecal sample to the plate. Stool samples can be frozen and thawed repeatedly without any diminution in antigen content for *Entamoeba histolytica* (Baumann and Gottstein, 1987), although this observation does not necessarily hold for every antigen preparation. Any antigen binding to the first antibody on the plate is then detectable (following suitable washing steps) using an enzyme-labelled second antibody (which usually binds to an exposed determinant antigenically different from that recognized by the capture antibody) and an appropriate substrate. The degree of antibody binding, dependent on the quantity of bridging antigen, is determined colorimetrically. Because of the highly technical nature of this assay, it might be inappropriate for use in field conditions and suitable adaptations are considered in section 19.2.3.

Specificity and sensitivity

Coproantigen detection is eventually expected to offer both specificity and sensitivity to the field of parasite diagnosis. This prediction is based on the fact that the coproantigen ELISA for *Giardia lamblia* is 98% specific and has 100% sensitivity (microscopy is only successful in 50% of cases) when detecting soluble, non-cyst associated antigen (Green, 1986). This ELISA was sensitive enough to detect 40 ng/ml of trophozoite protein and 25 ng/ml of cyst protein (Green, Miles and Warhurst, 1985). These figures were based on the processing of 1 g of host faeces in 10 ml saline. Therefore, by extrapolation, a minimum of 400 and 250 ng protein/g respectively would have to be present for the detection of faecal antigen.

In comparison, Baumann and Gottstein (1987) detected 400 ng of *Entamoeba histolytica* protein HK9/ml of stool, corresponding to 2000 amoebic trophozoites/ml.

With regard to the metazoa, the levels of sensitivity of detection have been largely recorded in cestode infections. Allan *et al.* (1990), using hyperimmune sera to whole worm extracts, were able to detect 35 ng/ml and 40 ng/ml of *T. solium* and *T. saginata* antigens respectively in human faeces, and prepatent detection was possible in experimental systems. This test was *Taenia*-specific and not species-specific, and the sensitivity of the test per gram of faeces was not recorded.

Allan and Craig (1989) detected 400 ng of *H. diminuta* antigen/ml of faeces, and were able to detect both single worm and prepatent infections. However, cross-reactivity with other cestode species was again seen, and these assays will no doubt now be refined using more specific antisera. It is also of interest to note here that these authors recorded a steep rise in antigen levels at patency (possibly due to increased metabolic activity, a break up of proglottids, or the appearance of ova), and a decrease in antigen concentrations following chemotherapy.

It is possible to extrapolate further from known data to predict the applicability of this technology to other intestinal parasitic infections. For example, we have determined in our laboratories that the human hookworm *Necator americanus* secretes approximately 1 μg/h of soluble antigen into culture medium. In a recent field study in Papua New Guinea, we determined that the mean worm burden in an endemic community was 40 worms/host (Pritchard *et al.*, 1990). Therefore, in the unlikely event that this quantity of antigen is produced by worms *in vivo*, and is evacuated in the faeces in its entirety, one might expect to find an average of 960 μg of antigen in faecal samples every day. As the mean faecal weight for the population was 200 g, each gram of faeces would be expected to contain 4.8 μg of soluble antigen. From the data presented above, this, albeit hypothetical, quantity of antigen would be detectable by antigen capture ELISA.

(b) Problems associated with this approach

The specificity and affinity of the capture antibody

Obviously, an ELISA assay is only as good as the reagents contained therein. Therefore, the capture antibody should be of high affinity, species-specific and directed against exogenous antigens excreted/secreted by the parasite or shed from its surface (Machnika and Krawczuk, 1988). The antibody should be directed against antigens which predominate in faeces, are chemically stable and lack epitopes which could possibly cross-react with antigens expressed by other faecal microflora. It could also be advantageous for the antigen in question to be non-immunogenic to the host, as this would avoid sequestration by components of the host immune system.

Antibody desorption by faecal extracts

Antibody desorption by faecal contents has been a problem experienced by a number of workers in this field (Hanvanich *et al.*, 1985). This problem has now been largely overcome by the addition of fetal calf sera (50%) to the assay (Viscidi *et al.*, 1984); its endogenous ability to inhibit protease activity presumably reduces faecal protease-induced desorption.

19.2.2 THE DETECTION OF CIRCULATING ANTIGEN

As stated above, diagnosis based on the presence of antibodies does not always give an accurate reflection of the state of infection existing at the time of blood sampling. The detection of circulating antigens derived from intestinal parasites therefore offers an alternative and sensitive method for the early diagnosis of infections, and possibly for estimating existing worm burdens.

(a) Methodology

The methodology for the detection of circulating antigen is generically identical to that already described for the detection of coproantigen, in that detection invariably involves the use of some form of antigen capture ELISA. For example, this technique was used to detect circulating *Toxocara canis* (CTA) antigens in dogs (Matsumara *et al.*, 1984) and CTA levels were significantly correlated with worm burdens. Similarly, Robertson *et al.* (1988) observed CTA during human infection, using a two-site assay with the sensitivity to detect 20 ng CTA/ml. The same authors, using an experimental system, demonstrated that CTA was detectable during the first week of infection, but became undetectable following the subsequent appearance of antibody in the circulation. The treatment of sera to disrupt immune complexes resulted in the redetection of antigen.

As a similar approach has also been used to detect circulating antigen in filarial and schistosome infections (Maizels, Denham and Sutarto, 1985; Forsyth *et al.*, 1985; de Jonge *et al.*, 1990; Fu and Carto, 1990), the applicability of this approach for the detection of truly gastrointestinal infections could be predicted, particularly as the sensitivity of the antigen capture assay for *S. mansoni* allows the detection of 1 ng of circulating cathodic antigen (CCA)/ml (de Jonge *et al.*, 1990). Interestingly, a good correlation was found between CCA titres in serum (or urine) and egg secretion.

(b) Problems associated with this approach

As with coproantigen detection, the specificity and affinity of the capture antisera are of paramount importance.

Immune complexes

It is well documented that communities living in areas where intestinal parasites are common are infected from a very early age and, as a consequence, soon develop significant levels of circulating antibodies (Pritchard *et al.*, 1990). Therefore, as it has already been demonstrated that complexed antigen may be undetectable in the circulation (Robertson *et al.*, 1988), it is probable that some form of sample manipulation would have to be performed prior to analysis. However, dissolution of antigen from immune complexes may be complicated. In addition, in immunocompetent individuals, complexed antigen will be removed rapidly from the circulation by the reticuloendothelial system and may not be available for detection.

Availability of circulating antigens

The figures presented above bear testament to the exquisite degree of sensitivity which can be achieved using capture techniques. However, although the most sensitive assay cited was able to detect 1 ng/ml of circulating *S. mansoni* antigen, it must be remembered that this is a systemic parasite, and intestinal parasite antigens, particularly those derived from relatively non-invasive species, may not be expected to gain such unrestricted access to the host circulation. A large proportion of these antigens would be evacuated in the faeces, whilst those gaining systemic access, for example from hookworms, would be largely sequestered by the gut-associated immune system of the host.

19.2.3 ADAPTATION OF EXISTING IMMUNOCHEMICAL TECHNIQUES FOR FIELD USE

Laboratory-based methods will undoubtedly be more sensitive than field-based assays but the benefits of being able to monitor samples at the time of sampling will probably outweigh the advantages of being able to monitor extremely low levels of antigen. For field tests or for regions with low technical infrastructure there exists a choice between direct agglutination assays and sandwich enzyme immunoassays on magnetic spheres or on membranes in the form of 'dip-sticks' The enzyme immunoassays are the more sensitive and straightforward to use and the dip-stick format will probably produce the most suitable 'on-site' assay. As the success of the assay will depend on the availability of antibodies with the appropriate characteristics (high affinity, species-specific) and having antibodies directed to different determinants, the following section will consider the source of antibodies for this purpose. In addition available detection systems and matrices, and currently used dip-stick formats are reviewed.

(a) Source and characteristics of antibodies

Monoclonal antibodies

Monoclonal antibodies have a homogeneous single specificity with defined, constant characteristics and are produced by immortal cells making supplies unlimited. In addition to their specificity and indefinite supply, monoclonal antibodies offer other advantages over polyclonal antibodies, including the following:

- affinity and fine specificity may be selected to suit application;
- availability of antibodies for multiple different and discrete epitopes on a given antigen (pertinent for the sandwich assay);
- rapid equilibration in binding of antigen, important in field assays (Siddle, 1985).

Monoclonal antibodies will thus be used in most of the assays developed in the future. If two monoclonal antibodies, rather than a monoclonal plus a polyclonal, are used in the sandwich approach, the specificity afforded is very high indeed.

The production of monoclonal antibodies is not technically difficult but is relatively demanding in terms of time, effort and money. Detailed accounts of the principles and methods of production can be obtained elsewhere (Mayer and Billett, 1985; Goding, 1986; Liddell and Cryer, 1991).

The two most critical variables that determine the success of hybridoma production are the immunization schedule and the screening method for detecting relevant antibodies. More recently an alternative approach to making monoclonal antibodies has evolved, involving gene technology. The work is being pioneered by Dr Greg Winter and his colleagues at the MRC Laboratory of Molecular Biology, Cambridge (Ward *et al.*, 1989; McCafferty *et al.*, 1990; Winter and Milstein, 1991). Using the polymerase chain reaction, multiple copies of lymphocyte DNA from immunized animals are produced and genes coding for antibody binding sites, the heavy and light chain variable domains, are isolated using primers designed from the sequences of the relatively invariant framework regions. These genes are then expressed in bacteria and the antibody products are screened for binding to antigen. With this approach, antibodies can be made in weeks rather than months.

Multiple monoclonal antibodies

To avoid long incubation times (hours or days) any enhancement in the avidity of the system is helpful. In order to increase the effective avidity of monoclonal-based systems for helminth antigens, two or more antibodies directed at different epitopes of the same antigen could be used for either the capture or the signal antibody in the sandwich assay. Indeed some mixtures of two monoclonal antibodies for different epitopes on a given antigen are known to show cooperativity in that the overall avidity of the mixture is considerably higher than that of the individual antibodies – a phenomenon dependent on antibody bivalency and attributed to the formation of multimeric heterocyclic complexes (Thompson and Jackson, 1984). Thus by the judicious mixing of defined monoclonal antibodies producing reproducible 'oligoclonals' (Siddle, 1985), high avidity reagents may be produced which achieve equilibrium very rapidly within two hours.

Antibody affinity

The affinity of monoclonal antibodies (or more correctly their avidity, if studied under conditions other than a simple bimolecular reaction) is frequently reported as being low, relative to their polyclonal counterparts (Siddle, 1985), although high affinity antibodies appear to have been more commonly reported for protein antigens (Siddle, 1985). This preponderance of low affinity monoclonals in part reflects the distribution of affinities seen *in vivo*, but it must be noted that even in polyclonal antibodies of apparent high avidity ($10^{10} - 10^{12}\,M^{-1}$), the effective antibodies may represent only a small proportion of the total binding activity. Thus it is presumed that, as the number of attempts to produce monoclonals to a given immunogen increases, the incidence with which such high affinity antibodies are recovered will also increase. Prolonging the course of immunizations and/or minimizing the amounts of immunogen used may also improve the frequency with which hybrids that produce high affinity antibodies are obtained (Tijssen, 1985). Of course, combining these procedures with the cloning approach may allow very rapid selection of suitable high affinity antibodies. Finally, the affinity of a single monoclonal antibody has been shown to increase dramatically after the reduction of inter-heavy chain disulphide bonds, a procedure which apparently increases molecular flexibility sufficiently to allow the formation of cyclic complexes of high avidity containing two dimeric antigen molecules and two identical antibody molecules (Jackson, Siddle and Thompson, 1983).

It is now recognized that two-site immunometric (i.e. antigen capture) assays have considerable advantages over competitive immunoassay methods, both in theory and practice (Weeks, Kemp and Woodland, 1981). Thus, sandwich assays offer a wider effective working range with good precision and a linear response for a considerable dose range, which allows single-point calibration for some applications. More importantly, these immunometric methods are capable of lower detection limits given a labelled antibody of sufficiently high activity and low non-specific binding. In theory this level of detection is not limited by the avidity of the labelled antibody as the reaction is favoured by excess reagent conditions. Thus an antibody of a given avidity will detect smaller amounts of antigen in an immunometric than in a competitive format, although it is always an advantage to use the antibody with the highest available avidity for both techniques.

(b) Detection system

The evaluation of assays that generate coloured products can simply be visual or can involve the use of simple colorimeters or reflectance spectrophotometers. Luminescence end-points can also be utilized in enzyme immunoassays and the end-points are extremely sensitive (routinely in the low pmole to fmole range) and involve the oxidation of a luminescent molecule during which light is emitted (Weeks and Woodland, 1988). Chemiluminescent labels, such as luminol and acridinium esters are used rather than bioluminescent ones, due to the lability of the latter. For example, Amersham International uses a peroxidase reagent which, on addition of excess luminescent substrate together with 4-iodophenol, produces a luminescent signal which lasts several minutes. The signal is often detected by a luminometer but, for on-site assays, it is possible to use photographic film as a qualitative recording medium.

(c) Matrices

Cellulose and microcrystalline celluloses have been used to provide concentrations of antibody or antigen that are sufficient to allow immunoreactions to occur in relatively short (<1–2 h) time periods, while maintaining a low level of background signal. They are, however, prone to surface irregularity resulting in a reduction in reproducibility. Modified cellulose, notably nitrocellulose, which has a higher loading capacity and binds macromolecules hydrophobically, has led to the development of dot-blot techniques for protein assays. Similarly, surface modified plastics, such as polylysine coated polystyrene or polyvinyl, have also been used as membranes. Although the load capacity of all these materials is a limiting factor, they appear to be in common use in commercially available dip-stick assays. The introduction of microporous membranes made from plastic or celluloid derivatives (Blankstein and Dorhman, 1985) with complex interior structures which serve dramatically to increase the surface area, has, however, solved the problem of load capacity. Other approaches to the issue of load capacity have utilized highly divided matrix particles of metal colloids (used by Kodak) and colloidal cellulose (used by Hybritech).

(d) Dip-stick formats

For field use, internally referenced end-point assays are the most suitable. Many formats are now available involving either diffusion or capillary migration. Although non-competitive sandwich assays are considered to be the most sensitive, competitive assays involving one antibody are also commercially available. Whatever type of assay is used, it needs to be robust, portable and, if possible, rapid, self-contained and independent of sophisticated instrumentation (Campbell, 1985).

A competitive (heterogeneous) assay involving capillary migration of antigen (essentially an antigen concentration-dependent migration system) through an immobilized antibody matrix was first published by Glad and Grubb (1978), refined by Zuk *et al.* (1985) and subsequently by Chen *et al.* (1987). The principle of the latter version is as follows. The assay strip (microporous membrane, cellulose, etc.) has the monoclonal anti-analyte antibody together with glucose oxidase attached covalently to it. This is immersed in a mixture of sample (or standard analyte) and horseradish peroxidase (HRP) conjugated to analyte. Migration is allowed to continue for about 10 min during which time free and conjugated analyte migrate up the strip in a concentration-dependent fashion: the more free analyte, the higher the extent of its migration. After migration, the strip is developed by immersion in a solution of glucose and a marker dye, for example 4-chloro-1-naphthol, and the coupled glucose oxidase–peroxidase reaction leads to the deposition of a blue-grey insoluble product over the position of the strip occupied by the analyte-HRP conjugate. The assay may be quantified by measuring the height of the coloured zone relative to a series of standards.

The above assay can be further streamlined by adding substrate to the sample-HRP conjugate in the presence of an inhibitor, e.g. ascorbic acid. The inhibitor acts as an internal 'chemical clock', inhibiting HRP during the migration period. By the end of the migration period the ascorbic acid will have been consumed, thus allowing colour development to occur.

A sandwich immunoassay involving radial diffusion chromotography is employed by Kodak in many of its Ektachem immunoassays for drugs. These assays are undertaken on postage stamp-sized layers (forming a 'chip') of membranes coated with finely divided metal oxides onto which reagents are immobilized. The detectable layer is illustrated in Figure 19.3. In these assays radial diffusion chromatography serves to separate antibody-bound antigen from unbound antigen. The initial incubation with sample is followed by a wash with a mixture of buffer

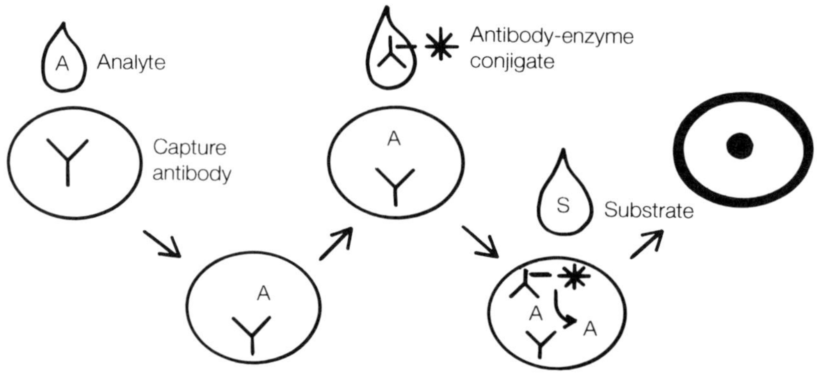

Figure 19.3 Radial diffusion chromatography: sandwich model detection layer (based on the Ektachem assays developed by Kodak). The capture antibody, ≻—, is immobilized at the centre of the detection device. Sample is applied and the analyte, A, allowed to bind. Buffer mixed with a reporting (second) antibody-enzyme conjugate (≻—*) is added next. This washes any unbound analyte to the periphery of the assay membrane. Finally buffer with enzyme substrate, S, is added and the deposition of coloured product at the centre of the membrane is used to quantify analyte.

and a reporting antibody-enzyme conjugate. Finally substrate is added and colour detected. Measurements are usually taken via reflectance spectroscopy (although visual reading is possible). Kodak offers a special portable analyser specifically for this purpose.

These types of assay can be further improved by the incorporation of colour development reagents (dye plus substrates) into the assay strip in microencapsulated forms, colour development being initiated by breaking the capsules. Alternatively the strip could be superimposed with the colour development reagents impregnated into a separate strip. These one-step assays have obvious advantages. The first of its type was launched in the UK by the British biotechnology company Unipath which produced the 'Clear-blue' pregnancy test system now familiar in most chemists. This kit avoids the use of droppers incorporating a hygienic urine sampling device, and measures human chorionic gonadotrophin (hCG). More recently Unipath have launched a 'Clearview' test for *Chlamydia* and hCG. An outline of the principle involved is shown in Figure 19.4.

For all these assays it is important to have an internal reference. The positive could involve an antibody directed against the reporting enzyme or the second antibody in the enzyme-second antibody conjugate or, preferably, a specified level of immobilized analyte. Hybritech for example, market a series of self-contained sandwich assays which contain both a negative control and a calibration reference.

19.3 NUCLEIC ACID TECHNIQUES

In a manner similar to the detection of coproantigens of intestinal parasites, identification of pathogenic organisms in faeces through the use of nucleic acid probes has evolved from the efforts of microbiologists, e.g. the detection of environmental contamination by enteric pathogens (Jain, Burlane and Sayler, 1988) and the identification of rotavirus serotypes from stool samples (Flores *et al.*, 1989). Subsequent adaptation of the technique to protozoan parasites such as *Entamoeba histolytica* (Samuelson *et al.*, 1989) and *Giardia lamblia* (Butcher and Farthing, 1989) indicated how nucleic acid-based systems could allow the sensitive, rapid

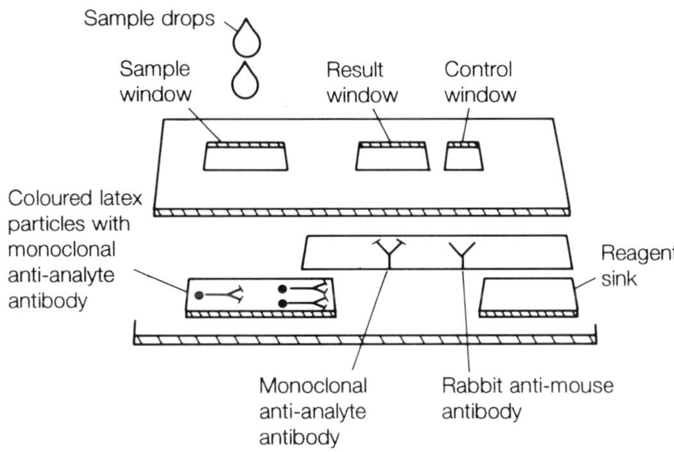

Figure 19.4 Clearview dip-stick sandwich format (based on Unipath's Clearview *Chlamydia* information). The sample pad on the test unit contains dried coloured latex particles sensitized with monoclonal antibodies directed to analyte. The sample pad is in contact with a membrane strip to which two bands of antibodies have been immobilized. The first immobilized zone, the Result Window zone, Control Window zone, contains polyclonal antibodies to mouse immunoglobulin. The upper end of the membrane strip is in contact with an inert pad which acts as a reagent sink. Addition of the sample extract to the sample pad hydrates the latex-labelled antibody. The extract-latex mixture moves chromatographically up the membrane strip to the zone of immobilized monoclonal antibodies to analyte antigen, onwards to the immobilized zone of anti-mouse immunoglobulin antibodies, and then beyond to the end of the strip, where remaining liquid is absorbed by the end of the reagent sink. If analyte antigen is present in the extract it will react with the antibody bound to the latex particles, forming a latex complex. This complex is carried up to the immobilized monoclonal antibodies to analyte antigen, where the antigen–latex complex is captured to form a classical sandwich, giving rise to a line in the Result Window. If analyte antigen is not present in the extract, no sandwich is built up and the Result Window remains clear. In either case, some antibody-sensitized latex is carried onwards to the test control zone, where it is bound by the immobilized zone of antibodies to mouse immunoglobulin, forming a line in the Control Window. The test takes 15 minutes.

detection and identification of intestinal parasites from faecal material. DNA hybridization probes are now available for numerous human parasites and their use has been reviewed by Rishi and McManus (1989). In addition, probes are now being assessed for the cestodes *Echinococcus granulosus* (McManus and Rishi, 1989) and *Taenia solium* (Flisser *et al.*, 1990). However, nematode probes have yet to make an appearance.

Nucleic acid detection methods have recently been improved in terms of assay sensitivity and specificity with the advent of the polymerase chain reaction or PCR (Saiki *et al.*, 1988) and the widespread availability of automated machines to perform this technique. The ability, in theory, specifically to amplify parasite DNA sequences 2^{30}-fold or more, *in vitro*, from a complex mixture, offers a powerful technique to the parasitologist for the accurate and rapid detection of infection. The enthusiasm with which this technique has been received is indicated by both the number of publications implicating PCR as the route of diagnostic detection, e.g. for the cestodes *Taenia saginata* (Gottstein *et al.*, 1991) and *Echinococcus multilocularis* (Gottstein and Mowatt, 1991), and by the number of publications on the detection of blood-borne parasites, which are outside the scope of this article. There are a number of recent reviews of the potential of the technique for diagnosis

(Rishi and McManus, 1989; Wright and Wynford-Thomas, 1990; Barker, 1990; Wilson, 1991).

19.3.1 METHODOLOGY

(a) Direct hybridization techniques

Direct hybridization with a DNA probe was originally all that was available for the molecular parasitologist. The technique involves isolating a parasite-specific cDNA, gene fragment or repetitive DNA sequence from the parasite of interest by standard cloning methods (Maniatis, Fritsch and Sambrook, 1982). This DNA sequence is then labelled, either with ^{32}phosphorus-dNTPs (Feinberg and Vogelstein, 1983) or preferably non-radioactively with biotin (McInnes *et al.*, 1987) or digoxigenin (Boehringer Mannheim). The latter non-radioactive methods are the only practical approach for use in remote areas or for large scale routine use.

A sample of stool is then treated to liberate genomic DNA from the parasite eggs or larvae present within it, by freeze-thawing or by boiling, for the more robust species, e.g. the cysts of *E. histolytica* (Samuelson *et al.*, 1989). There may also be a requirement for initial parasite concentration, protease/detergent treatment or sonication of the sample, depending on the parasite in question. A portion of each sample is then denatured with sodium hydroxide, applied to a nylon or nitrocellulose filter, and the filter probed with the labelled DNA in a standard DNA hybridization at a suitable temperature. After washing, probe DNA which has hybridized with filter-bound parasite DNA is detected either by autoradiography (if radiolabelled) or colorimetrically through the use of an enzyme-linked reporter system to detect the non-isotopic 'tag' on the probe, e.g. streptavidin or anti-digoxigenin conjugated to alkaline phosphatase.

(b) Amplification of parasite DNA by PCR

If DNA sequence information is available for specific parasite genes it is possible to have two synthetic oligonucleotides constructed, which hybridize to opposite strands and flank a region of the known DNA (100–2000 nucleotides). These oligonucleotide primers can be used to amplify the intervening region of DNA via the technique called the polymerase chain reaction (PCR) (Saiki *et al.*, 1988). For our purposes, PCR potentially offers a direct route to the development of sensitive, reproducible and transportable techniques.

The preparation of parasite DNA is essentially similar to that described above. However, additional purification of DNA in the resulting sample may be necessary as faecal contaminants may completely inhibit the amplification of specific DNA. Amplification of a target DNA sequence is performed on a small portion of the sample, determined empirically depending on the known range of parasite concentrations present in faecal samples. Briefly, 50–100 μl reactions containing the template (stool sample DNA), two oligonucleotide primers, dNTPs, an optimized buffer and a thermostable DNA polymerase, are cycled 25–40 times in an automated thermocycler, through a denaturation step (~94°C) and an annealing step (50–70°C), depending on the oligonucleotide melting temperatures required for specific hybridizations to occur, and a polymerization step (72°C) where the polymerase extends from each hybridized oligonucleotide 3′ end to generate new copies of the target sequence. Figure 19.5 shows the process graphically. Since the primers are extended along the DNA sequence towards the other priming site, new targets to which the primers can anneal are generated with each cycle, resulting in exponential amplification of the target sequence. Amplification products of a known size are then visualized by the simple process of agarose gel electrophor-

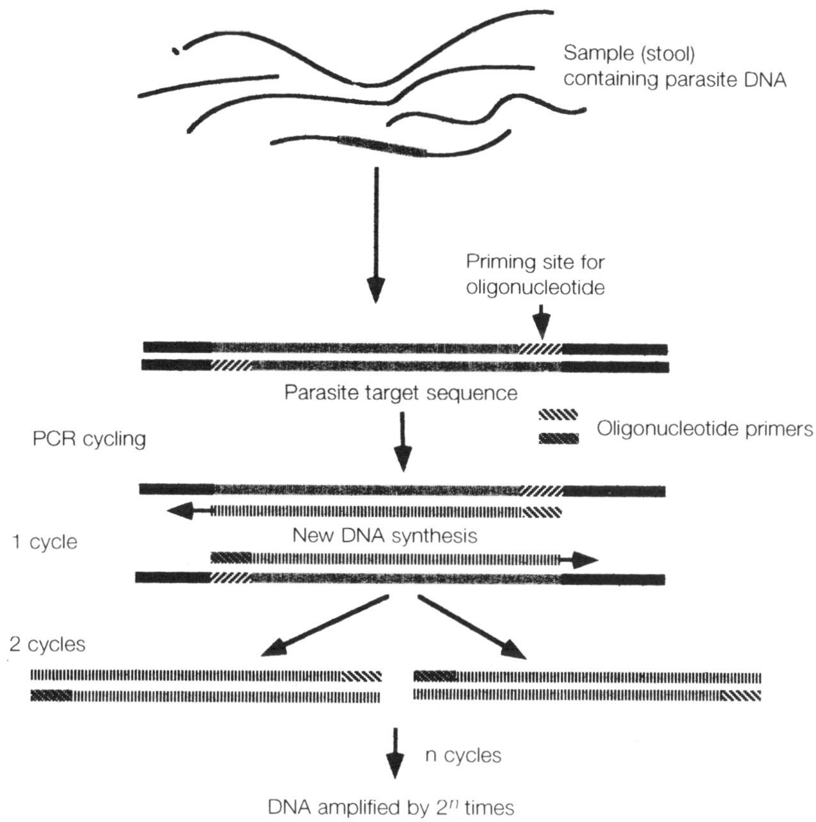

Figure 19.5 Basic polymerase chain reaction.

esis of the PCR reaction. Presence or absence of a DNA band of the correct size can be taken as an assessment of parasitological status.

Whilst the technology to perform this reaction is complex, it is possible to pre-optimize the procedure so that a technician unfamiliar with the technique is perfectly capable of processing the samples and using essentially a kit and an automated thermocycler to obtain satisfactory results.

19.3.2 SPECIFICITY AND SENSITIVITY OF NUCLEIC ACID TECHNIQUES AND PROBLEMS ASSOCIATED WITH THIS TECHNOLOGY

Detection of parasite DNA in faeces offers a high degree of sensitivity and specificity of detection, and it overcomes the problems of distinguishing species which might easily be confused by microscopic examination of eggs or larvae and may allow simultaneous strain differentiation important for epidemiological studies, given that suitable strain-dependent probe sequences are available. The use of DNA hybridization probes for the filarial parasite *Onchocerca volvulus*, for example, indicates the sensitivity and specific diagnostic potential of the technique, detecting DNA equivalent to that present in one tenth of a larva (about 100 pg of DNA; Shah *et al.*, 1987).

For faecal diagnosis, work with intestinal parasites such *Entamoeba histolytica* show that hybridization to faecally derived DNA can yield excellent results, with sensitivities in the range of 8 parasite cysts/g of faeces, and a specificity greater than that of currently used ELISA techniques (Samuelson *et al.*, 1989).

The sensitivity of the probes is paramount to the success of the technique and repetitive DNA sequences were used in both of the cases cited above, ensuring a maximal amount of target sequence (thousands of copies per parasite genome), and one could not expect the same sort of sensitivity with single copy gene probes.

With regard to the use of PCR techniques for faecal diagnosis of intestinal parasites, the polymerase chain reaction is quite capable of amplifying DNA from a single parasite egg to sufficient levels to visualize by gel electrophoresis (Gottstein *et al.*, 1991). However, the requirement for specific primers and suitable reaction conditions to avoid primer annealing to undesirable DNA, means that prior knowledge of the parasites' DNA has to be obtained. Also, the degree of contamination of the prepared sample could be problematic as this may affect the efficiency of PCR by interfering with the enzymic reaction, rather than with the annealing of primer and template.

If contaminants from faeces require extensive methods of removal, such as time-consuming DNA preparations, then the technique, whilst offering the ultimate in sensitivity, may be used for analytical and not large-scale clinical use. In addition, of the two techniques discussed here, PCR is by far the more expensive to operate routinely, and whilst both methods of detection are technically demanding, DNA hybridization offers the least complex of the two routes of diagnosis, especially with the development of non-isotopically labelled probes and colorimetric development which remove the dangers and time-span limitations of their radiolabelled counterparts.

19.3.3 ADAPTATION OF EXISTING TECHNIQUES FOR FIELD USE

Molecular techniques are obviously heavily reliant on good laboratory facilities. However, it is possible to perform at least some of the diagnostic techniques mentioned above in 'field' conditions. For instance, hybridization techniques require little more than pre-made solutions, appropriate DNA isolation techniques and small incubators for temperature control. Providing non-radioactive probes are used there should be few problems in the use of this approach; the problems which are present relate to the availability of suitable probe sequences, and whether on-site analysis is really worth the effort of setting up a field laboratory and processing samples under often difficult conditions.

The same general problems apply to the use of PCR as a diagnostic tool, but other difficulties arise. Whilst small, Peltier element driven thermocyclers, which will operate irrespective of water supplies as coolant and using a portable generator for power, are commonly available, the ancillary reagents (Taq polymerase, dNTPs, oligonucleotides, etc.) require careful handling to avoid failure due to improper storage. More importantly, extreme care is required to avoid false positive results due to contamination of stock solutions. At the very least, these techniques require rooms free from general environmental contamination, such as found in local community hospitals in many areas. In addition to the problems associated with PCR itself, the requirement of relatively clean DNA for PCR, with associated time-consuming preparation, would preclude PCR techniques from use in immediate analysis of samples during short-term field studies but possibly not for more longitudinal studies, where time may be available, and where loss of unaccompanied samples during transport home for analysis is entirely possible!

ACKNOWLEDGEMENTS

The authors would like to thank the following for their expert advice: Drs Jim Allan and Phil Craig of The Liverpool School of Tropical Medicine, and Drs Amanda Goldin and Michael Miles of The London School of Hygiene and Tropical Medicine. The authors' own work is supported by the Wellcome Trust.

REFERENCES

Allan, J. C. and Craig, P. S. (1989) Coproantigen in gut tapeworm infections: *Hymenolepis diminuta* in rats. *Parasit. Res.*, **76**, 68–73.

Allan, J. C., Avila, G., Garcia Noval, J. *et al.* (1990) Immunodiagnosis of taeniasis by coproantigen detection. *Parasitology*, **101**, 473–7.

Barker, R. H. Jr (1990) DNA probe diagnosis of parasitic infections. *Exp. Parasit.*, **70**, 494–9.

Baumann, D. and Gottstein, B. (1987) A double-antibody sandwich ELISA for the detection of *Entamoeba histolytica* antigen in stool samples of humans. *Trop. Med. Parasit.*, **38**, 81–5.

Blankstein, L. A. and Dorhman, L. (1985) An advanced affinity membrane for immunodiagnostic tests. *Amer. Clin. Prod. Rev.*, **4**, 33–41.

Butcher, P. D. and Farthing, M. J. G. (1989) DNA probes for the fecal diagnosis of *Giardia lamblia* infections in man. *Trans. Biochem. Soc.*, **17**, 363–4.

Campbell, K. L. (1985) Solid state assays: reagents and film technology for dip-stick assays, in *Non-radiometric Assays: Technology and Application in Polypeptide and Steroid Hormone Detection* (eds B. D. Albertson and F. P. Haselture), Alan R. Liss, New York, pp. 237–87.

Carr, A. and Pritchard D. I. (1987) Antigen expression during the development of the human hookworm *Necator americanus* (Nematoda). *Parasite Immun.*, **9**, 219–34.

Chen, R., Li, T. M., Merrick, H. *et al.* (1987) Use of an internal clock reaction to provide a one-step, visual enzyme immunochromatographic assay for theophylline in whole blood. *Clin. Chem.*, **33**, 1521–5.

de Jonge, N., Kremsner, P. G., Krijger, F. W. *et al.* (1990) Detection of the schistosome circulating cathodic antigen by enzyme immunoassay using biotinylated monoclonal antibodies. *Trans. Roy. Soc. Trop. Med. Hyg.*, **84**, 815–18.

Deplazes, P., Gottstein, B., Stingelin, Y. and Eckert, J. (1990) Detection of *Taenia hydatigena* copro-antigens by ELISA in dogs. *Vet. Parasit.*, **36**, 91–103.

Ellens, D. J. and de Leeuw, P. W. (1977) Enzyme-linked immunosorbent assay for the diagnosis of Rotavirus infections in calves. *J. Clin. Microbiol.*, **6**, 530–2.

Feinberg, A. P. and Vogelstein, B. (1983) A technique for the radiolabelling of restriction endonuclease fragments to high specific activity. *Anal. Biochem.*, **132**, 6–13.

Flisser, A., Plancarte, A., Correa, D. *et al.* (1990) New approaches in the diagnosis of *Taenia solium* cystercercosis and taeniasis. *Ann. Parasit. Hum. Comp.*, **65**, 95–8.

Flores, J., Green, K., Garcia, D. *et al.* (1989) Dot hybridization assay for distinction of rotavirus serotypes. *J. Clin. Microbiol.*, **27**, 29–34.

Forsyth, K. P., Spark, R., Kazura, J. *et al.* (1985) A monoclonal antibody-based immunoradiometric assay for detection of circulating antigen in Bancroftian filariasis. *J. Immun.*, **134**, 1172–7.

Fu, C. and Carter, C. E. (1990) Detection of circulating antigen in human schistosomiasis japonica using a monoclonal antibody. *Am. J. Trop. Med. Hyg.*, **42**, 347–51.

Glad, C. and Grubb, A. O. (1978) Immunocapillary migration – a new method for immunochemical quantitation. *Anal. Biochem.*, **85**, 180–7.

Goding, J. W. (1986) *Monoclonal Antibodies: Principles and Practice*, Academic Press.

Gottstein, B. and Mowatt, M. R. (1991) Sequencing and characterisation of an *Echinococcus multilocularis* DNA probe and its use in the polymerase-chain reaction. *Mol. Biochem. Parasit.*, **44**, 183–94.

Gottstein, B., Deplazes, P., Tanner, I. and Skaggs, J. S. (1991) Diagnostic identification of *Taenia saginata* with the polymerase chain reaction. *Trans. Roy. Soc. Trop. Med. Hyg.*, **85**, 248–9.

Green, E. L. (1986) Immunological detection of parasite antigen in faeces. *Parasitol. Today*, **2**, 198–200.

Green, E. L., Miles, M. A. and Warhurst, D. C. (1985) Immunodiagnostic detection of Giardia antigen in faeces by rapid visual enzyme-linked immunosorbent assay. *Lancet*, (September 28), 691–4.

Hanvanich, M., Viscidi, R., Laughon, B. E. *et al.* (1985) Stool desorbing activity: a possible cause of false positive reactions in competitive enzyme immunoassays. *J. Clin. Microbiol.*, **21**, 184–8.

Jackson, A. P., Siddle, K. and Thompson, R. J. (1983) A monoclonal antibody to human brain-type creatine kinase: increased avidity with mercaptans. *Biochem. J.*, **215**, 505–12.

Jackson, S. G., Yip Chuck, D. A. and Brodsky, M. H. (1985). A double antibody sandwich enzyme immunoassay for *Clostridium perfringens* Type A enterotoxin detection in stool specimens. *J. Immun. Methods*, **83**, 141–50.

Jain, R. K., Burlane, R. S. and Sayler, G. S. (1988) Methods for detecting recombinant DNA in the environment. *Crit. Rev. Biotechnol.*, **8**, 33–84.

Kennedy, M. W. and Qureshi F. (1986) Stage-specific secreted antigens of the parasitic larval stages of the nematode *Ascaris*. *Immunology*, **58**, 515–22.

Kennedy, M. W., Qureshi, F., Haswell–Elkins, M. and Elkins, D. B. (1987) Homology and heterology between the secreted antigens of the parasitic larval stages of *Ascaris lumbricoides* and *Ascaris suum*. *Clin. Exp. Immun.*, **67**, 20–30.

Liddell, J. E. and Cryer, A. (1991) *A Practical Guide to Monoclonal Antibodies*, Wiley and Sons, Chichester, UK.

McCafferty, J., Griffiths, A. D., Winter, G. and Chiswell, D. J. (1990). Phage antibodies: filamentous phage displaying antibody variable domains. *Nature*, **348**, 552–4.

Machnicka, B. and Krawczuk, S. (1988) *Hymenolepis diminuta* antigen: detection in faeces of rats. *Bull. Polish Acad. Sci. Biol. Sci.*, **36**, 103–6.

McInnes, J. L., Dalton, S., Vize, P. D. and Robins, A. J. (1987) Non-radioactive photobiotin-labelled probes detect single copy genes and low abundance messenger RNA. *Biotechnology*, **5**, 269–72.

McManus, D. P. and Rishi, A. K. (1989) Genetic heterogeneity within *Echinococcus granulosus*: isolates from different hosts and geographical areas characterised with DNA probes. *Parasitology*, **99**, 17–20.

Maizels, R. M., Denham, D. and Sutanto, I. (1985) Secreted and circulating antigens of the filarial parasite *Brugia pahangi*: analysis of *in vitro* released components and detection of parasite-derived products *in vivo*. *Mol. Biochem. Parasit.*, **17**, 277–88.

Maniatis, T., Fritsch, E. F. and Sambrook, J. (1982) *Molecular Cloning*: a *Laboratory Manual*, Cold Spring Harbor Laboratory Press, New York.

Martin, L. H. and Pasternak, J. J. (1986) *Ascaris lumbricoides*: monoclonal antibodies against the major cuticular collagen. *Exp. Parisit.*, **61**, 281–3.

Matsumara, K., Kazuta, Y., Endo, R. and Taraka, K. (1984) Detection of circulating toxocaral antigens in dogs by sandwich enzyme immunoassay. *Immunology*, **51**, 609–21.

Mayer, R. J. and Billett, E. E. (1985) Techniques in the production and application of monoclonal antibodies, in *Techniques in Life Science*, B1/11, (Suppl.) *Protein and Enzyme Biochemistry*, BS 111, Elsevier/North Holland Scientific Publishers Ltd, pp. 1–55.

Pritchard, D. I., McKean, P. G. and Schad, G. A. (1990) An immunological and biochemical comparison of hookworm species. *Parasit. Today*, **6**, 154–6.

Pritchard, D. I., Quinnell, R. J., Slater, A. F. G. *et al.* (1990) Epidemiology and immunology of *Necator americanus* infection in a community in Papua New Guinea: humoral responses to excretory – secretory and cuticular collagen antigens. *Parasitology*, **100**, 317–26.

Rishi, A. K. and McManus, D. P. (1989) DNA probes for the detection of human parasites. *Curr. Sci.*, **58**, 103–11.

Robertson, B. D., Burkot, T. R., Gillespie, S. H. *et al.* (1988) Detecting circulating parasite antigen and specific antibody in *Toxocara canis* infections. *Clin. Expl. Immunol.*, **74**, 236–41.

Saiki, R., Gelfand, D. H., Stoffel, S. *et al.* (1988) Primer-directed enzymatic amplification of DNA with a thermostable DNA polymerase. *Science*, **239**, 487–91.

Samuelson, J., Acuna-Soto, R., Reed, S. *et al.* (1989) DNA hybridization probe for clinical diagnosis of *Entamoeba histolytica*. *J. Clin. Microbiol.*, **27**, 671–6.

Shah, J., Karam, M., Piessens, W. F. and Wirth, D. F. (1987) Characterization of an *Onchocerca*-specific DNA clone from *Onchocerca volvulus*. *Am. J. Trop. Med. Hyg.*, **37**, 376–84.

Siddle, K. (1985) Properties and applications of monoclonal antibodies, in *Alternative Immunoassays* (ed. W. P. Collins) Wiley and Sons, Chichester, UK, pp. 13–37.

Smith, J. W. (1983) Identification of fecal parasites in the special parasitology survey of the college of American pathologists. *Am. J. Clin. Pathol.*, **80**, 858–60.

Thompson, R. J. and Jackson, A. P. (1984) Cyclic complexes and high avidity antibodies. *Trends Biochem. Sci.*, **9**, 1–3.

Tijssen, P. (1985) *Practice and Theory of Enzyme Immunossays*. Elsevier Science Publications BV (Biomedical Division), N. Y.

Viscidi, R., Laughon, B. E., Hanvanich, M. and Bartlett, R. H. (1984) Improved enzyme immunoassays for the detection of antigens in fecal specimens. Investigation and correction of interfering factors. *J. Immun. Methods*, **67**, 129–43.

Ward, E. S., Güssow, D., Griffiths, A. O. *et al.* (1989) Binding activities of a repertoire of single immunoglobulin variable domains secreted from *Escherichia coli*. *Nature*, **341**, 544–6.

Weeks, I. and Woodland, J. S. (1988) Chemiluminescence immunoassays, in *ELISA, and Other Solid Phase Immunoassays* (eds D. M. Kemeny and S. J. Challacombe), Wiley and Sons, pp. 265–78.

Weeks, I., Kemp, H. A. and Woodland, J. S. (1981) Two-site assay of human-fetoprotein using 125-I labelled monoclonal antibodies. *Biosci. Reports*, **1**, 785–91.

Wilson, S. M. (1991) Nucleic acid techniques and the detection of parasitic diseases. *Parasit. Today*, **7**, 255–9.

Winter, G. and Milstein, C. (1991) Man-made antibodies. *Nature*, **349**, 293–9.

Wright, P A. and Wynford-Thomas, D. (1990) The polymerase-chain reaction, miracle or mirage? A critical review of its uses and limitations in diagnostic research. *J. Path.*, **162**, 99–117.

Yolken, R. H., Kim, H. W., Clem, T. *et al.* (1977) Enzyme-linked immunosorbent assay (ELISA) for the detection of human reovirus-like agent of infantile gastroenteritis. *Lancet*, **ii**, 263–6.

Zuk, R. J., Ginsberg, U. K., Houts, T. *et al.* (1985) Enzyme immunochromatography – a quantitative immunoassay requiring no instrumentation. *Clin. Chem.*, **31**, 1144–50.

TWENTY

Principles of anthelmintic chemotherapy

H. Vanden Bossche

20.1 HISTORICAL ASPECTS

Since ancient times men have tried to rid themselves of worms. The Egyptian papyrus (Papyrus Ebers, also called Papyrus Leipzig), dating from about 1550 BC, and discovered by Georg Moritz Ebers in 1872, prescribed infusion of the bark or roots of the pomegranate tree (*Pucinia granatum* L.) (Ghalioungui, 1983) for the evacuation of a worm, probably the beef tapeworm, *Taenia saginata*.

Powdered rhizomes of *Dryopteris filix-mas* (male fern) and extracts of the plants have been used for millenia (Rüneberg, 1963). The efficacy of the extracts against tapeworm infections had already been recorded by Theophrastus of Eresus some 2300 years ago (Grove, 1990). The dried rhizome is called aspidium. For several decades oil of aspidium was the standard preparation against the tapeworm *Diphyllobothrium latum* (Bylund, Bång and Wikgren, 1977).

One of China's most successful remedies comes from ground pumpkin seeds. Their taeniafugal properties have been known for centuries and in Mexico minced seeds from *Cucurbita pepo* (calabazas) have been used in the treatment of *Ascaris* and *Taenia* (Maximo Martinez, 1969).

In the USA, *Chenopodium ambrosioides* var. *anthelminticum* (American wormseed plant) is a common plant from which the extracted oil is highly toxic for *Ascaris* and hookworm. This plant was introduced into Europe in 1723 (Grove, 1990). The active constituent, a terpenic peroxide, ascaridole (1-methyl-4-(1-methylethyl)-2, 3-di-oxabicyclo [2.2.2.] oct-5-ene), causes *in vitro* first a rise in muscle tone, then paralysis and death of *Ascaris* (Goodwin, 1958; Cavier, 1973). Chenopodium oil can be administered together with tetrachloroethylene in castor oil (Janssens, 1985). Although it is an effective ascaricide it is no longer used because of its marked action on the human nervous and gastrointestinal systems (del Castillo, 1969).

Berries from *Diospyros mollis* (Maklua), crushed to pulp while still green, show activity against hookworm. The anthelmintic activity originates from diospyrol (1, 1′, 8, 8′-tetrahydroxy-6, 6′-dimethyl-2, 2′-binaphthalene) (Sen *et al.*, 1974).

Semen-contra-vermes consists of the dried flower heads of *Artemisia cina*. It had already been mentioned in the first century AD as being indicated for the treatment of ascariasis and enterobiasis (Grove, 1990). The active principle is santonine, a sesquiterpene lactone (del Castillo, 1969). Goodwin (1958) suggested that santonine interferes with the coordinating nerve impulses which originate at the main nerve ring of *Ascaris*. However, it

Enteric Infection 2. Intestinal helminths. Edited by M.J.G. Farthing, G.T. Keusch and D. Wakelin. Published in 1995 by Chapman and Hall, London. ISBN 0 412 39140 6

also affects the mammalian nervous system. Therefore, the drug was abandoned as soon as less toxic anthelmintics became available.

These and other traditional drugs are merely of historical interest and cannot match the 'modern' anthelmintics in efficacy and selectivity. However, their active principles and mode of action can still be of help in the search for new tools to control parasitic infections.

It is the aim of this chapter to discuss the properties of the presently available anthelmintics of use in the treatment of gastrointestinal nematodiasis, intestinal tapeworm infections and intestinal trematodiasis. More details on the anthelmintics discussed here can be found in the following reviews and books: Davis, 1973; Stürchler, 1982; Vanden Bossche, Rochette and Hörig, 1982; Vanden Bossche, Thienport and Janssens, 1985; Vanden Bossche, 1978, 1985, 1990; Campbell and Rew, 1986; WHO, 1990.

20.2 CHEMOTHERAPY OF GASTROINTESTINAL NEMATODIASIS

The well used piperazine and its different salts are still good standard drugs against ascariasis and have been for a long time the standard treatment for *Enterobius vermicularis* (Janssens, 1985). In low-income countries it is still the cheapest anthelmintic available. Therefore, a summary of piperazine's properties is included. Pyrvinium pamoate is used only in the treatment of *E. vermicularis* infections. However, it has been replaced by the newer anthelmintics.

The era of broad-spectrum and orally active antinematodal agents started in 1961 with the introduction of the benzimidazole derivative thiabendazole (Brown *et al.*, 1961). Thiabendazole was the beginning of a long list of potent benzimidazoles of which albendazole, mebendazole and flubendazole are used in the treatment of intestinal human nematode infections. In 1966, the imidazothiazoles, tetramisole and levamisole were introduced (Thienpont *et al.*, 1966). The modern armamentarium of human medicine also contains pyrantel, oxantel and bephenium hydroxynaphthoate. The latter has been used mainly in the treatment of infections with *Ancylostoma duodenale*. Its clinical use has been extensively reviewed by Davis (1973) and Janssens (1985). Considering that there are more potent and better-tolerated broad-spectrum anthelmintics available, the use of bephenium hydroxynaphthoate will decline (Botero, 1986). Therefore, it will not be included in this overview.

Table 20.1 summarizes the doses used.

20.2.1 PIPERAZINE SALTS

The diethyldiamine or hexahydropyrazine is an alkaline crystalline compound which has been used since the end of the nineteenth century against gout. The story of the discovery of piperazine's anthelmintic activity has been described by Goodwin (1980): M. Boismare, a pharmacist of Rouen, made the observations that the citizens of Rouen after taking his piperazine preparation for their gout, had on occasion delivered themselves of roundworms in their stools.

Now, piperazine is available as an adipate, citrate, phosphate and tartrate. Their properties have been discussed in excellent survey articles (e.g. Davis, 1973; Cavier, 1973; Janssens, 1985).

(a) Pharmacological properties

Piperazine is readily absorbed from the gastrointestinal tract: in 24 h, about 30% of the dose is excreted unchanged via the urine. After administration of piperazine syrup (480 mg) to four fasting, healthy, non-smoking, male volunteers, 0.36–0.59 μg/ml of *N*-mononitrosopiperazine (a carcinogen) were found in the gastric fluid (Bellander,

Hagmar and Österdahl, 1981). However, the yield of *N*-mononitrosopiperazine is much lower than the dose demonstrated to be carcinogenic in rats on long-term administration of *N*-mononitrosopiperazine in the drinking water (50 and 200 mg/l) (Garcia, Keefer and Lijinsky, 1970).

Piperazine initiated important studies on the neuromuscular system of *Ascaris* (for reviews see Vanden Bossche, 1985; Martin, 1987). It has been shown that piperazine acts as an agonist at the extrasynaptic GABA receptor on *Ascaris* muscle. This increases the conductance of the membrane to chloride ions and hyperpolarizes muscle cells, with accompanying paralysis. Piperazine does not act on rat sympathetic neurons.

(b) Spectrum of activity and dosage

In man, the efficacy of this inexpensive drug is limited to the cosmopolitan worms, *Ascaris lumbricoides* and *Enterobius vermicularis* (pinworm). Piperazine salts are available as tablets containing 500 mg and as syrups containing 100 mg/ml, calculated as the hexahydrate.

Piperazine preparations are always taken orally. In ascariasis the single-dose treatment is 75 mg/kg (Janssens, 1985). A treatment regimen of 50–75 mg/kg on two consecutive days increases the cure rate to over 90% (Janssens, 1985). For children under 2 years, 50 mg/kg should be administered under medical supervision (WHO, 1990).

In enterobiasis a dose of 50 mg/kg is given for 7 days and the course is repeated after an interval of 2–4 weeks (WHO, 1990). It should be noted that in most countries piperazine is no longer the drug of choice. However, in low-income countries it is still the cheapest anthelmintic available.

(c) Adverse effects

The wide range between therapeutic and toxic doses makes piperazine a safe drug. Adverse reactions are uncommon and transient. Gastrointestinal upset is occasionally seen. Some individuals are or can become hypersensitive to the drug (reactions including skin rashes, fever and joint pains). Transient neurological effects may also occur. In case of overdosage, toxic central nervous system disturbances may occur.

(d) Precautions and contraindications

Treatment should be discontinued if hypersensitivity or if neurological signs occur (WHO, 1990). Epilepsy, liver and renal disease, and pregnancy in the first semester are conditions in which piperazine is contraindicated.

20.2.2 BENZIMIDAZOLES: THIABENDAZOLE

Thiabendazole [2–(4-thiazolyl)-1*H*-benzimidazole], the first so-called broad-spectrum anthelmintic (Brown *et al.*, 1961) and a well known systemic fungicide used in crop protection (Staron and Allard, 1964), has a molecular weight of 201.26 and is only slightly soluble in alcohols, esters and chlorinated hydrocarbons. Its maximum solubility in water at pH 2.2 is 3.8%. Thiabendazole is soluble in dimethylformamide.

(a) Pharmacokinetics

The absorption, metabolism and excretion have been studied in sheep by Toco *et al.* (1964, 1965). Peak plasma levels were found about 4 h after oral administration of 50 mg/kg/body weight. The greater part is eliminated in 48 h: 75% of the dose is found in the urine and about 15% in the faeces. Metabolites isolated from urine were identified as free 5-hydroxythiabendazole or as its glucuronide or sulfate. Wilson, Parke and Cawthorne (1973) proved that the 5-hydroxylation is cytochrome P450-dependent. In man thiabendazole is rapidly absorbed

Table 20.1 Anthelmintics used in the treatment of gastrointestinal nematodiasis*

Generic name	*Species*	*Dosages*	*Remarks*
Albendazole	*Ancylostoma duodenale; Necator americanus*	1 × 400 mg (200 mg tablets)	Adults and children over 2 years of age At moderate to heavy infections with *N. americanus* a longer treatment period may be required
	Ascaris lumbricoides	1 × 400 mg	Adults and children over 2 years of age
	Enterobius vermicularis	1 × 400 mg	Adults and children over 2 years of age
	Strongyloides stercoralis	1 × 400 mg for 3 days	Adults and children over 2 years of age 1 × 800 mg for 3 days may give higher cure rates (adults)
	Trichuris trichiura	1 × 400 mg	Better results at 1 × 400 mg for 3 days
Flubendazole	*Ancylostoma duodenale; Necator americanus*	2 × 100 mg/day for 3 days (100 mg tablets)	
	Ascaris lumbricoides	2 × 100 mg/day for 3 days	A single dose of 500 mg can be used
	Enterobius vermicularis	1 × 100 mg	To be repeated after 2 weeks
	Trichuris trichiura	2 × 100 mg/day for 3 days	
Levamisole	*Ancylostoma duodenale; Necator americanus*	2.5 mg/kg	Adults: 1 tablet of 150 mg levamisole base Children: tablets containing 50 mg levamisole base Dosages <10 kg: ½ tablet 10–20 kg: 1 tablet 20–30 kg: 1½ tablets 30–40 kg: 2 tablets
	Ascaris lumbricoides	2.5 mg/kg	see *Ancylostoma*
	Trichostrongylus spp.	2.5 mg/kg	see *Ancylostoma*
Mebendazole	*Ancylostoma duodenale; Necator americanus*	2 × 100 mg/day for 3 days (100 mg tablets)	Adults and children ≥ 2 years: for mass treatment: 1 tablet of 500 mg
	Ascaris lumbricoides	2 × 100 mg/day for 3 days	Adults and children ≥ 2 years: for infections with *A. lumbricoides* only: 1 × 200 mg for mass treatment of mixed infections (*Ascaris*, hookworm, *Trichuris*): 1 tablet of 500 mg

	Capillaria philippinensis	4 × 100 mg/day for 20–30 days	
	Enterobius vermicularis	1 × 100 mg	see flubendazole
	Gnathostoma spinigerum	200 mg 4 times daily for 6 days	or 200 mg t.i.d. for 28 days
	Strongyloides stercoralis	2 × 200 mg/day for 3–5 days	Adults and children ≥ 2 years
	Trichinella spiralis enteral phase	200 mg b.i.d. for 5 days	To control the muscle stage: initial dose 200 mg t.i.d. for 4 days, followed by a stepwise increase to 400–500 mg t.i.d. for 10 days (total amount 15 g) + prednisolone (40–60 mg daily)
	Trichostongylus spp.	2 × 100 mg/day for 3 days	Adults and children ≥ 2 years:
	Trichuris trichiura	2 × 100 mg/day for 3 days	For mass treatment: 1 tablet of 500 mg
Oxantel pamoate	*Trichuris trichiura*	10–20 mg/kg for 2 days	Oxantel in combination with pyrantel is available as an oral suspension (50 mg of each per ml). Doses 10–20 mg/kg of each constituent
Piperazine citrate	*Ascaris lumbricoides*	75 mg/kg	Tablets contain 500 mg hydrate Elixir contains 500 mg hydrate/5 ml Adults to a maximum of 3.5 g Children 2–12 years max. 2.5 g Children < 2 years: 50 mg/kg (under medical supervision)
	Enterobius vermicularis	50 mg/kg for 7 days	To be repeated after 2 weeks
Pyrantel pamoate	*Ancylostoma duodenale; Necator americanus*	1 × 10 mg/kg	Heavy hookworm infections: 10 mg/kg for 3 days 1 tablet = 250 mg base suspension: 50 mg base/ml
	Ascaris lumbricoides	as above	
	Enterobius vermicularis	as above	To be repeated after 2 weeks
Thiabendazole	*Angiostrongylus cantonensis*	25 mg/kg b.i.d. for 3 days	(max. 3 g/day)
	Strongyloides stercoralis	2 × 25 mg/kg/day for 3 to 5 days	or 25 mg/kg in three divided doses/day for 3 days. Max. dose for adults = 3 g

Sources: * doses listed are partly taken from Stürchler (1982); Janssens (1985); Pawlowski (1988); WHO (1990) and *Medical Letter on Drugs and Therapeutics* (1986), **28**, 9–18.
b.i.d. = twice daily, t.i.d. = three times daily.

and excreted via the urine. It is also absorbed from the skin.

(b) Mode of action

Optical and electron microscopy studies suggest that benzimidazoles interfere with the formation and/or functioning of microtubules. Biochemical studies of Davidse and Flach (1978) proved that thiabendazole binds to fungal tubulin. These results indicate that the antifungal activity of thiabendazole is based on an antimicrotubule mode of action. The anthelmintic activity of thiabendazole and the other benzimidazole anthelmintics is also based on the interaction with parasite tubulin (for a review see Lacey, 1988). Indeed, Dawson, Gutteridge and Gull (1984) proved that thiabendazole inhibits the *in vitro* polymerization of purified tubulin from *Ascaridia galli*. At 5 μM, 50% inhibition of nematode microtubule assembly was achieved, whereas more than 950 μM (limit of solubility) thiabendazole is needed to reach 50% inhibition of sheep brain microtubule assembly. Binding of thiabendazole to *Ascaris suum* tubulin has been demonstrated by the inhibition of intestinal extracts of the nematode to bind [^{3}H]colchicine (Barrowman, Marriner and Bogan, 1984). In addition, thiabendazole also inhibits the polymerization of *A. suum* intestinal tubulin into microtubules *in vitro* (Barrowman, Marriner and Bogan, 1984).

(c) Spectrum of activity and dosage

Thiabendazole has a broad spectrum of activity against such helminths as *A. lumbricoides*, *E. vermicularis* and *Angiostrongylus costaricencis* (intestinal angiostrongyliasis) but has moderate activity against *Ancylostoma duodenale* and *Necator americanus*. This benzimidazole has interesting activity against cutaneous larva migrans (*Ancylostoma braziliensis* and *A. caninum*) and at 10 mg/kg is also active against *Ternidens deminutus*, the 'false hookworm' (Goldsmid, 1972a,b). Thiabendazole is still a drug of choice for strongyloidiasis. For the treatment of strongyloidiasis 25 mg/kg is given (preferably after meals) divided into two or three doses daily for 3–5 consecutive days (Stürchler, 1982; Janssens, 1985; WHO, 1990). The maximum daily dose for adults is 3 g (Stürchler, 1982).

(d) Adverse effects

Dizziness, anorexia, nausea and vomiting, pruritus and headache are common. Transient leukopaenia, liver dysfunction, hypotension, crystalluria (sometimes with haematuria) and rashes have also been related to thiabendazole (Janssens, 1985; WHO, 1990).

(f) Precautions and contraindications

Thiabendazole should not be given during the first trimester of pregnancy. Patients should be cautioned not to drive or operate machinery.

20.2.3 BENZIMIDAZOLES: MEBENDAZOLE

Mebendazole (R 17635) or methyl [5-(benzoyl)-1*H*-benzimidazol-2-yl]carbamate has a molecular weight of 295.3. It is almost insoluble in water and most organic solvents but soluble in dimethyl sulfoxide. The partition coefficient between octanol and water (log P) is 3.10.

(a) Pharmacokinetics

In humans, the plasma concentrations of mebendazole and metabolites are low. After an oral dose of 200 mg/day for 3 days plasma concentrations never exceeded 30 ng/ml mebendazole and 90 ng/ml of the amino derivative, 2-amino-benzimidazol-5-yl-phenyl-methanone, which has no anthelmintic activity (Schantz, Vanden Bossche and Eckert, 1982). Plasma concentrations of 5–39.5

ng/ml are found if mebendazole tablets are swallowed during a meal. In a patient with cholestasis a plasma concentration of 112 ng/ml was found (Münst, Karlaganis and Bircher, 1980). In 22 patients with alveolar hydatid disease and in 5 patients with cystic hydatid disease, who received long-term mebendazole treatment at doses between 16 and 48 mg/kg/day, mebendazole plasma concentrations varied from the lower limit of detection (HPLC method) up to 295 ng/ml (Witassek *et al.*, 1981).

(b) Mode of action

Mebendazole shares with thiabendazole and the other benzimidazole anthelmintics, such as albendazole and flubendazole, the ability to bind to tubulin, the subunit protein of microtubules, and to inhibit the assembly of these microtubules (Borgers *et al.*, 1975; Vanden Bossche, 1976, Friedman and Platzer, 1978, 1980a,b; Köhler and Bachmann, 1980, 1981; Barrowman, Marriner and Bogan, 1984: Dawson, Gutteridge and Gull, 1984; Gull *et al.*, 1987; Lacey, 1988; Roos *et al.*, 1990). Mebendazole and other benzimidazole anthelmintics exert a number of effects which taken together, may account for its broad spectrum anthelmintic activity (for reviews see Vanden Bossche, 1976, 1980, 1985, 1986; Lacey, 1988). For example, mebendazole has been shown to inhibit glucose uptake both *in vitro* and *in vivo*, in *A. suum*, *Syphacia muris* and *Syngamus trachea* (Vanden Bossche, 1972a, 1976). This inhibition is associated with a compensatory depletion of glycogen stores. Thiabendazole also inhibits the fumarate reductase in *Haemonchus contortus* (Prichard, 1970) and *Trichinella spiralis* (Fornelio, Caabeiro and Gonzalez, 1987). Benzimidazoles have also been shown to inhibit the secretion of acetylcholinesterase in *Nippostrongylus brasiliensis* (Watts *et al.*, 1982). Recently McCracken and Stillwell (1991) suggested that benzimidazole anthelmintic activity, in part may be due to bioenergetic disruptions resulting from transmembrane proton discharge. Lacey (1988) collected data that support the concept of a primary microtubule action leading to a series of biochemical effects that may contribute to the anthelmintic activity of the benzimidazole derivatives.

(c) Spectrum of activity and dosage

Mebendazole is the anthelmintic with the broadest spectrum of activity. It is active against a long list of nematodes, including *Ascaris lumbricoides*; the ancylostomidae *Ancylostoma duodenale, Necator americanus, A. tubaeforme* and *A. caninum; Capillaria philippinensis, Enterobius vermicularis, Gnathostoma, Strongyloides stercoralis, Trichinella spiralis, Trichostrongylus* spp. and *Trichuris trichiura* (for reviews see Vanden Bossche, Rochette and Hörig 1982; Janssen and Vanden Bossche, 1982; Janssens, 1985).

Probably the most common nematode of man, *E. vermicularis*, is also the most sensitive to mebendazole. A single oral dose of 100 mg is virtually 100% effective. However, since reinfection is common, treatment should be repeated 2–4 weeks later. Furthermore, it is advisable to treat all members of the household.

In strongyloidiasis, mebendazole, at the usual dosage of 100 mg twice daily for 3 days, provides cure rates varying between 40 and 100%. Thus, in contrast with thiabendazole, mebendazole is not the drug of choice for strongyloidiasis. However, mebendazole (400 mg day for 20 to 30 days) is still the drug of choice for intestinal capillariasis (Janssens, 1985; Botero, 1986, WHO, 1990). Although less potent against *Trichostrongylus* spp. than levamisole (see below), mebendazole may be the best choice for mass therapy in countries where trichostrongyliasis is a problem.

Clinical studies have shown that even single doses of 100 or 200 mg of mebendazole give cure rates between 93 and 100% for ascariasis (Janssens, 1985). The most used regimen is 100 mg twice daily for 3 consecutive days. This dosage regimen has been selected for its high efficacy in the treatment of individual patients infected with the triad *Ascaris*, hookworm and *Trichuris*. In over 25 therapeutic studies, covering 864 patients with hookworm infections, this treatment regimen resulted in cure rates ≥90%; in many studies 100% cure rate was reached (Janssens, 1985). This treatment schedule also gives cure rates of 100% in patients infected with *Ternidens deminutus* (Goldsmid, 1974). A dose of 100 mg twice daily for 3 days has also been found to be highly effective in *Trichuris trichiura* infections; the cure rate often reaches 100% and falls only exceptionally under the 70% figure. It should be noted that sometimes uncommon results are found in the literature.

It is not always possible to find an explanation for these diverging results. However, in a number of studies mebendazole tablets or suspensions, manufactured without authorization, may have been used. For example a study of Rodriguez-Caabeiro *et al.* (1987) revealed that different polymorphic forms, e.g. the almost inactive polymorph A, can be found in Spain. According to these investigators discrepancies in results among workers who believe they are employing the same compound, may be due to their using drug forms with different physicochemical properties. This warning is, of course, not limited to mebendazole. The use of compounds manufactured by 'pirate' companies may lead to regrettable confusion and more important, the patient may have less or no benefit from the treatment.

Mebendazole is frequently used in mass treatment of mixed infections with soil-transmitted nematodes. It has been shown to be highly effective against mixed infections in adults and children, irrespective of age and body weight at the dosage of 100 mg twice daily for 3 consecutive days. However, for community-wide treatment single doses are better indicated. Many investigators have tried single dose treatment with varying doses which yielded relatively high cure and egg reduction rates (Abadi, 1985; Cabrera Valdez and Go, 1980; Crouch-Chivers, 1985; Evans, Hollmann and Du Preez, 1987; Feldmeier *et al.*, 1982; Kan, 1983; Muttalib, Kha'n and Haq, 1981). For example, among 156 subjects who were given 500 mg mebendazole in a single dose, treatment resulted in cure rates of 93.4%, 77.6% and 91.1%, and average egg-count reduction rates of 99%, 92.8% and 98.3% for ascariasis, trichuriasis and hookworm infections, respectively (Abadi, 1985). Evans, Hollmann and Du Preez (1987) administered single 500 mg doses to 211 children with single or mixed infections of *A. lumbricoides*, hookworm and *T. trichiura*. Apart from a combined cure rate of 71.5%, the overall eggs per gram (epg) rates were considerably reduced in the 'treatment failures'.

(d) Adverse effects

Mebendazole's safety margin is extremely broad. At the normal treatment schedule, no real adverse reactions have been reported, except some complaints of transient abdominal discomfort (Janssens, 1985). Mebendazole, given orally in a high dose of 100–200 mg/kg/day (maximum daily dose of 6 g) for 12 weeks to 29 children with cystic hydatidosis, did not induce serious side-effects (Messaritakis *et al.*, 1991). Seven children had a low grade fever, two had gastric discomfort and two had a transient moderate rise of transaminase activity.

(e) Precautions

Mebendazole (40 mg/kg), when given to rats on the 7th or 10th day of gestation, induces some skeletal abnormalities. Therefore, the potential risk to the fetus should be made known to women taking mebendazole during the first trimester of pregnancy.

20.2.4 BENZIMIDAZOLES: FLUBENDAZOLE

Flubendazole (R 17889) or methyl [5-(4-fluorobenzoyl)-1 *H*-benzimidazol-2-yl]carbamate has a molecular weight of 313.29. It is almost insoluble in water and most organic solvents but soluble in dimethyl sulfoxide. The partition coefficient between octanol and water (log P) is 3.22.

(a) Pharmacokinetics

The absorption of flubendazole in man is limited by the extremely poor solubility of the drug in the contents of the gastrointestinal tract (Michiels *et al.*, 1982). A peak concentration of 0.35 and 0.74 ng/ml plasma was obtained for dose of 100 or 2000 mg taken 2 h before a meal and 4.06 ng/ml for a dose of 2 g taken after a meal.

(b) Mode of action

Flubendazole has a similar mode of action to that of mebendazole.

(c) Spectrum of activity, dosage and administration

Clinical trials with flubendazole indicated a therapeutic potential and dosage requirements that are similar to those of mebendazole (for reviews see Vanden Bossche, Rochette and Hörig, 1982; Janssens, 1985). As in the case of mebendazole, a single oral dose of 100 mg is sufficient for enterobiasis; excellent results are obtained with 100 mg twice daily for 3 days in mixed infections with *A. lumbricoides*, hookworm and *T. trichiura*. In the treatment of *Ascaris* and hookworm, a single oral dose of flubendazole or mebendazole showed a similar efficacy; mebendazole seemed to be slightly superior in the treatment of trichuriasis (Feldmeier *et al.*, 1982). The therapeutic results indicate that flubendazole is not a good substitute for thiabendazole in the treatment of strongyloidiasis.

(d) Adverse effects

Tolerance is excellent and complaints are few and transient. No teratogenic effects were observed in rodents or rabbits (Vanden Bossche, Rochette and Hörig, 1982).

(e) Precautions

Although flubendazole is devoid of teratogenicity in rodents, it is advisable not to use flubendazole during pregnancy (at least not during the first trimester).

20.2.5 BENZIMIDAZIDES: ALBENDAZOLE

Albendazole (SKF 62979) is the generic name for methyl [5-(propylthio)-1*H*-benzimidazol-2-yl]carbamate and it has a molecular weight of 265.33. It is almost insoluble in water and only slightly soluble in most organic solvents.

(a) Pharmacokinetics

The proportion of albendazole that is absorbed is low but considerably higher than that of mebendazole. The absorbed albendazole is completely metabolized; the major metabolite is the anthelmintically active sulphoxide derivative. After a single oral dose of 400 mg, administered to 10 male volunteers, this metabolite reaches peak plasma concentrations of about 0.230 μg/ml after 2.5 h and has a half-life of 8.5 h (Penicaut *et al.*, 1983). The pharmacokinetics were also evaluated in 11 patients with hydatid disease. After 2–4 days of treatment with 10–14 mg/kg daily stable blood levels of 0.6–1.0 μg/ml (albendazole sulphoxide) were reached (Saimot *et al.*, 1983).

(b) Mode of action

Albendazole has a similar mode of action to that of mebendazole.

(c) Spectrum of activity and dosage

Albendazole shares with mebendazole and flubendazole high efficacy against *E. vermicu-*

laris. A single oral dose of 100 mg provides excellent results (Garin, 1980). However, doses up to 400 mg have also been used (Bastidas, 1982). In humans with ascariasis, a single dose of 400 mg gives cure rates of 80–100% (Janssens, 1985). The 400 mg dosage is also effective against hookworm (Botero, 1986) and light infections of the 'false hookworm' *Ternidens deminutus* (Bradley, 1990). However, in patients with moderate to heavy infections (epg 2000–10 000) with *Necator americanus* the egg reduction rate was 64–66% only (Janssens, 1985). The administration of 400 mg daily for 3 consecutive days provides a cure rate of 90% in the treatment of trichuriasis (Camilo-Coura, Velho Soli and Wilcox, 1981). However, at a single 400 mg dose, cure rates between 27 and 90.5% are obtained (Ramalingam, Sinniah and Krishnan, 1983; Pène *et al.*, 1982a,b; Camillo-Coura, Velho Soli and Wilcox, 1981; Janssens, 1985; Jagota, 1986). Albendazole also is much less active against *Strongyloides stercoralis*: a single oral dose of 800 mg/kg given for 3 consecutive days gives a cure rate of 77% (Coulaud *et al.*, 1982). A 45% cure rate is achieved following 400 mg once daily for 3 consecutive days (Pène *et al.*, 1982a).

(d) Adverse effects

Albendazole is very well tolerated. In a multinational clinical trial involving 1455 patients, mild and transient side effects had occurred in only 6% (Rossignol and Coulaud, 1983). No changes were seen in blood serum biochemistry. At a dose of 800 mg, there was an initial reduction of ±30% in the total leukocyte count (Ramalingam, Sinniah and Krishnan, 1983).

(e) Precautions

Since albendazole is known to produce embryotoxicity and teratogenicity in laboratory animals and sheep (Botero, 1986), it should not be administered during confirmed or suspected pregnancy (WHO, 1990).

20.2.6 IMIDAZOTHIAZOLES: LEVAMISOLE

Levamisole hydrochloride (R 12564), the levorotatory enantiomer of tetramisole hydrochloride (R 8299) [(±)-2,3,5,6-tetrahydro-6-phenylimidazo(2,1-b)thiazole monohydrochloride], is a stable white crystalline solid with a molecular weight of 240.75. The pKa of levamisole is 8. Levamisole is very soluble in water. It is stable in acidic aqueous solutions, but hydrolyses in alkaline solutions with the formation of the water-insoluble 2-oxo-3-(2-mercapto-ethyl)-5-phenyl-imidazolidine (OMPI), which was later found to be one of the major metabolites (Vanden Bossche and Janssen, 1967; Janssen, 1976; Symoens *et al.*, 1979).

Levamisole is effective against most gastrointestinal and pulmonary nematodes, but almost inactive against trematodes and cestodes (Thienpont *et al.*, 1966; Janssen, 1976). Next to its anthelmintic properties, levamisole also has immunomodulating properties (for reviews see Symoens *et al.*, 1979; Van Wauwe and Janssen, 1991). Recently the results of investigations using levamisole combined with 5-fluorouracil as post surgical adjuvant therapy have shown a reduction in rate of recurrence and death by one third in patients with Dukes C colon carcinoma (Laurie *et al.*, 1989; Moertel *et al.*, 1990).

(a) Pharmacokinetics

Levamisole is rapidly absorbed from the gastrointestinal tract. Peak plasma concentrations of ±0.7 μg/ml (i.e. ±2.9 μM) are reached within 1 to 2 h after a standard oral dose of 150 mg in adult human subjects (Graziani and de Martin, 1977). In man the drug has a plasma half-life of about 4 h, is extensively metabolized in the liver and is eliminated from the body in about 2 days.

(b) Mode of action

Levamisole causes a spastic contraction of nematode muscle by acting as a potent agonist at acetylcholine receptors on muscle bag membranes of *Ascaris suum* (Van Nueten, 1972; Harrow and Gration, 1985; Harris, 1987). Lewis *et al.* (1980) showed that levamisole-resistant strains of *Caenorhabditis elegans* lack normal cholinergic receptors indicating that nematode acetylcholine receptors are targets for levamisole. Levamisole is a much weaker agonist at vertebrate nicotinic receptors (Martin *et al.*, 1991). Martin *et al.* (1991) have shown that levamisole produces on the bag region of *Ascaris* muscle a dose-dependent increase in cation conductance and membrane depolarization which is blocked by tubocurarin. Patch-clamp studies using isolated muscle vesicles from *A. suum* show that both acetylcholine and levamisole (2–30 μM) activate non-selective cation channels with similar conductances and opening times (Martin *et al.*, 1991). This indicates that levamisole-activated channels have similar properties to the acetylcholine-activated channels.

(c) Spectrum of activity and dosage

Levamisole at 2.5 mg/kg is highly effective against *A. lumbricoides*. With single oral dosages of 2.5 mg/kg, a cure rate of 91% and egg reduction rate of 98% was produced (Moens *et al.*, 1978). Although a single dose of 2.5 mg/kg is likely to provide satisfactory results, levamisole is not a first choice for the treatment of ancylostomiasis in an individual patient (Janssens, 1985). However, since the egg reduction rate obtained with 2.5 mg/kg is quite satisfactory, levamisole can be considered as a tool in attempts at a mass reduction of soil-transmitted helminthiasis (ascariasis and ancylostomiasis) in a community. In five studies involving 203 patients with *S. stercoralis* infection, a single oral dose of 2.5 mg/kg levamisole provided cure rates > 70%. However, other investigators found cure rates of 32% only. Excellent results are obtained in the treatment of *Trichostrongylus* infections. In six studies involving 1289 patients the 2.5 mg/kg (for adults one 150 mg tablet) treatment regimen resulted in cure rates > 90%. The above listed results have been reviewed in detail by Janssens (1985).

(d) Adverse effects

Levamisole is very well tolerated. Abdominal pain, nausea, vomiting, headache and dizziness are occasionally reported as the only side-effects.

(e) Precautions

Contraindications are unknown. Studies in rats and rabbits did not show any embryotoxic or teratogenic effect. However, when the health of the mother and fetus is not compromised, levamisole should be withheld in pregnancy. Since levamisole and piperazine have antagonistic effects, they should never be used together.

20.2.7 TETRAHYDROPYRIMIDINES: PYRANTEL AND OXANTEL

Pyrantel is the generic name for (E)-1,4,5,6-tetrahydro-1-methyl-2-[2-(2-thienyl)vinyl]-pyrimidine. It has a molecular weight of 206.32 and is available as a pamoate salt (pyrantel emboate; (molecular weight 594.6). Pyrantel is almost insoluble in water.

Oxantel pamoate or (E)-3-[2-(1,4,5,6-tetrahydro-1-methyl-2-pyrimidinyl) ethenyl]-phenol (molecular weight 604.67) is a light yellow crystalline salt, practically insoluble in water. Pyrantel pamoate and oxantel pamoate were synthesized in order to provide anthelmintics that are poorly absorbed from the gut (Davis, 1973).

(a) Pharmacokinetics

Some 50–70% of the ingested dose of pyrantel pamoate is excreted in the faeces; blood levels are not higher than 1 μg/ml (Davis,

1973). After oral administration, oxantel pamoate is poorly absorbed so that high concentrations are reached in the caecum and colon (Garcia, 1976).

(b) Mode of action

The mode of action of pyrantel is similar to that of levamisole (see Harrow and Gration, 1985; Martin *et al.*, 1991).

(c) Spectrum of activity and dosage

Pyrantel pamoate is effective against enterobiasis and ascariasis in a single oral dose of 10 mg/kg. A dose of 10 mg/kg on 2 or 3 consecutive days is sufficient against most hookworm infections. However, for heavy infections, longer treatment schedules are required. Some authors prescribe 20 mg/kg for 3 days (see Janssens, 1985). Pyrantel is less active than levamisole in the treatment of *Trichostrongylus* infections. It is inactive against *T. trichiura*. However, its analogue, oxantel shows good activity in the treatment of trichuriasis. A combination of both tetrahydropyrimidines (available as an oral suspension containing 50 mg pyrantel and 50 mg oxantel per ml) resulted in a broadening of the anthelmintic spectrum. The recommended dose is 10–20 mg/kg of each constituent.

(d) Adverse effects

Side effects to both pyrantel and oxantel are mild and mostly limited to gastrointestinal complaints.

(e) Precautions

When the health of the mother and fetus is not compromised, both pyrantel and oxantel should be withheld in pregnancy. Since pyrantel (and oxantel) and piperazine have antagonistic effects they should not be used together.

20.3 CHEMOTHERAPY OF GASTROINTESTINAL CESTODIASIS

The tapeworm infections of man can be grouped in three categories:

- only adult worms are found in man: *Diphyllobothrium latum, D. pacificum, Dipylidium caninum* and *Taenia saginata;*
- both larvae and adults are present: *Taenia solium, T. saginata* (rarely) and *Hymenolepis nana (H. diminuta* is less frequently found in man);
- only larvae are present: *Echinococcus granulosus, E. multilocularis, E. vogeli, Spirometra mansonoides* and *S. prolifrum.*

Only the treatment of the intestinal tapeworms will be discussed in this overview.

A number of anticestodal drugs have been developed, some of which are only used in the treatment of cestode infections (e.g. niclosamide). Praziquantel is highly effective in the treatment of schistosomiasis and cestodiasis. The antinematodal benzimidazole carbamates have also been reported as effective in the treatment of taeniasis.

Table 20.2 summarizes the doses used and contains the most common tradenames.

20.3.1 BENZIMIDAZOLE CARBAMATES

(a) Spectrum of activity and dosage

Mebendazole is active against *Taenia saginata* and *T. solium*. However, at the normal therapeutic dose used in gastrointestinal infections with nematodes, i.e. 100 mg twice daily for 3 days, results were rated unsatisfactory. Cure rates between 90 and 95% were obtained with treatment regimens of 200 mg twice daily for 4 days or 300 mg twice daily for 3 days (for reviews see Vanden Bossche *et al.*, 1982; Kammerer, 1985). Mebendazole is more effective against *T. solium* than against *T. saginata*. For example, Vakil, Dalal and Enjetti (1975) reported no cures in patients with *T. saginata* infections treated with

Table 20.2 Anthelmintics used in the treatment of gastrointestinal cestodiasis*

Generic name	*Species*	*Dosages*	*Remarks*
Niclosamide	*Diphylobothrium latum*	1 × 2 g (adults) (4 tablets)	Children: < 10 kg: 0.5 g; 10–35 kg: 1g
	Hymenolepis nana	1 × 25 g on day 1 followed by 1 g daily for 6 days (adults)	To be repeated after 3–4 weeks; Children 10–35 kg: 1 g day 1, then 0.5 g/day for 6 days
	Taenia saginata	see *D. latum*	
	Taenia solium	see *D. latum*	see Precautions (see p. 280)
Praziquantel	*Diphylobothrium latum*	1 × 25 mg/kg	
	Hymenolepis nana	1 × 25 mg/kg	To be repeated after 4 days (see p. 281)
	Taenia saginata	1 × 10 mg/kg	
	Taenia solium	1 × 10 mg/kg	Also used to treat schistosomiasis

Sources: * Doses listed are partly taken from Sturchler (1982); Andrews *et al.* (1983); Kammerer (1985) and WHO (1990)

100–300 mg mebendazole twice daily for 4 days. In hymenolepiasis treatment schedules of 200 mg daily for 3 to 4 days gave cure rates of 40% (Goldsmid, 1974). Better results may be expected after a prolonged course of 7 days (Kammerer, 1985).

Single dose therapy with 400 mg of albendazole in patients with taeniasis resulted in cure rates of 57.2–64.9% (Misra *et al.*, 1983; Jagota, 1986). In patients with hymenolepiasis and/or taeniasis, treated with 400 mg daily for 3 consecutive days, cure rates were 63.4 and 86.1%, respectively (Jagota, 1986).

Although mebendazole and albendazole are not the drugs of choice in the treatment of tapeworm infections in man they may be suitable in the treatment of multiple infections with both nematodes and cestodes.

(b) Precautions

Because of the risks of cysticercosis associated with proglottid destruction and egg dissemination, the treatment of *Taenia solium* infections deserves special attention. Since it is not known whether albendazole and mebendazole have ovicidal properties for *T. solium* eggs, vomiting should be prevented.

20.3.2 NICLOSAMIDE

Niclosamide or 2′, 5-dichloro-4′-nitrosalicylanilide is practically insoluble in water and only moderately soluble in ethanol and ether. Its molecular weight is 327.1.

(a) Pharmacokinetics

Niclosamide is poorly absorbed from the gastrointestinal tract of the rat; 25–30% of the orally administered drug is excreted in the urine as glucoronide conjugates of niclosamide and metabolites (the main metabolite is the 4′-aminoderivative which is devoid of anthelmintic activity), the remainder is found unchanged in the faeces. In man 2–25% of the dose is excreted renally (for more details see Andrews, Thyssen and Lorke, 1983).

(b) Mode of action

Niclosamide and the other salicylanilides (e.g. closantel) disturb *in vitro* and/or *in vivo* mitochondrial phosphorylation. For example, niclosamide inhibits the anaerobic incorporation of inorganic phosphate (^{32}P) into ATP by intact *H. diminuta* and the ^{32}P-ATP exchange reaction in *H. diminuta* mitochondria (Scheibel *et al.*, 1968). This salicylanilide also inhibits the malate-induced ^{32}P incorporation into ATP by *Ascaris suum* mitochondria (Vanden Bossche, 1972b). The failure of niclosamide to affect intact *Ascaris* may be the result of a permeability barrier.

(c) Spectrum of activity and dosage

Numerous studies have demonstrated the efficacy and safety of niclosamide in the treatment of infections with *T. saginata*, *T. solium*, *H. nana* and *D. latum*. It is also active against *H. diminuta* and *Dipylidium caninum* (for reviews see Davis, 1973; Kammerer, 1985). Niclosamide is not active against the larval form of *T. solium* and has no ovicidal activity. The standard adult dose for all species (but not for infections with *Hymenolepis*) is 2 g, thoroughly chewed before swallowing with a little water, as a single oral dose. Children (< 10 kg) are given 500 mg as a single dose; older children (10–35 kg) are treated with 1.0 g (single dose).

H. nana infections should be treated for 7 consecutive days. According to WHO (1990) adults should receive 2 g followed by 1 g daily for 6 days. A similar treatment schedule is proposed for infections with *H. diminuta* (Kammerer, 1985). Young children receive smaller doses: 1 g on day 1, followed by 500 mg on days 2–7. According to Davis (1973) retreatment at 1 month to eliminate late-maturing larval forms will give optimal results.

There is no conclusive evidence that preliminary starvation is necessary, but it is wise to restrict the diet to fluids only, starting from the evening preceding treatment (Davis, 1973).

(d) Adverse effects

Few undesirable effects have been described. As with almost all other drugs, mild gastrointestinal disturbances, fever and pruritus have been reported.

(e) Precautions

Niclosamide has not been shown to be embryotoxic, mutagenic or teratogenic. It has been given to pregnant patients (Davis, 1973).

Since niclosamide is a taenicide and is nonovicidal, the treatment of *Taenia solium* infections deserves special attention. Vomiting should be prevented. An antiemetic before treatment and an adequate purge 1–2 h after treatment to rid the bowel of all dead segments before digestion can occur, may prevent cysticercosis.

20.3.3 PRAZIQUANTEL

Praziquantel (molecular weight 312.4) or 2-(cyclohexylcarbonyl)-1,2,3,6,7,11 *b*-hexa-hydro-4*H*-pyrazino [2,1*a*]isoquinolin-4-one is soluble in dimethylsulfoxide, ethanol and chloroform but almost insoluble in water. This acylated isoquinoline-pyrazine is available for the treatment of schistosomiasis (Bayer) and cestodiasis (E. Merck). For a review article see Andrews *et al.* (1983).

(a) Pharmacokinetics

After oral administration praziquantel is rapidly absorbed followed by an extensive metabolism (Andrews *et al.*, 1983). It is subjected to a pronounced first-pass metabolism; no unchanged drug is found in the urine, the major route of praziquantel elimination (in man 80% of the radioactivity derived from [^{14}C]praziquantel is found in the urine during the first 24 h after oral treatment). The major metabolite in serum of animals and man is the 4-hydroxycyclohexylcarbonyl analogue of praziquantel. After *in vitro* microsomal oxidation (rat liver) mainly monohydroxylated praziquantel derivatives are obtained. The main fraction contains 4-hydroxypraziquantel (35%) which consists of 80% *cis*-4-OH-praziquantel and 20% of *trans*-4-OH-praziquantel (Högemann *et al.*, 1990). Praziquantel is rapidly taken up by *Schistosoma mansoni* (and not transformed metabolically), *S. japonicum*, *H. nana* and encysted strobilocercus of *Taenia taeniaeformis* (Andrews *et al.*, 1983).

(b) Mode of action

The mode of action of praziquantel at the molecular level is still not well understood and what is known has been derived mainly from studies on schistosomes (for reviews see Andrews *et al.*, 1983; Andrews, 1985; Vanden Bossche, 1986; Sobhon and Upatham, 1990) and unilamellar vesicles (Schepers *et al.*, 1988). The latter studies revealed that praziquantel does not modify the lipid structure but acts as a spacer between lipid molecules.

Two striking effects are observed in trematodes and cestodes exposed to praziquantel: an almost instantaneous contraction of the parasite musculature and a rapid vacuolization of the syncytial tegument. For example a spastic paralysis of *Taenia pisiformis* and *Dipylidium caninum* was seen at 10 nM and 0.1 μM, respectively (Terada *et al.*, 1982). A rapid vacuolization of the tegumental region of the growth zone in the neck region of adult *Hymenolepis* spp., *E. multilocularis* and *Taenia taeniaeformis* has been described (Becker *et al.*, 1981). Both effects may originate from a praziquantel-induced release of Ca^{2+} from an intracellular Ca^{2+} pool (Prichard *et al.*, 1982). In contrast with cestodes, schistosomes showed in the presence of praziquantel an increased influx of exogenous Ca^{2+}. In schistosomes the praziquantel-induced muscle contraction is dependent on the uptake of external Ca^{2+} (reviewed by Sobhon and Upatham, 1990). It should be noted that effective chemotherapy of *S. mansoni* infections in mice requires the presence of host antiparasite antibodies. These antibodies bind to praziquantel-treated worms and may be involved in antibody-dependent cellular cytotoxicity reactions which result in the removal of worms from the vasculature (Brindley and Sher, 1987).

(c) Spectrum of activity and dosage

Praziquantel is active against all forms of schistosomiasis, numerous adult cestodes and cysticercosis cellulosae in man (Andrews *et al.*, 1983; Kammerer, 1985; Campbell and Garcia, 1986; WHO, 1990). Although praziquantel is active against the adult forms, it is inactive against hydatid cysts of *E. granulosus* and *E. multilocularis* (Andrews *et al.*, 1983). The drug has no ovicidal effect on the eggs of *Taenia hydatigena* or *E. granulosus*. Whether it is ovicidal for *T. solium* eggs is not clearly established (Kammerer, 1985).

For infections with *T. saginata* and *T. solium* a single oral dose of 10 mg/kg is recommended. The same dose is used against *Diphyllobothrium pacificum*. However, in infections with *Diphyllobothrium latum* or *H. nana* a single dose of 25 mg/kg is recommended (dosages are taken from Andrews *et al.*, 1983). Patients with cysticercoids of *H. nana* that are not fully developed (less than 48 h of development age) are not always cured by a single dose of 25 mg/kg. A second course of therapy (4 days after the first dose) is necessary in those patients (Andrews *et al.*, 1983; Kammerer, 1985). The doses listed are suitable for adults and children over 4 years (WHO, 1990).

A total dose of 50 mg/kg daily in three divided doses for 14–15 days is used in the treatment of neurocysticercosis (details on the clinical studies can be found in Sotelo *et al.*, 1984; Kammerer, 1985; Webbe, 1986). It is strongly recommended that additional corticosteroid (such as prednisolone) treatment is given in order to prevent immunological reactions to degenerating cysts in the central nervous system (Andrews *et al.*, 1983). A corticosteroid should be administered 2–3 days before and then during the period of treatment with praziquantel (WHO, 1990).

For dermal cysticercosis 20 mg/kg three times daily is used for 6 days (WHO, 1990).

(d) Adverse effects

Praziquantel is well tolerated. For the dosages used in the treatment of infections with adult cestodes the only adverse reactions reported are transient drowsiness, occasional abdominal cramps and nausea. Rarely praziquantel is reported to have induced pruritus or urticarial-type skin eruptions and fever (Webbe, 1986; WHO, 1990). In cysticercosis, degeneration of the cysts may result in local inflammation and oedema.

(e) Precautions

Praziquantel has not been shown to be embryotoxic, mutagenic or teratogenic. Because of the risk of cysticercosis, treatment of *T. solium* infection should always be instituted without delay.

As stated by Andrews *et al.* (1983) patients with neurocysticercosis should always be treated in hospital by expert neurologists; additional corticosteroid treatment is strongly recommended.

20.4 CHEMOTHERAPY OF GASTROINTESTINAL TREMATODIASIS

Intestinal trematode infections in humans generally do not cause significant clinical disease except in heavy infections. Of the three species of the fasciolidae that infect man only *Fasciolopsis buski* inhabits the intestinal tract. Fasciolopsiasis is endemic in Asia because of contamination of water by human and pig faeces containing eggs and the custom of eating fresh-water plants uncooked. In the areas endemic for fasciolopsiasis, gastrodisciasis (*Gastrodiscoides hominis*) also occurs. Heterophydiasis (*Heterophyes heterophyes, Metagonimus yokagawai*) is a zoonotic disease. Humans acquire infections from eating raw fish. *Heterophyes heterophyes* is reported from Asia, Mediterranean countries and parts of Africa. Prevalence rates for *Metagonimus yokagawai* in Korea and Japan vary from 0.5 to 29% and from 20 to 78%, respectively. Infections with *Echinostoma* spp. are rare except in a few areas of Asia where molluscan, amphibian and fish second intermediate hosts are eaten uncooked. (For more information on these and other human intestinal trematodiasis, see Cross, 1985.)

Many anthelmintics have been used to eliminate *F. buski, H. heterophyes, M. yokagawai, Echinostoma* spp. and *G. hominis* from the intestinal tract. Examples are oil of chenopodium, β-naphthol, thymol, carbon tetrachloride, powdered betel nut, dichlorophen and tetrachloroethylene. Dosages of 0.12 ml/kg (max. 5 ml) tetrachloroethylene are used in the treatment of fasciolopsiasis, heterophydiasis and gastrodisciasis (Cross, 1985). At present the drug of choice is certainly praziquantel. Harinasuta, Bunnag and Radomyos (1984) obtained cure rates of 100% in schoolchildren infected with *F. buski* treated with single doses of 40, 25 or 15 mg/kg. Unwanted side-effects were mild and transient. They were more frequent after the higher dosages. The authors recommend a single dose of 15 mg/kg of praziquantel at bed time for the treatment of fasciolopsiasis. For infections with *Echinostoma* spp. a single dose of 40 mg/kg or 25 mg/kg twice daily has also given good results (Campbell and Garcia, 1986). However, Katz (1986) recommends 75 mg/kg divided in 3 doses in one day. This is much higher than the doses listed by other investigators and even higher than that prescribed for *S. japonicum* (2 × 30 mg/kg). The most recently recommended dose for intestinal fluke infections is 25 mg/kg as a single dose (WHO, 1990).

REFERENCES

Abadi, K. (1985) Single dose mebendazole therapy for soil-transmitted nematodes. *Am. J. Trop. Med. Hyg.*, **34**, 129–33.

Andrews, P. (1985) Praziquantel: mechanisms of antischistosomal activity. *Pharmac. Ther.*, **29**, 129–56.

Andrews, P., Thyssen, J. and Lorke, D. (1983) The biology and toxicology of molluscicides, Bayluscide. *Pharmac. Ther.*, **19**, 245–95.

Andrews, P., Thomas, H., Pohlke, R. and Seubert, J. (1983) Praziquantel. *Med. Res. Rev.*, **3**, 147–200.

Barrowman, M. M., Marriner, S. E. and Bogan, J. A. (1984) The binding and subsequent inhibition of tubulin polymerization in *Ascaris suum* (in vitro) by benzimidazole anthelmintics. *Biochem. Pharmac.*, **33**, 3037–40.

Bastidas, G. (1982) Albendazol a dosis unica en nematodiasis intestinales multiples. *Invest. Med. Intern.*, **9**, 308–12.

Becker, B., Mehlhorn, H., Andrews, P. and Thomas, H. (1981) Ultrastructural investigations on the effect of praziquantel on the tegument of five species of cestodes. *Z. Parasietenkd.*, **64**, 257–69.

Bellander, B. T. D., Hagmar, L. E. and Österdahl, B. G. (1981) Nitrosation of piperazine in the stomach. *Lancet*, **ii**, 372.

Borgers, M., De Nollin, S., De Brabander, M. and Thienpont, D. (1975) Influence of the anthelmintic mebendazole on microtubules and intracellular organelle movement in nematode intestinal cells. *Am. J. Vet. Res.*, **26**, 1153–66.

Botero, D. (1986) Nematode infections of man – intestinal infections, in *Chemotherapy of Parasitic Diseases* (eds W. C. Campbell and R. S. Rew), Plenum Press, New York, pp. 267–76.

Bradley, M. (1990) Rate of expulsion of *Necator americanus* and the false hookworm *Ternidens deminutus* Railliet and Henry 1909 (Nematoda) from humans following albendazole treatment. *Trans. Roy. Soc. Trop. Med. Hyg.*, **84**, 720.

Brindley, P. J. and Sher, A. (1987) Anti-schistosomal drugs: observations on the mechanism of drug resistance to hycanthone and on the involvement of host antibodies in the mode of action of praziquantel. *Mem. Inst. Oswaldo Cruz*, Rio de Janeiro, **82** (suppl. IV), 157–61.

Brown, H. D., Matzuk, A. R., Ilves, I. R. *et al.* (1961) Antiparasitic drugs. IV. 2-(4'-thiazolyl)-benzimidazole, a new anthelmintic. *J. Am. Chem. Soc.*, **83**, 1764–5.

Bylund, G., Bång, B. and Wikgren, K. (1977) Tests with a new compound (praziquantel) against *Diphyllobotrium latum*. *J. Helminthol.*, **51**, 115–19.

Cabrera, B. D., Valdez, E. V. and Go, T. G. (1980) Clinical trials of broad spectrum anthelmintics against soil-transmitted helminthiasis. *S. Asian J. Trop. Med. Pub. Hlth.*, **11**, 502–6.

Camilo-Coura, L., Velho Soli A. De S. and Wilcox, H. P. F. (1981), Ensayo con albendazolen el tratamiento de las helminthiasis intestinales de los niños. Symp. latino americano geohelminthiasis y albendazol, in *Compendium de Investigaçiones Clinicos Latino Americaos*, Cancun, Mexico, pp. 75–81.

Campbell, W. C. and Garcia, E. G. (1986) Trematode infections of man, in *Chemotherapy of Parasitic Diseases* (eds. W. C. Campbell and R. S. Rew), Plenum Press, New York, pp. 385–99.

Campbell, W. C. and Rew, R. S. (1986) *Chemotherapy of Parasitic Diseases*, Plenum Press, New York.

Cavier, R. (1973) Chemotherapy of intestinal nematodes, in *Chemotherapy of Helminthiasis*, Vol. 1 (eds. R. Cavier and F. Hawking), Pergamon, Oxford, pp. 215–436.

Coulaud, J. P., Deluol, A. M., Cenac, J. and Rossignol, J. F. (1982) L'albendazole dans le traitement de la strongyloidose. A propos de 66 observations. *Bull. Soc. Pathol. Exot. Filiales*, **75**, 530–3.

Cross, J. H. (1985) Chemotherapy of intestinal trematodiasis, in *Chemotherapy of Gastrointestinal Helminths* (eds H. Vanden Bossche, D. Thienpont and P. G. Janssens), Springer-Verlag, Berlin, pp. 541–56.

Crouch-Chivers, P. R. (1985) Letter to the editor. *Am. J. Trop. Med. Hyg.*, **34**, 1239.

Davidse, L. C. and Flach, W. (1978) Interaction of thiabendazole with fungal tubulin. *Biochim. Biophys. Acta*, **543**, 82–90.

Davis, A. (1973) *Drug Treatment in Intestinal Helminthiasis*, World Health Organization, Geneva.

Dawson, P. J., Gutteridge, W. E. and Gull, K. (1984) A comparison of the interaction of anthelmintic benzimidazoles with tubulin isolated from mammalian tissue and the parasitic nematode *Ascaridia galli*. *Biochem. Pharmac.*, **33**, 1069–74.

del Castillo, J. (1969) Pharmacology of nematoda, in *Chemical Zoology*, Vol 3, (eds M. Florkin and B. T. Scheer), Academic Press, New York, pp. 521–54.

Evans, A. C., Hollmann, A. W. and Du Preez, L. (1987) Mebendazole 500 mg for single-dose treatment of nematode infestation. *S. Afr. Med. J.*, **72**, 665–7.

Feldmeier, H., Bienzle, U., Döhring, E. and Dietrich, M. (1982) Flubendazole versus mebendazole in intestinal helminthic infections. *Acta Trop.*, **39**, 185–9.

Fornelio, A. C., Caabeiro, F. R. and Gonzalez, J. (1987) The mode of action of some benzimidazole drugs on *Trichinella spiralis*. *Parasitology*, **95**, 61–70.

Friedman, P. A. and Platzer, E. G. (1978) Interaction of anthelmintic benzimidazoles and benzimidazole derivatives with bovine brain tubulin. *Biochim. Biophys. Acta*, **544**, 605–14.

Friedman, P. A. and Platzer, E. G. (1980a) The molecular mechanism of action of benzimidazoles with embryos of *Ascaris suum*, in *The Host*

Invader Interplay (ed. H. Vanden Bossche), Elsevier, Amsterdam, pp. 595–604.

Friedman, P. A. and Platzer, E. G. (1980b) Interaction of anthelmintic benzimidazoles with *Ascaris suum* embryonic tubulin. *Biochim. Biophys. Acta*, **630**, 271–8.

Garcia, E. G. (1976) Treatment for trichuriasis with oxantel. *Am. J. Trop. Med. Hyg.*, **25**, 914–15.

Garcia, H., Keefer, L. and Lijinsky, W. (1970) Carcinogenicity of nitrosothiomorpholine and 1-nitrosopiperazine in rats. *Z. Krebsforsch.*, **74**, 179–84.

Garin, J. P. (1980) L'Albendazole dans l'oxyurose. *Int. Clin. Res. Report Smith Kline French*, Lyon, France.

Ghalioungui, P. (1983) *La Médicine des Pharaons*, Édition Robert Laffont, Paris, p. 151.

Goldsmid, J. M. (1972a) Thiabendazole in the treatment of human infections with *Ternidens deminutus* (nematoda). *S. Afr. Med. J.*, **46**, 1046–7.

Goldsmid, J. M. (1972b) *Ternidens deminutus* and hookworm in Rhodesia and a review of the treatment of human infections with *T. deminutus*. *Centr. Afr. J. Med.* **18** (suppl.), 1–14.

Goldsmid, J. M. (1974) The use of mebendazole as a broad-spectrum anthelmintic in Rhodesia. *S.A. Med. J.*, (November), 2265–6.

Goodwin, L. G. (1958) A method for recording the effects of anthelmintics on the movements of *Ascaris lumbricoides*. *Brit. J. Pharmac.*, **13**, 197–201.

Goodwin, L. G. (1980) New drugs for old diseases. *Trans. Roy. Soc. Trop. Med. Hyg.*, **74**, 1–7.

Graziani, G. and de Martin, G. L. (1977) Pharmacrokinetic studies on levamisole: on the pharmacrokinetics and relative bioavailability of levamisole in man. *Drugs Exp. Clin. Res.*, **2**, 235–40.

Grove, D. I. (1990) *A History of Human Helminthology*, C.A.B. International, Wallingford, UK.

Gull, K., Dawson, P. J., Davis, C. and Byard, E. H. (1987) Microtubules as target organelles for benzimidazole anthelmintic chemotherapy. *Biochem. Soc. Trans.*, **15**, 59–60.

Harinsuta, T., Bunnag, D. and Radomyos, P. (1984) Efficacy of praziquantel on fasciolopsiasis. *Arzneimittelforsch.*, **34**, 1214–15.

Harris, B. G. (1987) Levamisole: mode of action. *Biochem. Soc. Trans.*, **15**, 61.

Harrow, I. D. and Gration, K. A. (1985) Mode of action of the anthelmintic morantel, pyrantel and levamisole on muscle cell membrane of the nematode *Ascaris suum*. *Pestic. Sci.*, **16**, 662–72.

Högemann, A., Kiec-Kononowicz, K., Westhoff, F. and Blaschke, G. (1990) Microsomal oxidation of praziquantel. *Arzneimittelforsch.*, **40**, 1159–62.

Jagota, S. C. (1986) Albendazole, a broad-spectrum anthelmintic, in the treatment of intestinal nematode and cestode infections: a multicenter study in 480 patients. *Clin. Therap.*, **8**, 226–31.

Janssen, P. A. J. (1976) The levamisole story, in *Progress Research*, Vol. 20 (ed. E. Jucker), Birkhäuser Verlag, Basel, pp. 347–383.

Janssen, P. A. J. and Vanden Bossche, H. (1982) Treatment of helminthiasis. *Scand. J. Infect. Dis.* (Suppl.) **36**, 52–57.

Janssens, P. G. (1985) Chemotherapy of gastrointestinal nematodiasis in man, in *Chemotherapy of Gastrointestinal Helminths* (eds. H. Vanden Bossche, D. Thienpont and P. G. Janssens), Springer-Verlag, Berlin, pp. 183–406.

Kammerer, W. S. (1985) Chemotherapy of tapeworm infections in man, in *Chemotherapy of Gastrointestinal Helminths* (eds. H. Vanden Bossche, D. Thienpont and P. G. Janssens), Springer-Verlag, Berlin, pp. 613–29.

Kan, S. P. (1983) Efficacy of single doses of mebendazole in the treatment of *Trichuris trichiura* infection. *Am. J. Trop. Med. Hyg.*, **32**, 118–22.

Katz, M. (1986) Anthelmintics. Current concepts in the treatment of helmintic infections. *Drugs*, **32**, 358–71.

Köhler, P. and Bachmann, R. (1980) The possible mode of action of mebendazole in *Ascaris suum*, in *The Host Invader Interplay* (ed. H. Vanden Bossche), Elsevier, Amsterdam, pp. 727–30.

Köhler, P. and Bachmann, R. (1981) Intestinal tubulin as possible target for the chemotherapeutic action of mebendazole in parasitic nematodes. *Mol. Biochem. Parasitol.*, **4**, 325–36.

Lacey, E. (1988) The role of the cytoskeletal protein, tubulin, in the mode of action and mechanism of drug resistance to benzimidazoles. *Int. J. Parasit.*, **18**, 885–936.

Laurie, J., Moertel, C., Fleming, T. *et al.* (1989) Surgical adjuvant therapy of large-bowel carcinoma: an evaluation of levamisole and the combination of levamisole and fluorouracil. *J. Clin. Oncol.*, **7**, 1447–56.

Lewis, J. A., Wu, C.-H., Levine, J. H. and Berg, H. (1980) Levamisole-resistant mutants of the nematode *Caenorhabitis elegans* appear to lack pharmacological acetylcholine receptors. *Neuroscience*, **5**, 967–89.

Martin, R. J. (1987) The γ-aminobutyric acid receptor of *Ascaris* as a target for anthelmintics. *Biochem. Soc. Trans.*, **15**, 61–5.

Martin, R. J., Pennington, A. J., Duittoz, A. H., *et al.* (1991) The physiology and pharmacology of neuromuscular transmission in the nematode parasite, *Ascaris suum. Parasitology*, **102**, S41–S58.

Maximino Martinez (1969) *Las Plantas Medicinales de Mexico*, 5th edn, Andres, Ediciones Botas, Mexico.

McCracken, M. O. and Stillwell, W. H. (1991) A possible biochemical mode of action for benzimidazole anthelmintics. *Int. J. Parasitol.*, **21**, 99–104.

Messaritakis, J., Psychou, P., Nicolaidou, P. *et al.* (1991) High mebendazole doses in pulmonary and hepatic disease. *Arch. Dis. Child.*, **66**, 532–3.

Michiels, M., Hendriks, R., Heykants, J. and Vanden Bossche, H. (1982) The pharmacokinetics of mebendazole and flubendazole in animals and man. *Archs. Int. Pharmacodyn. Thér.*, **256**, 180–91.

Misra, R. C., Dewan, R., Sachdev, S. *et al.* (1983) Albendazole, a new drug in the treatment of intestinal helminthiasis (nematodes and cestodes). *Curr. Ther. Res.*, **33**, 758–61.

Moens, M., Dom, J., Burke, W. E., *et al.*, (1978) Levamisole in ascariasis. A muticenter controlled evaluation. *Am. J. Trop. Med. Hyg.*, **27**, 897–904.

Moertel, C., Fleming, T., MacDonald, J. *et al.* (1990) Levamisole and fluorouracil for adjuvant therapy of resected colon carcinoma. *New Engl. J. Med.*, **322**, 352–8.

Münst, G. J., Karlaganis, G. and Bircher, J. (1980) Plasma concentrations of mebendazole during treatment of echinococcosis. Preliminary results. *Eur. J. Clin. Pharm.*, **17**, 375–8.

Muttalib, M. A., Khan, M. U. and Haq, J. A. (1981) Single dose regime of mebendazole in the treatment of polyparasitism in children. *J. Trop. Med. Hyg.*, **84**, 159–60.

Pawlowski, Z. S. (1988) Intestinal helminthiasis. *Med. Int.*, **55**, 2260–6.

Pène, P., Mojon, M., Garin, J. P. *et al.* (1982a) Albendazole: a new broad spectrum anthelmintic. Double blind multicenter clinical trial. *Am. J. Trop. Med. Hyg.*, **31**, 263–6.

Pène, P., Coulaud, J. P., Soula, G. *et al.* (1982b) Le Zentel® dans le traitement des helminthiases intestinales en Afrique de l'Ouest. *Med. Afr. Noire*, **29**, 43–8.

Penicaut, B., Maugein, Ph., Maisonneuve, H. and Rossignol, J. F. (1983) Pharmacocinétique et métabolisme urinaire de l'albendazole chez l'homme. *Bull. Soc. Path. Ex.*, **76**, 698–708.

Prichard, R. K. (1970) Mode of action of the anthelmintic thiabendazole in *Haemonchus contortus. Nature*, **228**, 684.

Prichard, R. K., Bachmann, R., Hutchinson, G. W. and Köhler, P. (1982). The effect of praziquantel on calcium in *Hymenolepis diminuta. Mol. Biochem. Parasit.*, **5**, 297–308.

Ramalingam, Sh., Sinniah, B. and Krishnan, U. (1983) Albendazole, an effective single dose, broad spectrum anthelmintic drug. *Am. J. Trop. Hyg.*, **32**, 984–9.

Rodriguez-Caabeiro, F., Criado-Fornellio, A., Jiminez-Gonzalez, A., *et al.* (1987) Experimental chemotherapy and toxicity in mice of three mebendazole polymorphic forms. *Chemotherapy*, **33**, 266–71.

Roos, M. H., Boersema, J. H., Borgsteede, F. H. M. *et al.* (1990) Molecular analysis of selection for benzimidazole resistance in the sheep parasite *Haemonchus contortus. Mol. Biochem. Parasit.*, **43**, 77–88.

Rossignol, J. F. and Coulaud, J. P (1983) Summary of clinical trials worldwide (evaluation of albendazole in Europe, West Africa and Asia as a single-dose anthelmintic: report on 1455 patients), in *Albendazole in Helminthiasis* (ed. M. Firth), International Congress Symposium Series, No. 57, Royal Society of Medicine, London, pp. 19–27.

Rüneberg, L. (1963) The effect of desaspidin and related chlorobutyrophenone derivatives from fern extract on oxidative phosphorylation and muscle adenosinetriphosphates. *Societas Scientiarum Fennica, Commentationes Biologicae, Helsinki*, **XXVL**, pp. 1–69.

Saimot, A. G., Cremieux, A. C., Hay, J. M. *et al.* (1983) Albendazole as a potential treatment for human hydatidosis. *Lancet*, (September 17), 652–6.

Schantz, P. M., Vanden Bossche, H. and Eckert, J. (1982) Chemotherapy of larval echinococcosis in animals and humans: report of a workshop. *Z. Parasitenkd.*, **67**, 5–26.

Scheibel, L. W., Saz, H. J. and Bueding, E. (1968) The anaerobic incorporation of ^{32}P into adenosine triphosphate by *Hymenolepis diminuta. J. Biol. Chem.*, **243**, 2229–35.

Schepers, H., Brasseur, R., Goormaghtigh, E. *et al.* (1988) Mode of insertion of praziquantel and derivatives into lipid membranes. *Biochem. Pharmacol.*, **37**, 1615–23.

Sen, H. G., Joshi, B. S., Parthasarathy, F. C. and Kamat V. N. (1974) Anthelmintic efficacy of diospyrol and derivatives. *Arzneimittelforsch.*, **24**, 2000–3.

Sobhon, P. and Upatham, E. S. (1990) *Snail Hosts, Life Cycle and Tegumental Structure of Oriental Schistosomes*. Published on behalf of the UNDP/World Bank/WHO Special Programme TDR, World Health Organization, Geneva.

Sotelo, J., Escobedo, F., Rodriguez–Carbajal, J., *et al.* (1984) Therapy of parenchymal brain cysticercosis with praziquantel. *N. Engl. J. Med.*, **310**, 1001–7.

Staron, T. and Allard, C. (1964) Propriétés antifongiques du 2-(4-thiazolyl)-benzimidazole ou thiabendazole. *Phytiat. Phytopharm.*, **13**, 163–8.

Stürchler, D. (1982) Chemotherapy of human intestinal helminthiasis: a review, with particular reference to community treatment. *Adv. Pharmac. Chemother.*, **19**, 129–54.

Symoens, J., De Cree, J., Van Bever, W. F. M. and Janssen, P. A. J. (1979) Levamisole, in *Pharmacological and Biochemical Properties of Drug Substances*, Vol. 2, (ed. M. E. Goldberg), American Pharmaceutical Association, Washinton, pp. 407–64.

Terada, M., Ishii, A. I., Kino, H. *et al.* (1982) Studies on chemotherapy of helminths (IX). Effects of praziquantel on the motility of various parasitic helminths and isolated host tissues. *Experientia*, **38**, 549–53.

Thienpont, D., Van Parijs, O. F. J., Raeymaekers, A. H. M. *et al.* (1966), Tetramisole (R 8299), a new, potent broad spectrum anthelmintic. *Nature*, **209**, 1084–5.

Toco, D. J., Buhs, R. P., Brown, M. D. *et al.* (1964) The metabolic fate of thiabendazole in sheep. *J. Med. Chem.*, **7**, 399–405.

Toco, D. J., Egerton, J. R., Bowers, W. *et al.* (1965) Absorption, metabolism and elimination of thiabendazole in farm animals and a method for the estimation in biological materials. *J. Pharm. Exp. Ther.*, **149**, 263–70.

Vakil, B. J., Dalal, N. J. and Enjetti, E. (1975) Clinical trials with mebendazole – a new broad spectrum anthelminticum. *J. Trop. Med. Hyg.*, **78**, 154–8.

Vanden Bossche, H. (1972a) Biochemical effects of the anthelmintic drug mebendazole, in *Comparative Biochemistry of Parasites* (ed. H. Vanden Bossche), Academic Press, New York, pp. 139–57.

Vanden Bossche, H. (1972b) Studies on the phosphorylation in *Ascaris* mitochondria in *Comparative Biochemistry of Parasites* (ed. H. Vanden Bossche), Academic Press, New York, pp. 455–68.

Vanden Bossche, H. (1976) The molecular basis of anthelmintic action, in *Biochemistry of Parasites and Host–Parasite Relationships* (ed. H. Vanden Bossche), Elsevier, Amsterdam, pp. 553–72.

Vanden Bossche, H. (1978) Chemotherapy of parasitic infections. *Nature*, **273**, 626–30.

Vanden Bossche, H. (1980) Peculiar targets in anthelmintic chemotherapy. *Biochem. Pharmac.*, **29**, 1981–90.

Vanden Bossche, H. (1985) Pharmacology of anthelmintics, in *Chemotherapy of Gastrointestinal Helminths* (eds, H. Vanden Bossche, D. Thienpont and P. G. Janssens), Springer-Verlag, Berlin, pp. 125–81.

Vanden Bossche, H. (1986) Mode of action of anticestodal drugs, in *Chemotherapy of Parasitic Diseases* (eds W. C. Campbell and R. S. Rew), Plenum Press, New York, pp. 495–503.

Vanden Bossche, H. (1990) Studies of the mode of action of anthelmintic drugs: tools to investigate the biochemical pecularities of helminths. *Ann. Parasitol. Hum. Comp.*, **65**, 99–102.

Vanden Bossche, H. and Janssen, P. A. J. (1967) The biochemical mechanism of action of the anthelmintic drug tetramisole. *Life Sciences*, **6**, 1781–92.

Vanden Bossche, H., Rochette, F. and Hörig, C. (1982) Mebendazole and related anthelmintics. *Adv. Pharmac. Chemother.*, **19**, 67–128.

Vanden Bossche, H., Thienpont, D. and Janssens, P. G. (1985) *Chemotherapy of Gastrointestinal Helminths*, Springer-Verlag, Berlin.

Van Nueten, J. M. (1972) Pharmacological aspects of tetramisole, in *Comparative Biochemistry of Parasites* (ed. H. Vanden Bossche), Academic Press, New York, pp. 101–15.

Van Wauwe, J. and Janssen, P. A. J. (1991) On the biochemical mode of action of levamisole: an update. *Int. J. Immunopharmac.*, **13**, 3–9.

Watts, S. D. M., Rapson, E. B., Atkins, A. M. and Lee, D. L. (1982) *Inhibition of acetylcholinesterase secretion from Nippostrongylus brasiliensis* by *benzimidazole anthelmintics. Biochem. Pharmac.*, **31**, 3035–40.

Webbe, G. (1986) Cestode infections of man, in *Chemotherapy of Parasitic Diseases* (eds W. C. Campbell and R. S. Rew), Plenum Press, New York, pp. 457–77.

WHO (1990) *WHO Model Prescribing Information. Drugs Used in Parasitic Diseases*, World Health Organization, Geneva.

Wilson, C. G., Parke, D. V., Cawthorne, M. A. (1973) Investigations of the 5-hydroxylation of thiabendazole in rat liver microsomal preparations. *Biochem. Soc. Trans.*, **1**, 195–6.

Witassek, F., Burkhardt, B., Eckert, J. and Bircher, J. (1981) Chemotherapy of alveolar echinococcosis. Comparison of plasma mebendazole concentrations in animals and man. *Eur. J. Clin. Pharm.*, **20**, 427–33.

TWENTY-ONE

Vaccines against intestinal helminths

D. Wakelin

Any consideration of this subject must firstly address two topics: the need for vaccination as a control measure against intestinal helminths, and the fact that, currently, there are very few such vaccines and none that can be used in humans.

Previous chapters have highlighted a number of important characteristics of intestinal worms that have bearing on the first of these topics:

- They are responsible for some of the commonest and most wide-spread intestinal infections.
- In the majority of cases their prevalence is closely related to climatic and socio-economic conditions and is highest in developing countries.
- Children are commonly the most heavily infected and most seriously affected members of the community.
- Infections can be long term and associated with a chronic pathology, which in children affects growth and development and in adults reduces work capacity.
- In endemic areas, removal of infections by anthelmintics has only a temporary effect on prevalence in the community. In the absence of continuing treatment prevalence returns rapidly to pre-treatment levels.
- Permanent control of infection requires effective interruption of transmission. This may well necessitate changes in social customs as well as improvements in sanitation and hygiene, all of which are costly and difficult to implement effectively.

It is quite clear from this summary that the option of controlling intestinal helminths by the use of well tolerated, easily administered vaccines, requiring only limited patient contact, is highly desirable. Vaccination would contribute immeasurably to improved public health in much of the third world and would improve the quality of life for many millions of people. Unfortunately such an option is not presently available. The only commercially successful vaccines for helminths of any kind are those used to control infections with lungworms (*Dictyocaulus* spp.) in cattle and sheep (Peacock and Poynter, 1980). The one vaccine to be used on any scale against an intestinal worm, that against the dog hookworm *Ancylostoma caninum*, was withdrawn, primarily because, although protecting against hookworm disease, it did not provide absolute protection against infection (Miller, 1971, 1978).

21.1 CONSTRAINING FACTORS TO VACCINE DEVELOPMENT

Many factors have contributed to the present failure to vaccinate successfully against any

Enteric Infection 2. Intestinal helminths. Edited by M.J.G. Farthing, G.T. Keusch and D. Wakelin. Published in 1995 by Chapman and Hall, London. ISBN 0 412 39140 6

of the species of helminths that parasitize the human intestine. Some of the most important are listed below:

- Intestinal helminths have been regarded as clinically insignificant and have been given low priority for research funding.
- For the major infections chemotherapy is simple and effective in the short term.
- Helminths have complex life cycles and are antigenically complex organisms.
- Immunity against infection, at least in certain individuals, appears absent or ineffective.
- Little is known of potential mechanisms of immunity to these parasites or about the origin, nature and function of target antigens.
- Characteristics of host-specificity and difficulties of *in vitro* culture impose severe limitations on the supply of candidate vaccine antigens.
- Vaccination against antigenically complex organisms, that elicit complex host responses, runs the risk of provoking immunopathological reactions.
- Vaccination against intestinally located organisms is more difficult than against systemic pathogens.
- Adjuvants shown to assist protective immune responses against helminths in experimental studies are unsuitable for use in humans.
- Parasites have evolved many strategies to avoid, inactivate or subvert host immune responses.
- There are difficulties in immunizing hosts subject to suboptimal nutrition, concurrent diseases and who may, in the case of young children, have immature immune systems and be exposed to high levels of maternal antiparasite antibodies.
- There are many logistic and financial problems to overcome in the successful use of any vaccine against infection in developing countries.

Some of these constraints on the development and use of vaccines (e.g. low research funding) require re-evaluation of the importance of helminth parasites in humans; others are inextricably linked with wider questions of public health in those countries where helminth infections are endemic; financial and logistic problems require political rather than scientific solutions. Of the remainder, there is optimism that some at least will be eliminated or significantly reduced by the progress that is now being made in the fields of immunoparasitology, intestinal immunology and vaccine development. In particular, the prospect that it will be possible to manufacture large amounts of vaccine material through recombinant or synthetic techniques removes one of the most important restrictions on eventual vaccine production (Fields and Chanock, 1989; Gamble and Zarlenga, 1986).

Much of the progress that will be reviewed in this chapter comes from experimental studies in model systems and from work directed towards the production of defined molecular vaccines against gastrointestinal parasites in domestic animals Both offer paradigms for the development of vaccines in humans and will be used to discuss 'what might be' in this field. Attention will be focused on data relevant to the immune control of those species against which vaccination is most necessary, namely the major gastrointestinal nematodes (*Ascaris*, hookworm, *Trichuris*). It is possible that vaccination might play a role in the control of strongyloidiasis, although the patients at risk from disease include those who have experienced immunosuppression after infection, and who are therefore unlikely to respond effectively to vaccination. Vaccination against *Trichinella spiralis* would be perhaps the easiest to achieve at the present time but, because of the distribution and epidemiology of the disease, is unlikely to be much in demand for humans, although it may well play a role in eliminating infection at source, i.e. in pigs.

21.2 IMMUNOPARASITOLOGICAL APPROACHES TO VACCINATION

There is an extensive literature dealing with existing approaches to vaccination, both in experimental models and in the target species for the lungworm and hookworm vaccines (Urquhart, 1977; Clegg and Smith, 1978; Lloyd, 1981; Miller, 1986). Much of this, although informative, is no longer wholly relevant to modern approaches. Many papers refer to attempts to immunize against intestinal nematodes using a wide variety of ill-defined antigen preparations, including: dead worms; live attenuated worms; crude, semi-purified or purified worm homogenates; dissected-out worm components; excretory – secretory (ES) antigens, or detergent-stripped surface antigens. All of these approaches are successful in raising immune responses against parasite antigens, but only in certain cases are these responses associated with an induced protective immunity against the parasite of origin; in a majority no significant protection is induced.

The most informative of these studies have been those where the material used for vaccination has come from life-cycle stages known to be a target for protective immunity under natural conditions of infection, and those where the source of protective material was known to contain antigens of critical importance to the parasite. In the case of both the lungworm and hookworm vaccines, the material selected was irradiation-attenuated infective larval stages. There is overwhelming evidence from many sources that living parasites are substantially more immunogenic than their inert components. The strategy of using attenuated stages allows a natural and prolonged release of antigen before the cumulative effects of irradiation result in the death of the worm. With *Dictyocaulus*, the irradiated infective larvae develop into the immunogenic fourth stage (L4), but die before maturing into the pathogenic adult stages (Poynter *et al.*, 1960). Although much of the development of this vaccine was empirical, it was known at an early stage that the L4 stage was a major target of protective immune responses. In the case of *Ancylostoma*, it is not known at which stage irradiated larvae die, or which stages are the major target(s) of immunity, but it is probable that immune attrition occurs systemically; pragmatically, the vaccine was successful because it reduced the numbers of worms that established in the intestine and minimized their pathological activity (Miller, 1964).

With intestinal worms the question of sites of attrition is an important one. In species that enter and establish directly in the intestine it is clear that vaccine-induced immunity must operate in that site. In those species which mature in the intestine after a period of somatic migration undertaken immediately after skin penetration (hookworm, *Strongyloides*) or after oral infection (*Ascaris*), attrition could occur in the tissues and/or within the intestine itself. The range of protective immune responses likely to be effective in each location is quite clearly different.

21.2.1 PROTECTIVE RESPONSES IN THE INTESTINE

Of the genera of helminths covered in this book, detailed experimental data about immune mechanisms operative in the intestine are restricted to a very few of the nematodes, primarily *Trichinella* and *Trichuris*, and one cestode, *Hymenolepis*; little is known about immunity to intestinal trematodes (Miller, 1984; Ito and Smyth, 1987; Rothwell, 1989; Wakelin, Harnett and Parkhouse, 1993). For those species located externally to the mucosa, protective immunity involving antibody (IgM, IgG, IgA) can be seen as acting against vulnerable tegumental surfaces (trematodes/cestodes), against sensory structures and receptors on tegument or cuticle (nematodes) or against feeding or penetration enzymes released from the worms. Complement-mediated activity has been implicated in resistance to tapeworms, but levels of complement in the intestine are low. Antibody-dependent cellular cytotoxicity (ADCC) mechanisms are equally unlikely to operate in the intestinal environment.

Inflammatory reactions, both immediate (involving IgE) and delayed, form an important element of the intestinal response to infection and undoubtedly have a protective role in bringing about worm expulsion (Moqbel and MacDonald, 1990). Precisely how this is achieved remains obscure. Realistic possibilities include release of harmful mediators from inflammatory cells (e.g. oxygen radicals, prostaglandins, leukotrienes, amines, leucocyte enzymes, basic proteins, cytokines); structural and functional changes induced in the mucosa by the inflammatory response, and physicochemical changes in the immediate environment of parasites. Whatever the ultimate cause, there can be no doubt that this type of protective response is, like the antibody responses mentioned earlier, T cell-dependent in origin, locally-mediated and can be enhanced by prior immunization.

21.2.2 PROTECTIVE RESPONSES IN THE TISSUES

Species that migrate through tissues do so as relatively small larvae. Because of their size, and their intimate contact with cellular and humoral effectors, they should be susceptible to immune-mediated destruction, especially ADCC. Although it can be shown that such destruction occurs *in vitro* and that a variety of antibody isotypes (IgM, IgG, IgE) and of cells (macrophages, neutrophils, eosinophils) can be involved (Butterworth, 1984; McLaren, 1985), evidence that these responses operate effectively *in vivo* remains circumstantial, and is based largely on histopathological data (e.g. Moqbel, 1980; Dawkins, Muir and Grove, 1981). Local mucosal destruction of invading larvae of certain nematodes (Behnke, Hannah and Pritchard, 1983; Ito and Smyth, 1987) and of the cestode *H. nana* can provide an effective protective response, and there is good evidence that this occurs more readily in immunized hosts.

21.3 ANTIGENS ELICITING PROTECTIVE RESPONSES

It will be apparent from the summary given of protective responses that there can be two approaches to the question of incorporating 'protective' antigens within vaccines. Where targeted antiparasite responses are involved, i.e. where there are antibody- or cell-mediated responses directed specifically against molecules whose structural or functional integrity is crucial to parasite survival, it is necessary to identify the particular molecules and to include them within vaccine material in order to prime specifically for the response concerned. These may be immunodominant molecules, and therefore easily identified, or may be relatively minor components. Where protective responses are induced specifically, but function non-specifically (as in the case of intestinal inflammation), it is still necessary to identify the antigens concerned, but it may be possible to make use of a wider spectrum of parasite molecules, each capable of triggering the necessary non-specific response. In a majority of cases it is probably true that, at the present time, no clear-cut equivalence is possible between particular antigens and protective immunity. One way of dealing with this problem is the systematic screening of antigen preparations by sera or cells from hosts known to express immunity or to have the genetic capacity so to do.

21.3.1 IMMUNODOMINANT ANTIGENS

Progress in identifying protective antigens in intestinal helminths is limited, but important observations have been made in a number of species (Almond and Parkhouse, 1985).

Perhaps the most thoroughly investigated of these is *Trichinella spiralis* (Appleton *et al.*, 1991). Work with this species has provided an insight into the nature and origins of molecules relevant to the induction of host immune responses, both protective and pathological. The data now available allow the construction of models in which the relative importance of target, immunodominant molecules and those involved in the generation of non-specific responses can be evaluated and vaccination strategies defined.

Protective antigens have been identified in worm homogenates, in ES material and on the cuticular surface. A major source of ES antigens is the glandular stichosome. Analysis has shown more than 20 immunogenic components in this material, but it is clear that particular components are of greater importance than others. A small number, with molecular weights between 43 and 60 kD, have been shown to immunize experimental animals very effectively, 1 μg of antigen providing more than 60% protection (Silberstein and Despommier, 1984). Immunization has also been achieved in the pig, although less successfully than in the mouse (Murrell and Despommier, 1984; Vernes, 1976). Some of these molecules have now been sequenced and their genes cloned. The role of these antigens in eliciting protective responses during vaccination is undefined. In rodents, but to a lesser degree in the pig, it is known that immunity operates against the worms in the intestine, and it seems likely that these antigens may act to prime T cell-dependent inflammatory responses and to initiate formation of antibodies capable of interfering with their normal biological function.

Similar, although less detailed, studies have been carried out on protective antigens of *Trichuris muris* and *Nippostrongylus brasiliensis*, and these, in essence, reinforce the picture provided by data from *T. spiralis*. In the first, stichosomal secretions are again of major importance (Jenkins and Wakelin, 1983) and specific MW components from these cells, e.g. a 43 kD molecule, can be used to generate protective immunity in mice. Secreted antigens of *N. brasiliensis* are equally effective in immunization of the rat host (Day *et al.*, 1979; Poulain, Pery and Luffau, 1976) In neither case is the mechanism of immunity known in detail. Antibody responses involving IgG and IgA are thought to be active components of immunity to *T. muris* (Else and Wakelin, 1989; Roach *et al.*, 1991), possibly because they interfere with functionally important ES molecules, and there is circumstantial evidence to suggest that this may be true also of the human whipworm *T. trichiura* (Lillywhite *et al.*, 1991). In *N. brasiliensis*, IgG (and possibly IgA) antibody-mediated responses are known to play a role in protective immunity, together with immunologically-mediated inflammatory changes in the intestinal environment (Miller, 1984; Rothwell, 1989).

Almost nothing is known about the antigens of *Dictyocaulus* that provide the major immunological stimulus in the irradiated vaccine, and nothing is known about the protective mechanisms involved, although studies are now in progress to define both of these. The protective antigens responsible for the effectiveness of the irradiated hookworm vaccine are similarly undefined. However, in this case, the early work of Thorson (1956) had implicated secreted feeding enzymes as one target of antibody-mediated immunity, and more recent data provide some indirect support for this view (Hotez, Le Trang and Cerami, 1987).

21.3.2 CRYPTIC ANTIGENS

The focus of the research briefly summarized in the previous paragraphs has been on antigens that are readily available to the immune system of the host, either because they are expressed on the worm surface or are released during metabolism. Indeed it is logical to examine these antigens because they are most likely to elicit immunity during initial exposure to a parasite and to be available to restimulate primed cells during challenge infections. This approach has to some extent been validated by the experimental work described above, but it is undeniable that there are many systems involving intestinal helminths where very little success has been obtained in vaccinating hosts with similar antigen preparations.

The view has been expressed, for example by Waksman (quoted by Sher, 1988) that, for well-adapted parasites, it may be futile to look for candidate antigens among those that are immunodominant, i.e. those readily presented to, and recognized by, the host. The argument is that, if these molecules were critical to the survival of the parasite, they would not be immunodominant in this way; indeed immunodominance may be a form of immunological smoke-screen to divert the immune response.

An alternative approach is therefore to look for cryptic antigens, i.e. antigens not normally available to the immune system because of their location in the parasite, but which nevertheless provide vulnerable targets for immune effectors because they play important roles in the structure or function of the parasite. Included within this category are structural molecules present within the cuticle in nematodes or the tegument in trematodes and cestodes, and structural or functional molecules (enzymes, hormones) located on the intestinal surfaces or within the somatic tissues. There are some significant precedents for this approach, notably the successful vaccines against ectoparasitic ticks, which are designed to raise antibodies in the host against molecules critical to the arthropod's ability to feed and to digest host blood (Morrison, 1989).

The view that hidden cuticular components of intestinal nematodes may provide suitable vaccine targets has been discussed by Pritchard, McKean and Rogan (1988). Nematodes are, despite the metabolic and immunologic activity of the cuticle, relatively well protected by this layer from the host's immune effector mechanisms. If it were possible to breach the integrity of this layer, then vaccine-induced antibody responses against cuticular components such as collagen might well prove destructive. Some support for this approach is provided by the evidence for the presence of antinematode collagen antibodies in populations exposed to infection in endemic areas (Pritchard *et al.*, 1990). These antibodies imply that the host is exposed to these molecules naturally, as a result of worm moulting or worm death, and is therefore primed against them.

Many groups are actively working on cryptic antigens located within the somatic tissues or the intestinal epithelia of those gastrointestinal trichostrongyle nematodes that are of major economic importance in sheep and cattle, with a view to the development of effective vaccine strategies. Although much of the latter work is subject to commercial confidentiality, it is clear that molecules located at the intestinal surface can be used as vaccine antigens to raise substantial levels of protective immunity. One such molecule that has been described is the polymeric protein contortin from the intestinal microvilli of *Haemonchus contortus*; another is the glycoprotein H11 (Smith and Munn, 1990). Similar molecules have subsequently been identified in other species and also shown to be protective. Other publications have described the identification of nematode tropomyosin as a candiate vaccine antigen in *Trichostrongylus colubriformis* (O'Donnell *et al.*, 1989), which has been shown to protect guineapigs against infection with this parasite. This approach is similar in concept to the earlier studies on the use of paramyosin as a vaccine antigen for schistosomiasis (Pearce *et al.*, 1988). Paramyosin also exists in nematodes and has been used to elicit protective immunity against the filarial worm *Brugia malayi* (Nanduri and Kazura, 1989). Although both of these molecules are widely distributed among helminths (and therefore are not 'parasite-specific' in the sense that other immunodominant antigens are), neither would normally be considered as an obvious target for immune responses, because of their location within the body of the worm. There is evidence, however, that molecules of this type are released *in vivo* and made available to the immune system; for example, there are natural responses to these components when worms die in the host. This fact is of some importance, because one possible drawback to the use of cryptic antigens in vaccines might be that vaccine-induced responses would not be boosted during natural infection. If dying worms do release the cryptic antigen it is possible that boosting may be adequate to maintain levels of protection.

21.4 ADMINISTRATION OF VACCINES AGAINST HELMINTHS

As has been pointed out earlier, it is possible in the case of two of the three major gastrointestinal helminths (*Ascaris* and hookworms) to think in terms of using vaccines to raise protective immune responses that operate systemically against migrating larvae, as well as responses focused against the intestinal stages of infection. Systemically administered vaccines can achieve both, as has been demonstrated in many experimental models and in the work concerned with current molecular vaccines against veterinary parasites. At the present time this remains the simplest approach to vaccination against intestinal worms, but even were vaccines available for humans there would still be an urgent need to improve antigen administration in order to make mass vaccination practicable and acceptable.

One of the most important problems concerns the need to provide safe, effective adjuvants. The majority of adjuvants used in experimental antiworm vaccines could not be used in people. The choice of adjuvants is increasing (Eppstein, Byars and Allison, 1990; Warren and Chedid, 1988) and there are many which offer a suitable combination of adjuvanticity and safety (e.g. liposomes, ISCOMS, solid matrix-antibody-antigen (SMAA) complexes, biodegradable polymers). The first of these has already been used successfully in experimental vaccines against intestinal helminths (Rhalem *et al.*, 1988). In addition it is now recognized that the choice of adjuvant can be critical in determining the nature of the immune response stimulated (Kenney *et al.*, 1989; Karagouni and Hadjipetrou–Kourounakis, 1990). In those instances where it is crucial to elicit antibodies of a specific isotype, such a response may be selectively stimulated by an appropriate antigen-adjuvant regimen.

Despite this progress, many factors still suggest that orally administered vaccines would be preferable for programmes concerned with control of intestinal helminths. These include, in addition to logistic difficulties, the very real possibility that systemic antiparasite responses may initiate pathogenesis. The fact that the target parasites all have intestinal stages focuses attention on the desirability of immunizing orally in order selectively to raise protective responses in the intestine itself. A great deal of current research is directed to the development of orally given, long-acting vaccines that would be suitable for administering to populations in developing countries. Many of the approaches being used are of direct relevance to the concept of anti-helminth vaccines.

One sophisticated possibility is the use of recombinant vectors to colonize the intestine and to release *in situ* the antigens necessary for immunization. The bacterium *Salmonella* is one potential vector (Hackett, 1990). Virulent forms can be attenuated and rendered avirulent by deletion of genes controlling specific metabolic pathways and by deletion of virulence-conferring plasmids. Genes coding for vaccine antigens can then be introduced into the bacterial genome. Vaccines of this kind have already been tested against a variety of microbial pathogens, including hepatitis B, tetanus and influenza A as well as the intestinal species *Vibrio*, *Shigella*, and *Escherichia coli* (Hormaeche, Dougan and Maskell, 1990). A combined *Salmonella* vaccine has also been used to immunize orally against *Plasmodium berghei* in mice (Sadoff *et al.*, 1988). A similar approach, using *Escherichia coli* as a vector, has been tested in chickens to immunize against the intestinal protozoans responsible for coccidiosis (Kim, Jenkins and Lillihoj, 1989). Bacterial vectors of this kind offer the possibility of producing multivalent vaccines, by inserting genes for protective antigens derived from a number of parasite species. Of course, if particular antigens were effective in raising protective immune responses against several parasites (as might well be the case with some of the conserved cryptic molecules), multivalency of action would also be achieved.

A second possibility is the use of microcapsules or microparticles of biodegradable polymers. These can be given orally and are taken up across the specialized epithelia of the Peyer's patches. Antigens incorporated into these microparticles stimulate the gut-associated lymphoid tissues directly and elicit mucosal responses (Eldridge *et al.*, 1989, 1990; O'Hagan *et al.*, 1991). The composition of the polymer can be altered to give controlled release of antigen over a period of time, effectively allowing restimulation (boosting) of the response primed by the initial antigen delivery, and a number of antigens can be incorporated into the same microparticles, allowing multiple vaccination. Although this system of oral vaccination has not been tested for an intestinal helminth, the potential advantages for mass campaigns in endemic areas are obvious.

21.5 RESTRICTIONS ON THE USE OF VACCINES

If the future of vaccines against intestinal helminths lies in the development and production of synthetic subunit vaccines it will be important to consider some of the difficulties that have been encountered with other pathogens. One concerns the possibilities of genetic restriction in ability to respond to small peptides as a consequence of polymorphism in the Class II loci of the major histocompatibility complex (MHC). Humans are genetically heterogeneous, as are all 'random-bred' species, and individuals carry only a part of the population repertoire of MHC genes. Immune recognition of antigenic determinants (epitopes) requires presentation of the processed antigen in the context of the correct Class II molecules on the surface of antigen-presenting cells. Individuals lacking the MHC molecules necessary for presentation of a particular epitope will fail to recognize or respond to that epitope. One danger of subunit vaccines is that small peptides may carry only a small number of epitopes, and some recipients of a vaccine will therefore fail to respond, as occurred during some early trials of the circumsporozoite malaria vaccine (Good, Berzofsky and Miller, 1988). This particular problem can easily be overcome by producing cocktails of immunogenic peptides, but other genetic restrictions may still operate, even with complex vaccines. For example it is well known that the effectiveness of BCG vaccination varies quite remarkably among different racial and geographic groups (World Health Organization, 1979).

Still other restrictions may operate in individuals who show a genetically determined, low or non-responsiveness to a particular parasite. There are many reasons for genetically determined deficiencies in response, and such deficiences may arise in both the efferent and afferent arms of the immune system (Wakelin and Blackwell, 1988). They may include defects in antigen processing or recognition, in lymphocyte proliferation, in qualitative and quantitative aspects of antibody responses, in complement components and so on. In addition, protective responses to helminths may be reduced in effectiveness because necessary components of the inflammatory response are deficient. It has been well documented in murine models that there are strong genetic influences on responsiveness to vaccination (Wakelin *et al.*, 1986; Else and Wakelin, 1990), and a similar picture has emerged from experimental studies on responses to irradiated larval vaccines in lambs exposed to *T. colubriformis* (Dineen, Gregg and Lascelles, 1978); it can safely be assumed that a similar situation would arise in human populations vaccinated against helminths, given the overwhelming evidence for variation in immune responsiveness to these parasites.

With all vaccines, efficiency of immunization is reduced if the recipient is malnourished or carries other infections, and vaccines against helminths are no exception. Several papers have recorded an impaired response to vaccination against parasites when the host is subject to protein-calorie restriction (Slater and Keymer, 1988; Wagland *et al.*, 1984). Perhaps more significantly, it has been shown that infection with the immunosuppressive stages of intestinal nematodes dramatically interferes with subsequent attempts to vaccinate against the same species (Behnke, Hannah and Pritchard, 1983; Else and Wakelin, 1990). It is very likely that the ability of parasites to suppress immune responses reflects their production of immunomodulatory factors, or the release of antigens that bear immunosuppressive epitopes (Roitt, 1989). Both of these contingencies have to be borne in mind when selecting candidate antigens.

The restrictions posed by genetic variation, by undernutrition and by concurrent infections are precisely those that will have to be faced if antihelminth vaccines are ever to be used in the developing world. These constraints are likely to be severest in the case of children who, being the most heavily infected with gastrointestinal parasites, are both the prime targets for vaccination and the group in whom effective antiparasite responses will be the most difficult to evoke by vaccination. The achievement of effective immunity against these ubiquitous and debilitating infections remains a major challenge for contemporary immunoparasitology.

REFERENCES

Almond, N. M. and Parkhouse, R. M. E. (1985) Nematode antigens. *Curr. Top. Microbiol. Immun.*, **120**, 173–203.

Appleton, J. A., Bell, R. G., Homan, W. and van Knapen, F. (1991) Consensus on *Trichinella spiralis* antigens and antibodies. *Parasit. Today*, **7**, 190–2.

Behnke, J. M., Hannah, J. and Pritchard, D. I. (1983) *Nematospiroides dubius* in the mouse: evidence that adult worms depress the expression of homologous immunity. *Parasite Immun.*, **5**, 397–408.

Butterworth, A. E. (1984) Cell-mediated immunity to helminths. *Adv. Parasit.*, **23**, 143–235.

Clegg, J. A. and Smith, M. A. (1978) Prospects for the development of dead vaccines against helminths. *Adv. Parasit.*, **16**, 165–218.

Dawkins, H. J. S., Muir, G. M. and Grove, D. I. (1981) Histopathological appearances in primary and secondary infections with *Strongyloides ratti* in mice. *Int. J. Parasit.*, **11**, 97–103.

Day, K. P., Howard, R. J., Prowse. S. J. *et al.* (1979) Studies on chronic versus transient intestinal nematode infections in mice. I. A comparison of responses to excretory/secretory (ES) products of *Nippostrongylus brasiliensis* and *Nematospiroides dubius* worms. *Parasite Immun.*, **1**, 217–39.

Dineen, J. K., Gregg, G. F. and Lascelles, A. K. (1978) The response of lambs to vaccination at weaning with irradiated *Trichostrongylus colubriformis* larvae: segregation into 'responders' and 'non-responders'. *Int. J. Parasit.*, **8**, 59–63.

Eldridge, J. H., Gilley, R. M., Staas, J. K. *et al.* (1989) Biodegradable microspheres. *Curr. Top. Microbiol. Immun.*, **146**, 59–68.

Eldridge, J. H., Hammond, C. J., Meulbroek, J. A. *et al.* (1990) Controlled vaccine release in the gut-associated lymphoid tissues. 1. Orally administered biodegradable microspheres target the Peyer's patches. *J. Contr. Rel.*, **11**, 205–14.

Else, K. J. and Wakelin, D. (1989) Genetic variation in the humoral immune responses of mice to the nematode *Trichuris muris*. *Parasite Immun.*, **11**, 77–90.

Else, K. J. and Wakelin, D. (1990) Genetically determined influences on the ability of poor responder mice to respond to immunization against *Trichuris muris*. *Parasitology*, **100**, 479–89.

Eppstein, D. A., Byars, N. E. and Allison, A. C. (1990) New adjuvants for vaccines containing purified protein antigens. *Adv. Drug Deliv. Rev.*, **4**, 233–53.

Fields, B. N. and Chanock, R. M. (1989) What biotechnology has to offer vaccine development. *Rev. Inf. Dis.*, **11** (suppl. 3), 5519–23.

Gamble, H. R. and Zarlenga, D. S. (1986) Biotechnology in the development of vaccines for animal parasites. *Vet. Parasit.*, **20**, 237–50.

Good, M. F., Berzofsky, J. A. and Miller, L. H. (1988) The T cell response to the malaria circumsporozoite protein: an immunological approach to vaccine development. *Ann. Rev. Immun.*, **6**, 663–88.

Hackett, J. (1990) Salmonella based vaccines. *Vaccine*, **8**, 5–11.

Hormaeche, C. E., Dougan, G. and Maskell, D. J. (1990) *Salmonella* vaccines and their potential as carriers of recombinant antigens, in *Basic Research in Helminthiases* (eds R. Ehrlich, A. Nieto and L. Yarbazal), Editiones Logos, Montivideo, pp. 175–87.

Hotez, P. J., Le Trang, N. and Cerami, A. (1987) Hookworm antigens: the potential for vaccination. *Parasit. Today*, **3**, 247–9.

Ito, A. and Smyth, J. D. (1987) Adult cestodes. Immunology of the lumen-dwelling cestode infections, in *Immune Responses in Parasitic Infections: Immunology, Immunopathology and Immunoprophylaxis* (ed. E. J. L. Soulsby), CRC Press, Boca Raton, pp. 115–63.

Jenkins, S. N. and Wakelin, D. (1983) Functional antigens of *Trichuris muris* released during *in vitro* maintenance: their immunogenicity and partial purification. *Parasitology*, **86**, 73–82.

Karagouni, E. E. and Hadjipetrou-Kourounakis, L. (1990) Regulation of isotype immunoglobulin production by adjuvants *in vivo*. *Scand. J. Immun.*, **31**, 745–51.

Kenney, J. S., Hughes, B. W., Masada, M. P. and Allison, A. C. (1989) Influence of adjuvants on the quantity, affinity, isotype and epitope specificity of murine antibodies. *J. Immun. Methods*, **121**, 157–62.

Kim, K. S., Jenkins, M. C. and Lillihoj, H. S. (1989) Immunization of chickens with live *Escherichia coli* expressing *Eimeria acervulina* merozoite recombinant antigen induces partial protection against coccidiosis. *Infect. Immun.*, **57**, 2434–40.

Lillywhite, J. E., Bundy, D. A. P., Didier, J. M. *et al.* (1991) Humoral immune responses in human infection with the whipworm *Trichuris trichiura*. *Parasite Immun.*, **13**, 491–507.

Lloyd, S. (1981) Progress in immunization against parasitic helminths. *Parasitology*, **83**, 225–42.

McLaren, D. J. (1985) Parasite defence mechanisms, in *Inflammation, Basic Mechanisms, Tissue Injuring Principles, and Clinical Models* (eds P. Venge and A. Lindbom), Almquist and Wiksell International, Stockholm, pp. 219–54.

Miller, H. R. P. (1984) The protective response against gastrointestinal nematodes in ruminants and laboratory animals. *Vet. Immun. Immunopath.*, **6**, 167–259.

Miller, H. R. P. (1986) Vaccination against intestinal parasites. *Int. J. Parasit.*, **17**, 43–51.

Miller, T. A. (1964) Effect of X-irradiation upon the infective larvae of *Ancylostoma caninum* and the immunogenic effect in dogs of a single infection with 40 Kr-irradiated larvae. *J. Parasit.*, **50**, 735–42.

Miller, T. A. (1971) Vaccination against the canine hookworm diseases. *Adv. Parasit.*, **9**, 153–83.

Miller, T. A. (1978) Industrial development and field use of the canine hookworm vaccine. *Adv. Parasit.*, **16**, 333–42.

Moqbel, R. (1980) Histopathological changes following primary, secondary and repeated infections of rats with *Strongyloides ratti*, with special reference to tissue eosinophils. *Parasite Immun.*, **2**, 11–27.

Moqbel, R. and MacDonald, A. J. (1990) Immunological and inflammatory responses in the small intestine associated with helminthic infections, in *Parasites: Immunity and Pathology* (ed. J. M. Behnke), Taylor and Francis, London, pp. 249–82.

Morrison, W. I. (1989) Immunological control of ticks and tick-borne parasitic diseases of livestock. *Parasitology*, **98**, S69–S85.

Murrell, K. D. and Despommier D. D. (1984) Immunization of swine against *Trichinella spiralis*. *Vet. Parasit.*, **15**, 263–70.

Nanduri, J., and J. W. Kazura (1989) Paramyosin-enhanced clearance of *Brugia malayi* microfilaremia in mice. *J. Immun.*, **143**, 3359–63.

O'Donnell, I. J., Dineen, J. K., Wagland, B. M. *et al.* (1989) A novel host-protective antigen from *Trichostrongylus colubriformis*. *Int. J. Parasit.*, **19**, 327–35.

O'Hagan, D. T., Rahman, D., McGee, J. P. *et al.* (1991) Biodegradable microparticles as controlled release antigen delivery systems. *Immunology*, **73**, 239–42.

Peacock, R. and Poynter, D. (1980) Field experience with a bovine lungworm vaccine. *Symp. Br. Soc. Parasit.*, **18**, 141–8.

Pearce, E. J., James, S. L., Hieny, S. *et al.* (1988) Induction of protective immunity against *Schistosoma mansoni* by vaccination with schistosome paramyosin (Sm 97), a nonsurface parasite antigen. *Proc. Natl Acad. Sci. USA*, **85**, 5678–82.

Poulain, J., Pery, P. and Luffau, G. (1976) Protection of rats against *Nippostrongylus brasiliensis* with worm antigens by oral administration. *Ann. Immun. (Inst. Pasteur)*, **127C**, 201–13.

Poynter, D., Jones, B. V., Peacock, A. M. R. *et al.* (1960) Recent experiences with vaccination. *Vet. Rec.*, **72**, 1078–90.

Pritchard, D. I., McKean, P. G. and Rogan, M. T. (1988) Cuticular collagens: a concealed target for immune attack in hookworms. *Parasit. Today*, **4**, 239–41.

Pritchard, D. I., Quinnell, R. J., Slater, A. F. G. *et al.* (1990) Epidemiology and immunology of *Necator americanus* infection in a community in Papua New Guinea: humoral responses to excretory-secretory and cuticular collagen antigens. *Parasitology*, **100**, 317–26.

Rhalem, A., Bourdieu, C., Luffau, G. and Pery, P. (1988) Vaccination of mice with liposome-entrapped adult antigens of *Nippostrongylus brasiliensis*. *Ann. Immun. (Inst. Pasteur)*, **139**, 157–66.

Roach, T. I. A., Else, K. J., Wakelin, D. *et al.* (1991) *Trichuris muris*: antigen recognition and transfer of immunity in mice by IgA monoclonal antibodies. *Parasite Immun.*, **13**, 1–12.

Roitt, I. M. (1989) Basic concepts and new aspects of vaccine development. *Parasitology*, S7–S12.

Rothwell, T. L. W. (1989) Immune expulsion of parasitic nematodes from the alimentary tract. *Int. J. Parasit.*, **19**, 139–68.

Sadoff, J. C., Ballou, W. R., Baron, L. S. *et al.* (1988) Oral *Salmonella typhimurium* vaccine expressing circumsporozoite protein protects against malaria. *Science*, **240**, 336–8.

Sher, A. (1988) Vaccination against parasites: special problems imposed by the adaptation of parasitic organisms to the host immune response, in *The Biology of Parasitism* (eds P. T. Englund and A. Sher), Alan R. Liss, New York, pp. 169–82.

Silberstein, D. S. and Despommier, D. D. (1984) Antigens from *Trichinella spiralis* that induce a protective response in the mouse. *J. Immun.*, **132**, 898–904.

Slater, A. F. G. and Keymer, A. E. (1988) The influence of protein deficiency on immunity to *Heligmosomoides polygyrus* (Nematoda) in mice. *Parasite Immun.*, **10**, 507–22

Smith, T. S. and Munn, E. A. (1990) Strategies for vaccination against gastro-intestinal nematodes. *Rev. Sci. Tech. Off. Int. Epiz.*, **9**, 577–95.

Thorson, R. E. (1956) Proteolytic activity in extracts of the esophagus of adult *Ancylostoma caninum* and the effect of immune serum on this activity. *J. Parasit.*, **42**, 21–30.

Urquhart, G. M. (1977) Irradiated vaccines. *INSERM*, **72**, 263–74.

Vernes, A. (1976) Immunization of the mouse and minipig against *Trichinella spiralis*, in *Biochemistry of Parasites and Host–Parasite Relationships* (ed. H. van den Bossche), Elsevier/North-Holland Biomedical Press, Amsterdam, pp. 319–24.

Wagland, B. M., Steel, J. W., Windon, R. G. and Dineen, J. K. (1984) The response of lambs to vaccination and challenge with *Trichostrongylus colubriformis*: effect of plane of nutrition on, and the inter-relationship between, immunological responsiveness and resistance. *Int. J. Parasit.*, **14**, 39–44.

Wakelin, D., and Blackwell, J. M. (eds) (1988) *Genetics of Resistance to Bacterial and Parasitic Infection*, Taylor and Francis, London.

Wakelin, D., Harnett, W. and Parkhouse, R. M. E. (1993) Nematodes, in *Immunology and Molecular Biology of Parasitic Infections* (eds K. S. Warren and N. Agabian), Academic Press, New York, pp. 496–526.

Wakelin, D., Mitchell, L. A., Donachie, A. M. and Grencis, R. K. (1986) Genetic control of immunity to *Trichinella spiralis* in mice. Response of rapid- and slow- responder strains to immunization with parasite antigens. *Parasite Immun.*, **8**, 159–70.

Warren, H. S. and Chedid, L. A. (1988) Future prospects for vaccine adjuvants. *CRC Crit. Rev. Immun.*, **8**, 83–101.

World Health Organization (1979) Trial of BCG vaccines in South India for tuberculosis prevention: first report. *Bull. WHO*, **57**, 819–27.

TWENTY-TWO

Global control of helminth-induced disease

K. S. Warren

After Anu made the heavens, the heavens made the earth, the earth made the rivers, the rivers made the canals, the canals made the marsh, the marsh made the worm . . .

Asurburnipal Library, 5th century BC

The first great attempt at global control of a major human helminth infection was initiated by The Rockefeller Foundation at the time of its inauguration in 1913. The Rockefeller Sanitary Commission, which had been working on the control of hookworm in the southern USA, was merged with the Foundation and christened the International Health Board. 'In the years that followed, [this] daring enterprise was extended to 52 countries, to six continents and to twenty-nine islands of the seas' (Fosdick, 1952).

Seventy-five years later, in Bellagio, Italy, a meeting was held to commemorate this first global public health campaign and to report on progress since then (Schad and Warren, 1990). While research on hookworm continues to enhance our knowledge of these organisms and their inter-relationships with the environment and their human hosts, at least 750 million people remain infected in the world today. It was clear, therefore, that the campaigns in the early part of this century had no lasting effect on the prevalence of infection. The inevitable question then arose: what is being done about it? This led to the realization that it was no longer necessary to deal with hookworm alone, because several broad-spectrum anthelmintics were available which were also effective against the other major intestinal helminths – *Ascaris*, *Trichuris*, and *Enterobius*. Furthermore, these drugs were single-dose, oral and non-toxic. Then it was observed that another similar drug, praziquantel, will treat virtually all cestodes and trematodes (Warren, 1988), and that yet another such drug, ivermectin, was available for the treatment of the mosquito-borne filariae. Thus, a new strategy was determined in order to control virtually all of the human disease caused by helminth infections.

22.1 HUMAN HELMINTH PARASITES

Most helminth infections involve the gastrointestinal tract and liver in one way or another: through oral ingestion of infective forms, development within the lumen, wall or blood vessels of the gut, or excretion of reproductive forms (eggs and larvae), The major human helminth parasites are shown in Table 22.1. Helminths are among the most prevalent of human infectious agents; over four decades ago, in *This Wormy World*, Norman Stoll (1947) observed that there were

Enteric Infection 2. Intestinal helminths. Edited by M.J.G. Farthing, G.T. Keusch and D. Wakelin. Published in 1995 by Chapman and Hall, London. ISBN 0 412 39140 6

Table 22.1 Major helminth infections of humans

Organism	*Common name*	*Means of infection*	*Prevalence (millions)*	*Major disease manifestation*	*Morbidity (thousands)*	*Mortality (thousands)*	*Oral, single-dose chemotherapy*
NEMATODES (Roundworms)							
Ancylostoma duodenale, Necator americanus	Hookworm	Skin	750	Anemia	1400	50	Albendazole
Ascaris lumbricoides	Giant roundworm	Oral	1000	Intestinal obstruction	1000	25	Albendazole; ivermectin
Dracunculus medinensis	Guinea worm	Oral	140	Cutaneous lesions	?	?	
Enterobius vermicularis	Pinworm	Oral	400	Anal pruritus	low	–	Albendazole
Onchocerca volvulus	River blindness	Insect	18	Blindness	330	–	Albendazole
Strongyloides stercoralis	Strongyloidiasis	Skin	80	Autoinfection	?	?	Ivermectin
Trichinella spiralis	Trichinosis	Oral	11	Myositis	940	?	
Trichuris trichiura	Whipworm	Oral	750	Rectal prolapse	500	–	Albendazole; ivermectin
Wuchereria bancrofti	Filariasis	Insect	295	Elephantiasis	3000	–	Ivermectin
TREMATODES (Flukes)							
Clonorchis sinensis, Opisthorchis viverrini, O. felineus	Liver fluke	Oral	32	Biliary obstruction	?	?	Praziquantel
Fasciola hepatica	Liver fluke	Oral	?	Hepatomegaly	?	?	
Fasciolopsis buski	Intestinal fluke	Oral	17	Diarrhea	?	?	Praziquantel
Paragonimus westermani	Lung fluke	Oral	6	Cough	?	?	Praziquantel
Schistosoma haematobium	Blood fluke	Skin	100	Hydronephrosis	4900	120	Praziquantel
Schistosoma japonicum	Blood fluke	Skin	95	Hepatosplenomegaly	4750	120	Praziquantel
Schistosoma mansoni	Blood fluke	Skin	65	Hepatosplenomegaly	3350	80	Praziquantel
CESTODES (Tapeworms)							
Diphyllobothrium latum	Fish tapeworm	Oral	9	Anemia	low	–	Praziquantel
Taenia saginata	Beef tapeworm	Oral	70	None	low	?	Praziquantel
Taenia solium	Pork tapeworm	Oral	5	Cysticercosis	400	?	Praziquantel
Echinococcus granulosus	Hydatid cyst	Oral	?	Cyst	?	?	

as many worm infections as people on the Earth. Today, the situation is relatively unchanged, with an overall prevalence of almost four billion infections. All but the filariae, which are transmitted by biting insects, and the urinary tract form of schistosomiasis caused by *Schistosoma haematobium*, involve the intestinal tract via transmission, pathology or both. While the morbidity and mortality rates are low, the prevalence and chronicity of helminth infections leads to overt disease in tens of millions of individuals throughout the developing world of the southern hemisphere.

All helminths have complicated life cycles including free-living stages and those in intermediate hosts such as insects or snails. Hookworm, for instance, has only free-living infective larvae which penetrate intact skin, from which they pass to the lungs and thence to the gut. Fertilized female worms attached to the gut wall ingest blood and produce large numbers of eggs which pass out into the external environment where they in turn develop into infective larvae. It is essential to note that neither the larvae nor the adult worms multiply within the human host, that their mean life span is only 2.5 years, and that intensity of infection is related to frequent exposure to infective larvae. Disease, such as anemia, is due to blood loss caused by these hematophagous parasites, and occurs only in those with heavy infections.

Schistosomiasis is an example of a helminth which requires an intermediate snail host within which the parasite undergoes asexual multiplication. Free-living forms emitted into the snail's watery habitat infect their human definitive hosts by direct penetration of the skin. The schistosomula pass to the lungs, then the liver where they develop into mature male or female worms which mate, move down into the venules of the intestines (*S. mansoni* and *S. japonicum*) where they produce large numbers of eggs. These enter the lumen of the gut, pass out, hatch in fresh water and penetrate into snails. The adult worms do not multiply within their human definitive hosts, their life span is less than five years, and disease is due to inflammatory and fibrotic reactions to schistosome eggs trapped in the tissues which cause obstructive lesions in the portal venous system. Heavy infection is also a necessary condition for disease.

Thus, as stated in an editorial (Warren, 1970):

> Worms are unique among infectious agents – they appear to follow the precepts of guerilla warfare as outlined by Chairman Mao, repeatedly infiltrating host defenses as individuals or in small groups and gradually building up into large forces; warfare is usually by attrition and tends to be prolonged. Virtually all the major worm parasites of man are guerillas. . . . Infection is not synonymous with disease. Many patients invaded by schistosomes, trichinellae, ascarides, filariae and hookworms never had and never will have overt signs or symptoms of disease. The respective manifestations caused by these worms – liver fibrosis, myositis, intestinal obstruction, elephantiasis and anemia – occur only when there is an unusually heavy attacking force or when large numbers of parasites have accumulated.

While the above concepts deal with the individual patient, crucial population-based factors have been considered (Warren, 1973). The basic idea came from the recently published concepts of Crofton (1971) who observed that 'parasitism is an ecological relationship which must be expressed quantitatively in terms of populations'. He noted that parasites do not follow the normal or bell-shaped distribution curve within the host population, but characteristically have an overdispersed distribution, which is best expressed by the negative binomial distribution. Thus, while the few with heavy parasite burdens get sick and can die, the many with infections of low intensity suffer little or no morbidity.

In 1979, Anderson and May published a

seminal paper on parasitism in general, in which they grouped viruses, bacteria and protozoa into *microparasites*, and helminths and arthropods into *macroparasites*. The former

> . . . are characterized by small size, short generation times, extremely high rates of direct reproduction within the host, and a tendency to induce immunity to reinfection in those that survive the initial onslaught. The duration of infection is typically short in relation to the expected life span of the host, and therefore is of a transient nature . . . Macroparasites tend to have much longer generation times than the microparasites, and direct multiplication within the host is either absent or occurs at a low rate. The immune responses elicited by these metazoans generally depend on the number of parasites present in a given host, and tend to be of relatively short duration. Macroparasitic infection, therefore, tends to be of a persistent nature, with the host being continually reinfected.

22.2 STRATEGY

A unique and cost-effective approach to the control of helminth infections is based on three simple principles:

- Parasitologically, helminths, with rare exceptions such as *Strongyloides* and *Echinococcus*, do not multiply within their definitive human hosts.
- Pathogenetically, disease occurs largely in heavily infected hosts.
- Epidemiologically, only a small proportion of hosts develop heavy infections.

22.3 CONTROL

There are three levels of control of infectious diseases: eradication, control of infections and control of disease. Each requires drastically different levels of stringency and cost. In the first quarter of this century The Rockefeller Foundation began at the most stringent level with its attempt at the global eradication of hookworm; this was followed by a similar attack on yellow fever. In the third quarter of the century the World Health Organization's exceedingly costly attempt to eradicate malaria failed. Its later attack on smallpox culminated with the first eradication of a major disease in 1979. At the moment two more eradication campaigns are being waged, against polio and Guinea worm. The lessons learned are that eradication is very costly in terms of both money and manpower, and that failure has a very serious backlash effect. Further candidates for eradication must be selected very carefully with respect to the likelihood of success, based on the epidemiology of the infection and the quality of the weapons available.

Control itself can be related to infection or disease. Examples might be taken from immunization: while the oral polio vaccine prevents both infection and transmission of the wild virus, tetanus toxoid does not prevent infection by the bacillus but inactivates the toxin which causes lockjaw. With many infectious agents the control of infection, i.e. transmission, is complex, costly and, at the moment, impossible. If disease could be prevented without specifically attacking transmission it is likely to be simpler, much less expensive and may become possible. Among all infectious agents, helminths are particularly amenable to this form of control since only the small proportion of hosts which bear heavy worm burdens develop disease.

The principal means of controlling helminth infections have been health education, water and food control, sanitation and vector control (both arthropods and molluscs). It was little more than a decade ago that the World Health Organization was recommending the use of multiple control measures in order to decrease transmission. In a 16-year study on the transmission and control of schistosomiasis on the island of St Lucia (Jordan, 1985), the effectiveness and cost of the three main control measures – water supplies, molluscicides, chemotherapy – were compared. It was found that treatment was most cost-effective and that the marked decrease in worm burdens that resulted was sustained for many years. Studies on 'targetted mass treatment' in Kenya (Warren and Mahmoud, 1976; Mahmoud *et al.*, 1983) were in agreement with these results. Furthermore, the value of the chemotherapeutic approach was greatly enhanced by the development of new and more effective anthelmintics, such as praziquantel.

It is interesting to realize that many of the above concepts of the control of helminth infections were described by Smillie (1924) and others during The Rockefeller Foundation hookworm campaigns in the southern USA more than 60 years ago. 'A distinction must be made between hookworm infection and hookworm disease. Light hookworm infection may be and commonly is acquired casually by all classes of people in a zone infected with hookworms. Actual hookworm disease, that is, an infection which is severe enough to be of real harm to the individual, occurs only in that group of individuals in the infected area whose bare skin has long and continuous contact with infected soil' (Smillie, 1924). Smillie also noted that disease is 'found almost exclusively in the rural children of school age (6–16 years)'; that 'hookworm disease can best be controlled by mass treatment of the heavily infected individuals', and that 'new infection is slowly acquired'.

Warren and Mahmoud (1976) and Mahmoud *et al.* (1983) rediscovered the wheel in studies of schistosomiasis in Lower Nduu, Kenya. The earlier study revealed peak age-intensity in teenage children, and a relationship between heavy infections and the development of disease, as manifested by hepatosplenomegaly. Figure 22.1, taken from the latter paper, revealed that the age-

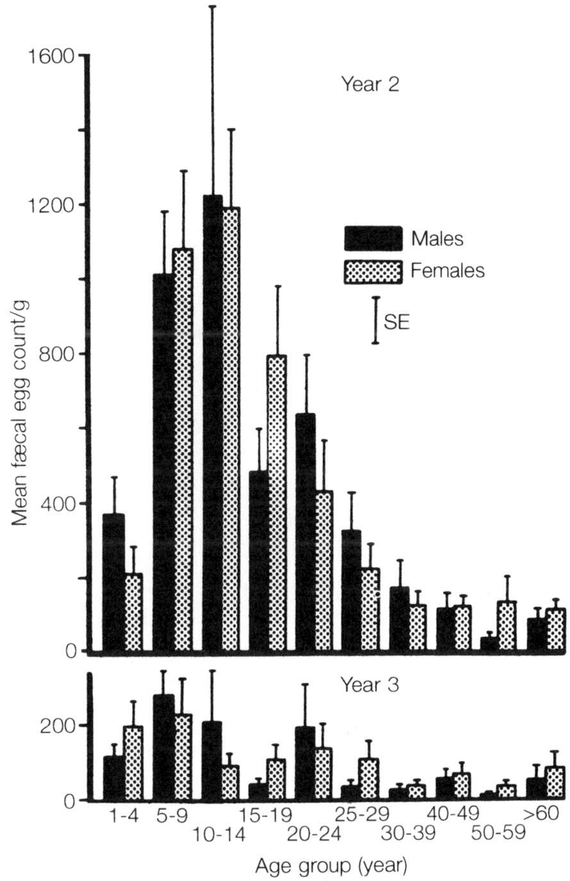

Figure 22.1 Effect of targeted mass treatment on age-specific intensity of *Schistosoma mansoni* infection. (Source: Mahmoud *et al.*, 1983.)

intensity profile was stable for two years, and that treatment of only the heavily infected individuals was followed by markedly lower intensities of infection, which were maintained for a least a year. This was in part related to the fact that treatment of less than 30% of the population led to a decrease of 80% in egg output into the environment and a possible fall in transmission. It is worthy of note that mass treatment of onchocerciasis with ivermectin clearly resulted in reduced transmission as determined by a marked reduction in incidence of infection (Taylor *et al.*, 1990).

22.3.1 INTEGRATED SYSTEM FOR THE CONTROL OF HUMAN HELMINTH DISEASE

A year after it was realized at the Bellagio hookworm meeting that three oral, single-dose, broad-spectrum anthelmintics given at intervals of a year or longer to school-age children could prevent most of the disease due to 18 of the 21 most common helminth infections, a paper was presented at the van Thiel lecture of the Institute of Tropical Medicine, Rotterdam-Leiden (Warren, 1990). This was followed by a detailed, multi-authored paper on the control of helminths for the World Bank's Health Sector Priorities Review (Warren, 1990).

Since we are dealing with an extremely prevalent problem in the developing world where populations are particularly large and finances are especially small it is essential to optimize strategies with respect to both effectiveness and cost. It is necessary to begin with the idea that eradication is impossible due to the ubiquitous nature of the infectious agents and the lack of general public health measures with respect to food, water, sanitation, housing, vector control, etc. Major control of transmission requires multiple public health measures which greatly multiply cost with little increment in effectiveness. Helminth infections, in particular, lend themselves to control of disease because of the factors described above, especially the relationship of disease to intensity of infection, the overdispersed distribution of infection with relatively low numbers of heavy infections, and the slow rate of reinfection. It is fortunate in terms of logistical ease that most heavy helminth infections are found in school-age children. Another positive factor is the recent development of a series of oral, broad-spectrum, single-dose, non-toxic anthelmintic drugs, three of which will treat the 18 major parasite species.

Further reason for focusing on school-age children is the evidence that they are particularly hard hit by helminth infections at the time when they are undergoing maximal growth and development. Studies after treatment of schistosomiasis, hookworm and ascaris have shown remarkable growth spurts (Stephenson *et al.*, 1989a,b). A review of the effects of parasitic infection on cognitive performance has revealed flaws in the design of previous studies and suggested new and more sensitive experimental approaches to elucidate this important problem (Kvalsvig, 1988). Finally, a meeting of experts convened by UNESCO has concluded that helminth infections are among the most important infectious disease problems of school-age children (Bundy, 1989).

The fundamental strategy, therefore, is to focus on school-age children, both those within and outside of the school system, by encouraging the latter to come to the schools during periods when treatment is being offered. Since the cost of the campaign would be almost doubled by performing diagnostic studies on each child, a better strategy is to treat all children on the basis of surveys showing moderate to high prevalence of infection. Concern has been expressed about the use of several different drugs simultaneously, but it must be realized that in many areas of the world only one drug is necessary, in others different combinations of two drugs are needed, and in a relative minority, three drugs (Figure 22.2). While praziquantel has a half-life of only 1 h, enabling the use of either of the other drugs on the same day, albendazole and ivermectin have half-lives of approximately 10 h which may require treatment at longer intervals. This might be done by having an annual health promotion week and giving the drugs at appropriate times therein. Studies are now in progress on the effects of various combinations of the drugs; at present, treatment with both praziquantel and albendazole seems innocuous. The question of drug resistance

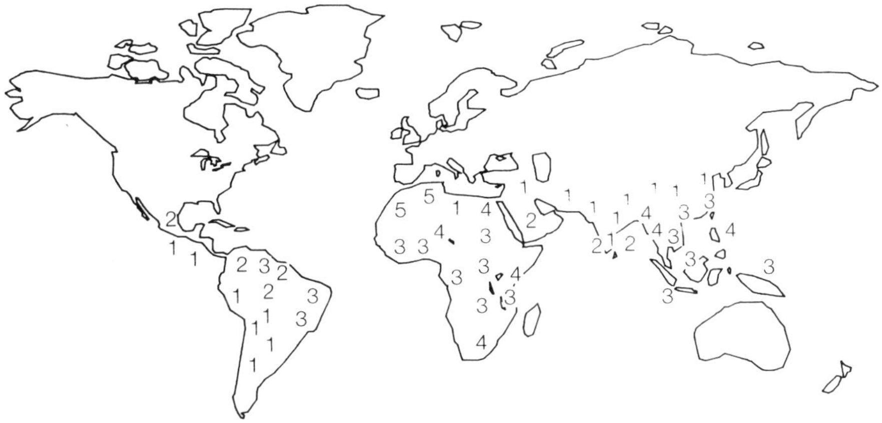

Figure 22.2 Estimated global requirements for anthelmintics. The figure was developed using secondary data on the global distribution of geohelminthiasis, schistosomiasis and filariasis. The numbers indicate a particular anthelmintic, or combination of anthelmintics, which would be appropriate for the treatment of the major helminthic infections occurring in that geographical area. 1 = albendazole; 2 = albendazole and ivermectin; 3 = albendazole and ivermectin and praziquantel; 4 = albendazole and praziquantel; 5 = praziquantel.

has been raised, but this is less likely with helminths than other infectious agents because of their far slower rates of reproduction. Furthermore, since albendazole and invermectin overlap in their spectrum of treatment, resistance after use of that combination would be even less likely.

Further logistical advantages are ease of transportation and storage of drugs (which do not require a cold chain), drastic price reductions with bulk purchase, and the possibility that teachers *in situ* can be trained to administer the drugs under reasonable surveillance. It has been suggested recently by Donald Hopkins that this program might be developed into an 'Expanded Program on Chemotherapy'. Oral micronutrients might be added as well as oral, single-dose drugs for the treatment of other diseases; for example, albendazole appears to be highly effective against *Giardia lamblia in vitro*, and might serve to control this prevalent and potentially debilitating chronic infection of children (Martinez Palomo, personal communication).

22.3.2 STATUS OF THE CAMPAIGN

In the short period since the idea of a campaign to control disease due to virtually all human helminth infections was broached in Bellagio in September 1988, similar concepts have arisen spontaneously among many of the key international organizations. Thus, in April 1989 a UNESCO meeting in Stockholm on improving primary school performance by better nutrition and health concluded that intestinal parasitoses were one of the most important problems of school-age children (Bundy, 1989). This was followed by a World Bank Health Sector Priorities Review in Woods Hole in May, and a UNICEF meeting on *Children and Parasites* in Florence in October. Two different divisions of the World Health Organization discussed this issue in 1990, the Special Programme for Tropical Diseases Research in May and the Communicable Diseases Division in July. It was also described at a meeting of the Task Force for Child Survival in Atlanta in August of that year, where Hopkins came up with the idea of an Expanded Program on Chemotherapy. It is a fitting conclusion to this odyssey of ideas all over Europe and the United States that the United Nations Development Programme and The Rockefeller Foundation hosted a conference in Bellagio (where the idea had its inception three years earlier), on *An Integrated System for the Control of Disease caused by the Major Human Helminth Parasites*. All of the multi-lateral agencies mentioned above were represented, as well as major bilateral donors and foundations. Parasitologists, ecologists, epidemiologists, pharmacologists, nutritionists and economists discussed the plan of action. Large-scale control programs are underway and it is hoped that sampling will reveal a positive effect on the well-being of school-age children throughout the world.

REFERENCES

Anderson, R. M. and May, R. M. (1979) Population biology of infectious diseases, Part I. *Nature*, **280**, 361–7.

Bundy, D. A. P. (1989) New UNESCO international project. *Parasit. Today*, **5**, 168.

Crofton, H. D. (1971) The quantitative approach to parasitism. *Parasitology*, **62**, 179–93.

Fosdick, R. B. (1952) *The Story of the Rockefeller Foundation*, Harper, New York.

Jordan, P. (1985) *Schistosomiasis: the St Lucia Project*, Cambridge University Press, Cambridge.

Kvalsig, N. D. (1988) The effects of parasitic infection on cognitive performance. *Parasit. Today*, **4**, 206–8.

Mahmoud, A. A. F., Ouma, J., Siongok, T. K. A. *et al.* (1983) Effect of targeted mass treatment on intensity of infection and morbidity in schistosomiasis mansoni: 3-year follow-up of a community in Machakos, Kenya. *Lancet*, **ii**, 849–51.

Schad, G. A. and Warren K. S. (1990) *Hookworm Disease: Current Status and New Directions*, Taylor and Francis, London.

Smillie, W. G. (1924) Control of hookworm disease in South Alabama. *South. Med. J.*, **17**, 494–9.

Stephenson, L. S., Latham, M. C., Kurz, K. M. *et al.* (1989a) Treatment with a single dose of albendazole improves growth of Kenyan schoolchildren with hookworm, *Trichuris trichiura*, and *Ascaris lumbricoides* infections. *Am. J. Trop. Med. Hyg.*, **41**, 78–87.

Stephenson, L. S., Lathem, M. C., Kurz, K. M. and Kinoti, S. N. (1989b) Single dose of metrifonate or praziquantel treatment in Kenyan schoolchildren II: Effects on growth in relation to *Schistosoma haematobium* and hookworm egg counts. *Am. J. Trop. Med. Hyg.*, **41**, 445–53.

Taylor, H. R., Pacque, M., Munoz, B. and Greene, B. M. (1990) Impact of mass treatment of onchocerciasis with ivermectin on the transmission of infection. *Science*, **250**, 116–18.

Warren, K. S. (1970) The guerilla worm (editorial). *New Engl. J. Med.*, **282**, 1494–5.

Warren, K. S. (1973) Regulation of the prevalence and intensity of schistosomiasis in man: immunology or ecology? *J. Infect. Dis.*, **127**, 595–609.

Warren, K. S. (1988) Conference on hookworm control, Bellagio, Italy. *Lancet*, 897–8.

Warren, K. S. (1990) An integrated system for the control of the major human helminth parasites. *Acta Leidensia*, **59**, 433–42.

Warren, K. S. and Mahmoud, A. A. F. (1976) Targeted mass treatment: a new approach to the control of schistosomiasis. *Trans. Assoc. Am. Physicians*, **89**, 195–204.

Warren, K. S., Bundy, D. A. P., Anderson, R. H. *et al.* (1993) Helminth infections, in Jamison, D. T., Mosky, Measham, A. R. *et al. Disease Control Priorities in Developing Countries*. Oxford University Press, Oxford, pp. 131–60.

Index

Note: page numbers in *italics* refer to tables; those in **bold** refer to figures.